EFFECTIVE TREATMENTS FOR PTSD

Effective Treatments for
PTSD

Practice Guidelines from
the International Society
for Traumatic Stress Studies

THIRD EDITION

edited by
David Forbes
Jonathan I. Bisson
Candice M. Monson
Lucy Berliner

THE GUILFORD PRESS
New York   London

Library of Congress Cataloging-in-Publication Data

Names: Forbes, David (Clinical psychologist), editor.
Title: Effective treatments for PTSD : practice guidelines from the
    International Society for Traumatic Stress Studies / edited by
    David Forbes, Jonathan I. Bisson, Candice M. Monson, Lucy Berliner.
Description: Third edition. | New York : The Guilford Press, [2020] |
    Includes bibliographical references and index.
Identifiers: LCCN 2019056124 | ISBN 9781462543564 (paperback) |
    ISBN 9781462543571 (hardback)
Subjects: LCSH: Post-traumatic stress disorder–Treatment–Standards. |
    Psychic trauma–Treatment–Standards. | Psychotherapy–Standards.
Classification: LCC RC552.P67 E35 2020 | DDC 616.85/21–dc23
LC record available at *https://lccn.loc.gov/2019056124*

About the Editors

David Forbes, PhD, is Director of Phoenix Australia Centre for Posttraumatic Mental Health and Professor in the Department of Psychiatry at the University of Melbourne. He began practicing as a clinical psychologist in the mid-1990s and has a strong research track record in the assessment and treatment of mental health problems in trauma survivors, with a speciality in military, veteran, emergency services, and post-disaster mental health. Dr. Forbes led the development of the Australian Guidelines for the Treatment of Acute Stress Disorder and PTSD and is Co-Chair of the 5-Eyes Mental Health Research and Innovation Collaboration.

Jonathan I. Bisson, DM, FRCPsych, is Professor of Psychiatry at Cardiff University School of Medicine, Wales, United Kingdom, and a practicing psychiatrist. He is Chair of the Treatment Guidelines Committee of the International Society for Traumatic Stress Studies and is currently developing an All Wales Traumatic Stress Quality Improvement Initiative. Dr. Bisson was Co-Chair of the first PTSD Guideline Development Group of the United Kingdom's National Institute for Health and Care Excellence. He is a past president of the European Society for Traumatic Stress Studies and led the development of Veterans NHS Wales. He has conducted widely cited research on the prevention and treatment of PTSD.

Candice M. Monson, PhD, is Professor of Psychology at Ryerson University in Toronto, Ontario, Canada. She is President-Elect of the International Society for Traumatic Stress Studies and is a Fellow of the American and Canadian Psychological Associations, the Association for Behavioral and Cognitive Therapies, and the Royal Society of Canada. Dr. Monson is a foremost expert on traumatic stress and the use of individual and conjoint therapies to treat PTSD. She is coauthor of *Cognitive Processing Therapy for PTSD* and *Cognitive-Behavioral Conjoint Therapy for PTSD* and coeditor of *Effective Treatments for PTSD, Third Edition*, among other books.

Lucy Berliner, MSW, is Director of the Harborview Center for Sexual Assault and Traumatic Stress at the University of Washington, where she is also Clinical Associate Professor in the School of Social Work and in the Department of Psychiatry and Behavioral Sciences. Her activities include clinical practice with child and adult victims of trauma and crime; research on the impact of trauma and the effectiveness of clinical and societal interventions; and participation in local and national social policy initiatives to promote the interests of trauma and crime victims.

Contributors

Eva Alisic, PhD, Child and Community Wellbeing Unit, School of Population and Global Health, University of Melbourne, Melbourne, Australia

Sudie E. Back, PhD, Department of Psychiatry and Behavioral Sciences, Medical University of South Carolina, Charleston, South Carolina

Lucy Berliner, MSW, Harborview Abuse and Trauma Center, Seattle, Washington

Jonathan I. Bisson, DM, FRCPsych, Department of Psychological Medicine and Clinical Neurosciences, School of Medicine, Cardiff University, Cardiff, Wales, United Kingdom

Chris R. Brewin, PhD, Department of Clinical, Educational, and Health Psychology, University College London, London, United Kingdom

Richard A. Bryant, PhD, School of Psychology, University of New South Wales, Sydney, Australia

Mark Burton, PhD, Department of Psychiatry and Behavioral Sciences, Emory University School of Medicine, Atlanta, Georgia

Kathleen M. Chard, PhD, Trauma Recovery Center, Cincinnati VA Medical Center and Department of Psychiatry and Behavioral Neuroscience, University of Cincinnati, Cincinnati, Ohio

Kelly Chrestman, PhD, Center for Deployment Psychology, Department of Medical and Clinical Psychology, Uniformed Services University of the Health Sciences, Bethesda, Maryland

Marylene Cloitre, PhD, National Center for PTSD, Palo Alto VA Health Care Services, Palo Alto, California; Department of Psychiatry and Behavioral Sciences, Stanford University, Stanford, California

Judith Cohen, MD, Department of Psychiatry, Drexel University College of Medicine, Pittsburgh, Pennsylvania

Zachary Cohen, PhD, National Center for PTSD, Palo Alto, California; Department of Psychiatry, University of California, Los Angeles, Los Angeles, California

Rowena Conroy, PhD, School of Psychological Sciences, University of Melbourne, Melbourne, Australia

Andrea Danese, MD, PhD, Department of Child and Adolescent Psychiatry, Institute of Psychiatry, Psychology and Neuroscience, King's College London, London, United Kingdom

JoAnn Difede, PhD, Department of Psychology, Weill Cornell Medicine, New York, New York

Shannon Dorsey, PhD, Department of Psychology, University of Washington, Seattle, Washington

Grete Dyb, MD, PhD, Norwegian Centre for Violence and Traumatic Stress Studies and Institute of Clinical Medicine, University of Oslo, Oslo, Norway

Anke Ehlers, PhD, Oxford Centre for Anxiety Disorders and Trauma, Department of Experimental Psychology, University of Oxford, Oxford, United Kingdom

Edna B. Foa, PhD, Center for the Study and Treatment of Anxiety, Department of Psychiatry, University of Pennsylvania, Philadelphia, Pennsylvania

David Forbes, PhD, Phoenix Australia Centre for Posttraumatic Mental Health and Department of Psychiatry, University of Melbourne, Melbourne, Australia

Julian D. Ford, PhD, ABPP, Center for Trauma Recovery and Juvenile Justice, Center for the Treatment of Developmental Trauma Disorders, and Department of Psychiatry, University of Connecticut Health Center, Farmington, Connecticut

Tara E. Galovski, PhD, National Center for PTSD, VA Boston Healthcare System, and Department of Psychiatry, Boston University School of Medicine, Boston, Massachusetts

Jaimie Gradus, DSc, MPH, Department of Epidemiology, Boston University School of Public Health; and Department of Psychiatry, Boston University School of Medicine, Boston, Massachusetts

Mathew D. Hoskins, MBBCh, MSc, MRCPsych, Division of Psychological Medicine and Clinical Neurosciences, School of Medicine, Cardiff University, Cardiff, Wales, United Kingdom

Lisa Jaycox, PhD, RAND Corporation, Arlington, Virginia

Tine Jensen, PhD, Department of Psychology, University of Oslo, and Norwegian Centre for Violence and Traumatic Stress Studies, Oslo, Norway

Tammy Jiang, MPH, Department of Epidemiology, Boston University School of Public Health, Boston, Massachusetts

Thanos Karatzias, PhD, School of Health and Social Care, Edinburgh Napier University, and NHS Lothian Rivers Centre for Traumatic Stress, Edinburgh, United Kingdom

Nancy Kassam-Adams, PhD, Department of Pediatrics, University of Pennsylvania Perelman School of Medicine, Philadelphia, Pennsylvania

Debra L. Kaysen, PhD, Department of Psychiatry and Behavioral Sciences, Stanford University Medical Center, Palo Alto, California

Justin Kenardy, PhD, School of Psychology, University of Queensland, Queensland, Australia

Karestan C. Koenen, PhD, Departments of Epidemiology and Social and Behavioral Sciences, Harvard T. H. Chan School of Public Health, Cambridge, Massachusetts

Kristina J. Korte, PhD, Department of Psychiatry, Massachusetts General Hospital, Boston, Massachusetts

Ariel J. Lang, PhD, MPH, VA San Diego Center for Excellence for Stress and Mental Health and Departments of Psychiatry and Family Medicine and Public Health, University of California, San Diego, San Diego, California

Christopher Lee, PhD, Faculty of Health and Medical Sciences, University of Western Australia, Perth, Australia

Catrin Lewis, PhD, Division of Psychological Medicine and Clinical Neurosciences, School of Medicine, Cardiff University, Cardiff, Wales, United Kingdom

Andreas Maercker, MD, PhD, Department of Psychopathology and Clinical Intervention, University of Zurich, Zurich, Switzerland

Sybil Mallonee, PhD, Department of Medical and Clinical Psychology, Uniformed Services University of the Health Sciences, Bethesda, Maryland

Jessica Maples-Keller, PhD, Department of Psychiatry and Behavioral Sciences, Emory University School of Medicine, Atlanta, Georgia

Ifigeneia Mavranezouli, MD, Research Department of Clinical, Educational and Health Psychology, University College London, London, United Kingdom

Richard Meiser-Stedman, PhD, Department of Clinical Psychology and Psychological Therapies, University of East Anglia, Norwich, United Kingdom

Cathrine Mihalopoulos, PhD, School of Health and Social Development, Deakin University, Geelong, Australia

Candice M. Monson, PhD, Department of Psychology, Ryerson University, Toronto, Ontario, Canada

Kim T. Mueser, PhD, Center for Psychiatric Rehabilitation, Boston University, Boston, Massachusetts

Laura K. Murray, PhD, Department of Mental Health, Johns Hopkins Bloomberg School of Public Health, Baltimore, Maryland

Barbara Niles, PhD, National Center for PTSD, VA Boston Healthcare System, and Department of Psychiatry, Boston University School of Medicine, Boston, Massachusetts

Reginald D. V. Nixon, PhD, College of Education, Psychology and Social Work, Flinders University, Adelaide, Australia

Meaghan L. O'Donnell, PhD, Phoenix Australia Centre for Posttraumatic Mental Health and Department of Psychiatry, University of Melbourne, Melbourne, Australia

Miranda Olff, PhD, Department of Psychiatry, Amsterdam University Medical Centers, University of Amsterdam, Amsterdam, Netherlands; ARQ National Psychotrauma Centre, Diemen, Netherlands

Belinda J. Pacella, MClinPsych, Phoenix Australia Centre for Posttraumatic Mental Health and Department of Psychiatry, University of Melbourne, Melbourne, Australia

Stephen Pilling, PhD, Division of Psychology and Language Sciences, University College London, London, United Kingdom

David S. Riggs, PhD, Center for Deployment Psychology, Department of Medical and Clinical Psychology, Uniformed Services University of the Health Sciences, Bethesda, Maryland

Neil P. Roberts, DClinPsy, Cardiff and Vale University Health Board and Division of Psychological Medicine and Clinical Neurosciences, School of Medicine, Cardiff University, Cardiff, Wales, United Kingdom

Craig Rosen, PhD, National Center for PTSD, VA Palo Alto Health Care System, Menlo Park, California

Rita Rosner, DPhil, DiplPsych, Department of Psychology, Catholic University of Eichstätt-Ingolstadt, Eichstätt, Germany

Barbara O. Rothbaum, PhD, ABPP, Emory Healthcare Veterans Program and Department of Psychiatry and Behavioral Sciences, Emory University School of Medicine, Atlanta, Georgia

Mark C. Russell, PhD, School of Applied Psychology, Counseling and Family Therapy, Antioch University, Seattle, Washington

Ulrich Schnyder, MD, Department of Consultation-Liaison Psychiatry and Psychosomatic Medicine, University Hospital, University of Zurich, Zurich, Switzerland

Sarah J. Schubert, PhD, private practice, Brentwood, Australia

Francine Shapiro, PhD (deceased), Mental Research Institute, Palo Alto, California; EMDR Institute, Watsonville, California

Marit Sijbrandij, PhD, Department of Clinical, Neuro, and Developmental Psychology and WHO Collaborating Centre for Research and Dissemination of Psychological Interventions, Vrije University Amsterdam, Amsterdam, Netherlands

Dan J. Stein, FRCPC, PhD, SA MRC Unit on Risk & Resilience in Mental Disorders, Department of Psychiatry and Neuroscience Institute, University of Cape Town, Cape Town, South Africa

Shannon Wiltsey Stirman, PhD, National Center for PTSD, VA Palo Alto Health Care System, Menlo Park, California; Department of Psychiatry and Behavioral Sciences, Stanford University, Palo Alto, California

Yilang Tang, MD, PhD, Department of Psychiatry and Behavioral Sciences, Emory University School of Medicine, and Atlanta VA Medical Center, Atlanta, Georgia

Larissa Tate, MS, MPS, Department of Medical and Clinical Psychology, Uniformed Services University of the Health Sciences, Bethesda, Maryland

Siri Thoresen, PhD, Norwegian Centre for Violence and Traumatic Stress Studies and Department of Psychology, University of Oslo, Oslo, Norway

Maegan M. Paxton Willing, BS, Department of Medical and Clinical Psychology, Uniformed Services University of the Health Sciences, Bethesda, Maryland

Laurence Astill Wright, MBBCH, Division of Psychological Medicine and Clinical Neurosciences, School of Medicine, Cardiff University, Cardiff, Wales, United Kingdom

Katarzyna Wyka, PhD, Department of Psychiatry, Weill Cornell Medicine, New York, New York

A Note from the Editors
of the Second Edition

Congratulations to Dave Forbes, Jon Bisson, Candice Monson, and Lucy Berliner on overseeing this new edition. They have masterfully synthesized the wide-ranging research on treating posttraumatic stress disorder that has been conducted since the publication of the second edition in 2009. Their editorial vision has brought a fresh perspective to the treatment guidelines of the International Society for Traumatic Stress Studies and offers the field an invaluable resource. We are thrilled to see the careful work in this arena continue, giving guidance to practitioners and researchers around the world.

EDNA B. FOA
TERENCE M. KEANE
MATTHEW J. FRIEDMAN
JUDITH A. COHEN

Preface

Clinical practice guidelines, which synthesize research evidence to generate specific treatment recommendations for a particular disorder, have been of crucial importance over the last decade in promoting a shift toward evidence-based care. Clinical practice guidelines for posttraumatic stress disorder (PTSD) are designed primarily to help clinicians achieve improved mental health outcomes for people affected by trauma. The secondary goal is to assist those people and their families, as well as policymakers and service delivery organizations, to develop a more sophisticated understanding of the range of available treatments and the evidence for their efficacy.

The recent *Posttraumatic Stress Disorder Prevention and Treatment Guidelines*, on which this book is based, were published by the International Society for Traumatic Stress Studies (ISTSS) in 2018, with earlier versions dating back to 2000 and 2009 (as well as guidelines for the treatment of complex PTSD in 2012). The latest guidelines build on the groundbreaking work of the initial guidelines through adopting a standardized rigorous systematic review of the available research literature across all the areas of focus. Similar evidence-driven guidelines for PTSD treatment have been published in several countries, including Australia, the United Kingdom, and the United States, with all arriving at largely similar conclusions. Although the high degree of consensus is reassuring, this methodological approach to guideline development comes at a price. A heavy reliance on randomized controlled trials means that other less rigorous but perhaps equally important sources of data, as well as the nuances of clinical practice, may not be considered in generating recommendations.

Perhaps more important, the challenge for clinicians is often one of how to apply the recommendations in the real world of clinical practice. It is one thing to know what the research evidence tells us about treatments that work. It is another thing altogether to implement those treatments in routine clinical practice, frequently in the context of significant clinical complexity, psychosocial disadvantage, and limitations in mental health delivery systems. Clinicians may question whether the findings from sophisticated research trials are translatable to their everyday clinical practice. They may question their own ability to deliver those evidence-based interventions and, perhaps, to contain any distress that might be triggered by trauma-focused psychological interventions.

Using the latest ISTSS PTSD guidelines as the starting point, each chapter of this book summarizes the research evidence base and resulting recommendations reported in those guidelines. While keeping the empirical findings front and center in driving the treatment recommendations, the book stands as a natural evolution of the science by explaining not only how the research foundations were derived but also how those findings were used to form the basis of the recommendations.

The book goes on to bridge the gap between evidence-based guidelines and routine practice in the real world. It is a unique contribution to the field, with each chapter going beyond the research evidence to explore the challenges of implementation. The authors, all specialists in their specific treatment approaches, were asked to build on the recommendations by considering the common difficulties encountered by clinicians across a diverse range of settings and with a broad range of trauma-affected populations. They were encouraged to explore when and why things go wrong in treatment, why some people do not respond, how we might decide to stop trying a particular approach, and what to do at that point. The treatment chapters are preceded by contextual chapters that outline recent developments in our understanding of the nature, epidemiology, and assessment of mental health responses to trauma exposure in adults, adolescents, and children, as well as the latest evidence on prevention. Following the treatment chapters, the book goes on to foreshadow future developments in areas such as transdiagnostic conceptualizations of posttraumatic mental health problems, tailoring treatment to the unique needs of the individual clinical presentation, dissemination challenges, and economic implications.

In focusing on the practical aspects of guideline implementation for clinicians, therefore, the authors recognize the limitations of the research and go beyond it to provide practical, clinically informed advice on how best to use and understand the recommendations in a way that is accessible and useful for clinicians and health service agencies.

After reading this book, clinicians will be clear about not only the specific treatment recommendations for PTSD, but also how to implement them in varying environments and with complex clinical presentations. They will understand where the field is heading in terms of clinical practice, research, and implementation science. By striving to adopt the advice provided by the expert clinicians who have authored each chapter, readers will become part of that journey as the field continues to develop. They will be up to date on the latest thinking in the treatment of PTSD, making them a point of reference for those who practice around them and leaders in the field among their clinical colleagues. In short, this book is essential reading for all clinicians working with survivors of trauma.

DAVID FORBES, PhD
JONATHAN I. BISSON, DM, FRCPsych,
CANDICE M. MONSON, PhD
LUCY BERLINER, MSW

Acknowledgments

We would like to acknowledge that this third edition of *Effective Treatments for PTSD* sits on the shoulders of the work of previous editors of the first and second editions of this book, Edna Foa, Terrence Keane, Matthew Friedman, and Judith Cohen. Without their field leadership and insight represented in the first two editions, this volume would not have been possible.

This book is founded on the *Posttraumatic Stress Disorder Prevention and Treatment Guidelines* of the ISTSS. We thank the entire PTSD Guidelines Committee for their work in developing the guidelines. The committee included Jonathon I. Bisson (Chair), David Forbes (Vice Chair), Lucy Berliner, Marylene Cloitre, Lutz Goldbeck, Tine Jensen, Catrin Lewis, Candice M. Monson, Miranda Olff, Stephen Pilling, David S. Riggs, Neil P. Roberts, and Francine Shapiro. The editors of this volume and the PTSD Guidelines Committee acknowledge the passing of our friends and colleagues in this work, Dr. Lutz Goldbeck and Dr. Francine Shapiro, both of whom contributed enormously through their work to reduce the suffering of people with PTSD.

Contents

II. EARLY INTERVENTION IN ADULTS

III. EARLY INTERVENTION IN CHILDREN AND ADOLESCENTS

IV. TREATMENTS FOR ADULTS

V. TREATMENTS FOR CHILDREN AND ADOLESCENTS

VI. APPLICATION, IMPLEMENTATION, AND FUTURE DIRECTIONS

PART I

INTRODUCTION AND BACKGROUND

CHAPTER 1

Effective Treatments for PTSD
Guiding Current Practice and Future Innovation

David Forbes, Jonathan I. Bisson, Candice M. Monson,
and Lucy Berliner

Empirically supported interventions to prevent and treat posttraumatic stress disorder (PTSD) and related conditions for people of all ages have been the focus of much attention over the last two decades, resulting in a substantial evidence base to inform clinical decisions. In this vein, there has been a significant accumulation of evidence since the last edition of *Effective Treatments for PTSD*; hence the timeliness of this third edition. This body of evidence has the potential to provide much-needed guidance to clinicians and mental health service systems, as well as to people with PTSD and their families. Concurrent with burgeoning empirical evidence on effective and ineffective interventions, there has been a substantial increase in awareness among the broader community regarding the psychological effects of trauma exposure. The mental health of our serving personnel, veterans and first responders, survivors of sexual and physical assault, family violence and childhood abuse, survivors of natural and man-made disasters, and other potentially traumatized people has become a high-profile issue in modern society. The topic receives widespread coverage in the media, both in current affairs and fictional drama. This high level of community attention has placed increasing pressure on clinicians, health service agencies, employers, and government to provide timely, accessible, and effective care.

Although increased recognition of the effects of trauma and a more robust knowledge base on interventions might seem optimistic, we face significant challenges in our field. Despite the evidence base—the existence of demonstrably effective interventions—most people at risk of or with PTSD still do not receive an evidence-based intervention. This is true not only in low- and middle-income countries (Tol et al., 2014), but also in developed

3

countries with comprehensive and sophisticated mental health systems (Rosen et al., 2017; Sripada, Pfeiffer, Rauch, Ganoczy, & Bohnert, 2018). There are several possible explanations for this, including poor practitioner access to clinical training and supervision in evidence-based practices, as well as the limited effectiveness and high cost of dissemination (Foa, Gillihan, & Bryant, 2013). An important related factor, however, remains a reticence by some clinicians to embrace these approaches. This may be due to a lack of confidence in their skills to deliver the intervention and, perhaps, to contain the potential distress that might accompany a trauma-focused psychological intervention. It may also be driven by misconceptions and misunderstandings about these evidence-based practices, and concerns about how translatable and generalizable the rigorous protocols used in research trials are for their own clinical practice. This book attempts to address some of those concerns, bridging the gap between (1) research protocols that form the basis of studies included in the evidence review that underpins the recommendations in the recently published *Posttraumatic Stress Disorder Prevention and Treatment Guidelines* (published by the International Society for Traumatic Stress Studies [ISTSS] in 2018) represented in this book and (2) delivery of evidence-based practices in routine clinical practice.

The purpose of this book, therefore, is not only to summarize the research evidence base and resulting recommendations reported in the ISTSS guidelines, but to expand upon that evidence and operationalize the recommendations to guide clinicians in implementing evidence-based practices. In doing so, the authors recognize the limitations of the research and go beyond it to provide practical, clinically informed advice on how best to use and understand the recommendations in a way that is accessible and useful for clinicians and health service agencies. Consequently, this book differs from both earlier evidence summaries and clinical treatment manuals by using the evidence base as a starting point, discussing the implementation of those treatments and practices that have been shown to work, and going beyond the evidence to discuss the challenges and limitations of delivering evidence-based practices in routine clinical practice. It is designed to be practical, useful, and applied, optimizing the value of the ISTSS guidelines for those tasked with delivering evidence-based practices. It aims to address the nuances of delivering those treatments with different populations and what to do when things do not go as planned or hoped.

The following chapters seek to improve our understanding of the nature, epidemiology, and assessment of traumatic stress, as well as patterns of recovery and long-term outcomes. Each of the prevention and treatment chapters aims to summarize, and improve our understanding of, the relevant guideline findings and recommendations, and in the case of chapters on combinations of psychological and pharmacological interventions and on complex PTSD and comorbidity, to consider important clinical presentations and approaches that were not covered by the scoping questions posed for the guidelines. These prevention and treatment chapters explore how the recommendations might be implemented in clinical practice, across diverse settings and with a broad range of trauma-affected populations. The authors endeavor to explore when and why things go wrong in treatment, why some people do not respond, when we might stop trying a particular approach, and what to do at that point. Later chapters draw out the common elements of effective evidence-based practices, the nuances of these common elements, and their implications for clinicians. The final chapters cover health economics, trying to address the question of "value for money," and consider what the future might hold in areas such as e-health, personalized medicine, and implementation and training.

Overview of the Contents of This Book

The introductory chapters of this book provide background information on the nature and epidemiology of PTSD and other mental health responses to trauma, as well as screening and assessment. Chapter 2 covers the nature of trauma and its sequelae, clinical presentations including comorbidity, and epidemiological issues in adults, and Chapter 3 explores clinical presentations, epidemiology, and developmental considerations in children and adolescents. It is clear from these contributions that the science is evolving as we continue to learn more about the nature and epidemiology of traumatic stress reactions. Increasingly large datasets, combined with expanding computational power, are providing opportunities to answer more complex and sophisticated questions about symptom profiles, risk and protective factors, and recovery trajectories. The fact that we can now devote a whole chapter in this area to children and adolescents is testament to our growing knowledge and understanding of developmental considerations in human responses to trauma exposure. Similarly, Chapter 4 covers screening, assessment, and diagnosis in adults, while Chapter 5 addresses those questions for children and adolescents, again highlighting the importance of paying appropriate attention to developmental issues. Both of these chapters explore a range of diagnostic issues, including those associated with the transition from the fourth edition of the *Diagnostic and Statistical Manual of Mental Disorders* (DSM-IV; American Psychiatric Association, 2000) to the fifth edition (DSM-5, American Psychiatric Association, 2013) and the differences between DSM-5 and the 11th revision of the *International Classification of Diseases* (ICD-11; World Health Organization, 2018). This latter comparison is important, since the ICD-11 has taken quite a different approach to defining the essential characteristics of a PTSD diagnosis and has introduced the new, parallel diagnosis of complex PTSD. Although it is, perhaps, too early to comment on the potential impact of these differences in diagnostic nomenclature for treatment recommendations, it is an important question to be addressed in future treatment outcome studies. Chapter 6 provides a summary of the guideline rationale, process, and methodology, before Chapter 7 outlines the specific guideline recommendations.

The next three chapters focus on prevention and early intervention. Chapters 8 and 9 discuss the guideline recommendations and implications for clinicians of psychological and pharmacological prevention and early interventions following trauma exposure for adults. Again, recognizing the importance of development, Chapter 10 addresses those issues in child and adolescent populations. These chapters highlight the current state of the evidence for preventive interventions and make recommendations for future directions. It is clear that prevention research in universally applied interventions is in its infancy and, at this stage, the data are not encouraging. Early psychological intervention for those who have developed symptoms, however, has a much more positive evidence base. These chapters provide an opportunity to explore the different theoretical models that underpin psychological and pharmacological early interventions, raising intriguing questions about the mechanisms that may underpin recovery.

The next section of the book discusses the guideline recommendations for the treatment of PTSD and related conditions in adults, along with the implications for clinicians. Trauma-focused psychological treatments have the strongest level of empirical support in the treatment of PTSD. The section begins with an overview chapter that highlights the commonalities across the four approaches with the largest body of research support: cognitive processing therapy (CPT; Resick, Monson, & Chard, 2017), cognitive therapy for PTSD (CT-PTSD; Ehlers, Clark, Hackmann, McManus, & Fennell, 2005), eye movement desensitization and reprocessing (EMDR) therapy (Shapiro, 2018), and prolonged exposure (PE; Foa, Hembree, & Rothbaum, 2007; Foa, Rothbaum, Riggs, & Murdock, 1991). The chapter also identifies some of the issues with which clinicians commonly struggle, as well as discussing when and why these interventions do not always seem to be effective. These and other clinical nuances are discussed in the subsequent chapters on each specific intervention, but this chapter aims to extract the common elements. It also addresses the implications for clinical practice of having four strongly recommended first-line psychological treatments.

Chapters 12, 13, 14, and 15 discuss the guideline recommendations and implications for clinicians of PE, CPT, EMDR therapy, and CT-PTSD in more detail. These chapters strive not only to describe the intervention and the available empirical support, but also to go beyond those factors to explore the challenges of implementation in routine, real-world clinical practice. The authors recognize that, although these remain the first-line treatments of choice for PTSD, there are limitations and that not everyone will achieve clinically significant benefits. The authors explore why that might be and, more importantly, what we as clinicians might do in those circumstances. These chapters are prefaced by Chapter 11, which outlines the psychological treatment recommendations overall and identifies the common ingredients among these four most strongly recommended treatments. The chapter examines the potentially shared putative mechanisms underlying these four recommended treatments and the implications of these mechanisms for other recommended psychological interventions.

Although trauma-focused psychological treatments have the strongest empirical support and remain the first-line treatment, pharmacological interventions have an important role to play in the comprehensive management of PTSD. Chapter 16 reviews the evidence for pharmacological approaches for adults and discusses the guideline recommendations. The authors recognize that clinicians do not always stick rigidly to the evidence base, with prescribing decisions often being made on the basis of the specific clinical presentation, response to initial pharmacotherapy, and personal preference. To assist clinicians in this difficult process, the authors provide an algorithm—a decision-making tree based on the available evidence, with advice on which medications to try in which order. In routine clinical practice, psychological therapy and pharmacotherapy are often provided concurrently, especially in more complex and chronic cases. Chapter 17 reviews the evidence on combining pharmacological and psychological treatment, discussing the guideline recommendations and their implications for treatment.

With the ubiquitous availability of technology and the Internet, including handheld devices, the field of "e-health" has received increasing attention in recent years. In the trauma field, several online intervention options and mobile "apps" have been proposed as both stand-alone and adjunct treatments. Chapter 18 reviews the emerging evidence on these approaches. Although the authors note the need for more research, it is clear that technological approaches provide intriguing possibilities for improving treatment options, especially for people in rural and remote locations, as well as in boosting the efficacy of more traditional approaches. The authors explore the issues and challenges faced by clinicians who wish to integrate technological approaches into their practice.

Increasing awareness of the mental health effects of trauma has resulted in much greater attention being paid to the quality and accessibility of treatment. Alongside a focus on mainstream approaches, a wide range of alternative interventions to treat PTSD and related conditions has been proposed. Some of these have a track record in the treatment of other conditions, strong theoretical underpinnings, and an emerging evidence base. Others are less well developed, but nevertheless have strong proponents. The challenge for the field is to be open to new ideas and innovations, while still adhering to scientific principles and a commitment to evidence-based treatment (EBT). Chapter 19 explores some of the alternative approaches that show early promise as treatments in their own right, or as adjuncts to first-line treatments with the aim of improving quality of life, and discusses the guideline recommendations in this area. Again, the challenge for clinicians is whether and how to incorporate some of these approaches into their treatment planning and practice.

Although the concept of complex PTSD has been discussed in the literature for many years, it was not until the advent of ICD-11 that the disorder was formally recognized in the diagnostic nomenclature. Chapter 20 discusses the diagnostic criteria and treatment recommendations, before considering the challenges faced by clinicians working in this area.

Chapter 21 discusses the evidence base for psychological and pharmacological treatments for PTSD in adolescents and children. Notably, there has been significant development in the evidence base since the last guidelines were published, and three psychosocial treatments receive strong recommendations. Psychopharmacological treatments have so far not been shown to be effective for children. Although not yet at the same level as interventions for adults, we can be more confident about the efficacy of some approaches now than we were previously.

The final group of chapters are more exploratory in nature. Chapter 22 explores the complex issue of comorbidity and transdiagnostics. A high degree of overlap in symptoms and clinical presentation exists across several of the high-prevalence conditions, and PTSD is no exception. The fact that the disorder is characterized by features of depression, anxiety, and (in many cases) dissociation raises the question of whether current diagnostic systems that conceptualize disorders as discrete categories represent the most useful model. The authors grapple with this issue and discuss the implications for clinicians. Chapter 23 takes this discussion to the next level, exploring the implications of different clinical presentations of PTSD on our conceptualizations of treatment models. The authors argue for a more personalized approach to intervention in the future, with the treatment plan better matched to the specific needs of the individual. They go on to discuss the challenges of progressing this individualized approach, while still retaining a commitment to the scientific method and EBT.

The best PTSD treatments in the world are of little use unless they are adopted by mental health practitioners working in routine clinical settings. Chapter 24 addresses the challenges of dissemination and implementation, exploring what needs to be done in order to improve the uptake of EBTs by clinicians. In a related vein, Chapter 25 reviews the economic implications of the guidelines. Drawing on international data, particularly from the United Kingdom and Australia, the authors highlight the potential economic benefits to be gained by widespread adoption of the guideline recommendations. Finally, Chapter 26 foreshadows future opportunities to advance more sophisticated approaches to understanding the nature and course of human responses to trauma, the mechanisms underlying those different trajectories, and how best to improve our treatments and implement best-practice interventions.

The ISTSS *Posttraumatic Stress Disorder Prevention and Treatment Guidelines* Process

Several clinical practice guidelines now exist to guide the treatment of PTSD and related conditions (American Psychological Association, 2017; Department of Veterans Affairs & Department of Defense Clinical Practice Working Group, 2017; National Institute for Health and Care Excellence, 2005;

Phoenix Australia—Centre for Posttraumatic Mental Health, 2013). Most of these are based on a systematic literature review process that uses clearly defined and internationally agreed-upon methods to collect and collate the research data, critically appraise research studies, and synthesize the findings to generate recommendations graded by the strength of the evidence. The recently published (2018) ISTSS guidelines represented in this book also adopted this approach (Bisson et al., 2019). As such, they embrace currently accepted gold standards for guideline development and represent a substantial change in methodology compared to the two earlier guidelines produced by ISTSS. The latest version provides an important addition to the growing body of evidence-based clinical practice guidelines in the trauma field and provides the platform upon which the chapters in this book build. The authors, who are not only leaders in their particular treatment approaches but also experienced clinicians, recognize that treatment guidelines alone do not change practice. They understand how hard it can be for clinicians to interpret and implement the guideline recommendations in their routine clinical work, and they are acutely aware of the clinical complexity that often confronts practitioners working with the mental health effects of trauma. The fact is that, despite substantial progress in the field of traumatic stress, many questions remain unanswered and many challenges confront those providing treatment.

As highlighted previously, Chapter 6 describes the rationale, process, and methodology used to develop the ISTSS guidelines (ISTSS, 2018), as well as summarizing the guideline recommendations themselves. Briefly, the process followed a rigorous systematic review approach, beginning with the development of explicit scoping questions. In developing the ISTSS guidelines, a systematic review identified 361 randomized controlled trials (RCTs) according to the a priori agreed inclusion criteria. There were 208 meta-analyses conducted, resulting in 125 recommendations (24 for children and adolescents and 101 for adults). An agreed-upon definition of clinical importance and strength of recommendation resulted in 8, *Strong*; 8, *Standard*; 5, *Intervention with Low Effect*; 26, *Intervention with Emerging Evidence*; and 78, *Insufficient Evidence to Recommend* recommendations. Narrative reviews were undertaken and two position papers (one for children and adolescents, and one for adults) were prepared to address current issues in complex PTSD and to make recommendations for further research. The draft recommendations were posted on the ISTSS website during August and September 2018 for a period of consultation by ISTSS members. Feedback from ISTSS members was reviewed and incorporated into the final recommendations, which were approved by the ISTSS Board in October 2018.

The adoption of a systematic review approach to developing clinical practice guidelines helps to ensure transparency and replicability by establishing key elements of the process prior to commencement: scoping questions, inclusion/exclusion criteria for papers, definition of clinical importance, and a recommendation generation algorithm. This rigorous approach helps to reduce the risk of inconsistency and conscious or implicit bias of committee members influencing the recommendations. It is consistent with an internationally accepted commitment to evidence-based practice and is a fundamental starting point in establishing first-line treatments.

Notwithstanding those benefits, adoption of a systematic review methodology in guideline development also has some limitations. For example, systematic reviews often limit the number of questions that can be addressed, either because they are not asked or because no solid data exist. This may result in some potentially important issues, especially around implementation in clinical practice—for example, in areas such as comorbidity—not being adequately explored. Despite rigorous selection criteria for inclusion, it is possible that methodological differences across studies may influence the interpretation of results and, therefore, the recommendations. Systematic reviews need to decide, a priori, on the primary outcomes of interest—in this case, PTSD symptom reduction. Clearly, in routine clinical practice, other outcomes might be equally (or more) important goals for intervention. Finally, and perhaps most importantly, a focus on RCTs in a systematic review may result in other important evidence being omitted (e.g., large observational cohort studies, nonrandomized controlled studies such as larger uncontrolled program evaluation studies, longer-term follow-ups, and "evidence from practice"). Despite the lack of methodological rigor, those pieces of evidence have the potential to contribute to a more accurate assessment of the effectiveness of a particular intervention in routine clinical practice. By going beyond the systematic review, this book allows the proponents of each approach to draw on that body of data and to recognize the importance of other, real-world factors that may be important to consider in the adoption and utilization of the guideline recommendations. This approach echoes the sentiments of the founders of evidence-based practice when they noted, "Good doctors use both individual clinical expertise and the best available external evidence, and neither alone is enough" (Sackett, Rosenberg, Muir Gray, Haynes, & Richardson, 1996, p. 72).

Summary

This book is designed to be a practical guide for those working with survivors of trauma. The starting point is the systematic review of the research evidence, and the resultant recommendations, contained in the ISTSS (2018) *Posttraumatic Stress Disorder Prevention and Treatment Guidelines*. That document illustrates just how far the field has come since the diagnosis of PTSD was first formally recognized in the diagnostic nomenclature in DSM-III (American Psychiatric Association, 1980) 40 years ago. Equally, we need to recognize the limitations of the research data for practicing clinicians and interpret the guideline recommendations to address the complexity that we routinely see in clinical practice. This book builds on the guidelines, going beyond the recommendations to make them useful for clinicians, service providers, and health and mental health service systems.

REFERENCES

American Psychiatric Association. (1980). *Diagnostic and statistical manual of mental disorders* (3rd ed.). Washington, DC: Author.

American Psychiatric Association. (2000). *Diagnostic and statistical manual of mental disorders* (4th ed., text rev.). Washington, DC: Author.

American Psychiatric Association. (2013). *Diagnostic and statistical manual of mental disorders* (5th ed.). Arlington, VA: Author.

American Psychological Association. (2017). *Clinical practice guideline for the treatment of posttraumatic stress disorder (PTSD) in adults.* Washington, DC: Author.

Bisson, J. I., Berliner, L., Cloitre, M., Forbes, D., Jensen, T. K., Lewis, C., et al. (2019). The International Society for Traumatic Stress Studies new guidelines for the prevention and treatment of PTSD: Methodology and development process. *Journal of Traumatic Stress, 32*(4), 475–483.

Department of Veterans Affairs & Department of Defense Clinical Practice Working Group. (2017). *VA/DoD clinical practice guideline for the management of posttraumatic stress disorder and acute stress disorder.* Washington, DC: VA Office of Quality and Performance.

Ehlers, A., Clark, D. M., Hackmann, A., McManus, F., & Fennell, M. (2005). Cognitive therapy for post-traumatic stress disorder: Development and evaluation. *Behaviour Research and Therapy, 43,* 413–431.

Foa, E. B., Gillihan, S. J., & Bryant, R. A. (2013). Challenges and successes in dissemination of evidence-based treatments for posttraumatic stress: Lessons learned from prolonged exposure therapy for PTSD. *Psychological Science in the Public Interest, 14*(2), 65–111.

Foa, E. B., Hembree, E. A., & Rothbaum, B. O. (2007). *Prolonged exposure therapy for PTSD: Emotional processing of traumatic experiences: Therapist guide.* New York: Oxford University Press.

Foa, E. B., Rothbaum, B. O., Riggs, D. S., & Murdock, T. B. (1991). Treatment of posttraumatic stress disorder in rape victims: A comparison between cognitive-behavioral procedures and counseling. *Journal of Consulting Clinical Psychology, 59*(5), 715–723.

International Society for Traumatic Stress Studies. (2018). New ISTSS prevention and treatment guidelines. Retrieved from *www.istss.org/clinical-resources/ treating-trauma/new-istss-prevention-and-treatment-guidelines.*

National Institute for Health and Care Excellence. (2005). *Post-traumatic stress disorder: The management of PTSD in adults and children in primary and secondary care.* Leicester, UK: Gaskell.

Phoenix Australia—Centre for Posttraumatic Mental Health. (2013). *Australian guidelines for the treatment of acute stress disorder and posttraumatic stress disorder.* Melbourne, Victoria, Australia: Author.

Resick, P., Monson, C., & Chard, K. (2017). *Cognitive processing therapy for PTSD: A comprehensive manual.* New York: Guilford Press.

Rosen, C. S., Eftekhari, A., Crowley, J., Smith, B. N., Kuhn, E., Trent, L., et al. (2017).

Maintenance and reach of exposure psychotherapy for posttraumatic stress disorder 18 months after training. *Journal of Traumatic Stress, 30,* 63–70.

Sackett, D. L., Rosenberg, W. M., Muir Gray, J. A., Haynes, R. B., & Richardson, W. S. (1996). Evidence based medicine: What it is and what it isn't. *British Medical Journal, 312,* 71–72.

Shapiro, F. (2018). *Eye movement desensitization and reprocessing (EMDR) therapy* (3rd ed.). New York: Guilford Press.

Sripada, R. K., Pfeiffer, P. N., Rauch, S. A., Ganoczy, D., & Bohnert, K. M. (2018). Factors associated with the receipt of documented evidence-based psychotherapy for PTSD in VA. *General Hospital Psychiatry, 54,* 12–17.

Tol, W. A., Barbui, C., Bisson, J., Cohen, J., Hijazi, Z., Jones, L., et al. (2014). World Health Organization guidelines for management of acute stress, PTSD, and bereavement: Key challenges on the road ahead. *PLOS Medicine, 11*(12), e1001769.

World Health Organization. (2018). *International statistical classification of diseases and related health problems* (11th rev.). Geneva, Switzerland: Author. Retrieved from *https://www.who.int/classifications/icd/en.*

CHAPTER 2

Trauma and PTSD

Epidemiology, Comorbidity, and Clinical Presentation in Adults

Kristina J. Korte, Tammy Jiang, Karestan C. Koenen, and Jaimie Gradus

Traumatic events, such as natural disasters, automobile and other accidents, sexual assault, and child abuse are common throughout the world and can take a tremendous psychological toll on individuals and communities. In this chapter, we present information about the global public health burden posed by trauma exposure. To accomplish this goal, we review the prevalence and distribution of traumatic events and trauma-related disorders from epidemiological studies, with a focus on posttraumatic stress disorder (PTSD). We also review the prevalence of disorders that commonly co-occur with PTSD and provide an overview of the clinical presentation of PTSD.

Epidemiology is the science of public health and focuses on the distribution and causes of disease in human populations, as well as developing and testing ways to prevent and control disease. Epidemiological studies provide empirical evidence on the high prevalence of trauma and the devastating effects of trauma-related disorders, and show that trauma is not equally distributed across populations. When presenting the results throughout this chapter, we note methodological considerations that make cross-study comparisons difficult. Although the focus in epidemiology is on populations and not individuals, to illustrate epidemiological findings we provide prototypical cases of trauma exposure and common trajectories observed (e.g., normal recovery and diagnosis of PTSD).

The Epidemiology of Trauma Exposure

Trauma exposure is common globally. A traumatic event is defined as exposure to actual or threatened death, serious injury, or sexual violence according to the fifth edition of the *Diagnostic and Statistical Manual of Mental Disorders* (DSM-5; American Psychiatric Association, 2013). Individuals can be exposed to a traumatic event by directly experiencing the traumatic event, witnessing in person the event as it occurred to others, learning that the traumatic event occurred to a close family member or close friend, or experiencing repeated or extreme exposure to aversive details of traumatic events (American Psychiatric Association, 2013). Approximately 70% of respondents in the World Health Organization's World Mental Health Surveys (WMHS) have experienced one or more traumas (Kessler et al., 2017). Globally, each person experiences an average of 3.2 lifetime traumas (Kessler et al., 2017). The most common traumatic events worldwide include witnessing death or serious injury, experiencing the unexpected death of a loved one, being mugged/assaulted, being in a life-threatening automobile accident, and experiencing a life-threatening illness or injury (Benjet et al., 2016). Combined, these five traumatic events account for over half of all instances of trauma exposure globally (Benjet et al., 2016). In the following material, we discuss factors that affect the prevalence of trauma exposure, including changes in the definition of a traumatic event, and heterogeneity in the people and places assessed.

Changes in the Definition of a Traumatic Event

The newest iteration of the DSM, the main diagnostic classification system used in the United States, resulted in three major changes in the definition of trauma from DSM-IV to DSM-5 that might impact the incidence and prevalence of trauma and PTSD. DSM-IV included a requirement of particular emotional responses to a traumatic event (Criterion A2). Thus, individuals who did not endorse fear, helplessness, or horror during a traumatic event could not receive a diagnosis of PTSD, even if they met the rest of the diagnostic criteria for PTSD (Pai, Suris, & North, 2017). In DSM-5, the requirement for emotional responses to a traumatic event is removed. A second change to the definition of trauma from DSM-IV to DSM-5 was that DSM-5 removed the term "threat to physical integrity" from the definition of trauma. Nonacute, noncatastrophic, life-threatening illness (e.g., terminal cancer) no longer qualifies as trauma, regardless of how stressful or severe it is (Pai et al., 2017). This change has been found to reduce the number of PTSD cases (Kilpatrick et al., 2013). A third change to the definition of trauma in the newest iteration of DSM was that DSM-IV-TR allowed for indirect exposure to trauma (without being present) at the time of the traumatic event, whereas DSM-5 added a new requirement for the witnessing of trauma to others to be "in person." Repeated or extreme exposure to aversive details of the traumatic event was added to DSM-5, but does not apply to exposure through electronic media, television, movies, or pictures, unless this exposure is work-related (American Psychiatric Association, 2013). Police officers, firefighters, ambulance personnel, and health care personnel often experience indirect traumatic events, such as witnessing the suffering of others as part of their work (Skogstad et al., 2013). The nature of the trauma witnessing may also be an important factor, such as dealing with child victims of abuse (North et al., 2002; Skogstad et al., 2013). More details about the diagnostic criteria for PTSD and the criteria as outlined in ICD-11 (which is used primarily outside of the United States) can be found in Bisson, Brewin, Cloitre, and Maercker (Chapter 4, this volume).

The Heterogeneity in the Prevalence of Trauma Exposure across Countries

The prevalence of trauma exposure varies across countries. According to the World Health Organization's WMHS, which are general population studies carried out throughout the world from 2001 until 2012 that used the DSM-IV definition of trauma, the prevalence of exposure to any traumatic event ranged from a high of 83% in the United States and Colombia to a low of 29% in Bulgaria (Benjet et al., 2016). Varying prevalence estimates of trauma exposure across countries may be due to true differences, differences in willingness to disclose traumatic events, and measurement error (Benjet et al., 2016). For example, sexual violence is highly stigmatized in many settings and the fear of being blamed and a perceived lack of support lead to underreporting of sexual violence (Abrahams et al., 2014).

Risk Factors for Trauma Exposure

Predictors of Trauma Exposure

Trauma exposure varies by individual and contextual factors that include sex, age, race/ethnicity, sexual orientation, educational attainment, marital status, genetics, risk-taking behavior, and neighborhood of residence (Benjet et al., 2016; Kessler et al., 2017; Roberts, Austin, Corliss, Vandermorris, & Koenen, 2010). Women are more likely than men to be exposed to intimate partner violence, whereas men are more likely than women to experience physical violence and unintentional injuries (Benjet et al., 2016). Traumas related to interpersonal violence have the earliest median age of occurrence (age 17), followed by intimate partner violence (age 18), war-related traumas (age 20), and unintentional injuries, unexpected deaths of loved ones, and other traumas with later median ages of occurrence (ages 24–31). The pattern of trauma exposure across age may reflect differences in life circumstances and lifestyles (Kessler et al., 2017). There are also racial/ethnic differences in types of traumas experienced. For example, blacks and Hispanics have a higher risk of child maltreatment and witnessing domestic violence than whites. Asians, black men, and Hispanic women are more likely to be exposed to war-related traumatic events than whites (Roberts et al., 2010). Assessments of sexual orientation disparities in exposure to violence and other traumatic events in a representative U.S. sample found that lesbians, gay men, bisexuals, and heterosexuals who reported any same-sex sexual partners during their lifetime had an increased risk of childhood maltreatment, interpersonal violence, trauma to a close friend or relative, and unexposed death of someone close, compared to heterosexuals without same-sex attractions or partners (Roberts et al., 2010). Low educational attainment is associated with elevated risk of some traumas (e.g., violence, unintentional injuries, and natural disasters) but not all traumas (e.g., unexpected death of a loved one). Higher levels of educational attainment are associated with a lower risk of being raped, being beaten up by a spouse or romantic partner, or stalked, but is associated with increased risk of non-penetrative sexual assault and traumatic event to a loved one (Kessler et al., 2017). Married individuals have a reduced risk of experiencing most trauma types compared to the never married, perhaps due to married individuals spending less time outside the home at later hours, unaccompanied, and in potentially vulnerable situations (Benjet et al., 2016). Genetic factors may affect the risk of exposure to trauma, possibly through individual differences in personality that influence environmental choices (Stein, Jang, Taylor, Vernon, & Livesley, 2002). Individual traits such as impulsivity and risk taking may increase the risk of traumatic events such as injuries (Romer, 2010). Neighborhoods that are highly disorganized (i.e., neighborhoods with high levels of poverty, family disruption, and residential mobility) are associated with higher levels of exposure to violence and crime, which could potentially be traumatic (Butcher, Galanek, Kretschmar, & Flannery, 2015).

Trauma Exposure Increases Risk of Subsequent Exposure to Trauma

Having experienced trauma increases one's risk of experiencing additional traumas later in life (Benjet et al., 2016; Gradus, Antonsen, et al., 2015). Over 30% of respondents to the WMHS were exposed to four or more traumatic events (Kessler et al., 2017). Exposure to childhood abuse is strongly associated with additional trauma exposure later in adulthood, and exposure to interpersonal violence is strongly associated with subsequent exposure to interpersonal violence (Benjet et al., 2016; Coid et al., 2001). Potential mechanisms underlying this association include perpetrators targeting individuals who have low self-esteem, are socially isolated, feel powerless, or have other psychological sequelae of previous victimization (Benjet et al., 2016; Coid et al., 2001; Grauerholz, 2000). Furthermore, impulsivity and risk taking, which may be both predictors and outcomes of trauma exposure, may also increase the risk of experiencing multiple traumatic events (e.g., injuries; Benjet et al., 2016).

Trauma Exposure and Natural Recovery

It is common to experience some psychological distress and PTSD-related symptoms immediately after enduring a traumatic event, such as fear, somatic symptoms, and sleeping disturbances (Sayed, Iacoviello, & Charney, 2015). However, many individuals experiencing a traumatic event will not develop PTSD (Atwoli, Stein, Williams, McLaughlin, & Koenen, 2015). Of those experiencing some PTSD-related symptoms most, if not all of the symptoms will dissipate within a month for a majority of individuals (Littleton, Axsom, & Grills-Taquechel, 2011), reflecting a course of natural recovery.

CASE EXAMPLE: Anne Marie—Normal Recovery

Anne Marie is a 27-year-old Hispanic female. She works as a pediatric nurse at a local hospital. One night, after finishing a long shift at midnight, Anne Marie said goodbye to her colleagues and left the pediatric ward, heading toward her car in the outside parking lot. She was parked in her usual parking spot in the back corner. As Anne Marie headed out to her car, she noted it was quite dark because the light post above her car appeared to have gone out. Once she got to her car, she unlocked the door and started to climb inside when she felt something pressed to her side and a low voice say, "Give me your car keys and I will not hurt you." Anne Marie quickly realized that someone was holding a gun to her side and that she was being robbed. As she moved to give the perpetrator her keys, he grabbed her arm, took her car keys, threw her to the ground, and kicked her in her stomach. The man sped away in her car, and after a few minutes Anne Marie was able to stumble to the hospital emergency room for an evaluation and to receive treatment for her injuries. Although she did not have any serious injuries, she experienced psychological distress from her assault and felt fearful and more cautious than usual as she went about her daily activities. In the following days, Anne Marie dreaded driving to work so much that she had her boyfriend drive her to and from work for the first week after the assault. The following week, Anne Marie knew she could not depend on her boyfriend to continue to drive her to work, so she began driving to work again, making sure that she was parking in spaces closest to the entrance of the hospital. When leaving work, she would also scan the parking lot for "suspicious"-looking men. After a few weeks, however, Anne Marie began to feel more secure as she realized that the likelihood of being assaulted in the parking lot again was low, her experience was the only assault reported in the last decade, and her symptoms began to dissipate. By the end of the month, she no longer scanned parking lots for "suspicious" males and began parking in her usual parking space at the hospital again. Anne Marie's reaction to her assault represents a typical reaction to experiencing a traumatic event.

Epidemiology of PTSD and Other Psychological Consequences of Trauma Exposure

As reviewed in the prior section, exposure to traumatic events is a common occurrence throughout the world. Although most people exposed to traumatic events will not go on to experience clinical levels of psychological distress, there is a significant portion of individuals who develop problems. Exposure to traumatic events can have a significant impact on psychological functioning and, in some cases, lead to mental health disorders. Although there is a variety of psychological consequences that can emerge after exposure to a traumatic event, such as acute stress disorder, adjustment disorders, and complicated grief—to name a few—PTSD is one of the most common and tends to receive the most attention as a psychological consequence of trauma exposure.

In general, PTSD is among the most prevalent mental health disorders in the United States, with approximately 2.5% of the general population meeting diagnostic criteria in any given year (Karam et al., 2014). This prevalence is significantly higher in the U.S. veteran population, with up to 15% of veterans meeting diagnostic criteria for PTSD (Seal et al., 2009). Approximately 8% of the population in the United States (Kessler, Petukhova, Sampson, Zaslavsky, & Wittchen, 2012), 4.4% in the United Kingdom (Fear, Bridges, Hatch, Hawkins, & Wessely, 2014), and 4.4% in Australia (McEvoy, Grove, & Slade, 2011) will be diagnosed with PTSD in their lifetime, which is second only to the prevalence of depression in these countries (Kessler et al., 2012; McEvoy et al., 2011). More generally, a pattern of PTSD prevalence across countries reveals that high-income countries report higher prevalence estimates of lifetime PTSD (6.9%) than those in middle- (3.9%) and low-income countries (3%; Koenen et al., 2017). Past 30-day prevalence follows a similar pattern, with high-income countries reporting the highest prevalence (1.9%) and middle- (0.7%) and low-income (0.6%) countries reporting lower prevalence of PTSD. Although these differing prevalence estimates may reflect true differences in the prevalence of PTSD across cultures, they may also be partially due to low reporting related to cultural factors such as mental health stigma, less understanding of mental health issues, and measurement error (Wang et al., 2007). Age of onset of PTSD tends to be younger in high-income countries than in low- and middle-income countries. The age of onset in high-income countries is generally before the age of 30, whereas the age of onset in low- and middle-income countries is generally before the age of 43 (Koenen et al., 2017). Moreover, despite questions of whether the changes in the PTSD diagnostic criteria from DSM-IV to DSM-5 would impact prevalence estimates, recent investigations have shown comparable prevalence estimates of PTSD when using DSM-IV versus DSM-5 criteria (Hoge, Riviere, Wilk, Herrell, & Weathers, 2014; Kilpatrick et al., 2013; Stein et al., 2014). When expanding beyond the DSM classification system, there tends to be an overlap between those meeting criteria for PTSD using DSM-5 and ICD-11; however, a substantial portion of those meeting criteria using one diagnostic system did not meet criteria using the other system (O'Donnell et al., 2014).

Correlates and Risk Factors of PTSD

Research demonstrates that socioeconomic and psychological factors predict PTSD diagnosis. Sociodemographic factors—including lower levels of educational attainment and income, prior exposure to trauma, preexisting psychopathology, white ethnicity (although these findings have been inconsistent), and female sex—are associated with a higher risk of PTSD. For example, women have twice the risk of PTSD as men (Kessler et al., 2005; Perrin et al., 2014). Also, personality variables such as being high in neuroticism and having poor coping responses are also associated with greater risk of PTSD (Perrin et al., 2014).

In addition to individual characteristics associated with PTSD, type of trauma itself has also been shown to be associated with this disorder. The psychological consequences of trauma exposure tend to be more severe and disabling subsequent to some types of trauma such as sexual assault and other forms of interpersonal violence (Breslau, 2009; Pietrzak, Goldstein, Southwick, & Grant, 2011). Events viewed to be "intentional" (e.g., assault) are associated with greater persistence of PTSD symptoms than those exposed to "nonintentional" traumatic events (e.g., natural disorders; Santiago et al., 2013). Number of traumatic events experienced is also associated with elevated risk. Experiencing four or more events significantly increases one's risk for PTSD compared to experiencing three or fewer traumatic events (Karam et al., 2014). Posttrauma variables also increase risk for PTSD. In particular, low perceived social support and subsequent life stressors (e.g., ongoing financial problems) are associated with greater severity of PTSD symptoms (Ozer, Best, Lipsey, & Weiss, 2003) and PTSD diagnosis (Brewin, Andrews, & Valentine, 2000; Bryant et al., 2018; Ozer et al., 2003).

Course and Impact on Functioning

PTSD is a disabling mental health disorder (Smith, Schnurr, & Rosenheck, 2005) associated with substantial societal costs and burden (Breslau, Lucia, & Davis, 2004; Kessler, 2000). Greater impairment among persons with PTSD appears to be associated with the number of traumatic events experienced. Findings from 20 population surveys (11 from high-income countries and nine from low- and middle-income countries) from the WMHS found that, of individuals reporting PTSD symptoms, approximately 20% reported that their symptoms were associated with multiple traumatic events (Karam et al., 2014). Moreover, the 12-month PTSD cases that reported experiencing four or more traumatic events also had greater functional impairment, earlier age of onset, more enduring PTSD symptoms, and more comorbidity with other mental disorders, such as mood and anxiety disorders. Thus, it appears that individuals with PTSD who have experienced four or more traumatic events may reach a "risk threshold" that sets these patients on a more severe and impairing PTSD course (Karam et al., 2014), and possibly a more chronic trajectory than those experiencing fewer traumatic events.

Treatment Seeking

Without treatment, PTSD tends to be chronic, although it is typical for individuals to experience a fluctuation in symptoms, including the remitting and reemergence of symptoms over time (Solomon & Mikulincer, 2006). Early research on the lifetime course of PTSD found that approximately two-thirds of those with PTSD will remit from the disorder over time; however, the remaining one-third will not remit from PTSD without treatment (Kessler, Sonnega, Bromet, Hughes, & Nelson, 1995). Research data from WMHS indicate that 20–440% of PTSD cases will remit within 1 year. Of those cases, most will remit within the first 6 months (Kessler et al., 2017). Despite the generally chronic course and disability associated with PTSD, rates of treatment seeking remain low. Respondents to the WMHS report that less than 50% of those individuals with PTSD received some form of treatment (Koenen et al., 2017). Treatment is most common among persons living in high-income countries where the probability of treatment seeking is twice that of lower economic regions (Koenen et al., 2017). Even among patients who receive treatment, there may be a significant delay in treatment initiation. Data collected by the National Epidemiologic Survey on Alcohol and Related Conditions–III (NESARC-III) from 36,309 adults showed that, of those with PTSD, approximately 59% sought treatment, with an average delay of 4.5 years before receiving treatment (Goldstein et al., 2016). NESARC-III respondents reported most commonly talking to a therapist or mental health counselor (54.6%), receiving prescribed psychiatric medications (33.7%), or being involved in support groups (17.2%; Goldstein et al., 2016).

The gap between diagnosis and seeking treatment is largest in low-income counties, where less than 25% of individuals with PTSD receive treatment (Koenen et al., 2017; Wang et al., 2007). The decreased availability of treatment resources in low-income countries has led to a global effort to improve screening for mental health problems, including trauma exposure and PTSD, and to provide treatments using novel approaches, such as telehealth approaches (Nasland et al., 2017) and the use of "task sharing" (i.e., providing treatments in nontraditional settings administered by lay providers, such as nurses in primary care centers; Eaton et al., 2011; Patel, Chowdhary, Rahman, & Verdeli, 2011). Although this line of research is nascent, preliminary findings show that the use of task sharing and other novel treatment approaches is effective (Hanlon et al., 2014; Patel et al., 2011) and may help in the scaling up of effective treatments in low-resource settings worldwide (Eaton et al., 2011).

Comorbidity of PTSD

Comorbidity of PTSD and Other Mental Health Disorders

Approximately 78% of individuals diagnosed with PTSD also meet criteria for at least one additional mental health disorder in their lifetime (Koenen et al., 2017). Co-occurrence of PTSD with mood disorders, and in particular unipolar depression, is especially high, with over half of those with PTSD also meeting criteria for depression (Kessler et al., 2005). The co-occurrence of PTSD and anxiety disorders is also common (Gradus, Antonsen, et al., 2015; Kaufman & Charney, 2000; Kessler et al., 2005). Epidemiological findings from the NESARC-III data showed that individuals with PTSD had greater odds (odds ratio = 4.3, 95% confidence interval = 3.8, 4.8) of being diagnosed with an anxiety disorder than those without PTSD (Pietrzak et al., 2011). Mood and anxiety disorders tend to be preexisting conditions before the onset of PTSD and in some cases may represent a risk factor for PTSD (Bromet, Sonnega, & Kessler, 1998; Perkonigg, Kessler, Storz, & Wittchen, 2000), although the alternative has also been found, in which mood and anxiety disorders tend to have an onset that follows a PTSD diagnosis (Gradus, Antonsen, et al., 2015). It has been argued that the high prevalence of comorbidity among mood and anxiety disorders and PTSD may be attributed to underlying vulnerability factors shared across the disorders (i.e., shared genetic vulnerability: Duncan et al., 2018; neuroticism: Brown & Barlow, 2009), or shared diagnostic symptom clusters across the disorders (e.g., dysphoric symptoms in both depression and PTSD; Simms, Watson, & Doebbeling, 2002), or may actually represent a distinct phenotype (Flory & Yehuda, 2015).

Comorbid substance use disorders (SUDs) are highly prevalent among those with PTSD, with approximately 40% of individuals with PTSD also meeting criteria for a co-occurring SUD (Blanco et al., 2013; Pietrzak et al., 2011). Interestingly, SUDs tend to emerge after a PTSD diagnosis (Kessler et al., 2005), and likely reflect a tendency for those with PTSD to use substances as a self-medicating strategy to mitigate the distressing symptoms of PTSD (Gradus, Antonsen, et al., 2015; Stewart & Conrod, 2003). This suggests that PTSD may serve as a risk factor for the later development of SUDs.

PTSD is also associated with increased risk for suicide. Epidemiological studies report that individuals with PTSD have approximately a sixfold increase in risk for suicidal ideation and suicide attempts (Kessler, Borges, & Walters, 1999; Sareen, Cox, & Asmundson, 2005). For example, in a Danish cohort study, patients with PTSD had 13 times the rate of death by suicide than patients without PTSD (Gradus, Antonsen, et al., 2015). The high prevalence of PTSD and co-occurring mental disorders, such as depression and SUDs, paired with increased rates of suicidality, problematic anger (McHugh, Forbes, Bates, Hopwood, & Creamer, 2012; Olatunji, Ciesielskil, & Tolin, 2010), guilt (Lee, Scragg, & Turner, 2001), and dissociation (Bryant, 2007; Stein et al., 2013) make this clinical profile a particularly important target for efforts aimed at the prevention and treatment of these often comorbid clinical problems.

Comorbidity of PTSD and Physical Health Problems

Although PTSD has long been implicated in the development of various physical health disorders, such as gastrointestinal disorders (Gradus et al., 2017; Kessler, 2000; Schnurr & Jankowski, 1999) and other somatic disorders (Pacella, Hruska, & Delahanty, 2013), findings have been relatively mixed for these disorders (Pacella et al., 2013). There is stronger evidence for an association between PTSD and cardiovascular disease (CVD). Support for the link between PTSD and CVD has been found in veteran samples (Beristianos, Yaffe, Cohen, & Byers, 2016; Vaccarino et al., 2013) and in the general population (Gradus et al., 2015). Individuals with PTSD have greater odds (odds ratio = 3.4, 95% confidence interval = 1.9, 6.0) of heart failure than those without PTSD (Spitzer et al., 2009). It is unclear whether having PTSD increases the risk of CVD or if the two disorders share an underlying vulnerability, but there is some evidence of a dose–response relationship, in which those with a greater number of PTSD symptoms have higher levels of hypertension (Sumner et al., 2016). Similarly, there is a strong association between PTSD and pain disorders (Otis, Keane, & Kerns, 2003), with 30% of the general population suffering from PTSD and a co-occurring pain disorder (Asmundson, Coons, Taylor, & Katz, 2002). Possible explanations for the comorbidity of PTSD and chronic pain include a shared underlying vulnerability, such as elevated levels of anxiety sensitivity (Asmundson et al., 2002), and mutual maintenance models, whereby the presence of PTSD symptoms increases pain-related distress, and vice versa (Asmundson & Katz, 2009; Sharp & Harvey, 2001).

CASE EXAMPLE: Michael—PTSD and Co-Occurring Alcohol Use Disorder

Michael is a 24-year-old combat veteran. As a child, he was exposed to frequent physical fights between his mother and father and was often the victim of physical abuse. After completing high school at 18 years of age, Michael left home and enlisted in the military. He was stationed in Afghanistan and worked in transportation for 4 years. One morning, while transporting materials in a convoy, an improvised explosive device (IED) went off in the road. As Michael was swerving to miss the explosion, he saw that the IED hit the truck ahead of him, and he knew his fellow soldiers were injured. He later found out that one of them died in the explosion. Immediately after the event, Michael began having difficulty sleeping and had nightmares related to the explosion. Within a few weeks, he also began to have daily intrusions, was easily startled, began to withdraw from social activities, and reported feeling very little connection with others. Two months later, Michael was discharged from the military and returned home. Upon his return, he continued to suffer from his symptoms of PTSD. He began drinking, first to help him sleep at night, but over the years, he began drinking during the day. One day, when Michael was in a doctor's appointment with his primary care physician, his doctor began to inquire about his experiences in the military and his drinking habits. The doctor then referred him to the mental health clinic, where he completed an intake evaluation and was diagnosed with PTSD and co-occurring alcohol dependence. During the intake, Michael denied needing treatment, and it was not until 2 years later, after his employer reported concerns about his mental health, that he finally engaged in treatment.

Michael's case is a prototypical example of an individual with PTSD and a co-occurring substance use disorder. After encountering a traumatic event, he began experiencing symptoms of PTSD, including having trouble sleeping, nightmares, intrusions, and withdrawing from others. To help cope with his symptoms, Michael began to use alcohol. His symptoms remained undiagnosed for 4 years, until a medical professional recognized a potential psychological issue. Despite receiving an intake evaluation, it took another 2 years before Michael actually enrolled in treatment.

Conclusion

The epidemiology of trauma and PTSD is relatively new, with the first national general population-based studies published only in the early 1990s (e.g., Resnick, Kilpatrick, Dansky, Saunders, & Best, 1993). Since that time, epidemiology has made at least four major contributions to our understanding of the population burden of trauma and PTSD. First, trauma exposure is common and not randomly distributed in the population. Factors both within the individual and the social context contribute to exposure. Second, some persons exposed to trauma will go on to have PTSD and this, also, is dependent on individual and contextual risk factors. Third, PTSD is a highly prevalent, chronic, and debilitating disorder that is not only often comorbid with other mental and behavioral disorders such as depression, anxiety, and SUDs, but also increases the risk of adverse physical health outcomes such as CVD (Gradus et al., 2019). Fourth, the majority of individuals with PTSD, whether in high- or low-income countries, goes untreated. This is particularly tragic, given the major strides that have been made in our knowledge of how to treat PTSD—and even prevent PTSD among the trauma-exposed—as is evidenced in this volume. The challenge ahead for epidemiology is to develop tools to improve our ability to identify persons at risk of PTSD to target prevention and treatment efforts (Shalev et al., 2019).

REFERENCES

Abrahams, N., Devries, K., Watts, C., Pallitto, C., Petzold, M., Shamu, S., et al. (2014). Worldwide prevalence of non-partner sexual violence: A systematic review. *Lancet, 383,* 1648–1654.

American Psychiatric Association. (2013). *Diagnostic and statistical manual of mental disorders* (5th ed.). Arlington, VA: Author.

Asmundson, G. J. G., Coons, M. J., Taylor, S., & Katz, J. (2002). PTSD and the experience of pain: Research and clinical implications of shared vulnerability and mutual maintenance models. *Canadian Journal of Psychiatry, 47,* 930–937.

Asmundson, G. J. G., & Katz, J. (2009). Understanding the co-occurrence of anxiety disorders and chronic pain: State-of-the-art. *Depression and Anxiety, 26,* 888–901.

Atwoli, L., Stein, D. J., Williams, D. R., Mclaughlin, K. A., & Koenen, K. C. (2015). Epidemiology of posttraumatic stress disorder: Prevalence, correlates, and consequences. *Current Opinion in Psychiatry, 28,* 307.

Benjet, C., Bromet, E., Karam, E. G., Kessler, R. C., McLaughlin, K. A., Ruscio, A. M., et al. (2016). The epidemiology of traumatic event exposure worldwide: Results from the World Mental Health Survey Consortium. *Psychological Medicine, 46*(2), 327–343.

Beristianos, M. H., Yaffe, K., Cohen, B., & Byers, A. L. (2016). PTSD and risk of incident cardiovascular disease in aging veterans. *American Journal of Geriatric Psychiatry, 24,* 192–200.

Blanco, C., Xu, Y., Brady, K. T., Pérez-Fuentes, G., Okuda, M., & Wang, S. (2013). Comorbidity of posttraumatic stress disorder with alcohol dependence among US adults: Results from National Epidemiological Survey on Alcohol and Related Conditions. *Drug and Alcohol Dependence, 132,* 630–638.

Breslau, N. (2009). The epidemiology of trauma, PTSD, and other posttrauma disorders. *Trauma, Violence, and Abuse, 10,* 198–210.

Breslau, N., Lucia, V. C., & Davis, G. C. (2004). Partial PTSD versus full PTSD: An empirical examination of associated impairment. *Psychological Medicine, 34,* 1205–1214.

Brewin, C. R., Andrews, B., & Valentine, J. D. (2000). Meta-analysis of risk factors for posttraumatic stress disorder in trauma-exposed adults. *Journal of Consulting and Clinical Psychology, 68,* 748–766.

Bromet, E., Sonnega, A., & Kessler, R. C. (1998). Risk factors for DSM-III-R posttraumatic stress disorder: Findings from the National Comorbidity Survey. *American Journal of Epidemiology, 147,* 353–361.

Brown, T. A., & Barlow, D. H. (2009). A proposal for a dimensional classification system based on the shared features of the DSM-IV anxiety and mood disorders: Implications for assessment and treatment. *Psychological Assessment, 21*(3), 256–271.

Bryant, R. A. (2007). Does dissociation further our understanding of PTSD? *Journal of Anxiety Disorders, 21*, 183–191.

Bryant, R. A., Gibbs, L., Gallagher, H. C., Pattison, P., Lusher, D., MacDougall, C., et al. (2018). Longitudinal study of changing psychological outcomes following the Victorian Black Saturday bushfires. *Australian and New Zealand Journal of Psychiatry, 52*, 542–551.

Butcher, F., Galanek, J. D., Kretschmar, J. M., & Flannery, D. J. (2015). The impact of neighborhood disorganization on neighborhood exposure to violence, trauma symptoms, and social relationships among at-risk youth. *Social Science and Medicine, 146*, 300–306.

Coid, J., Petruckevitch, A., Feder, G., Chung, W.-S., Richardson, J., & Moorey, S. (2001). Relation between childhood sexual and physical abuse and risk of revictimisation in women: A cross-sectional survey. *Lancet, 358*, 450–454.

Duncan, L. E., Ratanatharathorn, A., Aiello, A. E., Almli, L. M., Amstadter, A. B., Ashley-Koch, A. E., et al. (2018). Largest GWAS of PTSD (N = 20,070) yields genetic overlap with schizophrenia and sex differences in heritability. *Molecular Psychiatry, 23*, 666–673.

Eaton, J., McCay, L., Semrau, M., Chatterjee, S., Baingana, F., Araya, R., et al. (2011). Scale up of services for mental health in low-income and middle-income countries. *Lancet, 378*, 1592–1603.

Fear, N., Bridges, S., Hatch, S., Hawkins, V., & Wessely, S. (2014). Posttraumatic stress disorder. In S. McManus, P. Bebbington, S. Jenkins, & T. Brugha (Eds.), *Mental health and wellbeing in England: Adult Psychiatric Morbidity Survey 2014* (pp. 106–130). Leeds, UK: NHS Digital. Retrieved from *https://assets.publishing. service.gov.uk/government/uploads/system/uploads/attachment_data/file/556596/ apms-2014-full-rpt.pdf.*

Flory, J. D., & Yehuda, R. (2015). Comorbidity between post-traumatic stress disorder and major depressive disorder: Alternative explanations and treatment considerations. *Dialogues of Clinical Neuroscience, 17*, 141–150.

Goldstein, R. B., Smith, S. M., Chou, S. P., Saha, T. D., Jung, J., Zhang, H., et al. (2016). The epidemiology of DSM-5 posttraumatic stress disorder in the United States: Results from the National Epidemiologic Survey on Alcohol and Related Conditions–III. *Society of Psychiatry and Psychiatric Epidemiology, 51*, 1137–1148.

Gradus, J. L., Antonsen, S., Svensson, E., Lash, T. L., Resick, P. A., & Hansen, J. G. (2015). Trauma, comorbidity, and mortality following severe stress and adjustment disorder diagnoses: A nationwide cohort study. *American Journal of Epidemiology, 182*, 451–458.

Gradus, J. L., Farkas, D. K., Svensson, E., Ehrenstein, V., Lash, T. L., Milstein, A., et al. (2015). Associations between stress disorders and cardiovascular events in the Danish population. *BMJ Open, 5*, e009334.

Gradus, J. L., Farkas, D. K., Svensson, E., Ehrenstein, V., Lash, T. L., & Sorensen, T. (2017). Posttraumatic stress disorder and gastrointestinal disorders in the Danish population. *Epidemiology, 28*, 354–360.

Gradus, J. L., Horváth-Puhó, E., Lash, T. L., Ehrenstein, V., Tamang, S., Adler, N. E., et al. (2019). Stress disorders and dementia in the Danish population. *American Journal of Epidemiology, 188*(3), 493–499.

Grauerholz, L. (2000). An ecological approach to understanding sexual revictimization: Linking personal, interpersonal, and sociocultural factors and processes. *Child Maltreatment, 5*, 5–17.

Hanlon, C., Luitel, N. P., Kathree, T., Murhar, V., Shrivasta, S., Medhin, G., et al. (2014). Challenges and opportunities for implementing integrated mental health care: A district level situation analysis from five low- and middle-income countries. *PLOS ONE, 9*(2), e88437.

Hoge, C. W., Riviere, L. A., Wilk, J. E., Herrell, R. K., & Weathers, F. W. (2014). The prevalence of post-traumatic stress disorder (PTSD) in US combat soldiers: A head-to-head comparison of DSM-5 versus DSM-IV-TR symptom criteria with the PTSD checklist. *Lancet Psychiatry, 1*, 269–277.

Karam, E. G., Friedman, M. J., Hill, E. D., Kessler, R. C., McLaughlin, K. A., Petukhova, M., et al. (2014). Cumulative traumas and risk thresholds: 12-month PTSD in the World Mental Health (WMH) surveys. *Depression and Anxiety, 31*, 130–142.

Kaufman, J., & Charney, D. (2000). Comorbidity of mood and anxiety disorders. *Depression and Anxiety, 12*, 69–76.

Kessler, R. C. (2000). Posttraumatic stress disorder: The burden toAv the individual and to society. *Journal of Clinical Psychiatry, 61*(Suppl. 5), 4–12; discussion 13–14.

Kessler, R. C., Aguilar-Gaxiola, S., Alonso, J., Benjet, C., Bromet, E. J., Cardoso, G., et al. (2017). Trauma and PTSD in the WHO World Mental Health Surveys. *European Journal of Psychotraumatology, 8*(Suppl. 5).

Kessler, R. C., Berglund, P., Demler, O., Jin, R., Merikangas, K. R., & Walters, E. E. (2005). Lifetime prevalence and age-of-onset distributions of DSM-IV disorders in the National Comorbidity Survey Replication. *Archives of General Psychiatry, 62*, 593–602.

Kessler, R. C., Borges, G., & Walters, E. E. (1999). Prevalence of and risk factors for lifetime suicide attempts in the National Comorbidity Survey. *Archives of General Psychiatry, 56*, 617–626.

Kessler, R. C., Petukhova, M., Sampson, N. A., Zaslavsky, A. M., & Wittchen, H. U. (2012). Twelve-month and lifetime prevalence and lifetime morbid risk of anxiety and mood disorders in the United States. *International Journal of Methods and Psychiatric Research, 21*, 169–184.

Kessler, R. C., Sonnega, A., Bromet, E., Hughes, M., & Nelson, C. B. (1995). Posttraumatic stress disorder in the National Comorbidity Survey. *Archives of General Psychiatry, 52*, 1048–1060.

Kilpatrick, D. G., Resnick, H. S., Milanak, M. E., Miller, M. W., Keyes, K. M., & Friedman, M. J. (2013). National estimates of exposure to traumatic events and PTSD prevalence using DSM-IV and DSM-5 criteria. *Journal of Traumatic Stress, 26*, 537–547.

Koenen, K. C., Ratanatharathorn, A., Ng, L., McLaughlin, K. A., Bromet, E. J., Stein, D. J., et al. (2017). Posttraumatic stress disorder in the World Mental Health Surveys. *Psychological Medicine, 47*, 2260–2274.

Lee, D. A., Scragg, P., & Turner, S. (2001). The role of shame and guilt in traumatic events: A clinical model of shame-based and guilt-based PTSD. *British Journal of Medical Psychology, 74*, 451–466.

Littleton, H., Axsom, D., & Grills-Taquechel, A. E. (2011). Longitudinal evaluation of the relationship between maladaptive trauma coping and distress:

Examination following the mass shooting at Virginia Tech. *Anxiety, Stress, and Coping, 24,* 273–290.

McEvoy, P. E., Grove, R., & Slade, T. (2011). Epidemiology of anxiety disorders in the Australian general population: Findings of the 2007 Australian National Survey of Mental Health and Wellbeing. *Australian and New Zealand Journal of Psychiatry, 45,* 957–967.

McHugh, T., Forbes, D., Bates, G., Hopwood, M., & Creamer, M. (2012). Anger in PTSD: Is there a need for a concept of PTSD-related posttraumatic anger? *Clinical Psychology Review, 32,* 93–104.

Nasland, J. A., Aschbrenner, K. A., Araya, R., Marsch, L. A., Unutzer, P. V., & Bartels, S. J. (2017). Digital technology for treating and preventing mental disorders in low and middle-income countries: A narrative review of the literature. *Lancet Psychiatry, 4,* 486–500.

North, C. S., Tivis, L., McMillen, J. C., Pfefferbaum, B., Cox, J., Spitznagel, E. L., et al. (2002). Coping, functioning, and adjustment of rescue workers after the Oklahoma City bombing. *Journal of Traumatic Stress, 15,* 171–175.

O'Donnell, M. L., Alkemade, N., Nickerson, A., Creamer, M., McFarlane, A., Silove, D., et al. (2014). The impact of the diagnostic changes to posttraumatic stress disorder for DSM-5 and the proposed changes to ICD-11. *British Journal of Psychiatry, 205,* 230–235.

Olatunji, B. O., Ciesielskil, B. G., & Tolin, D. F. (2010). Fear and loathing: A meta-analytic review of the specificity of AIP. *Behavior Therapy, 41,* 93–105.

Otis, J. D., Keane, T. M., & Kerns, R. D. (2003). An examination of the relationship between chronic pain and post-traumatic-stress disorder. *Journal of Rehabilitation Research and Development, 40,* 397–405.

Ozer, E. J., Best, S. R., Lipsey, T. L., & Weiss, D. S. (2003). Predictors of posttraumatic stress disorder and symptoms in adults: A meta-analysis. *Psychological Bulletin, 129,* 52–73.

Pacella, M. L., Hruska, B., & Delahanty, D. L. (2013). The physical health consequences of PTSD and PTSD symptoms: A meta-analytic review. *Journal of Anxiety Disorders, 27,* 33–46.

Pai, A., Suris, A. M., & North, C. S. (2017). Posttraumatic stress disorder in the DSM-5: Controversy, change, and conceptual considerations. *Behavioral Sciences, 7.* [Epub ahead of print]

Patel, V., Chowdhary, N., Rahman, A., & Verdeli, H. (2011). Improving access to psychological treatments: Lessons from developing countries. *Behavior Research and Therapy, 49*(9), 523–528.

Perkonigg, A., Kessler, R. C., Storz, S., & Wittchen, H.-U. (2000). Traumatic events and post-traumatic stress disorder in the community: Prevalence, risk factors and comorbidity. *Acta Psychiatrica Scandinavica, 101,* 46–59.

Perrin, M., Vandeleur, C. L., Castelao, E., Rothen, S., Glaus, J., Vollenweider, P., et al. (2014). Determinants of the development of post-traumatic stress disorder in the general population. *Social Psychiatry and Psychiatric Epidemiology, 49,* 447–457.

Pietrzak, R. H., Goldstein, R. B., Southwick, S. M., & Grant, B. F. (2011). Prevalence and Axis I comorbidity of full and partial posttraumatic stress disorder in the United States: Results from Wave 2 of the National Epidemiologic Survey on Alcohol and Related Conditions. *Journal of Anxiety Disorders, 25,* 456–465.

Resnick, H. S., Kilpatrick, D. G., Dansky, B. S., Saunders, B. E., & Best, C. L. (1993). Prevalence of civilian trauma and posttraumatic stress disorder in a representative national sample of women. *Journal of Consulting and Clinical Psychology, 61,* 984–991.

Roberts, A. L., Austin, S. B., Corliss, H. L., Vandermorris, A. K., & Koenen, K. C. (2010). Pervasive trauma exposure among US sexual orientation minority adults and risk of posttraumatic stress disorder. *American Journal of Public Health, 100,* 2433–2441.

Romer, D. (2010). Adolescent risk taking, impulsivity, and brain development: Implications for prevention. *Developmental Psychobiology, 52,* 263–276.

Santiago, P. N., Ursano, R. J., Gray, C. L., Pynoos, R. S., Spiegel, D., Lewis-Fernandez, R., et al. (2013). A systematic review of PTSD prevalence and trajectories in DSM-5 defined trauma exposed populations: Intentional and non-intentional traumatic events. *PLOS ONE, 8*(4), e59236.

Sareen, J., Cox, B. J., & Asmundson, G. J. G. (2005). Anxiety disorders and risk for suicidal ideation and suicide attempts: A population-based longitudinal study of adults. *Archives of General Psychiatry, 62,* 1249–1257.

Sayed, S., Iacoviello, B. M., & Charney, D. S. (2015). Risk factors for the development of psychopathology following trauma. *Current Psychiatry Reports, 17,* 70–76.

Schnurr, P., & Jankowski, M. (1999). Physical health and post-traumatic stress disorder: Review and synthesis. *Seminars in Clinical Neuropsychiatry, 4,* 295–304.

Seal, K. H., Metzler, T. J., Gima, K. S., Bertenthal, D., Maguen, S., & Marmar, C. R. (2009). Trends and risk factors for mental health diagnoses among Iraq and Afghanistan veterans using Department of Veterans Affairs health care, 2002–2008. *American Journal of Public Health, 99,* 1651–1658.

Shalev, A., Gevonden, M., Ratanatharathorn, A., Laska, E., van der Mei, W., Qi, W., et al. (2019). Estimating the risk of PTSD in recent trauma survivors: Results from the International Consortium to Predict PTSD (ICCP). *World Psychiatry, 18,* 77–87.

Sharp, T. J., & Harvey, A. G. (2001). Chronic pain and posttraumatic stress disorder: Mutual maintenance? *Clinical Psychology Review, 21,* 857–877.

Simms, L. J., Watson, D., & Doebbeling, B. N. (2002). Confirmatory factor analyses of posttraumatic stress symptoms in deployed and non-deployed veterans of the Gulf War. *Journal of Abnormal Psychology, 111,* 637–647.

Skogstad, M., Skorstad, M., Lie, A., Conradi, H. S., Heir, T., & Weisæth, L. (2013). Work-related post-traumatic stress disorder. *Occupational Medicine, 63*(3), 175–182.

Smith, M. W., Schnurr, P. P., & Rosenheck, R. A. (2005). Employment outcomes and PTSD symptom severity. *Mental Health Services Research, 7,* 89–101.

Solomon, Z., & Mikulincer, M. (2006). Trajectories of PTSD: A 20-year longitudinal study. *American Journal of Psychiatry, 163,* 659–666.

Spitzer, C., Barnow, S., Volzke, H., John, U., Freyberger, H. J., & Grabe, H. J. (2009). Trauma, posttraumatic stress disorder, and physical illness: Findings from the general population. *Psychosomatic Medicine, 71,* 1012–1017.

Stein, D. J., Koenen, K. C., Friedman, M. J., Hill, E., McLaughlin, K. A., Petukhova, M., et al. (2013). Dissociation in posttraumatic stress disorder: Evidence from the World Mental Health Surveys. *Biological Psychiatry, 73,* 302–312.

Stein, D. J., McLaughlin, K. A., Koenen, K. C., Atwoli, L., Freidman, M. J., Hill, E. D., et al. (2014). DSM-5 and ICD-11 definitions of posttraumatic stress disorder:

Investigating "narrow" and "broad" approaches. *Depression and Anxiety, 31,* 494–505.

Stein, M. B., Jang, K. L., Taylor, S., Vernon, P. A., & Livesley, W. J. (2002). Genetic and environmental influences on trauma exposure and posttraumatic stress disorder symptoms: A twin study. *American Journal of Psychiatry, 159,* 1675–1681.

Stewart, S. H., & Conrod, P. J. (2003). Psychosocial models of functional associations between posttraumatic stress disorder and substance use disorder. In P. Ouimette & P. J. Brown (Eds.), *Trauma and substance abuse: Causes, consequences, and treatment of comorbid disorders* (pp. 29–55). Washington, DC: American Psychological Association.

Sumner, J. A., Kubzansky, L. D., Roberts, A. L., Gilsanz, P., Chen, Q., Winning, A., et al. (2016). Post-traumatic stress disorder symptoms and risk of hypertension over 22 years in a large cohort of younger and middle-aged women. *Psychological Medicine, 46,* 3105–3116.

Vaccarino, V., Goldberg, J., Rooks, C., Shah, A. J., Veledar, E., Faber, T. L., et al. (2013). Post-traumatic stress disorder and incidence of coronary heart disease: A twin study. *Journal of the American College of Cardiology, 62,* 970–978.

Wang, P. S., Aguilar-Gaxiola, S., Alonso, J., Angermeyer, M. C., Borges, G., Bromet, E. J., et al. (2007). Use of mental health services for anxiety, mood, and substance disorders in 17 countries in the WHO World Mental Health Surveys. *Lancet, 370,* 841–850.

CHAPTER 3

Epidemiology, Clinical Presentation, and Developmental Considerations in Children and Adolescents

Eva Alisic, Rowena Conroy, and Siri Thoresen

A majority of children worldwide are exposed to at least one traumatic experience while growing up. Although exposure can happen anywhere, for certain trauma types there are strong ties to children's characteristics and context. In addition, just as the *types of traumatic exposure* are diverse and multifaceted, children's *responses* to trauma exposure are widely varying as well. Although the focus of this book is on posttraumatic stress disorder (PTSD), children may also develop other disorders and difficulties, including depression, anxiety, and externalizing behavior problems, with a wide range of adverse developmental and functional outcomes. In the present chapter, we give a brief overview of current knowledge regarding trauma exposure and its consequences among children and adolescents; consider how developmental, systemic, and other contextual factors can affect children's exposure and reactions to trauma; and close with considerations regarding the limitations of our current evidence base.

Exposure to Traumatic Events

According to DSM-5 (American Psychiatric Association, 2013, p. 271), a traumatic event for a child or adolescent is a threat-related event(s). The event may involve death, assault, community or family violence, child abuse, any form of sexual assault, accidental or natural disaster, war, or terrorism. It may be experienced directly, witnessed, or happen to a close loved one. An often-cited study from the United States (Copeland, Keeler, Angold, &

Costello, 2007) found that 68% of 16-year-olds in a large population sample had experienced at least one traumatic event. McLaughlin and colleagues (2013) similarly found that 62% of over 6,000 U.S. adolescents had experienced trauma. In both studies, about half of the trauma-exposed youth had experienced two or more events. In other countries, exposure rates are substantial as well. For example, 31% of young people in England and Wales reported trauma exposure by age 18 years (Lewis et al., 2019), and among Swiss adolescents the exposure rate was 56% (Landolt, Schnyder, Maier, Schoenbucher, & Mohler-Kuo, 2013).

Although exposure to trauma is a common experience in childhood, it comes in many substantially different forms. A key distinction made in the literature is between noninterpersonal and interpersonal types of trauma. Noninterpersonal trauma includes experiences such as accidents, disaster, sudden loss of a loved one due to accidental injury, and other unintentional harm. Sudden loss of a loved one, particularly the death of a parent or sibling, is a frequently reported potentially traumatic life event in childhood (Landolt et al., 2013; see also Gunaratnam & Alisic, 2017, for an overview). McLaughlin and colleagues (2013) found that 28% of their sample had experienced the unexpected death of a loved one. Serious accidental injury is also common, often caused by motor vehicle crashes, drowning, burns, or falls (Elklit & Frandsen, 2014; Ghazali, Elklit, Balang, Sultan, & Kana, 2014; World Health Organization, 2014). Disasters are another example of a noninterpersonal trauma, the frequency, scale, and impact of which are all expected to increase in the next few decades (United Nations Office for Disaster Risk Reduction, 2015).

Interpersonal types of trauma include experiences of intentional harm such as physical violence experienced and/or witnessed within family and community contexts, sexual violence and abuse, terrorism, and war. The extent of children's exposure to violence in peacetime situations is probably substantially underreported, especially with regard to sexual violence (Saunders & Adams, 2014). Nevertheless, the reported exposure rates are high. For example, in the National Survey of Children's Exposure to Violence in the United States, 24.5% of the children and adolescents had witnessed violence, 37.3% had experienced a physical assault, 15.2% had been exposed to any type of maltreatment by caregivers (including physical abuse, emotional abuse, neglect, and custodial interference), and 1.4% had been sexually assaulted *in the past year* (Finkelhor, Turner, Shattuck, & Hamby, 2015). By late adolescence, 26.6% of U.S. girls and 5.1% of boys report sexual abuse or assault (Finkelhor, Shattuck, Turner, & Hamby, 2014). A Swiss study showed that 40.2% of female and 17.2% of male adolescents reported at least one incident of (contact or no-contact) child sexual assault (Mohler-Kuo et al., 2014). Adolescents ages 15–19 years in major cities in South Africa, Nigeria, India, and China reported high rates of physical and sexual violence, with the prevalence of past-year intimate partner violence ranging from 10.2% in Shanghai to 36.6% in Johannesburg (among female adolescents who ever had a partner; Decker et al., 2014). When considering rates of exposure to other forms of interpersonal trauma, terrorism, and war, these involve high rates of exposure in specific groups or regions. The number of forcibly displaced people is nearing 71 million worldwide (United Nations High Commissioner for Refugees, 2019), with about 50% of all refugees being children.

Although any child may be exposed to trauma, not every child is at equal risk; exposure is related to a range of factors. On an *individual* level, several factors stand out. For example, looking at demographics, trauma exposure varies with developmental stage. Overall, older children show higher lifetime, and in many cases higher 12-month, exposure rates than younger children, likely because they are more likely to participate in independent activities and have had more time to have been exposed (Alisic, van der Schoot, van Ginkel, & Kleber, 2008; Copeland et al., 2007; Finkelhor, Ormod & Turner, 2009). A few types of trauma, however, such as accidental burn injuries, are more common among younger children (Stoddard et al., 2006). Girls are more at risk of certain types of trauma exposure, such as sexual violence, compared to boys (Finkelhor et al., 2015; Landolt et al., 2013; Salazar, Keller, Gowen, & Courtney, 2013), who are more at risk of experiencing community physical violence and accidental injury (Landolt et al., 2013; McLaughlin et al., 2013). Children with externalizing behavior problems, disabilities, and other "otherness" (i.e., ways in which children may be different in terms of appearance, behavior, or background) appear to be at higher risk of accidents and violent exposure (McLaughlin et al., 2013; Owens, Fernando, & McGuinn, 2005). At a *family* level, low socioeconomic status and/or difficulties related to family functioning, such as mental health problems, drug abuse, or marital conflict, may put a child at increased risk of exposure (e.g., due to lack of supervision, Morrongiello & House, 2004; Schwebel & Gaines, 2007). At the *community and country* level, socioeconomic disadvantage also represents a risk factor: neighborhoods with high crime rates involve, logically, higher risk for children of exposure to violence (Irie, Lang, Kaltner, Le Brocque, & Kenardy, 2012), and children living in low-income countries are at higher risk of disaster and conflict (e.g., see Demyttenaere et al., 2004).

Moreover, exposure appears to come in clusters: initial exposure, in particular to violence, increases the risk of further exposure, both in the near and distant future (Aakvaag, Thoresen, Wentzel-Larsen, & Dyb, 2017; Finkelhor et al., 2015; Updegrove & Muftic, 2019). Childhood physical and sexual abuse commonly co-occur with other types of child maltreatment— namely, emotional abuse and neglect—and with other forms of dysfunction or difficulty within the home (e.g., parental intimate partner violence, caregiver mental health problems or substance abuse, criminal activity; see Dong et al., 2004; Finkelhor, Ormond, & Turner, 2007; Hamby, Finkelhor, Turner, & Ormrod, 2010). Indeed, exposure to multiple types of trauma and adversity is the norm for children who have been maltreated (e.g., Dong et al., 2004). The range of adversities to which maltreated children are exposed do not always fulfill the above-mentioned criteria for a traumatic stressor but are nonetheless associated with adverse psychological and developmental outcomes (e.g., Taillieu, Brownridge, Sareen, & Afifi, 2016) that may compound the effects of exposure to traumatic stressors.

Consequences of Trauma Exposure

Although this book focuses on PTSD, it is critical to acknowledge that there is a range of potential consequences of traumatic exposure for children. In this chapter, we discuss the negative mental health consequences that have received most empirical attention, and some of the associated functional difficulties that children and adolescents can experience. In terms of mental health, we discuss PTSD, acute stress disorder (ASD), depression, prolonged grief disorder, anxiety, and externalizing behavior problems. With regard to associated difficulties, we focus on physical health problems and academic difficulties. Importantly, there are high levels of comorbidity: children and adolescents often experience multiple difficulties at the same time (e.g., Copeland et al., 2007).

Mental Health Problems

The range of documented mental health problems in youth after trauma is vast. Over the past few decades, there has been increased recognition of differences between children and adults in terms of the nature and expression of trauma-related mental health difficulties (e.g., Scheeringa, Zeanah, & Cohen, 2011). There is substantial debate about the extent to which current diagnostic classification systems adequately capture the wide range of difficulties that children experience (e.g., Cohen & Scheeringa, 2009; D'Andrea, Ford, Stolbach, Spinazzola, & van der Kolk, 2012; Goldbeck & Jensen, 2017). Here, we focus largely on those mental difficulties currently described by the major classification systems (i.e., the DSM and ICD).

Posttraumatic Stress Disorder

In DSM-5, diagnostic criteria for PTSD in *older children* (ages 6 years and over) are the same as they are for adults, with PTSD conceptualized and diagnosed as a four-factor model of symptoms: reexperiencing of the trauma, persistent avoidance of trauma-related stimuli, negative alterations in cognition and mood, and hyperarousal and reactivity. There are some developmental specifiers within the text of DSM-5 in recognition of the fact that children's traumatic stress reactions can manifest differently from those of adults. For example, it is noted that intrusive memories may be shown via repetitive, trauma-themed play, and that nightmares may not have recognizable content (American Psychiatric Association, 2013).

For *younger children* (under the age of 6 years), there is a separate set of diagnostic criteria, developed in response to research showing marked developmental differences in how posttraumatic stress reactions are manifest in the preschool period (see Scheeringa et al., 2011). This represents the first developmental subtype of a disorder of any kind in the DSM. In this "preschool" subtype, avoidance and negative alterations in cognition/mood combine into a single symptom cluster. In addition, some symptoms that appear in the criteria for older children and adults are excluded (e.g., cognitive symptoms that preschoolers are unlikely to display or describe, such as negative beliefs about the self/world/future, and persistent blame of self/others). Furthermore, within the preschool subtype criteria there is explicit recognition that some symptoms may present differently in this age group than in older children/adults. For example, it is noted that "spontaneous and intrusive memories may not necessarily appear distressing" and that "diminished interest in significant activities" may be reflected in "constriction of play."

ICD-11 (World Health Organization, 2018) uses a three-factor model for PTSD, such that to meet criteria, an individual (child or adult) must show core symptoms of reexperiencing of the trauma, avoidance of trauma reminders, and arousal/reactivity. In ICD-11, a diagnosis of *complex PTSD* can also be made when an individual meets the aforementioned criteria for PTSD and also shows prominent features of affect dysregulation, negative self-concept (accompanied by feelings of shame, guilt, or failure related to the trauma), and interpersonal problems.

Current estimates are that, overall, approximately 16% of children and adolescents exposed to trauma develop PTSD (Alisic et al., 2014), with higher rates for interpersonal trauma compared to noninterpersonal trauma. Children typically follow one of three to four trajectories (e.g., Le Brocque, Hendrikz, & Kenardy, 2010; Miller-Graff & Howell, 2015; although see also Nugent et al., 2009). The first trajectory ("resilience") is one of consistently low levels of distress. The second ("recovery") group experiences acute stress, which resolves over time. The third ("chronic") experiences consistent and persistent high levels of distress. The fourth ("delayed" onset) experiences subclinical initial levels of distress but develops clinically significant symptoms over time. This fourth trajectory (Punamäki, Palosaari, Diab, Peltonen, & Qouta, 2015) does not always appear in studies among children, in contrast to studies among adults (e.g., see Smid, Mooren, van der Mast, Gersons, & Kleber, 2009). Over half of children fall into the resilient group, a quarter to a third into the recovery group, and a small percentage into the chronic group. This pattern is very similar to trajectories seen in adults (e.g., see Bonanno, 2005). Importantly, while on average, symptom levels in trauma-exposed children decline over the first 6 months posttrauma, there is little evidence that natural recovery occurs beyond 6 months, suggesting that it is unlikely a child would recover from PTSD without intervention at that point (Hiller et al., 2016).

It is still difficult to predict which children will end up on which trajectory (see also Gunaratnam & Alisic, 2017). In terms of *preexisting* factors, in contrast to their role in risk for exposure, demographic factors, such as gender, age, race, and socioeconomic status, do not seem to play particularly important roles in predicting a child's level of distress posttrauma (Alisic, Jongmans, Van Wesel, & Kleber, 2011; Scheeringa et al., 2011; Trickey, Siddaway, Meiser-Stedman, Serpell, & Field, 2012). Prior exposure to trauma does, however, play an important role (Catani, Jacob, Schauer, Kohila, & Neuner, 2008; Cox, Kenardy, & Hendrikz, 2008; McLaughlin et al., 2013). Similarly, prior mental health difficulties and family functioning are predictors of PTSD (e.g., see Cox et al., 2008; McLaughlin et al., 2013). In terms of *peritrauma* factors, a key predictor of PTSD is the nature of the exposure; interpersonal trauma is much more likely to lead to PTSD than noninterpersonal trauma (pooled PTSD rates of 25% vs. 10% in a meta-analysis; Alisic et al., 2014), and separation from family is a risk factor as well (McFarlane, 1987; McGregor, Melvin, & Newman, 2015). Biological variables during or shortly after exposure, such as increased heart rate and cortisol levels, appear to be predictive (Nugent, Christopher, & Delahanty, 2006; Pervanidou, 2008), although the effect sizes found have been small. Cognitions during or after the exposure, such as the experience of life threat or the feeling of permanent and disturbing change, show much stronger associations with subsequent PTSD (Meiser-Stedman, Dalgleish, Gluckman, Yule, & Smith, 2009; Trickey et al., 2012). In terms of *posttrauma* factors, those related to parental adjustment—namely, parents' own posttrauma coping, stress reactions, and mental health—seem to matter a great deal for the child's ability to heal (Alisic et al., 2011; Cox et al., 2008; Landolt, Ystrom, Sennhauser, Gnehm, & Vollrath, 2012; Marsac, Donlon, Winston, & Kassam-Adams, 2013). Social support seems to be protective against PTSD for children and adolescents (e.g., Langley et al., 2013; Trickey et al., 2012).

Acute Stress Disorder

ASD, according to DSM-5 criteria, is diagnosed if a child/adolescent displays a high level of symptomatology (associated with impairment in functioning) between 3 days and 1 month following a trauma, with symptoms in the following domains: reexperiencing, avoidance, negative alterations in cognition/mood, arousal/reactivity, and/or dissociation. ICD-11 does not include an equivalent classification; acute stress is instead considered a normal reaction to a traumatic event. Research on ASD in children and adolescents has occurred mostly within the accidental injury context. In this setting, concerns have been raised about the sensitivity of DSM criteria for children. For example, Kassam-Adams and colleagues (2012) combined data from 15 hospital-based studies in the United States, the United Kingdom, Australia, and Switzerland; they found that 41% of children and adolescents experienced clinically relevant impairment, yet only 12% met criteria similar to the current ASD criteria. Recent data suggest that ASD does not function as a "catch-all" for identifying those at risk of persistent posttraumatic mental health difficulties (e.g., see Meiser-Stedman et al., 2017). A more broad-based assessment that includes depression may be a more effective approach to identifying young people at risk of later difficulties, though this is yet to be fully tested.

Prolonged Grief Disorder

Increased attention has been given in recent years to understanding the bereavement-related psychological difficulties experienced by youth when their trauma exposure involves the death of someone close to them (e.g., Kaplow, Layne, Pynoos, Cohen, & Lieberman, 2012). Indeed, in response to a traumatic death, approximately 10% of children develop prolonged or "complicated" grief reactions that are distinct from bereavement-related PTSD, anxiety, and depression (e.g., Dillen, Fontaine, & Verhofstadt-Deneve, 2009; Melhem, Moritz, Walker, Shear, & Brent, 2007; Melhem, Porta, Shamseddeen, Walker Payne, & Brent, 2011; Spuij et al., 2012). These responses are associated with significant functional impairment and are typically characterized by intense yearning, difficulty accepting the loss, prominent anger, and a sense that life is meaningless. The DSM does not yet recognize such difficulties by way of a formal diagnostic category, but "persistent complex bereavement disorder" has been listed in the "conditions for further study" section of DSM-5 (American Psychiatric Association, 2013). In ICD-11, a formal diagnostic category has been introduced to describe bereavement-related reactions that warrant clinical attention—namely, prolonged grief disorder (PGD). Core symptoms include longing for and preoccupation with the deceased, together with emotional distress and impaired functioning that persist beyond 6 months after the person's death and go beyond what is normal in one's culture.

Depression

Research with children exposed to a range of trauma types has shown that clinically significant levels of depression frequently co-occur with PTSD (see Goenjian et al., 2009; Lai, Auslander, Fitzpatrick, & Podkowirow, 2014; Scheeringa, 2015). Studies reveal wide variability in rates of depression, but with rates often found to be greater than those in the general population. Lai and colleagues (2014), for example, found that studies examining depression in youth following natural disasters reported rates of depression from 2 to 69% compared to typical ranges of 1–9% in general population studies. In an accidental injury sample, Kassam-Adams, Bakker, Marsac, Fein, and Winston (2015) found that 13% of 8- to 17-year-old participants displayed clinically significant levels of depression. Meiser-Stedman and colleagues (2017) found that 23.4% of children exposed to a single-incident trauma resulting in emergency department visits experienced substantial depression symptoms that were largely stable and persistent across time.

Anxiety

Symptoms of anxiety, as indexed via continuous symptomatology measures, have been shown to co-occur with PTSD in trauma-exposed youth across several studies (e.g., La Greca, Danzi, & Chan, 2017; La Greca et al., 2013). Questions remain, though, regarding whether such findings are best conceptualized as capturing symptom overlap with PTSD, or representing the presence of a distinct form of psychopathology (see Cohen & Scheeringa, 2009; Scheeringa, 2015). In a preschool sample, Scheeringa (2015) found that 11% of those exposed to Hurricane Katrina, 18% of those exposed to other single-incident traumas, and 16% of those exposed to repeated trauma (mainly domestic violence) developed an anxiety disorder (either separation anxiety disorder, generalized anxiety disorder, or social phobia). Very few, however, had anxiety disorders in the absence of PTSD, raising important questions about the mechanisms underlying development of anxiety following trauma.

Relatively limited empirical data are available regarding the prevalence of specific anxiety disorders in trauma-exposed youth. Hoven and colleagues (2005) studied the mental health of children living in New York City in the aftermath of September 11, 2001, and found that, 6 months after the terrorist attack, probable agoraphobia (14.8%) and separation anxiety disorder (12.3%) were most prevalent, even more than PTSD (10.6%). Generalized anxiety disorder was also quite frequently reported among this group of children (10.3%). Kim and colleagues (2009) conducted a study 6 months after a fire escape drill that resulted in a fatal accident and found that agoraphobia was the most prevalent DSM-IV anxiety disorder (22.4%), followed by generalized anxiety disorder (GAD; 13.8%), separation anxiety disorder (SAD; 6.9%), PTSD (5.2%), and social phobia (5.2%). Using subclinical cutoff points, however, SAD was the most common (41.4%), followed by agoraphobia (34.5%), obsessive–compulsive disorder (OCD; 22.4%), PTSD (20.7%), and social phobia (20.7%).

Externalizing Behavior

Whereas PTSD, depression, and anxiety are examples of internalizing problems, trauma-exposed children may also exhibit externalizing behavior problems (Whitson & Connell, 2016), such as defiant or oppositional behavior (Li et al., 2016), conduct problems (Reigstad & Kvernmo, 2016), and symptoms of attention-deficit/hyperactivity disorder (Hunt, Slack, & Berger, 2017). In adolescence, interpersonal violence and child maltreatment are associated not exclusively with PTSD and depression, but as well with delinquency, substance abuse, and risky sexual behaviors (Cisler et al., 2012; Jones et al., 2010;

Yoon, Kobulsky, Yoon, & Kim, 2017). In line with these behaviors, level of drinking among adolescents has been related to maltreatment and violence during childhood, and externalizing behavior may represent a pathway between the two (Cornelius, De Genna, Goldschmidt, Larkby, & Day, 2016; Proctor et al., 2017).

Regarding the pathway from maltreatment to behavior problems, physical abuse may be more closely linked with behavioral problems and emotional abuse more closely with emotional problems (Li et al., 2016), but this is uncertain, and emotional abuse may also increase the risk of externalizing symptoms, for both girls and boys (Hagborg, Tidefors, & Fahlke, 2017). Several studies of children make use of both child self-report and parental report, and the relationship between maltreatment and adjustment seems to vary with the informant (Sternberg et al., 1993). Fortunately, there are indications that safe relationships with teachers (or other "safe adults") and other children can protect against the development of behavior problems in abused children (Ban & Oh, 2016). In addition, improvement in behavioral problems over time is likely with proper care (Whitson & Connell, 2016).

Other Difficulties: Functional Outcomes

Revictimization as an Outcome

An alarming finding is that children and adolescents exposed to interpersonal violence are at increased risk of experiencing new violence (revictimization), not only later in their childhood but also as adults (Finkelhor et al., 2007). The risk of sexual revictimization following child sexual abuse has long been known (Arata, 2002), but more recently it has been shown that victimization by any child violence leads to substantial vulnerability for revictimization through other types of trauma (Finkelhor et al., 2007). This risk of revictimization is not a very distant threat, and studies have found that about one-third of young people exposed to childhood violence experienced revictimization in a 12- to 18-month time frame (Strøm, Kristian Hjemdal, Myhre, Wentzel-Larsen, & Thoresen, 2017). This knowledge, combined with the well-documented cumulative health effects of trauma, calls for increased attention to the future safety of violence-exposed children. For adults and clinicians who try to help traumatized children, building safety may be just as important as alleviating current symptoms.

Physical Health Problems

Although there is compelling evidence that childhood maltreatment increases the risk of adult mental and physical health problems, little research has focused on children and adolescents' somatic complaints following trauma while they are still young. Nevertheless, headaches, migraines, and stomachaches have been associated with community violence (Bailey et al., 2005) and with interpersonal violence in childhood (Stensland, Dyb,

Thoresen, Wentzel-Larsen, & Zwart, 2013). Furthermore, trauma and interpersonal violence seems to increase the risk of eating disorders (Trottier & MacDonald, 2017), overweight (Oh et al., 2018; Stensland, Thoresen, Wentzel-Larsen, & Dyb, 2015), chronic pain (McLaughlin et al., 2016), and musculoskeletal problems (Dirkzwager, Kerssens, & Yzermans, 2006; Dorn, Yzermans, Spreeuwenberg, Schilder, & van der Zee, 2008). In a community study of preschool children experiencing poverty, exposure to domestic violence was one of the strongest predictors of somatic health problems (Graham-Bermann & Seng, 2005).

Adverse somatic outcomes following traumatic events have predominantly been considered products of posttraumatic stress (Pacella, Hruska, & Delahanty, 2013). However, it has also been argued that somatic problems in children are underrecognized because they are understood as secondary to psychological symptoms (Hensley & Varela, 2008). We do not yet fully understand the interplay between physical and mental health problems following trauma and violence in childhood. Nevertheless, somatic health problems in the aftermath of violence or trauma can affect the child's ability to attend school, take part in leisure activities, and engage in social relationships.

Difficulties in School or Academic Performance

Both acute and chronic traumatic events seem to have a negative impact on cognitive functioning, academic results, and social and emotional behavior in school (Perfect, Turley, Carlson, Yohanna, & Saint Gilles, 2016; Veltman & Browne, 2001). In the acute trauma context, for example, primary school children affected by disaster can show decreased academic performance over time, particularly in the domains of mathematics and reading (Gibbs et al., 2019). Childhood abuse has also been linked to problems with cognitive functioning and lower academic performance (Crozier & Barth, 2005; Kendall-Tackett & Eckenrode, 1996; Veltman & Browne, 2001), in terms of grades, test scores, and school absences (Leiter & Johnsen, 1994). Learning difficulties in abused or neglected children can relate to their behavior difficulties, which may also vary with the type of abuse to which they have been exposed. For example, neglected children may show less social interaction with their classmates, whereas physically abused children may display aggressive behavior (Hoffman-Plotkin & Twentyman, 1984). Likely, a child's potential problems at school will be influenced by the type of home environment they experience, including the type and intensity of maltreatment they have undergone (Pears, Kim, & Fisher, 2008). Long-term studies are few, but violence and abuse reported at age 15 has been found to prospectively predict high school dropout, work marginalization, and long-term welfare benefits 10 years later (Strøm, 2014). Maintaining school attendance and educational support over time seems to be of importance for children exposed to maltreatment and other forms of trauma, and a close cooperation between clinicians, educators, and parents seems warranted (Strøm, Schultz, Wentzel-Larsen, & Dyb, 2016).

Caveats about Current Epidemiological and Clinical Knowledge

Although it is well established that following trauma exposure, children of all ages can develop persistent difficulties, many aspects of child adaptation posttrauma are still underresearched or not well understood. For example, there is still a dearth of research on children in low- and middle-income countries, and on children from minority groups in high-income countries. We also have more knowledge of children in some age groups compared to other age groups: very young children are still underresearched, although research activity is increasing (e.g., De Young, Kenardy, & Cobham, 2011; Haag & Landolt, 2017). Similarly, when looking at family factors, we have substantially more knowledge that relates to children's mothers than to their fathers.

Although there is a substantial body of knowledge regarding child PTSD, research into other child health and well-being outcomes is sparse. Some prevalence data are available; future studies should generate insights regarding other aspects of posttrauma depression, grief, and other disorders among children, including their predictors and trajectories, and mechanisms underlying the high levels of comorbidity often seen (see also Cohen & Scheeringa, 2009; Scheeringa, 2015). Moreover, traditionally there has been a strong focus on disorders, whereas recently researchers have increasingly started to collect data on children's functioning in daily life.

Methodologically, a few caveats should be noted. First, a recurring question in child psychotraumatology is who serves as "informant" regarding a child's well-being: the child and/or the parent, or a third party, such as a teacher? Reports that build solely on parents' perspectives are known to underreport children's symptoms (e.g., Daviss et al., 2000), leading to recommendations to make use of combined parent and child reports when possible (Meiser-Stedman, Smith, Glucksman, Yule, & Dalgleish, 2007), and otherwise to use child reports as much as available. Second, much research has relied on self-report of mental health experiences and behaviors. Recent studies endeavor to broaden this type of evidence gathering by including both biological and behavioral data (e.g., Alisic et al., 2017; Bicanic et al., 2013; Marsac & Kassam-Adams, 2016). Finally, many studies are still cross-sectional, which makes it difficult to build an understanding of children's and families' trajectories of recovery, and the various factors that play a role in it.

Conclusion

Trauma is a common and painful experience for children and adolescents throughout the world. Although some trauma-exposed children remain healthy, such experiences leave lasting emotional footprints for other children, and the negative consequences for health and well-being have a high societal cost. Some trauma-exposed children and adolescents will carry a burden of emotional distress and physical health problems into adulthood and even into old age. Whereas a substantial knowledge base exists regarding exposure to, and consequences of, trauma among children and adolescents, the mechanisms involved in the development of these long-term adverse outcomes need more empirical attention. Most of our knowledge is currently based on a fraction of the children and adolescents around the world; as such, cultural and societal differences in how children react to trauma are still poorly understood. There is still a lot to discover regarding how children's and families' biological and behavioral characteristics predict their trajectories with respect to the wide range of posttrauma responses and their interactions. For clinicians, it is clear that staying open to a wide range of potential outcomes is important when working with trauma-exposed youth, so that relevant evidence-based assessments and interventions can be implemented.

REFERENCES

Aakvaag, H. F., Thoresen, S., Wentzel-Larsen, T., & Dyb, G. (2017). Adult victimization in female survivors of childhood violence and abuse: The contribution of multiple types of violence. *Violence Against Women, 23,* 1601–1619.

Alisic, E., Gunaratnam, S., Barrett, A., Conroy, R., Jowett, H., Bressan, S., et al. (2017). Injury talk: Spontaneous parent–child conversations in the aftermath of a potentially traumatic event. *Evidence-Based Mental Health, 20,* e19–e20.

Alisic, E., Jongmans, M. J., Van Wesel, F., & Kleber, R. J. (2011). Building child trauma theory from longitudinal studies: A meta-analysis. *Clinical Psychology Review, 31,* 736–747.

Alisic, E., van der Schoot, T. A., van Ginkel, J. R., & Kleber, R. J. (2008). Trauma exposure in primary school children: Who is at risk? *Journal of Child and Adolescent Trauma, 1,* 263–269.

Alisic, E., Zalta, A. K., Van Wesel, F., Larsen, S. E., Hafstad, G. S., Hassanpour, K., et al. (2014). Rates of post-traumatic stress disorder in trauma-exposed children and adolescents: Meta-analysis. *British Journal of Psychiatry, 204,* 335–340.

American Psychiatric Association. (2013). *Diagnostic and statistical manual of mental disorders* (5th ed.). Arlington, VA: Author.

Arata, C. M. (2002). Child sexual abuse and sexual revictimization. *Clinical Psychology: Science and Practice, 9,* 135–164.

Bailey, B. N., Delaney-Black, V., Hannigan, J. H., Ager, J., Sokol, R. J., & Covington, C. Y. (2005). Somatic complaints in children and community violence exposure. *Journal of Developmental and Behavioral Pediatrics, 26,* 341–348.

Ban, J., & Oh, I. (2016). Mediating effects of teacher and peer relationships between parental abuse/neglect and emotional/behavioral problems. *Child Abuse and Neglect, 61,* 35–42.

Bicanic, I. A., Postma, R. M., Sinnema, G., De Roos, C., Olff, M., Van Wesel, F., et al. (2013). Salivary cortisol and dehydroepiandrosterone sulfate in adolescent rape victims with post traumatic stress disorder. *Psychoneuroendocrinology, 38,* 408–415.

Bonanno, G. A. (2005). Resilience in the face of potential trauma. *Current Directions in Psychological Science, 14*(3), 135–138.

Catani, C., Jacob, N., Schauer, E., Kohila, M., & Neuner, F. (2008). Family violence, war, and natural disasters: A study of the effect of extreme stress on children's mental health in Sri Lanka. *BMC Psychiatry, 8,* 33–42.

Cisler, J. M., Begle, A. M., Amstadter, A. B., Resnick, H. S., Danielson, C. K., Saunders, B. E., et al. (2012). Exposure to interpersonal violence and risk for PTSD, depression, delinquency, and binge drinking among adolescents: Data from the NSA-R. *Journal of Traumatic Stress, 25*(1), 33–40.

Cohen, J. A., & Scheeringa, M. S. (2009). Post-traumatic stress disorder diagnosis in children: Challenges and promises. *Dialogues in Clinical Neuroscience, 11,* 91–99.

Copeland, W. E., Keeler, G., Angold, A., & Costello, E. J. (2007). Traumatic events and posttraumatic stress in childhood. *Archives of General Psychiatry, 64,* 577–584.

Cornelius, M. D., De Genna, N. M., Goldschmidt, L., Larkby, C., & Day, N. L. (2016). Prenatal alcohol and other early childhood adverse exposures: Direct and indirect pathways to adolescent drinking. *Neurotoxicology and Teratology, 55,* 8–15.

Cox, C. M., Kenardy, J. A., & Hendrikz, J. K. (2008). A meta-analysis of risk factors that predict psychopathology following accidental trauma. *Journal for Specialists in Pediatric Nursing, 13,* 98–110.

Crozier, J. C., & Barth, R. P. (2005). Cognitive and academic functioning in maltreated children. *Children and Schools, 27,* 197–206.

D'Andrea, W., Ford, J. D., Stolbach, B., Spinazzola, J., & van der Kolk, B. A. (2012). Understanding interpersonal trauma in children: Why we need a developmentally appropriate trauma diagnosis. *American Journal of Orthopsychiatry, 82,* 187–200.

Daviss, W., Racusin, R., Fleischer, A., Mooney, D., Ford, J. D., & McHugo, G. J. (2000). Acute stress disorder symptomatology during hospitalization for pediatric injury. *Journal of the American Academy of Child and Adolescent Psychiatry, 39,* 569–575.

De Young, A. C., Kenardy, J. A., & Cobham, V. E. (2011). Trauma in early childhood: A neglected population. *Clinical Child and Family Psychology Review, 14*(3), 231–250.

Decker, M. R., Peitzmeier, S., Olumide, A., Acharya, R., Ojengbede, O., Covarrubias, L., et al. (2014). Prevalence and health impact of intimate partner violence and non-partner sexual violence among female adolescents aged 15–19 years in vulnerable urban environments: A multi-country study. *Journal of Adolescent Health, 55,* S58–S67.

Demyttenaere, K., Bruffaerts, R., Posada-Villa, J., Gasquet, I., Kovess, V., Lepine, J. P., et al. (2004). Prevalence, severity, and unmet need for treatment of mental disorders in the World Health Organization World Mental Health Surveys. *Journal of the American Medical Association, 291,* 2581–2590.

Dillen, L., Fontaine, J. R., & Verhofstadt-Deneve, L. (2009). Confirming the distinctiveness of complicated grief from depression and anxiety among adolescents. *Death Studies, 33,* 437–461.

Dirkzwager, A. J., Kerssens, J. J., & Yzermans, C. J. (2006). Health problems in children and adolescents before and after a man-made disaster. *Journal of the American Academy of Child and Adolescent Psychiatry, 45,* 94–103.

Dong, M., Anda, R. F., Felitti, V. J., Dube, S. R., Williamson, D. F., Thompson, T. J., et al. (2004). The interrelatedness of multiple forms of childhood abuse, neglect, and household dysfunction. *Child Abuse and Neglect, 28,* 771–784.

Dorn, T., Yzermans, J. C., Spreeuwenberg, P. M., Schilder, A., & van der Zee, J. (2008). A cohort study of the long-term impact of a fire disaster on the physical and mental health of adolescents. *Journal of Traumatic Stress, 21,* 239–242.

Elklit, A., & Frandsen, L. (2014). Trauma exposure and posttraumatic stress among Danish adolescents. *Journal of Traumatic Stress Disorders and Treatment, 4,* 2.

Finkelhor, D., Ormrod, R. K., & Turner, H. A. (2007). Poly-victimization: A neglected component in child victimization. *Child Abuse and Neglect, 31*(1), 7–26.

Finkelhor, D., Ormrod, R. K., & Turner, H. A. (2009). Lifetime assessment of poly-victimization in a national sample of children and youth. *Child Abuse and Neglect, 33*(7), 403–411.

Finkelhor, D., Shattuck, A., Turner, H. A., & Hamby, S. L. (2014). The lifetime prevalence of child sexual abuse and sexual assault assessed in late adolescence. *Journal of Adolescent Health, 55*(3), 329–333.

Finkelhor, D., Turner, H. A., Shattuck, A., & Hamby, S. L. (2015). Prevalence of childhood exposure to violence, crime, and abuse: Results from the National Survey of Children's Exposure to Violence. *JAMA Pediatrics, 169*(8), 746–754.

Ghazali, S. R., Elklit, A., Balang, R. V., Sultan, M., & Kana, K. (2014). Preliminary findings on lifetime trauma prevalence and PTSD symptoms among adolescents in Sarawak Malaysia. *Asian Journal of Psychiatry, 11,* 45–49.

Gibbs, L., Nursey, J., Cook, J., Ireton, G., Alkemade, N., Roberts, M., et al. (2019). Delayed disaster impacts on academic performance of primary school children. *Child Development, 90*(4), 1402–1412.

Goenjian, A. K., Walling, D., Steinberg, A. M., Roussos, A., Goenjian, H. A., & Pynoos, R. S. (2009). Depression and PTSD symptoms among bereaved adolescents 6½ years after the 1988 Spitak earthquake. *Journal of Affective Disorders, 112*(1–3), 81–84.

Goldbeck, L., & Jensen, T. K. (2017). The diagnostic spectrum of trauma-related disorders in children and adolescents. In M. A. Landolt, M. Cloitre, & U. Schnyder (Eds.), *Evidence-based treatments for trauma related disorders in children and adolescents* (pp. 3–28). Cham, Switzerland: Springer.

Graham-Bermann, S. A., & Seng, J. (2005). Violence exposure and traumatic stress symptoms as additional predictors of health problems in high-risk children. *Journal of Pediatrics, 146*(3), 349–354.

Gunaratnam, S., & Alisic, E. (2017). Epidemiology of trauma and trauma-related disorders in children and adolescents. In M. A. Landoh, M. Cloitre, & V. Schnyder (Eds.), *Evidence-based treatments for trauma related disorders in children and adolescents* (pp. 29–47). Cham, Switzerland: Springer.

Haag, A. C., & Landolt, M. A. (2017). Young children's acute stress after a burn injury: Disentangling the role of injury severity and parental acute stress. *Journal of Pediatric Psychology, 42*(8), 861–870.

Hagborg, J. M., Tidefors, I., & Fahlke, C. (2017). Gender differences in the association between emotional maltreatment with mental, emotional, and behavioral problems in Swedish adolescents. *Child Abuse and Neglect, 67,* 249–259.

Hamby, S., Finkelhor, D., Turner, H., & Ormrod, R. (2010). The overlap of witnessing partner violence with child maltreatment and other victimizations in a nationally representative survey of youth. *Child Abuse and Neglect, 34,* 734–741.

Hensley, L., & Varela, R. E. (2008). PTSD symptoms and somatic complaints following Hurricane Katrina: The roles of trait anxiety and anxiety sensitivity. *Journal of Clinical Child and Adolescent Psychology, 37,* 542–552.

Hiller, R. M., Meiser-Stedman, R., Fearon, P., Lobo, S., MacKinnon, A., Fraser, A., et al. (2016). Changes in the prevalence and symptom severity of child PTSD in the year following trauma: A meta-analytic study. *Journal of Child Psychology and Psychiatry, 57,* 884–898.

Hoffman-Plotkin, D., & Twentyman, C. T. (1984). A multimodal assessment of behavioral and cognitive deficits in abused and neglected preschoolers. *Child Development, 55,* 794–802.

Hoven, C. W., Duarte, C. S., Lucas, C. P., Wu, P., Mandell, D. J., Goodwin, R. D., et al. (2005). Psychopathology among New York City public school children 6 months after September 11. *Archives of General Psychiatry, 62,* 545–551.

Hunt, T. K., Slack, K. S., & Berger, L. M. (2017). Adverse childhood experiences and behavioral problems in middle childhood. *Child Abuse and Neglect, 67,* 391–402.

Irie, F., Lang, J., Kaltner, M., Le Brocque, R., & Kenardy, J. (2012). Effects of gender, indigenous status and remoteness to health services on the occurrence of assault-related injuries in children and adolescents. *Injury, 43,* 1873–1880.

Jones, D. J., Runyan, D. K., Lewis, T., Litrownik, A. J., Black, M. M., Wiley, T., et al. (2010). Trajectories of childhood sexual abuse and early adolescent HIV/AIDS risk behaviors: The role of other maltreatment, witnessed violence, and child gender. *Journal of Clinical Child and Adolescent Psychology, 39*(5), 667–680.

Kaplow, J. B., Layne, C. M., Pynoos, R. S., Cohen, J., & Lieberman, A. (2012). DSM-V diagnostic criteria for bereavement-related disorders in children and adolescents: Developmental considerations. *Psychiatry, 75,* 242–265.

Kassam-Adams, N., Bakker, A., Marsac, M. L., Fein, J. A., & Winston, F. K. (2015). Traumatic stress, depression, and recovery: Child and parent responses after emergency medical care for unintentional injury. *Pediatric Emergency Care, 31*(11), 737–742.

Kassam-Adams, N., Palmieri, P. A., Rork, K., Delahanty, D. L., Kenardy, J., Kohser, K. L., et al. (2012). Acute stress symptoms in children: Results from an international data archive. *Journal of the American Academy of Child and Adolescent Psychiatry, 51,* 812–820.

Kendall-Tackett, K. A., & Eckenrode, J. (1996). The effects of neglect on academic achievement and disciplinary problems: A developmental perspective. *Child Abuse and Neglect, 20,* 161–169.

Kim, B. N., Kim, J. W., Kim, H. W., Shin, M. S., Cho, S. C., Choi, N. H., et al. (2009). A 6-month follow-up study of posttraumatic stress and anxiety/depressive symptoms in Korean children after direct or indirect exposure to a single incident of trauma. *Journal of Clinical Psychiatry, 70,* 1148–1154.

La Greca, A. M., Danzi, B. A., & Chan, S. F. (2017). DSM-5 and ICD-11 as competing models of PTSD in preadolescent children exposed to a natural disaster: Assessing validity and co-occurring symptomatology. *European Journal of Psychotraumatology, 8,* 1310591.

La Greca, A. M., Lai, B. S., Llabre, M. M., Silverman, W. K., Vernberg, E. M., & Prinstein, M. J. (2013). Children's postdisaster trajectories of PTS symptoms: Predicting chronic distress. *Child and Youth Care Forum, 42,* 351–369.

Lai, B. S., Auslander, B. A., Fitzpatrick, S. L., & Podkowirow, V. (2014). Disasters and depressive symptoms in children: A review. *Child and Youth Care Forum, 43,* 489–504.

Landolt, M. A., Schnyder, U., Maier, T., Schoenbucher, V., & Mohler-Kuo, M. (2013). Trauma exposure and posttraumatic stress disorder in adolescents: A national survey in Switzerland. *Journal of Traumatic Stress, 26*(2), 209–216.

Landolt, M. A., Ystrom, E., Sennhauser, F. H., Gnehm, H. E., & Vollrath, M. E. (2012). The mutual prospective influence of child and parental post-traumatic stress symptoms in pediatric patients. *Journal of Child Psychology and Psychiatry, 53,* 767–774.

Langley, A. K., Cohen, J. A., Mannarino, A. P., Jaycox, L. H., Schonlau, M., Scott, M., et al. (2013). Trauma exposure and mental health problems among school children 15 months post-Hurricane Katrina. *Journal of Child and Adolescent Trauma, 6,* 143–156.

Le Brocque, R. M., Hendrikz, J., & Kenardy, J. A. (2010). The course of posttraumatic stress in children: Examination of recovery trajectories following traumatic injury. *Journal of Pediatric Psychology, 35*(6), 637–645.

Leiter, J., & Johnsen, M. C. (1994). Child maltreatment and school performance. *American Journal of Education, 102,* 154–189.

Lewis, S. J., Arseneault, L., Caspi, A., Fisher, H. L., Matthews, T., Moffitt, T. E., et al. (2019). The epidemiology of trauma and post-traumatic stress disorder in a representative cohort of young people in England and Wales. *Lancet Psychiatry, 6*(3), 247–256.

Li, L., Lin, X., Chi, P., Heath, M. A., Fang, X., Du, H., et al. (2016). Maltreatment and emotional and behavioral problems in Chinese children with and without oppositional defiant disorder: The mediating role of the parent–child relationship. *Journal of Interpersonal Violence, 31*(18), 2915–2939.

Marsac, M. L., Donlon, K. A., Winston, F. K., & Kassam-Adams, N. (2013). Child coping, parent coping assistance, and post-traumatic stress following paediatric physical injury. *Child: Care, Health and Development, 39,* 171–177.

Marsac, M. L., & Kassam-Adams, N. (2016). A novel adaptation of a parent–child observational assessment tool for appraisals and coping in children exposed to acute trauma. *European Journal of Psychotraumatology, 7,* 31879.

McFarlane, A. C. (1987). The relationship between patterns of family interaction and psychiatric disorder in children. *Australian and New Zealand Journal of Psychiatry, 21,* 383–390.

McGregor, L. S., Melvin, G. A., & Newman, L. K. (2015). Familial separations, coping styles, and PTSD symptomatology in resettled refugee youth. *Journal of Nervous and Mental Disease, 203,* 431–438.

McLaughlin, K. A., Basu, A., Walsh, K., Slopen, N., Sumner, J. A., Koenen, K. C., et al. (2016). Childhood exposure to violence and chronic physical conditions in a national sample of US adolescents. *Psychosomatic Medicine, 78*(9), 1072–1083.

McLaughlin, K. A., Koenen, K. C., Hill, E. D., Petukhova, M., Sampson, N. A., Zaslavsky, A., et al. (2013). Trauma exposure and posttraumatic stress disorder in a national sample of adolescents. *Journal of the American Academy of Child and Adolescent Psychiatry, 52,* 815–830.

Meiser-Stedman, R., Dalgleish, T., Glucksman, E., Yule, W., & Smith, P. (2009). Maladaptive cognitive appraisals mediate the evolution of posttraumatic stress reactions: A 6-month follow-up of child and adolescent assault and motor vehicle accident survivors. *Journal of Abnormal Psychology, 118*(4), 778.

Meiser-Stedman, R., McKinnon, A., Dixon, C., Boyle, A., Smith, P., & Dalgleish, T. (2017). Acute stress disorder and the transition to posttraumatic stress disorder in children and adolescents: Prevalence, course, prognosis, diagnostic suitability, and risk markers. *Depression and Anxiety, 34*(4), 348–355.

Meiser-Stedman, R., Smith, P., Glucksman, E., Yule, W., & Dalgleish, T. (2007). Parent and child agreement for acute stress disorder, post-traumatic stress disorder and other psychopathology in a prospective study of children and adolescents exposed to single-event trauma. *Journal of Abnormal Child Psychology, 35*(2), 191–201.

Melhem, N. M., Moritz, G., Walker, M., Shear, M. K., & Brent, D. (2007). Phenomenology and correlates of complicated grief in children and adolescents. *Journal of the American Academy of Child and Adolescent Psychiatry, 46,* 493–499.

Melhem, N. M., Porta, G., Shamseddeen, W., Walker Payne, M., & Brent, D. A. (2011). Grief in children and adolescents bereaved by sudden parental death. *Archives of General Psychiatry, 68,* 911–919.

Miller-Graff, L. E., & Howell, K. H. (2015). Posttraumatic stress symptom trajectories among children exposed to violence. *Journal of Traumatic Stress, 28,* 17–24.

Mohler-Kuo, M., Landolt, M. A., Maier, T., Meidert, U., Schönbucher, V., & Schnyder, U. (2014). Child sexual abuse revisited: A population-based cross-sectional study among Swiss adolescents. *Journal of Adolescent Health, 54,* 304–311.

Morrongiello, B. A., & House, K. (2004). Measuring parent attributes and supervision behaviors relevant to child injury risk: Examining the usefulness of questionnaire measures. *Injury Prevention, 10,* 114–118.

Nugent, N. R., Christopher, N. C., & Delahanty, D. L. (2006). Emergency medical service and in-hospital vital signs as predictors of subsequent PTSD symptom severity in pediatric injury patients. *Journal of Child Psychology and Psychiatry, 47*(9), 919–926.

Nugent, N. R., Saunders, B. E., Williams, L. M., Hanson, R., Smith, D. W., & Fitzgerald, M. M. (2009). Posttraumatic stress symptom trajectories in children living in families reported for family violence. *Journal of Traumatic Stress, 22,* 460–466.

Oh, D. L., Jerman, P., Marques, S. S., Koita, K., Boparai, S. K. P., Harris, N. B., et al. (2018). Systematic review of pediatric health outcomes associated with childhood adversity. *BMC Pediatrics, 18,* 83.

Owens, J. A., Fernando, S., & McGuinn, M. (2005). Sleep disturbance and injury risk in young children. *Behavioral Sleep Medicine, 3,* 18–31.

Pacella, M. L., Hruska, B., & Delahanty, D. L. (2013). The physical health consequences of PTSD and PTSD symptoms: A meta-analytic review. *Journal of Anxiety Disorders, 27*(1), 33–46.

Pears, K. C., Kim, H. K., & Fisher, P. A. (2008). Psychosocial and cognitive functioning of children with specific profiles of maltreatment. *Child Abuse and Neglect, 32,* 958–971.

Perfect, M. M., Turley, M. R., Carlson, J. S., Yohanna, J., & Saint Gilles, M. P. (2016). School-related outcomes of traumatic event exposure and traumatic stress symptoms in students: A systematic review of research from 1990 to 2015. *School Mental Health, 8,* 7–43.

Pervanidou, P. (2008). Biology of post-traumatic stress disorder in childhood and adolescence. *Journal of Neuroendocrinology, 20*(5), 632–638.

Proctor, L. J., Lewis, T., Roesch, S., Thompson, R., Litrownik, A. J., English, D., et al. (2017). Child maltreatment and age of alcohol and marijuana initiation in high-risk youth. *Addictive Behaviors, 75,* 64–69.

Punamäki, R. L., Palosaari, E., Diab, M., Peltonen, K., & Qouta, S. R. (2015).

Trajectories of posttraumatic stress symptoms (PTSS) after major war among Palestinian children: Trauma, family- and child-related predictors. *Journal of Affective Disorders, 172,* 133–140.

Reigstad, B., & Kvernmo, S. (2016). Concurrent adversities among adolescents with conduct problems: The NAAHS study. *Social Psychiatry and Psychiatric Epidemiology, 51,* 1429–1438.

Salazar, A. M., Keller, T. E., Gowen, L. K., & Courtney, M. E. (2013). Trauma exposure and PTSD among older adolescents in foster care. *Social Psychiatry and Psychiatric Epidemiology, 48,* 545–551.

Saunders, B. E., & Adams, Z. W. (2014). Epidemiology of traumatic experiences in childhood. *Child and Adolescent Psychiatric Clinics of North America, 23,* 167–184.

Scheeringa, M. S. (2015). Untangling psychiatric comorbidity in young children who experienced single, repeated, or Hurricane Katrina traumatic events. *Child and Youth Care Forum, 44*(4), 475–492.

Scheeringa, M. S., Zeanah, C. H., & Cohen, J. A. (2011). PTSD in children and adolescents: Toward an empirically based algorithm. *Depression and Anxiety, 28,* 770–782.

Schwebel, D. C., & Gaines, J. (2007). Pediatric unintentional injury: Behavioral risk factors and implications for prevention. *Journal of Developmental and Behavioral Pediatrics, 28*(3), 245–254.

Smid, G. E., Mooren, T. T., van der Mast, R. C., Gersons, B. P., & Kleber, R. J. (2009). Delayed posttraumatic stress disorder: Systematic review, meta-analysis, and meta-regression analysis of prospective studies. *Journal of Clinical Psychiatry, 70,* 1572.

Spuij, M., Reitz, E., Prinzie, P., Stikkelbroek, Y., de Roos, C., & Boelen, P. A. (2012). Distinctiveness of symptoms of prolonged grief, depression, and post-traumatic stress in bereaved children and adolescents. *European Child and Adolescent Psychiatry, 21,* 673–679.

Stensland, S. Ø., Dyb, G., Thoresen, S., Wentzel-Larsen, T., & Zwart, J.-A. (2013). Potentially traumatic interpersonal events, psychological distress and recurrent headache in a population-based cohort of adolescents: The HUNT study. *BMJ Open, 3,* e002997.

Stensland, S. Ø., Thoresen, S., Wentzel-Larsen, T., & Dyb, G. (2015). Interpersonal violence and overweight in adolescents: The HUNT Study. *Scandinavian Journal of Public Health, 43,* 18–26.

Sternberg, K. J., Lamb, M. E., Greenbaum, C., Cicchetti, D., Dawud, S., Cortes, R. M., et al. (1993). Effects of domestic violence on children's behavior problems and depression. *Developmental Psychology, 29*(1), 44–52.

Stoddard, F. J., Saxe, G., Ronfeldt, H., Drake, J. E., Burns, J., Edgren, C., et al. (2006). Acute stress symptoms in young children with burns. *Journal of the American Academy of Child and Adolescent Psychiatry, 45,* 87–93.

Strøm, I. F. (2014). *Violence in adolescence and later work marginalization: A prospective study of physical violence, sexual abuse and bullying in 15-year-olds and marginalization from work in young adulthood.* Oslo, Norway: University of Oslo.

Strøm, I. F., Kristian Hjemdal, O., Myhre, M. C., Wentzel-Larsen, T., & Thoresen, S. (2017). The social context of violence: A study of repeated victimization in adolescents and young adults. *Journal of Interpersonal Violence.* [Epub ahead of print]

Strøm, I. F., Schultz, J.-H., Wentzel-Larsen, T., & Dyb, G. (2016). School performance

after experiencing trauma: A longitudinal study of school functioning in survivors of the Utøya shootings in 2011. *European Journal of Psychotraumatology, 7,*
31359.

Taillieu, T. L., Brownridge, D. A., Sareen, J., & Afifi, T. O. (2016). Childhood emotional maltreatment and mental disorders: Results from a nationally representative adult sample from the United States. *Child Abuse and Neglect, 59,* 1–12.

Trickey, D., Siddaway, A. P., Meiser-Stedman, R., Serpell, L., & Field, A. P. (2012). A
meta-analysis of risk factors for post-traumatic stress disorder in children and
adolescents. *Clinical Psychology Review, 32,* 122–138.

Trottier, K., & MacDonald, D. E. (2017). Update on psychological trauma, other
severe adverse experiences and eating disorders: State of the research and
future research directions. *Current Psychiatry Reports, 19,* 45.

United Nations High Commissioner for Refugees. (2019). *Global trends: Forced dis-
placement in 2018.* Geneva, Switzerland: Author.

United Nations Office for Disaster Risk Reduction. (2015). *Sendai framework for disaster risk reduction 2015–2030.* Geneva: Author.

Updegrove, A. H., & Muftic, L. R. (2019). Childhood polyvictimization, adult violent
victimization, and trauma symptomatology: An exploratory study of prostitu-
tion diversion program participants. *Journal of Family Violence, 34*(8), 733–743.

Veltman, M. W., & Browne, K. D. (2001). Three decades of child maltreatment
research: Implications for the school years. *Trauma, Violence, and Abuse, 2,* 215–
239.

Whitson, M. K., & Connell, C. M. (2016). The relation of exposure to traumatic
events and longitudinal mental health outcomes for children enrolled in systems of care: Results from a national system of care evaluation. *American Journal of Community Psychology, 57,* 380–390.

World Health Organization. (2014). Main messages from the world report [Fact
sheet]. Retrieved from *www.who.int/violence_injury_prevention/child/injury/
world_report/Main_messages_english.*

World Health Organization. (2018). ICD-11 for mortality and morbidity statistics.
Retrieved from *https://www.who.int/violence_injury_prevention/child/injury/
world_report/Main_messages_english.pdf?ua=1.*

Yoon, S., Kobulsky, J. M., Yoon, D., & Kim, W. (2017). Developmental pathways from
child maltreatment to adolescent substance use: The roles of posttraumatic
stress symptoms and mother–child relationships. *Children and Youth Services
Review, 82,* 271–279.

CHAPTER 4

Diagnosis, Assessment, and Screening for PTSD and Complex PTSD in Adults

Jonathan I. Bisson, Chris R. Brewin, Marylene Cloitre, and Andreas Maercker

Posttraumatic stress disorder (PTSD) was first formally recognized as a diagnosable condition in the third edition of the *Diagnostic and Statistical Manual of Mental Disorders* (DSM) classification system (American Psychiatric Association, 1980), with the *International Classification of Diseases and Related Health Problems* (ICD) following suit in 1992 (World Health Organization, 1992). The definition and conceptualization of PTSD have changed over the years, and this chapter considers the current situation with DSM-5 (American Psychiatric Association, 2013) and ICD-11 (World Health Organization, 2018). To facilitate understanding of many of the key issues concerning the classification of traumatic stress symptoms, a particular focus is on the development of the parallel diagnoses of PTSD and complex PTSD (CPTSD) in ICD-11, with the World Health Organization having taken an arguably more radical and innovative approach to its latest revision than the American Psychiatric Association. Commonly used instruments designed to assess DSM-5 PTSD and ICD-11 PTSD and CPTSD are also considered along with screening for PTSD/CPTSD.

DSM-5 PTSD

The fifth edition of DSM (DSM-5) was published in 2013 (American Psychiatric Association, 2013), replacing DSM-IV (American Psychiatric Association, 1994) and introducing some important changes to the previous requirements for diagnosis of PTSD. The symptom clusters comprising reexperiencing and hyperarousal have undergone minor amendments, with avoidance symptoms now included as a symptom cluster on their own. Other key changes include an increase in the total number of symptom criteria to be considered from 17 to 20, significant changes to the traumatic stressor criterion, and the introduction of a new cluster of symptoms defined as "negative alterations in cognitions and mood that are associated with the traumatic event(s)." There is also a greater emphasis on the symptoms being definitely related to the traumatic event(s), and PTSD is now described as a "trauma and stress-related disorder" as opposed to an anxiety disorder. The full criteria for DSM-5 PTSD are available in DSM-5 (American Psychiatric Association, 2013).

DSM-5 has introduced a "with dissociative symptoms" subtype if depersonalization or derealization is present; it allows classification of a "with delayed expression" subtype if the full symptom criteria are not met until at least 6 months after the event. PTSD symptoms usually arise soon after the event (e.g., Galatzer-Levy & Bryant, 2013; Peleg & Shalev, 2006), but in a minority of cases, the diagnostic threshold may not be met until beyond 6 months after the traumatic event ("delayed PTSD"). In these cases, clinically significant PTSD symptoms can emerge following strong reminders or other life stressors (Andrews, Brewin, Philpott, & Stewart, 2007). DSM-5 also includes a preschool (6 years or younger) PTSD subtype with separate symptom criteria, which are discussed by Berliner, Meiser-Stedman, and Danese (Chapter 5, this volume).

In DSM-IV, the traumatic stressor criterion required that individuals had to experience horror, helplessness, or fear at the time of the event. It has been removed in DSM-5, given concerns about its utility and its prevention of some individuals being diagnosed with PTSD despite clearly experiencing the full symptom criteria following severe traumatic events (Bedard-Gilligan & Zoellner, 2008). The description of qualifying traumatic events is more specific than in DSM-IV, resulting in greater clarity but also excluding a number of highly traumatic experiences that could previously have led to a diagnosis of PTSD (e.g., hearing about the unexpected death of a close family member as a result of a sudden medical event such as a heart attack). The reexperiencing and avoidance symptoms are relatively unchanged, but the two deliberate avoidance symptoms are now contained within a separate criterion, and avoidance is therefore an absolute requirement for the diagnosis.

The introduction of the new Criterion D symptom cluster was based on confirmatory factor analysis (Friedman, Resick, Bryant, & Brewin, 2011) and moves the DSM definition of PTSD away from being conceptualized primarily as a fear-based disorder, formally recognizing that other emotions such as shame and guilt may be prominent. More of the Criterion D symptoms overlap with the ICD-11 CPTSD disturbances in self-organization (DSO) symptoms than do the other DSM-5 symptom clusters. For example, D symptoms of persistent and exaggerated negative beliefs about oneself, others, or the world and of feelings of shame or guilt overlap with ICD-11 DSO cluster symptoms related to negative self-concept, and D symptoms of feelings of detachment or estrangement from others overlap with ICD-11 interpersonal disturbances regarding difficulties feeling close to others and maintaining relationships. The increased arousal criteria in DSM-5 are similar to those discussed in DSM-IV but now include "reckless or self-destructive behavior."

Despite considerable effort to improve on the DSM-IV classification of PTSD, the DSM-5 classification is still vulnerable to a number of the criticisms commonly leveled at DSM-IV, not least being that the composition of the symptom clusters is too broad, many thousands of different combinations of symptoms exist that could lead to a PTSD diagnosis, and there are high levels of comorbidity, all combining to reduce optimal clinical utility (Brewin, Lanius, Novac, Schnyder, & Galea, 2009; Galatzer-Levy & Bryant, 2013; Stein, Seedat, Iversen, & Wessely, 2007).

The DSM-5 criteria for PTSD can be considered a further iteration of DSM-IV, based on empirical evidence and the views of the work group that oversaw their development. The specification of DSM-5 and ICD-11 was seen by some as an opportunity to bring the American Psychiatric Association and World Health Organization definitions closer together (First, 2009; Jablensky, 2009; Kupfer, Regier, & Kuhl, 2008) or even to make them identical (Frances, 2009). Indeed, an ICD–DSM Harmonization Coordination Group was created to facilitate this goal. Interestingly, the two classification systems have, in fact, diverged with respect to PTSD, and the argument that the differences in the ICD-10 and DSM-IV classifications of PTSD were definitional as opposed to conceptual (First, 2009) is not the case for DSM-5 and ICD-11. Arguably, the fact the main classification systems now offer different conceptualizations of PTSD introduces unintended risks, such as interchangeable use depending on whether the presence or absence of a diagnosis of PTSD is desired, and confusion among people with PTSD and CPTSD, clinicians, and others (Bisson, 2013).

Assessment of DSM-5 PTSD

Validated and reliable instruments used to assess DSM-IV PTSD have been adapted to assess DSM-5 PTSD. For example, the widely used Clinician-Administered PTSD Scale (CAPS) for DSM-IV (Weathers, Keane, & Davidson, 2001) has been revised and developed as the CAPS-5 with psychometric data on it now becoming available (Weathers et al., 2018). Its sibling, self-administered measure, the PTSD Checklist (PCL; Blanchard, Jones Alexander, Buckley, & Forneris, 1996), is also now available for DSM-5 PTSD (PCL-5; Weathers et al., 2013). Both these instruments (their English-language versions) are available on request from the U.S. National Center for PTSD and can be used by appropriately trained clinicians and researchers free of charge (*www.ptsd.va.gov/professional/assessment/dsm-5_validated_measures. asp*).

Guiding Principles in the Development of ICD-11 Diagnoses

Clinical utility is a key principle that has guided the development of the ICD-11 diagnoses. It refers to the characteristics of a diagnostic system that make it useful at the level of a clinical encounter (Reed et al., 2019). Health data for the World Health Organization are collected at the level of the clinical encounter across all countries and communities. Thus, diagnostic systems with characteristics such as being overly complex, difficult to understand, or not clinically relevant are unlikely to be properly or routinely implemented, leading to underreporting or unreliable reports of diagnoses. For these reasons, ICD-11 guidelines urged that in addition to being scientifically valid, diagnoses have characteristics that support clinical utility, including that the diagnoses be limited in number of symptoms, be easily discriminated from one another, and translate into effective and resource-efficient treatment plans (Reed, 2010). The ICD-11 diagnoses that have emerged from this process, including PTSD and CPTSD, have been evaluated in clinical settings in 13 countries and have been assessed by clinicians as having high clinical utility (Reed, Keeley, et al., 2018). Moreover, the reliability of the ICD-11 diagnoses appear to be at least as high as that obtained by DSM-5 (Reed, Sharan, et al., 2018).

Rationale for a PTSD and CPTSD Distinction

The rationale for the development of two trauma-related disorders was primarily to account for and organize the heterogeneity of posttraumatic stress symptoms along conceptual and etiological lines and ultimately to direct treatment options in a resource-efficient way. PTSD is articulated as a trauma-generated disorder where symptoms focus on reactions to trauma-related stimuli as represented in three symptom clusters: reexperiencing of the traumatic event in the present, avoidance of traumatic reminders, and a sense of current threat. CPTSD includes not only the symptoms of PTSD but also problems in self-organization related to affective, self-concept and interpersonal domains that are typically associated with exposure to sustained, repeated, or multiple types of traumas (e.g., childhood sexual abuse, domestic violence, exposure to sustained civil war or community violence). CPTSD is composed of six clusters: the three PTSD clusters as well as three clusters related to disturbances in self-organization (DSO): affect dysregulation, negative self-concept, and disturbances in relationships.

The validity of the PTSD/CPTSD distinction has been demonstrated in several studies indicating that the two disorders consistently differ by the types of traumas that create risk, by comorbidity burden, and by level of impairment (see Brewin et al., 2017; Cloitre et al., 2019). Moreover, several latent class analyses have found that trauma-exposed populations fall into distinct classes by the types of symptoms they report, with one group reporting only PTSD symptoms and the other complex PTSD symptoms (Brewin et al., 2017). These data provide substantial evidence supporting the validity of the PTSD and CPTSD profiles as distinct disorders.

Certain characteristics of the ICD-11 diagnoses are important to note. First, diagnosis of PTSD and CPTSD occurs in an either/or fashion. An individual can have either one or the other diagnosis, not both. If a person receives the diagnosis of CPTSD, then the individual does not also receive a PTSD diagnosis. This distinction leads to consistent observations that those with PTSD have fewer comorbidities and less functional impairment. Some studies that have viewed CPTSD as a subtype of PTSD have combined both disorders under one "ICD-11 PTSD" umbrella and reported, misleadingly, that ICD-11 PTSD is associated with as high or higher rates of comorbidity as DSM-5. Second, the diagnosis of CPTSD requires functional impairment that is related to the PTSD as well as the DSO symptom clusters. Lastly, the diagnoses of PTSD and CPTSD are made by reference to symptoms, not to type of traumatic event. Type of event is viewed as a risk factor, not a requirement for each disorder. This recognizes the potential influence of predisposing factors such as personal and environmental resources (e.g., resilience, social support) or lack thereof on individual outcomes.

ICD-11 PTSD

ICD-11 diagnoses are presented in the *Clinical Descriptions and Diagnostic Guidelines* (CDDG), a document intended for general clinical, educational, and service use. The ICD-11 PTSD exposure and symptom description is shown in Figure 4.1. There is significant overlap with the DSM-5 A, B, C, and E criteria but also important differences, including the significantly lower number of symptoms required for the diagnosis and the emphasis on

---

Posttraumatic stress disorder (PTSD) is a disorder that may develop following exposure to an extremely threatening or horrific event or series of events that is characterized by all of the following: (1) reexperiencing the traumatic event or events in the present in the form of vivid intrusive memories, flashbacks, or nightmares. These are typically accompanied by strong or overwhelming emotions, particularly fear or horror, and strong physical sensations; (2) avoidance of thoughts and memories of the event or events, or avoidance of activities, situations, or people reminiscent of the event or events; and (3) persistent perceptions of a heightened current threat, as indicated by hypervigilance or an enhanced startle reaction to stimuli such as unexpected noises. The symptoms persist for at least several weeks and cause significant impairment in personal, family, social, educational, occupational, or other important areas of functioning.

FIGURE 4.1. Definition of ICD-11 PTSD. Used with permission from the World Health Organization.

fear and horror. The exposure criterion has been modified from ICD-10 to remove the statement that it would "cause distress in almost everyone."

There are context-dependent presentations and other symptoms typical of PTSD. In conditions where conscious memory of the event is reduced or absent, such as after head injury or very early childhood trauma, emotional or physiological reactivity to trauma reminders may be present instead of reexperiencing (cf. Harvey & Bryant, 2001). Accompanying the reexperiencing core symptoms, strong or overwhelming emotions typically appear. The most prominent themes are fear or horror in the case of witnessing traumatic events. Other emotions commonly present in PTSD can be anger, shame, sadness, humiliation, and guilt, including survivor guilt. The definition of PTSD requires "functional impairment" to differentiate it from normal-range reactions to extreme stressors (Rona et al., 2009) and a duration of at least several weeks.

Other symptoms that are not essential for the diagnosis of PTSD but commonly occur in people with it include dissociative symptoms such as memory disturbances (e.g., dissociative amnesia); pseudo-hallucinations (e.g., hearing one's own thoughts as voices); somatic complaints without a medical basis, including headache and dyspnea (cf. Somasundaram & Sivayokan, 1994); suicidal ideation and behavior; and excessive use of alcohol or drugs to avoid reexperiencing or to manage emotional reactions. The course of PTSD often fluctuates (Bryant, O'Donnell, Creamer, McFarlane, & Silove, 2013; Maercker, Gäbler, & Schützwohl, 2013) and may develop into ICD-11 complex PTSD.

Evidence Base for ICD-11 PTSD Changes

A major innovation in ICD-11 is the specification of *core features* rather than *explicit operationalized criteria and an explicit diagnostic algorithm* for PTSD. The specification of core features was based on empirical and theoretical grounds and was designed to most clearly distinguish PTSD from other disorders. In contrast, features that are *typical though not core* are commonly present but are likely to represent general distress or dysphoria rather than being specific to PTSD, such as irritability, lack of concentration, or feelings of detachment or estrangement from others (Gootzeit & Markon, 2011; Yufik & Simms, 2010).

Empirical evidence for defining ICD-11 PTSD was drawn primarily from studies investigating the symptom structure of previous PTSD definitions (e.g., Gootzeit & Markon, 2011; King, King, Fairbank, Keane, & Adams, 1998). In addition to intrusions, avoidance, and hyperarousal, a group of numbing symptoms (amnesia, loss of interest, detachment, and restricted affect) were found in many of the early factor analyses. For example, a comprehensive confirmatory factor analysis (CFA) was conducted with 3,700 U.S. veterans and found a four-factor solution of intrusions, avoidance, hyperarousal, and dysphoria using 17 DSM-IV-based PTSD symptoms

(Simms, Watson, & Doebbeling, 2002). The dysphoria factor consisted of three numbing symptoms and three hyperarousal symptoms. Further investigation determined that only the dysphoria factor correlated relatively highly with depression (r = 0.80) and generalized anxiety (r = 0.63), whereas all other factors were only moderately correlated with other disorders. The authors concluded that the dysphoria factor was nonspecific to PTSD, a finding supported by a subsequent meta-analysis of 41 studies conducted with a total of 61,000 participants (Gootzeit & Markon, 2011).

Evidence also exists that some single symptoms are more specific to PTSD than others. For example, intrusive memories have been found in clinical samples across a number of mental disorders, including obsessive compulsive disorder (Salkovskis, 1985), depression (Brewin, 1998), social phobia (Hackmann, Clark, & McManus, 2000), and agoraphobia (Day, Holmes, & Hackmann, 2004), and have also been noted in nonclinical samples (Brewin, Christodoulides, & Hutchinson, 1996). In contrast, flashbacks with their "here-and-now" quality have been confirmed in cross-sectional (Bryant, O'Donnell, Creamer, McFarlane, & Silove, 2011; Duke, Allen, Rozee, & Bommaritto, 2008) as well as prospective studies (Michael, Ehlers, Halligan, & Clark, 2005) to be a particularly sensitive and specific indicator of PTSD. Posttraumatic nightmares are another distinctive feature of PTSD, occurring in up to 70% of diagnosed individuals (Harvey, Jones, & Schmidt, 2003; Lamarche & de Koninck, 2007). In a clinical sample with various mental disorders, Swart, van Schagen, Lancee, and van den Bout (2013) found nightmares to be significantly more common in PTSD (67%) than in depressive disorders (37%), anxiety disorders (16%), personality disorders (31%), or psychotic and other disorders (27%).

These findings led to the current ICD-11 conceptualization of PTSD being developed and published (Maercker, Brewin, et al., 2013), with extensive research between 2013 and 2017 supporting the definition. Brewin and colleagues (2017) reviewed 27 studies from this period, the majority of which supported the proposed ICD-11 definition. In particular, the proposed three-factor structure of PTSD, operationalized with two core symptoms representing each factor, provides a very good fit to the data. Although the level of agreement between the presence or absence of a diagnosis using ICD-11 and the DSM is generally high, the prevalence of PTSD in adult samples is also consistently slightly lower when ICD-11, rather than the DSM, is used. This is consistent with the narrower definition of PTSD in ICD-11.

ICD-11 CPTSD

The ICD-11 definition of CPTSD and its essential or core features are presented in Figure 4.2. Core features are those symptoms or characteristics that "a clinician could reasonably expect to find in all cases of the disorder" (First, Reed, Hyman, & Saxena, 2015, p. 85). Problems in affect, negative self-concept, and interpersonal problems are described in some detail. Problems

---

Definition

Complex posttraumatic stress disorder (complex PTSD) is a disorder that may develop following exposure to an event or series of events of an extremely threatening or horrific nature, most commonly prolonged or repetitive events from which escape is difficult or impossible (e.g., torture, slavery, genocide campaigns, prolonged domestic violence, repeated childhood sexual or physical abuse). All diagnostic requirements for PTSD are met. In addition, complex PTSD is characterized by severe and persistent (1) problems in affect regulation; (2) beliefs about oneself as diminished, defeated, or worthless, accompanied by feelings of shame, guilt, or failure related to the traumatic event; and (3) difficulties in sustaining relationships and in feeling close to others. These symptoms cause significant impairment in personal, family, social, educational, occupational, or other important areas of functioning.

Diagnostic Guidelines

- Exposure to a stressor typically of an extreme or prolonged nature and from which escape is difficult or impossible, such as torture, concentration camps, slavery, genocide campaigns and other forms of organized violence, domestic violence, and childhood sexual or physical abuse

- Presence of the core symptoms of PTSD (reexperiencing the trauma in the present, avoidance of reminders of the trauma, and persistent perceptions of current threat)

- Following onset of the stressor event and co-occurring with PTSD symptoms, the development of persistent and pervasive impairments in affective, self, and relational functioning, including problems in affect regulation, persistent beliefs about oneself as diminished, defeated, or worthless, persistent difficulties in sustaining relationships

- The stressors associated with complex PTSD are typically of an interpersonal nature, that is, the result of human mistreatment rather than acts of nature (e.g., earthquakes, tornadoes, tsunamis) or accidents (train wrecks, motor vehicle accidents). In addition to the typical symptoms of PTSD, complex PTSD is characterized by more persistent long-term problems in affective, self, and relational functioning. Problems in all three areas often co-occur.

FIGURE 4.2. ICD-11 definition of and guidelines for complex PTSD. Used with permission from the World Health Organization.

in affect dysregulation include both hyperreactivity, such as heightened emotional reactivity, difficulty recovering from minor stressors, and violent outbursts, as well as hyporeactivity, such as numbing, difficulty experiencing pleasure or positive emotions, and tendency toward dissociative states when under stress. Problems in self-concept include persistent beliefs about oneself as diminished, defeated, or worthless accompanied by deep and pervasive feelings of shame, guilt, or failure. Interpersonal problems are characterized by persistent difficulties in sustaining relationships. Examples of such difficulties include problems feeling close to others, avoidance of relationships, ending relationships when difficulties or conflicts emerge, or even deriding the value or importance of relationships.

Associated features are symptoms and problems that may be observed in the individual with CPTSD but are not necessary to making the diagnosis. These symptoms and problems help the clinician in recognizing the full range of symptoms that may be present. In ICD-11 CPTSD, they include suicidal ideation and behavior and substance abuse, both of which have been related to difficulties regulating emotions, as well as significant depression and psychotic episodes. Somatic complaints may be present but vary by culture and might be the result of the trauma (torture, physical punishment, or inadequate food, clothing, or shelter).

Differential Diagnosis

One criticism of a complex PTSD diagnosis is that it would not be distinguishable from PTSD with borderline personality disorder (BPD). ICD-11 CPTSD and BPD do share conceptual overlap in the type of problems that are included in each diagnosis, namely, difficulties in affect regulation, self-concept, and interpersonal relationships. However, the specific nature of these difficulties is quite distinct. In BPD, self-concept difficulties reflect an unstable sense of self, whereas in CPTSD, they reflect a persistent, negative view of self. Relational difficulties in BPD are characterized by volatile patterns of interaction, whereas in CPTSD, they reflect a persistent tendency to avoid relationships. With regard to affect dysregulation, BPD is characterized by fears of abandonment and self-harming/suicidal behavior, and these symptoms are not part of the DSO profile in CPTSD. Other relevant features differentiate BPD and CPTSD, most notably the fact that CPTSD requires the presence of trauma-specific PTSD symptoms that are not a feature of BPD; BPD also does not require traumatic exposure for diagnosis. Three studies have tested and found support for the discriminant validity of ICD-11 CPTSD and BPD (Cloitre, Garvert, Weiss, Carlson, & Bryant, 2014; Frost, Hyland, Shevlin, & Murphy, 2018; Knefel, Tran, & Lueger-Schuster, 2016).

Assessment of ICD-11 PTSD and CPTSD

Even though ICD-11 CPTSD and PTSD are relatively newly formulated disorders, there are at least two measures that have been developed to identify them and for which there are validity and reliability data. In line with the ICD-11 goal of clinical utility, the International Trauma Questionnaire (ITQ; Cloitre et al., 2018), a self-report measure, was developed to be brief and easily implemented. The ITQ includes 12 symptom-related items, two for each of the six clusters of symptoms, and an additional six items measuring functional impairment (three associated with the PTSD cluster and three associated with the DSO cluster). An initial version of the measure included 24 symptom-related items to represent the wide range of symptoms described, particularly as related to the DSO symptoms. Through a repeated process of testing, including item response theory (IRT) modeling, the number of symptom-related items was reduced to 12 (Shevlin et al., 2018). In a recent survey of a nationally representative sample in the United States (Cloitre et al., 2019), the reliability (Cronbach's alpha) of the items was satisfactory for the full sample (PTSD alpha = 0.89 and DSO alpha = 0.89), among males (PTSD alpha = 0.88, DSO alpha = 0.89) and females (PTSD alpha = 0.88, DSO alpha = 0.89). The ITQ has been translated into several languages and is available for free at *www.traumameasuresglobal.com.*

An interview measure for ICD-11 PTSD and CPTSD, the International Trauma Interview (ITI; Roberts, Cloitre, Bisson, & Brewin, 2018), is in development and will be posted at the website just cited once testing is complete.

Cross-Cultural and Supra-Individual Contexts for DSM-5 PTSD and ICD-11 PTSD/CPTSD

With respect to the cross-cultural validity of DSM-5 PTSD and ICD-11 PTSD and CPTSD, the debate is ongoing as to whether the PTSD construct describes a universal trauma response or if its clinical utility lags behind that of more regional forms of expressing trauma-related psychopathology, including cultural syndromes (Maercker, Heim, & Kirmayer, 2019). Culturally shaped expressions of symptoms can include a spiritual component, for example, the sense of heightened current threat may result in distressing dreams that are interpreted as indicating spiritual insecurity or supernatural powers seeking out the person in distress (Hinton, Hinton, Pich, Loeum, & Pollack, 2009; Kwon, 2006, 2008). Several other symptoms seem to be prominent aspects of PTSD in certain cultural settings, in part because they are codified into cultural syndromes or "idioms of distress" (Hinton & Lewis-Fernandez, 2011; McFarlane & Hinton, 2009)—for example, *ohkum-lang* (tiredness) in Bhutanese; *susto* (fright) among Latino populations; and *kit chraen* (thinking too much) in Cambodia (Hinton & Lewis-Fernandez, 2010). Although not equivalent to PTSD symptoms, these manifestations could indicate the presence of traumatization that needs to be explored in a culture-sensitive assessment.

Health care professionals in some countries have developed concepts of supra-individual (collective, community, or societal) trauma aftereffects that are of relevance for mental health care interventions (Bhugra & Becker, 2005). In collectivistic or sociocentric cultures, the impact of traumatic events can be far-reaching through changes in family and community relationships, institutions, practices, and social resources, resulting in consequences such as loss of communality (Beiser, Wiwa, & Adebajo, 2010; Betancourt et al., 2012; Kirmayer, Kienzler, Afana, & Pedersen, 2010) and cultural bereavement (Bhugra & Becker, 2005; Eisenbruch, 1991; Somasundaram, 2007).

Such supra-individual effects can manifest in a variety of forms, including collective distrust; loss of motivation; loss of beliefs, values, and norms; learned helplessness; antisocial behavior; substance abuse; gender-based violence; child abuse; and suicidality (Abramowitz, 2005; Somasundaram, 2007).

Some cross-cultural studies indicate that an extended definition of PTSD with a broader range of symptoms may be a better way to delineate trauma-related disorder (de Jong, Komproe, Spinazzola, van der Kolk, & van Ommeren, 2005; Morina & Ford, 2008). One reason is the undeniable fact that torture, genocide, and severe adversity, as well as intergenerational and historical trauma, are common in some regions or countries of the world (Evans-Campbell, 2008; Gone, 2013; Hinton & Lewis-Fernandez, 2011).

Given that CPTSD is a new disorder, studies assessing DSO symptoms that might vary across cultures have yet to be conducted. Some of the symptoms and problems already identified in the cited studies of PTSD may fall into the CPTSD profile. For example, affect dysregulation might be expressed in somatic symptoms such as *perumuchu* (deep sighing in Tamil culture) or the bodily weakness associated with *Dhat* syndrome (see Humayun & Somasundaram, 2018). In more collective societies, a changed sense of identity and interpersonal relationships may be experienced through loss of communality, such as the outcast status of Yazidi women who were subjected to sexual slavery (Hoffman et al., 2018; Ibrahim, Ertl, Catani, Ismail, & Neuner, 2018) or cultural bereavement among those who have experienced violent conflict (Somasundaram, 2007).

Screening for DSM-5 PTSD and ICD-11 PTSD/CPTSD

Screening for PTSD has normally been conducted by asking people to rate a number of symptoms, with a cutoff score denoting that the diagnosis is probably present. It is perfectly possible to create screening instruments that take into account many other types of information, but these tend to be only useful for specific trauma populations, such as adults admitted to the hospital following injury (O'Donnell et al., 2008). The performance of screening instruments is usually assessed in terms of their sensitivity, the likelihood that a person with the diagnosis will score above the cutoff, and their specificity, the likelihood that a person without the diagnosis will score below the cutoff. Cutoff scores usually try to achieve an optimal balance of sensitivity and specificity, while recognizing that scores can be legitimately increased or decreased in specific contexts. For example, scores may be lowered if sensitivity is the most important criterion.

Screening is sometimes conducted with instruments that assess each PTSD symptom individually, such as the PTSD Checklist for DSM-5 (PCL-5; Blevins, Weathers, Davis, Witte, & Domino, 2015), or include larger numbers of items, such as the Impact of Event Scale–Revised (IES-R; Weiss, 2007).

However, because DSM-defined PTSD has a large number of symptoms, such a screening process is not necessarily efficient. Shorter instruments might be able to estimate the likely presence of PTSD with considerable savings in time and cost. Studies do indeed indicate that those with between four and ten items, simpler response scales, and simpler scoring methods often perform as well as, if not better than, longer and more complex instruments (Brewin, 2005; Freedy et al., 2010; Mouthaan, Sijbrandij, Reitsma, Gersons, & Olff, 2014). In contrast, a single screening item ("Were you recently bothered by a past experience that caused you to believe you would be injured or killed . . . not bothered, bothered a little, or bothered a lot?") performed more poorly (Gore, Engel, Freed, Liu, & Armstrong, 2008).

Screening Instruments

Among the most commonly used short screeners have been the Primary Care PTSD Screen (PC-PTSD; Prins et al., 2003) and the Trauma Screening Questionnaire (TSQ; Brewin et al., 2002), both answered with a simple yes/no response scale. The PC-PTSD includes four items covering nightmares and intrusive thoughts, active avoidance of thoughts or situations, hypervigilance/startle, and numbness/detachment from people and activities. A score of 3 or above generally reflects the best screening threshold. The TSQ has 10 items corresponding to the reexperiencing and hyperarousal questions from the PTSD Symptom Scale (PSS; Foa, Riggs, Dancu, & Rothbaum, 1993). A score of 6 or above generally reflects the best screening threshold. Another widely used brief screener is the SPAN self-report (derived from the Davidson Trauma Scale; Davidson et al., 1997), which has four items assessing startle, physiological arousal on reminders, anger, and numbness, each answered on a 5-point severity scale (Meltzer-Brody, Churchill, & Davidson, 1999). Recently, briefer versions of the PCL-5 containing only four or eight items have been investigated (Price, Szafranski, van Stolk-Cooke, & Gros, 2016). There has also been interest in using brief screeners within more specific populations where a high prevalence of PTSD is known to exist. Studies have confirmed the value of the TSQ in samples with severe mental illness (de Bont et al., 2015) and of the PC-PTSD in samples with substance use disorders (van Dam, Ehring, Vedel, & Emmelkamp, 2010).

The performance of brief screeners will not necessarily be affected by changes to diagnostic criteria, such as the three additional symptoms and one additional symptom cluster introduced in DSM-5 (American Psychiatric Association, 2013). However, a new version of the PC-PTSD, the PC-PTSD-5 (Prins et al., 2016), has been developed to better assess DSM-5 PTSD. The authors added one item on guilt or blame and found that the most sensitive threshold score was 3, whereas optimal efficiency was obtained at 4 and optimal specificity at 5.

ICD-11, in contrast, has introduced a distinction between PTSD and complex PTSD, the former being based on only six symptoms and the latter on the six PTSD symptoms plus a further six assessing aspects of disturbances in self-organization (Brewin et al., 2017). Diagnostic instruments such as the ITQ (Cloitre et al., 2018) additionally assess functional impairment and are able to determine an ICD-11 diagnosis while remaining relatively brief. Six items from the IES-R can also be used to approximate ICD-11 PTSD (Hyland, Brewin, & Maercker, 2017). Alternative instruments for assessing complex PTSD, such as the Complex Trauma Inventory (CTI; Litvin, Kaminski, & Riggs, 2017) and the German-language Screening for Complex PTSD (SkPTBS; Dorr, Sack, & Bengel, 2018), approximate the final ICD-11 formulation and are likely to become useful additional screening instruments.

General Issues

Psychometric studies on the performance of screening instruments are relatively uncommon, with cutoff scores not always independently validated. It is nevertheless clear that their performance is likely to vary depending on the setting and the population sampled (Dow, Kenardy, Le Brocque, & Long, 2012; McDonald & Calhoun, 2010). Translation into other languages may result in slightly different cutoff scores being optimal, even if overall performance remains good (Dekkers, Olff, & Näring, 2010).

These considerations need to be borne in mind when screening is implemented on a larger scale. For example, screening has recently begun to be regularly employed after major incidents in conjunction with active outreach to overcome the known failure of traditional mental health pathways to detect and provide evidence-based treatment to those affected. A positive screen is typically followed by a more detailed clinical assessment to determine whether treatment is required. This strategy has been employed successfully after incidents such as the 2005 terrorist bombings in London (Brewin, Fuchkan, Huntley, Robertson, et al., 2010) and the 2009 plane crash at Amsterdam Airport (Gouweloos-Trines et al., 2019).

A more detailed investigation of screening performance was conducted using the TSQ during the London bombings mental health program (Brewin, Fuchkan, Huntley, & Scragg, 2010). It showed, consistent with evidence supporting temporarily increased levels of general stress after terrorist incidents, that the specificity of the TSQ was low directly after the bombings but increased steadily over the two years following them. There was also evidence that members of ethnic minority groups tended to score more highly overall, reducing the specificity of the TSQ when the original cutoff score was used. Other studies have found that the TSQ had greater sensitivity than specificity shortly after major incidents, indicating that in these situations use of the TSQ maximizes the chance of identifying affected persons at the expense of some unnecessary clinical assessments (Gouweloos-Trines et al., 2019). It is likely that the performance of all screening instruments varies according to situational and personal factors, but this subject is rarely studied and should be a priority for future research.

Screening Summary

Relatively brief screening measures appear to be as effective as longer questionnaires. Their main value is detecting the presence of probable PTSD in large samples for whom more detailed assessment is not feasible, such as patients suffering from other disorders where a history of trauma is common or people being exposed to a major traumatic incident such as an earthquake, transportation accident, or terrorist attack. Research to date has suggested that existing measures are suitable for these purposes and can yield adequate sensitivity and specificity. Nevertheless, data on their performance in different settings and with different populations are insufficient, and considerable further research is needed to establish optimal screening procedures.

Concluding Remarks

The introduction of DSM-5 and ICD-11 highlights a significant divergence in the approach to diagnosis of PTSD by the principal classification systems, and the addition of a new diagnosis, CPTSD, to ICD-11. Early underpinnings of CPTSD can be seen in the disorders of extreme stress not otherwise specified (DESNOS) concept, but this is the first time that a formal parallel diagnosis to PTSD has been introduced. The divergence raises a number of issues; some people will meet diagnostic criteria according to one system but not the other, risking interchangeable use of the diagnostic systems and the potential for confusion—for example, how should we define PTSD to someone affected by a traumatic event(s)? The divergence also provides research opportunities to assess and compare the utility of the new systems, and to develop more personalized treatments designed to treat specific constellations of symptoms; very different approaches may be required to treat CPTSD, ICD-11 PTSD, and DSM-5 PTSD. Whatever we think about the divergence, it is here to stay, at least until the next DSM and ICD revisions, and it is important that we embrace the changes and use them to facilitate better approaches to the detection, assessment, prevention, and management of PTSD and CPTSD.

REFERENCES

Abramowitz, S. A. (2005). The poor have become rich, and the rich have become poor: Collective trauma in the Guinean Languette. *Social Science & Medicine, 61*(10), 2106–2118.

American Psychiatric Association. (1980). *Diagnostic and statistical manual of mental disorders* (3rd ed.). Washington, DC: Author.

American Psychiatric Association. (1994). *Diagnostic and statistical manual of mental disorders* (4th ed.). Washington, DC: Author.

American Psychiatric Association. (2013). *Diagnostic and statistical manual of mental disorders* (5th ed.). Alexandria, VA: Author.

Andrews, B., Brewin, C. R., Philpott, R., & Stewart, L. (2007). Delayed-onset post-traumatic stress disorder: A systematic review of the evidence. *American Journal of Psychiatry, 164*(9), 1319–1326.

Bedard-Gilligan, M., & Zoellner, L. A. (2008). The utility of the A1 and A2 criteria in the diagnosis of PTSD. *Behaviour Research and Therapy,* 46(9), 1062–1069.

Beiser, M., Wiwa, O., & Adebajo, S. (2010). Human-initiated disaster, social disorganization and post-traumatic stress disorder above Nigeria's oil basins. *Social Science and Medicine, 71*(2), 221–227.

Betancourt, T. S., Salhi, C., Buka, S., Leaning, J., Dunn, G., & Earls, F. (2012). Connectedness, social support and internalising emotional and behavioural problems in adolescents displaced by the Chechen conflict. *Disasters, 36*(4), 635–655.

Bhugra, D., & Becker, M. A. (2005). Migration, cultural bereavement and cultural identity. *World Psychiatry, 4*(1), 18–24.

Bisson, J. I. (2013). What happened to harmonisation of the PTSD diagnosis?: The divergence of ICD11 and DSM5. *Epidemiology and Psychiatric Sciences, 22,* 205–207.

Blanchard, E. B., Jones Alexander, J., Buckley, T. C., & Forneris, C. A. (1996). Psychometric properties of the PTSD Checklist (PCL). *Behaviour Research and Therapy, 34,* 669–673.

Blevins, C. A., Weathers, F. W., Davis, M. T., Witte, T. K., & Domino, J. L. (2015). The Posttraumatic Stress Disorder Checklist for DSM-5 (PCL-5): Development and initial psychometric evaluation. *Journal of Traumatic Stress, 28*(6), 489–498.

Brewin, C. R. (1998). Intrusive autobiographical memories in depression and post-traumatic stress disorder. *Applied Cognitive Psychology, 12*(4), 359–370.

Brewin, C. R. (2005). Systematic review of screening instruments for adults at risk of PTSD. *Journal of Traumatic Stress, 18*(1), 53–62.

Brewin, C. R., Christodoulides, J., & Hutchinson, G. (1996). Intrusive thoughts and intrusive memories in a nonclinical sample. *Cognition and Emotion, 10,* 107–112.

Brewin, C. R., Cloitre, M., Hyland, P., Shevlin, M., Maercker, A., Bryant, R. A., et al. (2017). A review of current evidence regarding the ICD-11 proposals for diagnosing PTSD and complex PTSD. *Clinical Psychology Review, 58,* 1–15.

Brewin, C. R., Fuchkan, N., Huntley, Z., Robertson, M., Thompson, M., Scragg, P., et al. (2010). Outreach and screening following the 2005 London bombings: Usage and outcomes. *Psychological Medicine, 40*(12), 2049–2057.

Brewin, C. R., Fuchkan, N., Huntley, Z., & Scragg, P. (2010). Diagnostic accuracy of the Trauma Screening Questionnaire after the 2005 London bombings. *Journal of Traumatic Stress, 23*(3), 393–398.

Brewin, C. R., Lanius, R. A., Novac, A., Schnyder, U., & Galea, S. (2009). Reformulating PTSD for DSM-V: Life after Criterion A. *Journal of Traumatic Stress, 22*(5), 366–373.

Brewin, C. R., Rose, S., Andrews, B., Green, J., Tata, P., McEvedy, C., et al. (2002). Brief screening instrument for post-traumatic stress disorder. *British Journal of Psychiatry, 181,* 158–162.

Bryant, R. A., O'Donnell, M. L., Creamer, M., McFarlane, A. C., & Silove, D. (2011). Posttraumatic intrusive symptoms across psychiatric disorders. *Journal of Psychiatric Research, 45*(6), 842–847.

Bryant, R. A., O'Donnell, M. L., Creamer, M., McFarlane, A. C., & Silove, D. (2013).

A multisite analysis of the fluctuating course of posttraumatic stress disorder. *JAMA Psychiatry, 70,* 839–846.

Cloitre, M., Garvert, D. W., Weiss, B., Carlson, E. B., & Bryant, R. A. (2014). Distinguishing PTSD, complex PTSD, and borderline personality disorder: A latent class analysis. *European Journal of Psychotraumatology, 5.*

Cloitre, M., Hyland, P., Bisson, J. I., Brewin, C. R., Roberts, N. P., Karatzias, T., et al. (2019). ICD-11 PTSD and complex PTSD in the United States: A population-based study. *Journal of Traumatic Stress, 32*(6), 833–842.

Cloitre, M., Shevlin, M., Brewin, C. R., Bisson, J. I., Roberts, N. P., Maercker, A., et al. (2018). The International Trauma Questionnaire: Development of a self-report measure of ICD-11 PTSD and complex PTSD. *Acta Psychiatrica Scandinavica, 138,* 536–546.

Davidson, J. R., Book, S. W., Colket, J. T., Tupler, L. A., Roth, S., David, D., et al. (1997). Assessment of a new self-rating scale for post-traumatic stress disorder. *Psychological Medicine, 27*(1), 153–160.

Day, S. J., Holmes, E. A., & Hackmann, A. (2004). Occurrence of imagery and its link with early memories in agoraphobia. *Memory, 12*(4), 416–427.

de Bont, P. A. J. M., van den Berg, D. P. G., van der Vleugel, B. M., de Roos, C., de Jongh, A., van der Gaag, M., et al. (2015). Predictive validity of the Trauma Screening Questionnaire in detecting post-traumatic stress disorder in patients with psychotic disorders. *British Journal of Psychiatry, 206*(5), 408–416.

de Jong, J. T., Komproe, I. H., Spinazzola, J., van der Kolk, B. A., & van Ommeren, M. (2005). DESNOS in three postconflict settings: Assessing cross-cultural construct equivalence. *Journal of Traumatic Stress, 18*(1), 13–21.

Dekkers, A. M. M., Olff, M., & Näring, G. W. B. (2010). Identifying persons at risk for PTSD after trauma with TSQ in the Netherlands. *Community Mental Health Journal, 46*(1), 20–25.

Dorr, F., Sack, M., & Bengel, J. (2018). Validation of the Screening for Complex PTSD (SkPTBS)–Revision. *Psychotherapie Psychosomatik Medizinische Psychologie, 68*(12), 525–533.

Dow, B. L., Kenardy, J. A., Le Brocque, R. M., & Long, D. A. (2012). The utility of the Children's Revised Impact of Event Scale in screening for concurrent PTSD following admission to intensive care. *Journal of Traumatic Stress, 25*(5), 602–605.

Duke, L. A., Allen, D. N., Rozee, P. D., & Bommaritto, M. (2008). The sensitivity and specificity of flashbacks and nightmares to trauma. *Journal of Anxiety Disorders, 22*(2), 319–327.

Eisenbruch, M. (1991). From post-traumatic stress disorder to cultural bereavement: Diagnosis of Southeast Asian refugees. *Social Science and Medicine, 33*(6), 673–680.

Evans-Campbell, T. (2008). Historical trauma in American Indian/Native Alaska communities: A multilevel framework for exploring impacts on individuals, families, and communities. *Journal of Interpersonal Violence, 23*(3), 316–338.

First, M. B. (2009). Harmonisation of ICD-11 and DSM-V: Opportunities and challenges. *British Journal of Psychiatry, 195,* 382–390.

First, M. B., Reed, G. M., Hyman, S. E., & Saxena, S. (2015). The development of the ICD-11 clinical descriptions and diagnostic guidelines for mental and behavioural disorders. *World Psychiatry, 14,* 82–90.

Foa, E. B., Riggs, D. S., Dancu, C. V., & Rothbaum, B. O. (1993). Reliability and validity of a brief instrument for assessing postraumatic stress disorder. *Journal of Traumatic Stress, 6*(4), 459–473.

Frances, A. (2009). Advice to DSM-V: Integrate with ICD-11. *Psychiatric Times, 26,* 1–2.

Freedy, J. R., Steenkamp, M. M., Magruder, K. M., Yeager, D. E., Zoller, J. S., Hueston, W. J., et al. (2010). Post-traumatic stress disorder screening test performance in civilian primary care. *Family Practice, 27*(6), 615–624.

Friedman, M. J., Resick, P. A., Bryant, R. A., & Brewin, C. R. (2011). Considering PTSD for DSM5. *Depression and Anxiety, 28,* 750–769.

Frost, R., Hyland, P., McCarthy, A., Halpin, R., Shevlin, M., & Murphy, J. (2019). The complexity of trauma exposure and response: Profiling PTSD and CPTSD among a refugee sample. *Psychological Trauma: Theory, Research, Pratice, and Policy, 11*(2), 165–175.

Galatzer-Levy, I. R., & Bryant, R. A. (2013). 636,120 ways to have posttraumatic stress disorder. *Perspectives on Psychological Science, 8*(6), 651–662.

Gone, J. P. (2013). Redressing First Nations historical trauma: Theorizing mechanisms for indigenous culture as mental health treatment. *Transcultural Psychiatry, 50*(5), 683–706.

Gootzeit, J., & Markon, K. (2011). Factors of PTSD: Differential specificity and external correlates. *Clinical Psychology Review, 31*(6), 993–1003.

Gore, K. L., Engel, C. C., Freed, M. C., Liu, X., & Armstrong, D. W., III. (2008). Test of a single-item posttraumatic stress disorder screener in a military primary care setting. *General Hospital Psychiatry, 30*(5), 391–397.

Gouweloos-Trines, J., te Brake, H., Sijbrandij, M., Boelen, P. A., Brewin, C. R., & Kleber, R. J. (2019). Evaluating a psychosocial support program for survivors of an airplane crash: Screening for PTSD and depression and assessment of self-reported treatment needs. *European Journal of Psychotraumatology, 10.*

Hackmann, A., Clark, D. M., & McManus, F. (2000). Recurrent images and early memories in social phobia. *Behaviour Research and Therapy, 38*(6), 601–610.

Harvey, A. G., & Bryant, R. A. (2001). Reconstructing trauma memories: A prospective study of "amnesic" trauma survivors. *Journal of Traumatic Stress, 14*(2), 277–282.

Harvey, A. G., Jones, C., & Schmidt, D. A. (2003). Sleep and posttraumatic stress disorder: A review. *Clinical Psychology Review, 23*(3), 377–407.

Hinton, D. E., Hinton, A. L., Pich, V., Loeum, J. R., & Pollack, M. H. (2009). Nightmares among Cambodian refugees: The breaching of concentric ontological security. *Culture, Medicine and Psychiatry, 33*(2), 219–265.

Hinton, D. E., & Lewis-Fernandez, R. (2010). Idioms of distress among trauma survivors: Subtypes and clinical utility. *Culture, Medicine and Psychiatry, 34*(2), 209–218.

Hinton, D. E., & Lewis-Fernandez, R. (2011). The cross-cultural validity of posttraumatic stress disorder: Implications for DSM-5. *Depression and Anxiety, 28*(9), 783–801.

Hoffman, Y. S., Grossman, E. S., Shrira, A., Kedar, M., Ben-Ezra, M., Dinnayi, M., et al. (2018). Complex PTSD and its correlates amongst female Yazidi victims of sexual slavery living in post-ISIS camps. *World Psychiatry, 17,* 112–113.

Humayun, A., & Somasundaram, D. (2018). Using International Classification of

Diseases 11 "mental disorders specifically associated with stress" in developing countries. *Indian Journal of Social Psychiatry, 34,* S23–S28.

Hyland, P., Brewin, C. R., & Maercker, A. (2017). Predictive validity of ICD-11 PTSD as measured by the Impact of Event Scale-Revised: A 15-year prospective study of political prisoners. *Journal of Traumatic Stress, 30*(2), 125–132.

Ibrahim, H., Ertl, V., Catani, C., Ismail, A. A., & Neuner, F. (2018). Trauma and perceived social rejection among Yazidi women and girls who survived enslavement and genocide. *BMC Medicine, 16,* 154.

Jablensky, A. (2009). Towards ICD-11 and DSM-V: Issues beyond harmonisation. *British Journal of Psychiatry, 195,* 379–381.

King, L. A., King, D. W., Fairbank, J. A., Keane, T. M., & Adams, G. A. (1998). Resilience-recovery factors in post-traumatic stress disorder among female and male Vietnam veterans: Hardiness, postwar social support, and additional stressful life events. *Journal of Personality and Social Psychology, 74*(2), 420–434.

Kirmayer, L. J., Kienzler, H., Afana, A. H., & Pedersen, D. (2010). Trauma and disasters in social and cultural context. In C. Morgan & D. Bhugra (Eds.), *Principles of social psychiatry* (pp. 155–177). Chichester, UK: Wiley.

Knefel, M., Tran, U. S., & Lueger-Schuster, B. (2016). The association of posttraumatic stress disorder, complex posttraumatic stress disorder, and borderline personality disorder from a network analytical perspective. *Journal of Anxiety Disorders, 43,* 70–78.

Kupfer, D., Regier, D. A., & Kuhl, E. (2008). On the road to DSM-V and ICD-11. *European Archives of Psychiatry and Clinical Neuroscience, 258,* 2–6.

Kwon, H. (2006). *After the massacre: Commemoration and consolation in Ha My and My Lai.* Berkeley: University of California Press.

Kwon, H. (2008). *Ghosts of war in Vietnam.* Cambridge, UK: Cambridge University Press.

Lamarche, L. J., & de Koninck, J. (2007). Sleep disturbance in adults with post-traumatic stress disorder: A review. *Journal of Clinical Psychiatry, 68*(8), 1257–1270.

Litvin, J. M., Kaminski, P. L., & Riggs, S. A. (2017). The Complex Trauma Inventory: A self-report measure of posttraumatic stress disorder and complex posttraumatic stress disorder. *Journal of Traumatic Stress, 30*(6), 602–613.

Maercker, A., Brewin, C. R., Bryant, R. A., Cloitre, M., van Ommeren, M., Jones, L. M., et al. (2013). Diagnosis and classification of disorders specifically associated with stress: Proposals for ICD-11. *World Psychiatry, 12*(3), 198–206.

Maercker, A., Gäbler, I., & Schützwohl, M. (2013). Verläufe von Traumafolgen bei ehemaligen politisch Inhaftierten der DDR [Course of trauma sequelae in ex-political prisoners in the GDR: A 15-year follow-up study]. *Nervenarzt, 84*(1), 72–78.

Maercker, A., Heim, E., & Kirmayer, L. J. (Eds.). (2019). *Cultural clinical psychology and PTSD.* Boston: Hogrefe.

McDonald, S. D., & Calhoun, P. S. (2010). The diagnostic accuracy of the PTSD Checklist: A critical review. *Clinical Psychology Review, 30*(8), 976–987.

McFarlane, A., & Hinton, D. (2009). Ethnocultural issues. In D. J. Nutt, M. B. Stein, & J. Zohar (Eds.), *Post traumatic stress disorder: Diagnosis, management, and treatment* (2nd ed., pp. 163–175). Boca Raton, FL: CRC Press.

Meltzer-Brody, S., Churchill, E., & Davidson, J. R. T. (1999). Derivation of the SPAN, a brief diagnostic screening test for post-traumatic stress disorder. *Psychiatry Research, 88*(1), 63–70.

Michael, T., Ehlers, A., Halligan, S. L., & Clark, D. M. (2005). Unwanted memories of assault: What intrusion characteristics are associated with PTSD? *Behaviour Research and Therapy, 43*(5), 613–628.

Morina, N., & Ford, J. D. (2008). Complex sequelae of psychological trauma among Kosovar civilian war victims. *International Journal of Social Psychiatry, 54*(5), 425–436.

Mouthaan, J., Sijbrandij, M., Reitsma, J. B., Gersons, B. P. R., & Olff, M. (2014). Comparing screening instruments to predict posttraumatic stress disorder. *PLOS ONE, 9*(5).

O'Donnell, M. L., Creamer, M. C., Parslow, R., Elliott, P., Holmes, A. C. N., Ellen, S., et al. (2008). A predictive screening index for posttraumatic stress disorder and depression following traumatic injury. *Journal of Consulting and Clinical Psychology, 76*(6), 923–932.

Peleg, T., & Shalev, A. Y. (2006). Longitudinal studies of PTSD: Overview of findings and methods. *CNS Spectrums, 11*(8), 589–602.

Price, M., Szafranski, D. D., van Stolk-Cooke, K., & Gros, D. F. (2016). Investigation of abbreviated 4 and 8 item versions of the PTSD Checklist 5. *Psychiatry Research, 239*, 124–130.

Prins, A., Bovin, M. J., Smolenski, D. J., Marx, B. P., Kimerling, R., Jenkins-Guarnieri, M. A., et al. (2016). The Primary Care PTSD Screen for DSM-5 (PC-PTSD-5): Development and evaluation within a veteran primary care sample. *Journal of General Internal Medicine, 31*(10), 1206–1211.

Prins, A., Ouimette, P., Kimerling, R., Cameron, R. P., Hugelshofer, D. S., Shaw-Hegwer, J., et al. (2003). The primary care PTSD screen (PC-PTSD): Development and operating characteristics. *Primary Care Psychiatry, 9*(1), 9–14.

Reed, G. M. (2010). Toward ICD-11: Improving the clinical utility of WHO's International Classification of mental disorders. *Professional Psychology: Research and Practice, 41*(6), 457–464.

Reed, G. M., First, M. B., Kogan, C. S., Hyman, S. E., Gureje, O., Gaebel, W., et al. (2019). Innovations and changes in the ICD-11 classification of mental, behavioural and neurodevelopmental disorders. *World Psychiatry, 18*, 3–19.

Reed, G. M., Keeley, J. W., Rebello, T. J., First, M. B., Gureje, O., Ayuso-Mateos, J. L., et al. (2018). Clinical utility of ICD-11 diagnostic guidelines for high-burden mental disorders: Results from mental health settings in 13 countries. *World Psychiatry, 17*, 306–315.

Reed, G. M., Sharan, P., Rebello, T. J., Keeley, J. W., Elena Medina-Mora, M., Gureje, O., et al. (2018). The ICD-11 developmental field study of reliability of diagnoses of high-burden mental disorders: Results among adult patients in mental health settings of 13 countries. *World Psychiatry, 17*, 174–186.

Roberts, N., Cloitre, M., Bisson, J. I., & Brewin, C. (2018). *PTSD and Complex PTSD Diagnostic Interview Schedule for ICD-11*. Unpublished interview.

Rona, R. J., Jones, M., Iversen, A., Hull, L., Greenberg, N., Fear, N. T., et al. (2009). The impact of posttraumatic stress disorder on impairment in the UK military at the time of the Iraq war. *Journal of Psychiatric Research, 43*(6), 649–655.

Salkovskis, P. M. (1985). Obsessional-compulsive problems: A cognitive-behavioural analysis. *Behaviour Research and Therapy, 23*(5), 571–583.

Shevlin, M., Hyland, P., Roberts, N. P., Bisson, J. I., Brewin, C. R., & Cloitre, M. (2018). A psychometric assessment of Disturbances in Self-Organization symptom indicators for ICD-11 complex PTSD using the International Trauma Questionnaire. *European Journal of Psychotraumatology, 9,* Article 1419749.

Simms, L. J., Watson, D., & Doebbeling, B. N. (2002). Confirmatory factor analyses of posttraumatic stress symptoms in deployed and nondeployed veterans of the Gulf War. *Journal of Abnormal Psychology, 111*(4), 637–647.

Somasundaram, D. J. (2007). Collective trauma in northern Sri Lanka: A qualitative psychosocial-ecological study. *International Journal of Mental Health Systems, 1*(1), 5.

Somasundaram, D. J., & Sivayokan, S. (1994). War trauma in a civilian population. *British Journal of Psychiatry, 165*(4), 524–527.

Stein, D. J., Seedat, S., Iversen, A., & Wessely, S. (2007). Post-traumatic stress disorder: Medicine and politics. *Lancet, 369,* 139–144.

Swart, M. L., van Schagen, A. M., Lancee, J., & van den Bout, J. (2013). Prevalence of nightmare disorder in psychiatric outpatients. *Psychotherapy and Psychosomatics, 82*(4), 267–268.

van Dam, D., Ehring, T., Vedel, E., & Emmelkamp, P. M. G. (2010). Validation of the Primary Care Posttraumatic Stress Disorder screening questionnaire (PC-PTSD) in civilian substance use disorder patients. *Journal of Substance Abuse Treatment, 39*(2), 105–113.

Weathers, F. W., Bovin, M. J., Lee, D. J., Sloan, D. M., Schnurr, P. P., Kaloupek, D. G., et al. (2018). The Clinician-Administered PTSD Scale for DSM-5 (CAPS-5): Development and initial psychometric evaluation in military veterans. *Psychological Assessment, 30*(3), 383–395.

Weathers, F. W., Keane, T. M., & Davidson, T. R. (2001). Clinician-administered PTSD scale: A review of the first ten years of research. *Depression and Anxiety, 13*(3), 132–156.

Weathers, F. W., Litz, B. T., Keane, T. M., Palmieri, P. A., Marx, B. P., & Schnurr, P. P. (2013). *The PTSD Checklist for DSM-5 (PCL-5)*. Washington, DC: National Center for PTSD, U.S. Department of Veterans Affairs.

Weiss, D. S. (2007). The Impact of Event Scale–Revised. In J. P. Wilson & T. M. Keane (Eds.), *Assessing psychological trauma and PTSD: A practitioner's handbook* (2nd ed., pp. 168–189). New York: Guilford Press.

World Health Organization. (1992). *The ICD-10 classification of mental and behavioural disorders: Clinical descriptions and diagnostic guidelines*. Geneva, Switzerland: Author.

World Health Organization. (2018). *International classification of diseases and related health problems* (11th rev.). Geneva, Switzerland: Author. Retrieved February 2, 2019, from *https://icd.who.int/browse11/l-m/en*.

Yufik, T., & Simms, L. J. (2010). A meta-analytic investigation of the structure of posttraumatic stress disorder symptoms. *Journal of Abnormal Psychology, 119*(4), 764–776.

CHAPTER 5

Screening, Assessment, and Diagnosis in Children and Adolescents

Lucy Berliner, Richard Meiser-Stedman, and Andrea Danese

Trauma Exposure and Impact

Children are exposed to potentially traumatic events (PTEs) at high rates. Population-based studies directly interviewing children and young adults about PTE show that a majority of children throughout the world experience threat-related events, including child abuse, rape, family and community violence, natural disasters, serious accidents, the sudden or violent loss of loved one, and war (Finkelhor, Turner, Shattuck, & Hamby, 2015; Lewis et al., 2019; Saunders & Adams, 2014; Sumner et al., 2015). Rates are even higher in clinical populations that include children in psychiatric inpatient settings, child welfare, and juvenile justice (Dierkhising et al., 2013; Havens et al., 2012; Salazar, Keller, Gowen, & Courtney, 2013). Not all children who experience a PTE will develop posttraumatic stress disorder (PTSD) or clinically significant posttraumatic stress symptoms. In trauma-exposed samples of youth, Alisic and colleagues (2014) found that, on average, 16% met diagnostic criteria for PTSD; higher rates were found for girls and for interpersonal trauma. About a third of girls with interpersonal trauma developed PTSD. Trauma-exposed young people are not only at risk for PTSD but can also develop the full range of emotional and behavioral disorders (Lewis et al., 2019).

Predisposing Factors

Since only a fraction of trauma-exposed young people develop PTSD, it is important to characterize which factors may increase risk for PTSD in young people who are exposed. Research indicates several potential characteristics

69

of the trauma, the child, and the family that could increase risk of PTSD in trauma-exposed young people. For example, interpersonal traumas (e.g., child physical or sexual abuse) are associated with greater PTSD risk compared to public events (disasters) and single-event traumas (e.g., road traffic crashes; Alisic et al., 2014; Cisler et al., 2012). Prior victimization, previous psychiatric history, family psychopathology, and social disadvantage may increase risk of PTSD. Trickey, Siddaway, Meiser-Stedman, Serpell, and Field (2012) found that factors related to the subjective experience during the event (e.g., fear, life threat) and posttrauma responses (e.g., low social support, family dysfunction, avoidance) had more influence than pretrauma risk factors and severity of the event. All these factors have been shown to identify groups of trauma-exposed young people at greater risk of PTSD. However, only an initial understanding exists of their clinical utility in estimating individualized risk prediction in any particular young person (Lewis et al., 2019).

At this time, identification of children with clinical need due to trauma exposure and trauma impact is the most critical task. There are effective treatments for PTSD and trauma impact in children (Gilles, Taylor, Gray, O'Brien, & D'Abrew, 2013; Gutermann et al., 2016; Jensen, Holt, Mørup Ormhaug, Fjermestad, & Wentzel-Larsen, 2018; Morina, Koerssen, & Pollet, 2016), but without identification, the children in need will not receive the benefit of these therapies. Trauma exposure and trauma impact assessment are the primary strategies for increasing identification of trauma-exposed and affected children in need of trauma-specific mental health services and for ensuring they get access to effective care.

This chapter will review trauma screening and trauma impact assessment procedures. In some cases, trauma screening will already have been done in another often nonclinical setting (e.g., school, child welfare, primary care, child advocacy centers, juvenile justice). We focus primarily on screening and assessment of children and families in the clinical context. In some cases, these activities will take place in specialty clinics for trauma. However, most children with mental health needs receive behavioral health care in nonspecialty settings that provide clinical services for the full range of childhood disorders (e.g., Medicaid Behavioral Health Services in the United States; Child and Adolescent Mental Health Services in the United Kingdom and Australia). There are also some circumstances where a population approach to trauma screening may be indicated, and it will take place in a nonclinical setting. For example, children in a school where there has been a school shooting or a community that has suffered a major natural disaster may be best served by screening in a more natural setting.

For children affected by trauma, we are not just concerned with making a PTSD diagnosis. We want to ensure that all children exposed to potentially traumatic events are identified and, once identified, are assessed to determine if they are safe or might be experiencing ongoing risk, even before they are assessed for PTSD and other behavioral health need. Our primary focus in this chapter will be PTSD, but we will consider other common disorders such as depression that occurs even more frequently in exposed children than PTSD. We will follow the flow that typically would occur, especially in nonspecialty settings where most affected children will receive care. The chapter will proceed from screening for trauma exposure to brief screening for trauma impact, diagnosis-based self-report measures, structured diagnostic interviews, and finally diagnosis including addressing comorbidities. The goal is to ensure that all affected children are identified and receive appropriate care.

The chapter will cover both comprehensive trauma screening and assessment procedures as might be the standard of care in specialty clinics, as well as the more basic trauma screening and assessment that can be carried out in primary care and general child mental health programs. The emphasis will be on procedures and measures that can be implemented at low or no cost.

Routine Screening for Trauma Exposure and Impact

Screening as an Opportunity

Screening for exposure to trauma is the first and necessary step for identifying children at risk for ongoing harm and at risk for behavioral health concerns because children do not typically volunteer their trauma experiences. Exposure to potentially traumatic events by itself or in combination with other adversities substantially increases risk for psychopathology (Lewis et al., 2019; McLaughlin et al., 2012). McLaughlin and colleagues (2012) found that exposure to trauma and other adversities accounted for a substantial portion of childhood (45%) and adolescent (32%) onset of all psychiatric disorders.

Trauma exposure screening and/or brief trauma impact screening can be undertaken in primary care or nonspecialty behavioral health settings. This will be the best method of identifying children with PTSD. Children, even those receiving behavioral health services, frequently do not report their trauma experiences or are not seeking care for a trauma-specific disorder such as PTSD. Many children exposed to trauma and other adversities and suffering from PTSD are likely receiving care in nonspecialty behavioral health settings. In the absence of routine trauma exposure and trauma impact screening, their trauma histories may never be uncovered; they may remain in danger or be misdiagnosed.

However, routine screening in health settings, especially for exposure to adverse events and behavioral health conditions, must be undertaken thoughtfully. Recommendations to screen in primary care settings have become more common for adverse experiences (e.g., DV, ACEs) or behavioral health conditions such as depression in adults and adolescents (*www.uspreventiveservicestaskforce.org/Page/Document/UpdateSummaryFinal/ depression-in-children-and-adolescents-screening*).   However,   controversies remain about the value of routine screening. For example, screening for exposure to domestic violence has not proven helpful for patients (e.g., McLennan & MacMillan, 2018). Finkelhor (2018) raised the issue of caution for screening for childhood adversities as recommended by the American Academy of Pediatrics (Garner et al., 2012). Screening is not always helpful and may even be harmful (e.g., create negative expectancies, cause worry, lead to unnecessary services). Therefore, if trauma screening is to be done, procedures to review results and facilitate access to trauma therapy must be in place for children who screen in.

The purpose of behavioral health screening is to help patients with clinical need. Unfortunately, even when clinical need is identified, most children with mental health need do not receive mental health services (Kovess-Masfety et al., 2017; Lewis et al., 2019; Merikangas et al., 2011; Sawyer et al., 2018; Simon, Pastor, Reuben, Huang, & Goldstrom, 2015). Children with the internalizing disorders that are most associated with trauma-specific impact such as PTSD, depression, and anxiety are less likely than youth with disruptive disorders to be referred or access needed services even when identified. Therefore, simply identifying children exposed to trauma or with elevated trauma-related symptoms is insufficient without a commitment to ensure that a benefit accrues to the patients. For example, care should be taken to convey a message that while having a trauma history increases risk for deleterious outcomes, not all exposed children develop trauma or other disorders and effective treatments are available. Providers who screen and identify children with trauma-specific or other mental health need must be prepared to offer services or facilitate access to services.

We contend that administration of trauma exposure and impact measures and review of the results with the client can be conceptualized as a therapeutic clinical encounter. First, it gives a message to children that professionals are aware trauma exposure occurs, are interested to learn about it from clients, and can handle hearing about trauma. Second, going over the results of the screen creates an opportunity for validation ("I'm sorry that happened to you"), normalization ("you are not alone, traumas are common in children's lives"), and psychoeducation regarding impact ("traumas are threat events that can cause reactions"), and instills hope ("we have a treatment that works for posttraumatic stress"). Screening can also initiate the core elements of effective trauma treatments, such as exposure and identifying unhelpful thoughts to target in therapy.

Trauma Screening Concerns

There has been significant concern that screening for trauma exposure is distressing for children. The evidence does not bear that out. Population-based studies that screen youth regarding victimization history typically use lay interviewers. They are able to elicit reports of victimization and trauma from youth as young as 10 years old without having mental health training or a therapeutic relationship with the respondent. Several such studies have directly asked children about distress and find that very few children report the interviews as even mildly upsetting (Finkelhor, Vanderminden, Turner, Hamby, & Shattuck 2014; Landolt, Schnyder, Maier, Schoenbucher, & Mohler-Kuo, 2013; Zajac, Ruggiero, Smith, Saunders, & Kilpatrick, 2011). In a clinical context, Skar and colleagues (Skar, Ormhaug, & Jensen, 2019) incorporated routine trauma exposure and impact screening into an implementation study of trauma-focused cognitive-behavioral therapy (TF-CBT) in mental health clinics across Norway. To identify children eligible for TF-CBT, clinics were expected to screen all children. They have assessed thousands of service-seeking children and youth. Overall, only a small minority report distress at screening. Talking about trauma does not cause distress in young people without trauma exposure and only leads to minimal distress among children with trauma exposure but without PTSD. Children with PTSD are somewhat more likely to be distressed, but this should be expected. The distress of disclosure is unlikely to be experienced as more overwhelming than their everyday experience of living with PTSD; and the relief at being taken seriously may more than compensate for any short-lived upset. It is essential to identify children who have been exposed and have developed PTSD, in order to plan further assessment and treatment.

Potential Screening Impact

Although many children who are exposed to trauma will report their experiences and the impact if given a direct opportunity, it should always be kept in mind how difficult young people can find acknowledging and talking about trauma. Even with direct questioning, children may not initially report trauma as they might fear upsetting parents, being stigmatized, and causing trouble for themselves or others. They may worry about being believed and supported. In certain cases of interpersonal violence, especially when it occurs within the home, revealing information may lead to negative outcomes such as family separations or breakup. And clinically, children may want to actively avoid discussing these experiences because it is upsetting to recall the events or triggers distressing reliving symptoms.

It is also important to bear in mind that young people may not be prepared initially to provide the full details of the trauma they acknowledge during screening. Clinicians have an important role to play in facilitating facing up to and talking about trauma by creating a safe environment and trusting relationship. Clinicians should reassure young people that it is helpful to talk about bad experiences and encourage candor, but stress that whatever level of detail the young person is willing to share initially will be accepted.

Clinicians must consider confidentiality when asking children about trauma experiences, especially those that may occur within the family, such as sexual or physical abuse or domestic violence. In some countries, there are mandatory child abuse reporting laws that would be triggered if a child discloses maltreatment. Clinicians should be familiar with the laws in their country or jurisdiction as well as the procedures that must be followed and what clients can anticipate in any child protection systems. Clinicians can actively support children in sharing their traumas with their parents or in contacting authorities to mitigate the potential negative fallout of a report of maltreatment.

In addition, other legal considerations can come into play. Clinicians should avoid asking many leading questions, especially with younger children. Extensive direct questioning can cause children to acquiesce or in some cases even change aspects of their memories. This could be harmful, including undermining young peoples' credibility and disqualifying their account during legal proceedings. Open-ended approaches tend to produce the most complete and accurate accounts.

It is not clinically necessary to know all the facts; what is clinically important is to learn if a trauma has happened and how it has affected the young people from their perspective. Elicitation-oriented questioning, acceptance, nonjudgmental approaches, and encouragement to focus on thoughts and feelings versus specific facts can reduce the risk of memory error or misstatements and be more clinically meaningful.

Overall, research and clinical experience support the idea that the benefits of routine screening in clinical settings outweigh any drawbacks as long as it is done in a sensitive, clinical way. Routine screening is feasible and does not induce distress in nonexposed children, and when distress occurs, it is mostly in the children with clinically significant posttraumatic stress who are the very children that need to be identified in order to be helped. Thus, we recommend trauma exposure and impact screening as a standard part of intake or initial assessment procedures in clinical settings, provided it is accompanied by supportive, clinically oriented feedback.

Screening and Assessment Questionnaires and Checklists

Questionnaires and checklists are essential tools for assessing trauma exposure and PTSD in children and young people. For individual assessment, they offer a brief and time-efficient way of determining whether a child has been exposed to trauma and, if exposed, the presence of posttraumatic stress symptoms and whether symptoms are clinically significant. Administration of questionnaires does not require a young person to discuss a trauma with a clinician, possibly reducing distress around assessment.

Screening measures also allow for population-level approaches with groups of trauma-exposed young people for whom individual assessment would not be feasible. They can provide an approximate assessment of PTSD symptom severity. For cases with only mild symptoms, this then gives clinicians a convenient way of reassuring parents and caregivers that although *some* symptoms may be present, they are of a level that would not normally warrant treatment.

Standard measures provide clinicians with an important tool for indexing trauma exposure, which may be particularly important when a child or young person is only just beginning to disclose a long and complicated history of trauma or when a child or young person finds the process of disclosure very difficult. There are a wide range of well-validated measures available with subtly different structures and purposes, facilitating clinicians across settings.

Of course, questionnaires and checklists also have their limitations that clinicians need to keep in mind. Reading comprehension is critical to assess; it may be necessary to read the checklists to younger children or explicitly encourage them to ask questions if they do not understand. Questionnaires can be scored or interpreted incorrectly. Questionnaire administration may allow fewer opportunities for children and young persons to ask questions or clarify the meaning of some items. To our knowledge, no measure has complete accuracy, and cutoffs are produced based on the responses from certain groups in particular contexts.

Completing a questionnaire can be an upsetting activity for some children, and efforts should be made to ensure that appropriate care and support are available if needed. On occasion, questionnaires may be viewed with some distrust, although with proper explanation, we find their value can be understood by children. Care must also be taken when considering the environment for completing questionnaires; while the clinic generally offers a suitable setting for this activity, a school classroom may require additional measures to ensure privacy and support. Though comparatively "cheap," the interpretation and processing of questionnaires in situations where a large number of youth are completing them at the same time still require considerable diligence and attentiveness.

Given these concerns, it is important to recognize that questionnaires, while remaining an essential tool, are an aid for good clinical work rather than authoritative or beyond reproach. It is our experience that in the clinic, questionnaires and checklists are frequently useful as a prompt for further, more detailed discussion of trauma histories and particular symptoms.

Trauma Exposure Screening

One important consideration with trauma screening and assessment checklists is the distinction between exposure and trauma symptoms. Exposure screeners simply ask the young person whether or not an event has happened. They are not scored and conclusions cannot be drawn about the accuracy of the response. Sometimes children are confused, conflate events, or omit mention of actual traumas. Exposure screening per se should be considered the explicit clinical invitation to acknowledge trauma experiences, not the definitive means of establishing a complete trauma history.

Knowing about trauma exposure is necessary before assessing for posttraumatic stress symptoms since there must be a traumatic stressor that is tied to the symptoms. For diagnostic purposes, the symptoms have to have developed or been exacerbated following the event. Sometimes the trauma is known (e.g., emergency room visit or hospitalization for injury, exposure to public disaster) and only impact screening is necessary. For example, the Child Stress Disorders Checklist Short Form (CSDC) is designed for injured children and includes only four items (e.g., "child gets very upset if reminded of the trauma"; Bosquet Enlow, Kassam-Adams, & Saxe, 2010). In cases where the trauma is not already known, most trauma exposure screens comprise the first section of screening measures for trauma impact. Typically, these checklists include both a trauma screen and an assessment of PTSD symptoms. There are very brief psychometrically sound exposure and impact screeners in the public domain, such as the Child Trauma Screen (CTS; e.g., Lang & Connell, 2017). The trauma exposure screen consists of four items (e.g., "Have you ever seen people pushing, hitting, and throwing things at each other, or stabbing, shooting, or trying to hurt each other?"). Several more in-depth measures include both a trauma screen and assessment of PTSD symptoms consistent with DSM-5 (Child and Adolescent Trauma Screen [CATS]: Sachser, Berliner, et al., 2017; Child PTSD Symptom Scale for DSM-5 [CPSS-5]: Foa, Asnaani, Zang, Capaldi, & Yeh, 2018; UCLA PTSD Reaction Index [UCLA PTSD-RI]: Kaplow et al., 2020). The trauma exposure screen sections contain 14 possible traumas and an option for another as perceived by the respondent (child or parent). The Trauma Event Screening Instrument for Children (TESI-C; Ribbe, 1996) only assesses the trauma events but in great detail.

Assessing Trauma Impact

If young people report trauma exposure or are known to have been exposed to trauma, it is important to assess for the presence of trauma-related psychopathology. Although most children show emotional and behavioral symptoms in the aftermath of a traumatic experience, these symptoms are often transient, and most trauma-exposed young people do not develop clinically significant, persistent psychopathology due to the event. Therefore, screening for trauma-related psychopathology is often only undertaken a few weeks after trauma.

Screening in generic child and adolescent mental health settings can be brief, for example, with the support of a short, validated screening measure for PTSD (e.g., Child Revised Impact of Event Scale [CRIES]). When possible, the screening should also include brief assessment of other types of psychopathology or overall psychopathology, as psychiatric disorders with a higher base rate in the general population (e.g., depression) also have higher prevalence in trauma-exposed young people.

When trauma-exposed young people screen positive for PTSD or clinically distressing posttraumatic stress, more detailed assessment of symptoms is required. The intensity and duration of this assessment will necessarily vary based on the setting. In general clinical settings, PTSD assessment may be undertaken through more detailed trauma-specific questionnaires (e.g., CATS, CPSS, UCLA PTSD-RI) and/or unstructured interviews focusing on cardinal symptom dimensions (e.g., reexperiencing, avoidance, arousal). Functional impairment should also be routinely assessed. In specialist settings, PTSD assessment is typically more in-depth and includes structured or semistructured interviews and may include direct observation of behavior in nonclinical settings. Specialty clinics also often use repeated assessments of posttraumatic stress to provide a way of monitoring session-by-session recovery or, occasionally, deterioration. Regardless of setting, it is essential that children and young people be screened and assessed directly and on their own. Questionnaires should be completed by children as soon as they are developmentally able (e.g., around 7 years).

Parents or other caregivers should be actively involved in the assessment. They are critical for gaining a comprehensive impression because they know more about their children and see them under many more circumstances. They can contribute important collateral information on the young person's clinical presentation, in addition to essential historical details (e.g., pretrauma functioning, timeline of symptoms' presentation, psychiatric history, developmental history) and information on family functioning (e.g., family composition and functioning, family history of psychopathology, family reaction and adaptation to the trauma).

However, it is important to bear in mind that parents may under- or over-report PTSD symptoms and other psychiatric symptoms after trauma. On the one hand, this may be due to the difficulties in detecting internalized symptoms, framing clinical-level symptoms as normal reactions to difficult experiences. Or, parents may withhold information on symptoms they have observed because of fears, worries, stigma, or in some cases the minimization of trauma impact on their child. On the other hand, some parents may overattribute symptoms and behaviors to trauma (e.g., parents with their own trauma history; parents seeking to externalize the cause of their child's difficulties).

Checklists and Questionnaires

Quite a number of questionnaires and subscales are available for trauma exposure screening and/or assessment of trauma-related impact. Some are very brief screeners, whereas others produce a probable PTSD diagnosis. We have opted to consider two broad classes of measures separately: questionnaires and checklists that are not specific to a particular diagnostic model, and diagnosis-specific scales. We also consider scales that may be useful for informing the psychological formulation of an individual child or young person's posttraumatic stress response.

Non-Diagnosis-Specific Questionnaires and Checklists

We outline several measures of this type in Table 5.1. We list those measures that are most widely used and have the most robust psychometric validation. This is not a systematic review of all available measures, and although we have sought to provide the most up-to-date information about each one, we would encourage clinicians to stay alert to the publication of further data on each scale. We also make the following observations about these measures. First, the breadth of available measures in this group should ensure that clinicians can identify an instrument specific to the needs of their own client group and setting or context. Second, the strength of using one of the following measures is that all are unlikely to be made redundant with further diagnostic innovations—they are likely to withstand further iterations of the PTSD diagnosis (e.g., DSM-6, ICD-12). Third, this list is specific to measures based on the responses of children or young persons or responses from their parents or caregivers. Other screening tools that also incorporate demographic, medical, or other trauma-related information are available (e.g., the Screening Tool for Early Predictors of PTSD [STEPP]).

The Child Trauma Screen (CTS), the Child Stress Disorders Checklist–SS (CSDC), and the Child Trauma Screening Questionnaire (CTSQ) are brief tools for screening children and young people exposed to trauma; the Young Child PTSD Screen performs the same function but specifically for young children. Each measure provides a clear cutoff for identifying children and young people at high risk of having PTSD, and therefore deserving of further attention. The CTS also includes a trauma exposure screen.

The Child Revised Impact of Event Scale (CRIES) may function as both a screening instrument (particularly in its brief eight-item format) and a severity/intensity measure. A particular strength of the CRIES is its availability in numerous languages (see *www.childrenandwar.org/measures*). The Pediatric Emotional Distress Scale (PEDS) is aimed at preschool and younger children, addressing many "core" PTSD symptoms and symptoms considered specific to this age group (e.g., clinginess, loss of developmentally appropriate skills, bedwetting).

Diagnosis-Specific Questionnaires

We list diagnosis-specific instruments for children and young people in Table 5.2. Several options exist for questionnaires that address PTSD as defined by DSM-5, while the DSM-IV acute stress disorder diagnosis is addressed by the Acute Stress Checklist for Children (ASC-Kids; Kassam-Adams, 2006). To our knowledge, there are no published measures for ICD-10 or ICD-11 PTSD, or the newly introduced ICD-11 complex PTSD (CPTSD) diagnosis. Where these constructs have been investigated, researchers have used the items from DSM-5-focused measures; given the subtle differences in wording between DSM and ICD PTSD symptoms, this approach may be problematic.

TABLE 5.1. Checklists and Self-Report Questionnaire Measures, Not Diagnosis-Based

Measure	Reference	Respondent	Type	Cutoffs?	Age range (years)	Items	Published psychometrics?	Free to use?
Child Revised Impact of Events Scale (CRIES)	Dyregrov & Yule (1995)	CYP	Intensity/ severity	17+ for 8 item; 30+ for 13 item	8–18	8 or 13	Yes	Yes
Child Stress Disorders Checklist ASD/PTSD (CSDC)	Saxe et al. (2003)	CG/ Par	Screening	No	5–17	36	Yes	Yes
Child Stress Disorders Checklist–Short Form (CSDC-SF)	Bosquet Enlow, Kassam-Adams, & Saxe (2010)	CG/ Par	Screening	No	6–18	4	Yes	Yes
Child Trauma Screen (CTS)	Lang & Connell (2017)	CG/ Par, CYP	Screening	CG/Par 8+, CYP 6+	3–18	10	Yes	Yes
Pediatric Emotional Distress Scale (PEDS)	Saylor, Swenson, Stokes Reynolds, & Taylor (1999)	CG/ Par	Intensity/ severity	No	2–10	21	Yes	Yes
Trauma Symptom Checklist for Children (TSCC)	Briere (1996)	CYP	Intensity/ severity	Yes (*T*-scores)	8–16	54	Yes	No
Trauma Symptom Checklist for Young Children (TSCYC)	Briere (2005)	CG/ Par	Intensity/ severity	Yes (*T*-scores)	3–12	90	Yes	No
Young Child PTSD Screen (YCPS)	Scheeringa & Haslett (2010)	CG/ Par	Screening	Yes	3–6	6	No	Yes
Child Trauma Screening Questionnaire (CTSQ)	Kenardy, Spence, & Macleod (2006)	CYP	Screening	Yes (5+)	7–16	10	Yes	Yes

Note. CYP, child or young person; CG/Par, caregiver or parent.

TABLE 5.2. Self-Report Questionnaire Measures, Diagnosis-Based

Measure	Reference	Respondent	Cutoffs?	Age range (years)	Items	Published psychometrics?	Free to use?
Acute Stress Checklist for Children (ASC-Kids)	Kassam-Adams (2006)	CYP	Nov	8–17	29	Yes	Yes
Child and Adolescent Trauma Screen (CATS)	Sachser, Berliner, et al. (2017)	CG/Par; CYP	Yes (21+)	3–17	20 (7–17 years); 16 (3–6 years)	Yes	Yes
Child PTSD Symptom Scale for DSM-5 (CPSS-5)	Foa, Asnaani, Zang, Capaldi, & Yeh (2018)	CYP	Yes (31+)	8–18	20 PTSD symptoms	Yes	Yes
UCLA PTSD Reaction Index (UCLA PTSD-RI)	Kaplow et al. (2020)	CG/Par; CYP	Yes (38+, DSM-IV version)	7–18	31	Yes (DSM-IV version)	No

Note: CYP, child or young person; CG/Par, caregiver or parent.

Three measures—CATS, CPSS-5, and UCLA PTSD-RI—offer a comprehensive assessment of DSM-5 PTSD symptomatology. They include the traumatic stressor screen; the four symptom clusters of intrusion, avoidance, negative alteration in cognitions and mood, and alterations in arousal and reactivity; and impairment. It is also important to note that the DSM-IV forms of the CPSS and UCLA PTSD-RI have been widely used, including in clinical trials, and that such data may still be useful in certain contexts.

With the advent of ICD-11 and its new conceptualizations and definitions for PTSD and CPTSD, new measures are currently in development. With some adjustments to the intrusion symptoms to capture "nowness" in reexperiencing, it is possible to crosswalk from DSM-5 to ICD-11 PTSD. The "negative alternations in cognitions and mood" symptom cluster included in the DSM-5 PTSD criteria may to some extent address the "complexity" that is encapsulated within the CPTSD diagnosis. Currently, one study finds support for the existence of CPTSD in children using a DSM-5 measure and selected items from other measures used in a TF-CBT randomized trial (Sachser, Keller, & Goldbeck, 2017). However, at this time, there is no alternative treatment for young people with CPTSD, and some evidence exists that CPTSD can benefit from standard evidence-based CBTs for trauma. Treatment for PTSD and CPTSD in children and adolescents is expanded on by Jensen, Cohen, Jaycox, and Rosner (Chapter 21, this volume).

Structured and Semistructured Interview Assessments for PTSD in Children and Young People

There are instances where a structured or semistructured interview assessment for PTSD is essential, such as when a formal diagnostic process is required to access health care; to establish unequivocally that PTSD is present and its importance relative to other needs; for medicolegal assessment; and where self-report measures are inappropriate (e.g., if a child or young person lacks the appropriate literacy skills). A structured assessment has several advantages over self-report measures. Although more intrusive and time-consuming, an interview potentially allows for a far more thorough understanding of a child or young person's symptoms and how they occur in their familial and developmental context, their onset and impact. Clinically, a well-conducted, empathic comprehensive interview assessment may help to build a therapeutic relationship and establish a solid platform for psychological therapy. Of course, a clinician may simply use a given diagnostic framework (e.g., DSM-5, ICD-11) to direct his or her clinical assessment. However, a structured interview assessment typically supports the interviewer by providing follow-up questions and points of clarification, and support for children and young people in framing their responses (e.g., by offering several options for time period or frequency). A structured interview may also be very useful for non-mental health professionals or paraprofessionals, for example, more junior staff who conduct initial assessment, or research assistants working in the context of a clinical trial.

Several structured interview assessments are available for assessing PTSD in children and young people (see Table 5.3). As with diagnosis-specific questionnaire measures, these were produced to assess DSM-IV or DSM-5 PTSD. Although several PTSD-specific interviews are available, the Anxiety Disorders Interview Schedule (ADIS), Kiddie Schedule for Affective Disorders and Schizophrenia (K-SADS), and Diagnostic Infant and Preschool Assessment (DIPA) include PTSD as part of a broader assessment of different psychiatric diagnoses. These interviews involve some initial probe or screening questions, with additional questions then asked to confirm the presence of a particular diagnosis or class of diagnoses. At least two interview assessments are interview-formatted versions of other questionnaires (CPSS5; UCLA RI). (See Table 5.2.)

Other Measures for Use with Trauma-Exposed Children and Adolescents

Assessing trauma-related appraisals or beliefs is extremely important. They are considered a key etiological factor in cognitive behavioral models of PTSD. Multiple recent studies (Hiller et al., 2019; Jensen et al., 2018; McLean, Yeh, Rosenfield, & Foa, 2015; Pfeiffer, Sachser, de Haan, Tutus, & Goldbeck,

2017) have found that trauma-related cognitions mediate PTSD symptoms and symptom reduction. Therefore, it is critical to assess cognitions that may be perpetuating the PTSD symptoms. The Child Post-Traumatic Cognitions Inventory (CPTCI; Meiser-Stedman et al., 2009) is validated for older children and adolescents, and has been translated into multiple languages. An abbreviated 10-item form of the CPTCI has also been validated and may support its brief administration in therapy sessions (McKinnon et al., 2016).

TABLE 5.3. Structured Interview Assessments for Children and Young People

Interview	Reference	Respondent	Diagnostic system	Type	Proposed age range (years)	Published psychometrics?	Free to use?
Clinician-Administered PTSD Scale for DSM-5–Child/Adolescent Version (CAPS-CA-5)	Pynoos et al. (2015)	CYP	DSM-5	PTSD-specific	7+	Yes (DSM-IV version)	Yes
Child PTSD Symptom Scale for DSM-5, interview (CPSS-5-I)	Foa, Asnaani, Zang, Capaldi, & Yeh (2018)	CYP	DSM-5	PTSD-specific	8–18	Yes	Yes
Children's Posttraumatic Stress Disorder Inventory (CPTSDI)	Saigh (2004)	CYP	DSM-IV	PTSD-specific	6–18	Yes	No
Anxiety Disorders Interview Schedule (ADIS-IV): Child and Parent Interview Schedules	Silverman & Albano (1996)	CYP, CG/Par	DSM-IV	Multi-disorder	7–16	Yes (for full schedule)	Yes
Kiddie Schedule for Affective Disorders and Schizophrenia (K-SADS)	Kaufman et al. (1997)	CYP	DSM-5	Multi-disorder	7–17	Yes	Yes
Diagnostic Infant and Preschool Assessment (DIPA)	Scheeringa & Haslett (2010)	CG/Par	DSM-IV	Multi-disorder	9 months–6 years	Yes	Yes

Note. CYP, child or young person; CG/Par, caregiver or parent.

With respect to family context and potential maintaining factors within that system, two measures have recently been proposed: the Parent Trauma Response Questionnaire (Williamson et al., 2018) and the Thinking about Recovery Scale (Schilpzand, Conroy, Anderson, & Alisic, 2018). Each includes items that address multiple behavioral and cognitive processes (e.g., child vulnerability, permanent psychological harm to the child, over-protectiveness and avoidance) that are considered maladaptive in the parent or caregiver whose child has been subjected to trauma. Assessing parental PTSD and mood may be clinically indicated; we would encourage the use of any measure endorsed in the adult section of this volume.

For assessing dissociation, the Child Dissociation Checklist (Putnam, Helmers, & Trickett, 1993) and Adolescent Dissociative Experiences Scale (Farrington, Smerden, & Faupel, 2001) have been developed; they offer a wide-ranging assessment of a child or young's person experience of such phenomena, including depersonalization, derealization, and identity confusion. For *peritraumatic* dissociative experiences, the child version of the Peritraumatic Dissociative Experiences Questionnaire (PDEQ-C; Bui et al., 2011) and ASC-Kids are available.

Formulation and Treatment Recommendations

Diagnosis

A diagnosis of PTSD based on the current World Health Organization definition (ICD-11; World Health Organization, 2018) is made when children and young people have core symptoms in the dimensions of reliving experiences, active avoidance, and physiological hyperreactivity. Criteria for a diagnosis of PTSD in the fifth edition of the *Diagnostic and Statistical Manual of Mental Disorders* (DSM-5; American Psychiatric Association, 2013) are broader; children and young people have the above core symptoms and negative alterations in mood and cognition that are trauma-related. DSM-5 also includes a separate, developmentally appropriate set of symptoms for diagnosing PTSD in children who are 6 years old or younger.

Differential Diagnosis

Differential diagnosis is important because PTSD is not the most common condition observed in the aftermath of trauma, as psychiatric disorders with a higher base rate in the general population (e.g., depression) also have higher prevalence in trauma-exposed young people (Lewis et al., 2019). PTSD symptoms can resemble symptoms of other psychiatric conditions, which should be carefully investigated. For example, inattention and restlessness seen in trauma-exposed young people may be explained by pre-existing ADHD; sleep problems and negative cognitions may be explained by a depressive episode; avoidance may be explained by anxiety disorders (e.g., agoraphobia, social phobia); affect dysregulation may be explained by substance use or bipolar disorder; and dissociation may be explained by psychosis. These conditions should therefore be directly assessed.

Comorbidity

In addition to identifying alternative explanations for the clinical presentation, in a diagnostic assessment, it is also important to describe psychiatric disorders that co-occur with PTSD. A wide range of possible comorbid conditions exist, and those commonly observed in young people with PTSD include depression, generalized anxiety disorder, conduct disorder, and alcohol misuse. Comorbidity is the rule rather than the exception in patients with PTSD (Lewis et al., 2019), and the type of comorbidity may inform treatment targets and the overall prognosis. In particular, it is helpful to clarify the timeline for the onset of various symptoms in order to characterize pretrauma functioning and to understand if trauma-focused treatment might also relieve secondary symptoms (e.g., depressive symptoms).

Precipitating Factors

PTSD is unique in comparison to other types of psychopathology because the disorder is unambiguously linked to a causal risk factor, namely, the index trauma. PTSD diagnosis requires endorsement of an index trauma. If symptoms of PTSD are present in the absence of an established or reported trauma exposure, the diagnosis cannot be given. Instead, clinicians should consider the differential diagnoses discussed previously. This is especially true because many of the nonspecific symptoms in DMS-5 PTSD could result from other disorders. Exploring the specific symptoms the youth endorsed in depth, especially the core PTSD symptoms of intrusion and avoidance, can clarify if there is an eligible stressor that accounts for them (e.g., what are the upsetting thoughts or memories that are popping into your head?"). If the youth is reporting distress, he or she should receive care, but it would not be appropriate to deliver a trauma-focused therapy without an identified stressor and clinically significant posttraumatic stress. During treatment for the distress, a reluctant child may later report trauma once clinicians are able to build a trusting relationship.

Perpetuating Factors

To identify relevant treatment targets, it is important to understand the mechanisms that maintain PTSD symptoms. Common mechanisms identified map onto key PTSD symptoms' dimensions. Avoidance is cardinal in PTSD. It leads young people to avoid facing up to the trauma or avoid places or people that remind them of the trauma but are not dangerous. Avoidance prevents desensitization and can interfere with normal development activities. Another key mechanism is likely untrue or unhelpful negative cognitions about themselves, such as guilt, shame, and helplessness. Family factors can also be important as parents may accommodate the young person's avoidance strategies in an attempt to reduce distress and may at times contribute to establishing or perpetuating negative cognitions.

Risk and Opportunity

Trauma exposure and PTSD diagnosis are associated with a substantial increase in risk for psychiatric disorders, health problems, and impaired functioning later on. Unlike most other psychiatric disorders, PTSD must be precipitated by a traumatic stressor. When the stressor is known (e.g., car crash, earthquake) or is discovered through trauma-specific screening and assessment, a unique opportunity is created to intervene early if needed, to identify high-risk children, and to make sure that children are accurately diagnosed so they can receive effective treatments.

This volume and the International Society for Traumatic Stress Studies' *Posttraumatic Stress Disorder Prevention and Treatment Guidelines* (*www. istss.org/getattachment/Treating-Trauma/New-ISTSS-Prevention-and-Treatment-Guidelines/ISTSS_PreventionTreatmentGuidelines_FNL.pdf.aspx*) resulted in strong recommendations for several treatments for children and young people with posttraumatic stress. The goal of routine screening and assessment for PTSD in children is to ensure that children and youth with need are identified and that access to effective treatments is facilitated.

REFERENCES

Alisic, E., Zalta, A. K., Van Wesel, F., Larsen, S. E., Hafstad, G. S., Hassanpour, K., et al. (2014). Rates of post-traumatic stress disorder in trauma-exposed children and adolescents: Meta-analysis. *British Journal of Psychiatry, 204,* 335–340.

American Psychiatric Association. (2013). *Diagnostic and statistical manual of mental disorders* (5th ed.). Arlington, VA: Author.

Bosquet Enlow, M., Kassam-Adams, N., & Saxe, G. (2010). The Child Stress Disorders Checklist—Short Form: A four-item scale of traumatic stress symptoms in children. *General Hospital Psychiatry, 32*(3), 321–327.

Briere, J. (1996). *Trauma Symptom Checklist for Children (TSCC): Professional manual.* Odessa, FL: Psychological Assessment Resources.

Briere, J. (2005). *Trauma Symptom Checklist for Young Children (TSCYC): Professional manual.* Odessa, FL: Psychological Assessment Resources.

Bui, E., Brunet, A., Olliac, B., Very, E., Allenou, C., Raynaud, J., et al. (2011). Validation of the Peritraumatic Dissociative Experiences Questionnaire and Peritraumatic Distress Inventory in school-aged victims of road traffic accidents. *European Psychiatry, 26,* 108–111.

Cisler, J., Begle, A., Amstadter, A., Resnick, H., Kmett Danielson, K., Saunders, B., et al. (2012). Exposure to Interpersonal Violence and Risk for PTSD, depression, delinquency, and binge drinking among adolescents: Data from the NSA-R. *Journal of Traumatic Stress, 25,* 33–40.

Dierkhising, C., Ko, S., Woods-Jaeger, B., Briggs, E., Lee, R., & Pynoos, S. (2013). Trauma histories among justice-involved youth: Findings from the National Child Traumatic Stress Network. *European Journal of Psychotraumatology, 4*(1).

Dyregrov, A., & Yule, W. (1995, May). *Screening measures: The development of the UNICEF screening battery.* Paper presented at the Fourth European Conference on Traumatic Stress, Paris.

Farrington, A., Smerden, J., & Faupel, A. (2001). The adolescent dissociative experiences scale: Psychometric properties and difference in scores across age groups. *Journal of Nervous and Mental Disease, 10,* 722–727.

Finkelhor, D. (2018). Screening for adverse childhood experiences (ACEs): Cautions and suggestions. *Child Abuse and Neglect, 85,* 174–179.

Finkelhor, D., Turner, H., Shattuck, A., & Hamby, S. (2015). Prevalence of childhood exposure to violence, crime, and abuse: Results from the national survey of children's exposure to violence. *JAMA Pediatrics, 169*(8), 746–754.

Finkelhor, D., Vanderminden, J., Turner, H., Hamby, S., & Shattuck, A. (2014). Upset among youth in response to questions about exposure to violence, sexual assault and family maltreatment. *Child Abuse and Neglect, 38,* 217–223.

Foa, E. B., Asnaani, A., Zang, Y., Capaldi, S., & Yeh, R. (2018). Psychometrics of the Child PTSD Symptom Scale for DSM-5 for trauma-exposed children and adolescents. *Journal of Clinical Child and Adolescent Psychology, 47*(1), 38–46.

Garner, A. S., Shonkoff, J. P., Committee on Psychosocial Aspects of Child and Family Health, Committee on Early Childhood, Adoption, and Dependent Care, & Section on Developmental and Behavioral Pediatrics. (2012). Early childhood adversity, toxic stress, and the role of the pediatrician: Translating developmental science into lifelong health. *Pediatrics, 129*(1), e224–e231.

Gilles, D., Taylor, F., Gray, C., O'Brien, L., & D'Abrew, N. (2013). Psychological therapies for the treatment of post-traumatic stress disorder in children and adolescents (Review). *Evidence-Based Child Health: A Cochrane Review Journal, 8*(3), 1004–1116.

Gutermann, J., Schreiber, F., Matulis, S., Schwartzkopff, L., Deppe, J., & Stell, R. (2016). Psychological treatments for symptoms of posttraumatic stress disorder in children, adolescents, and young adults: A meta-analysis. *Clinical Child and Family Psychology Review, 19,* 77–93.

Havens, J., Gudiño, O., Biggs, E., Diamond, U., Weis, J., & Cloitre, M. (2012). Identification of trauma exposure and PTSD in adolescent psychiatric inpatients: An exploratory study. *Journal of Traumatic Stress, 25*(2), 171–178.

Hiller, R., Creswell, C., Meiser-Stedman, R., Lobo, S., Cowdrey, F., Lyttle, M., et al. (2019). A longitudinal examination of the relationship between trauma-related cognitive factors and internalising and externalising psychopathology in physically injured children. *Journal of Abnormal Child Psychology, 47*(4), 683–693.

Jensen, T., Holt, T., Mørup Ormhaug, S., Fjermestad, K., & Wentzel-Larsen, T. (2018). Change in post-traumatic cognitions mediates treatment effects for traumatized youth—A randomized controlled trial. *Journal of Counseling Psychology, 65*(2), 166–177.

Kaplow, J., Rolon-Arroyo, B., Layne, C., Rooney, E., Oosterhoff, B., Hill, R., et al. (2020). Validation of the UCLA PTSD Reaction Index for *DSM-5:* A developmentally-informed assessment tool for youth. *Journal of the American Academy of Child and Adolescent Psychiatry, 59*(1), 186–194.

Kassam-Adams, N. (2006). The Acute Stress Checklist for Children (ASC-Kids): Development of a child self-report measure. *Journal of Traumatic Stress, 19*(1), 129–139.

Kaufman, J., Birmaher, B., Brent, D., Rao, U. M. A., Flynn, C., Moreci, P., et al. (1997). Schedule for Affective Disorders and Schizophrenia for School-Age Children-Present and Lifetime Version (K-SADS-PL): Initial reliability and validity data. *Journal of the American Academy of Child and Adolescent Psychiatry, 36*(7), 980–988.

Kenardy, J. A., Spence, S. H., & Macleod, A. C. (2006). Screening for posttraumatic stress disorder in children after accidental injury. *Pediatrics, 118*(3), 1002–1009.

Kovess-Masfety, V., Van Engelen, J., Stone, L., Otten, R., Carta, M., Bitfoi, A., et al. (2017). Unmet need for specialty mental health services among children across Europe. *Psychiatric Services, 68*(8), 789–795.

Landolt, M., Schnyder, U., Maier, T., Schoenbucher, V., & Mohler-Kuo, M. (2013). Trauma exposure and posttraumatic stress disorder in adolescents: A national survey in Switzerland. *Journal of Traumatic Stress, 26*(2), 209–216.

Lang, J. M., & Connell, C. M. (2017). Development and validation of a brief trauma screening measure for children: The Child Trauma Screen. *Psychological Trauma: Theory, Research, Practice, and Policy, 9*(3), 390–398.

Lewis, S., Arseneault, L., Caspi, A., Fisher, H. L., Matthews, T., Moffitt, T. E. et al. (2019). The epidemiology of trauma and post-traumatic stress disorder in a representative cohort of young people in England and Wales. *Lancet Psychiatry, 6*(3), 247–256.

McKinnon, A., Smith, P., Bryant, R., Salmon, K., Yule, W., Dagleish, T., et al. (2016). An update on the clinical utility of the Children's Post-Traumatic Cognitions Inventory. *Journal of Traumatic Stress, 29*(3), 253–258.

McLaughlin, K., Green, J., Gruber, M., Sampson, N., Zaslavsky, A., & Kessler, R. (2012). Childhood adversities and first onset of psychiatric disorder in a national sample of US adolescents. *Archives of General Psychiatry, 69*(11), 1151–1160.

McLean, C., Yeh, R., Rosenfield, D., & Foa, E. (2015). Changes in negative cognitions mediate PTSD symptom reductions during client-centered therapy and prolonged exposure for adolescents. *Behaviour Research and Therapy, 68,* 64–69.

McLennan, J. D., & MacMillan, H. L. (2016). Routine primary care screening for intimate partner violence and other adverse psychosocial exposures: What's the evidence? *BMC Family Practice, 17.* [Epub ahead of print]

Meiser-Stedman, R., Smith, P., Bryant, R., Salmon, K., Yule, W., Dagleish, T., et al. (2009). Development and validation of the Child Post-Traumatic Cognitions Inventory (CPTCI). *Journal of Child Psychology and Psychiatry, 50*(4), 432–440.

Merikangas, K., He, J., Burstein, M., Swendsen, J., Avenevoli, S., Case, B., et al. (2011). Service utilization for lifetime mental disorders in US adolescents: Results of the National Comorbitidy Survey—Adolescent supplement (NCS-A). *Journal of the American Academy of Child and Adolescent Psychiatry, 50*(1), 32–45.

Morina, N., Koerssen, R., & Pollet, T. (2016). Interventions for children and adolescents with posttraumatic stress disorder: A meta-analysis of comparative outcome studies. *Clinical Psychology Review, 47,* 41–54.

Pfeiffer, E., Sachser, C., de Haan, A., Tutus, D., & Goldbeck, L. (2017). Dysfunctional posttraumatic cognitions as a mediator of symptom reduction in trauma-focused cognitive behavioral therapy with children and adolescents: Results of a randomized controlled trial. *Behaviour Research and Therapy, 97,* 178–182.

Putnam, F., Helmers, K., & Trickett, P. (1993). Development, reliability, and validity of a child dissociation scale. *Child Abuse and Neglect, 16*(6), 731–741.

Pynoos, R. S., Weathers, F. W., Steinberg, A. M., Marx, B. P., Layne, C. M., Kaloupek, D. G., et al. (2015). Clinician-Administered PTSD Scale for DSM-5—Child/Adolescent Version. Retrieved from the National Center for PTSD at *www.ptsd.va.gov/professional/assessment/documents/CAPS-CA-5.pdf.*

Ribbe, D. (1996). Psychometric review of Traumatic Event Screening Instrument for Children (TESI-C). In B. H. Stamm (Ed.), *Measurement of stress, trauma, and adaptation* (pp. 386–387). Lutherville, MD: Sidran Press.

Sachser, C., Berliner, L., Holt, T., Jensen, T. K., Jungbluth, N., Risch, E., et al. (2017). International development and psychometric properties of the Child and Adolescent Trauma Screen (CATS). *Journal of Affective Disorders, 210,* 189–195.

Sachser, C., Keller, F., & Goldbeck, L. (2017). Complex PTSD as proposed for ICD-11: Validation of a new disorder in children and adolescents and their response to trauma-focused cognitive therapy. *Journal of Child Psychology and Psychiatry, 58*(2), 160–168.

Saigh, P. A. (2004). *The Children's Posttraumatic Stress Disorder Inventory.* San Antonio, TX: Psychological Corp.

Salazar, A., Keller, T., Gowen, L., & Courtney, M. (2013). Trauma exposure and PTSD among older adolescents in foster care. *Social Psychiatry and Psychiatric Epidemiology, 58*(4), 545–551.

Saunders, B., & Adams, Z. (2014). Epidemiology of traumatic experiences in childhood. *Child and Adolescent Psychiatric Clinics of North America, 23,* 167–184.

Sawyer, M., Reece, C., Sawyer, A., Johnson, S., Hiscock, H., & Lawrence, D. (2018). Access to health professionals by children and adolescents with mental disorders: Are we meeting their needs? *Australian and New Zealand Journal of Psychiatry, 52*(10), 972–982.

Saxe, G., Chawla, N., Stoddard, F., Kassam-Adams, N., Courtney, D., Cunningham, K., et al. (2003). Child Stress Disorders Checklist: A measure of ASD and PTSD in children. *Journal of the American Academy of Child and Adolescent Psychiatry, 42*(8), 972–978.

Saylor, C. F., Swenson, C. C., Stokes Reynolds, S., & Taylor, M. (1999). The Pediatric Emotional Distress Scale: A brief screening measure for young children exposed to traumatic events. *Journal of Clinical Child Psychology, 28*(1), 70–81.

Scheeringa, M. S., & Haslett, N. (2010). The reliability and criterion validity of the Diagnostic Infant and Preschool Assessment: A new diagnostic instrument for young children. *Child Psychiatry & Human Development, 41*(3), 299–312.

Schilpzand, E., Conroy, R., Anderson, V., & Alisic, E. (2018). Development and evaluation of the Thinking About Recovery Scale: Measure of parent posttraumatic cognitions following children's exposure to trauma. *Journal of Traumatic Stress, 31,* 71–78.

Silverman, W. K., & Albano, A. M. (1996). *The Anxiety Disorders Interview Schedule for Children (ADIS-C/P).* San Antonio, TX: Psychological Corp.

Simon, A., Pastor, P., Reuben, C., Huang, L., & Goldstrom, E. (2015). Use of mental health services by children ages six to 11 with emotional or behavioural difficulties. *Psychiatric Services, 66*(9), 930–937.

Skar, A-M. S., Ormhaug, S., & Jensen, T. (2019). Reported levels of upset following routine trauma screening at mental health services. *JAMA Network Open, 2*(5), e194003.

Sumner, S., Mercy, J., Saul, J., Motsa-Nzuza, N., Kwesigabo, G., Buluma, R., et al. (2015). Prevalence of sexual violence against children and use of social services—Seven countries, 2007–2013. *Morbidity and Mortality Weekly Report, 64*(21), 565–569.

Trickey, D., Siddaway, A., Meiser-Stedman, R., Serpell, L., & Field, A. (2012). A meta-analysis of risk factors for post-traumatic stress disorder in children and adolescents. *Clinical Psychology Review, 32,* 122–138.

Williamson, V., Hiller, R., Meiser-Stedman, R., Creswell, C., Dalgleish, T., Fearon, P., et al. (2018). The Parent Trauma Response Questionnaire (PTRQ): Development and preliminary validation. *European Journal of Psychotraumatology, 9,* 1478583.

World Health Organization. (2018). *International statistical classification of diseases and related health problems* (11th rev.). Geneva, Switzerland: Author. Retrieved February 2, 2019, from *https://icd.who.int/browse11/l-m/en.*

Zajac, K., Ruggiero, K., Smith, D., Saunders, B., & Kilpatrick, D. (2011). Adolescent distress in traumatic stress research: Data from the National Survey of Adolescents-Replication. *Journal of Traumatic Stress, 24,* 226–229.

CHAPTER 6

ISTSS PTSD Prevention and Treatment Guidelines
Methodology

Jonathan I. Bisson, Catrin Lewis, and Neil P. Roberts

This chapter outlines the methodology and the subsequent recommendations for the *Posttraumatic Stress Disorder Prevention and Treatment Guidelines* of the International Society for Traumatic Stress Studies (ISTSS). Important issues that should be considered when interpreting the recommendations, and translating them into practice, are highlighted.

Introduction and Methodology Overview

The recommendations and position papers were developed through a rigorous process that was overseen by the ISTSS Guidelines Committee (listed in Appendix 6.1). The methodology involved the development of scoping questions and undertaking systematic reviews to identify randomized controlled trials (RCTs) that could answer them (Appendix 6.2). Meta-analyses were then conducted with usable data from included studies, and the results used to generate recommendations for prevention and treatment interventions. A definition of clinical importance and an algorithm for determining the recommendation level of a given intervention were agreed upon before the meta-analyses were undertaken.

Given the limited resources available, it was not possible to commission new comprehensive systematic reviews in every area. It was, however, possible to develop a robust and replicable process that systematically gathered and considered the RCT evidence currently available for any intervention in a standardized manner. A process adapted from approaches taken by the Australian Centre for Posttraumatic Mental Health (2007; now the Phoenix Australia–Centre for Posttraumatic Mental Health), the Cochrane Collaboration (Higgins & Green, 2011), the United Kingdom's National Institute for Health and Care Excellence (NICE; 2005), and the World Health Organization (WHO; 2013) was used.

The Committee agreed on general scoping questions in a PICO (population, intervention, comparator, outcomes) format (e.g., "For adults with PTSD [posttraumatic stress disorder], do psychological treatments, when compared to treatment as usual, waiting list, or no treatment, result in a clinically important reduction of symptoms, improved functioning/quality of life, presence of disorder, or adverse effects?") for the prevention and treatment of PTSD in children, adolescents, and adults. Prior to finalization, the Committee sought and integrated feedback from the ISTSS membership around these scoping questions.

High-quality systematic reviews developed through the Cochrane Collaboration, NICE, and WHO were identified that addressed the scoping questions. RCTs from these reviews were used as the basis of the evidence to be considered and reevaluated according to the criteria agreed upon for the ISTSS guidelines. Existing reviews were supplemented with additional systematic searches for more recent RCTs and by asking experts in the field and the ISTSS membership to determine if there were any missing studies.

The evidence for each of the scoping questions was summarized and its quality assessed using the Cochrane Collaboration's risk of bias rating tool (Higgins & Green, 2011) to assess for potential methodological concerns within identified studies. The Cochrane Collaboration's risk of bias criteria determine low-, uncertain-, or high-risk ratings for random sequence generation (selection bias); allocation concealment (selection bias); blinding of participants and personnel (performance bias); blinding of outcome assessment (detection bias); incomplete outcome data (attrition bias); selective reporting (reporting bias); and other bias. The GRADE Working Group Grades of Evidence system (see *www.gradeworkinggroup.org*) was used to determine the level of confidence that the estimate of the effect of an intervention is correct. There are four possible ratings: high quality (further research is very unlikely to change our confidence in the estimate of effect); moderate quality (further research is likely to have an important impact on our confidence in the estimate of effect and may change the estimate); low quality (further research is very likely to have an important impact on our confidence in the estimate of effect and is likely to change the estimate); and very low quality (we are very uncertain about the estimate).

The evidence summaries and quality assessments were then used to generate draft recommendations using the algorithm described. The draft recommendations were posted on the ISTSS website during August and September 2018, for a period of consultation by ISTSS members. Feedback was incorporated before the recommendations were finalized and approved by the ISTSS Board in October 2018.

Scoping Questions

Following consultation with the ISTSS membership and reference groups of practitioners and nonpractitioner consumers, the ISTSS Guidelines Committee proposed 20 scoping questions that were passed by the ISTSS Board. Inclusion of separate scoping questions on treatments for complex presentations of PTSD for children, adolescents, and adults was considered. Concerns were raised, however, that due to definitional issues and the virtual absence of studies specifically designed to answer possible scoping questions on treatments for complex presentations of PTSD, their inclusion would be unlikely to provide clear answers.

It was concluded that, rather than systematically reviewing the evidence for the treatment of complex presentations of PTSD, it would likely be more beneficial to undertake a narrative review of the current situation with respect to complex PTSD, what it is, and how it should be defined to enable the development of an evidence base of how best to treat it. Facilitated by the publication of the ICD-11 diagnosis of complex PTSD during the course of the Committee's operation, position papers (one for children and adolescents, and one for adults) were developed that consider the current issues around complex PTSD and make recommendations to facilitate further research. The position papers were drafted by members of the ISTSS Guidelines Committee and in consultation with the rest of the Committee, the ISTSS Board, and ISTSS membership before being finalized.

Systematic Reviews and Meta-Analyses

New systematic searches were undertaken by the Cochrane Collaboration for the period from January 1, 2008, until March 31, 2018, using their comprehensive search strategies, to identify RCTs of any intervention designed to prevent or treat PTSD. Additional RCTs were identified through consultation with experts in the field, including the ISTSS Board and the entire ISTSS membership.

The new searches identified 5,500 potential new studies. These and the studies included in existing systematic reviews were assessed against the inclusion criteria agreed upon for the ISTSS guidelines. The inclusion criteria were designed to focus on reduction in symptoms of PTSD as the primary outcome and differed slightly for early intervention and treatment studies (i.e., as opposed to early intervention studies, treatment studies required a defined severity of PTSD symptoms to be included).

The inclusion criteria for early intervention studies were:

- Any RCT (including cluster and crossover trials) evaluating the efficacy of interventions aimed at preventing, treating, or reducing symptoms of PTSD.
- Study participants have been exposed to a traumatic event, as specified by PTSD diagnostic criteria for DSM-III, DSM-III-R, DSM-IV, DSM-5, ICD-9, ICD-10, or ICD-11.
- Intervention is not provided pretrauma.
- Intervention begins no later than 3 months after the traumatic event.
- Eligible comparator interventions for psychosocial interventions: waitlist, treatment as usual, symptom monitoring, repeated assessment, other minimal-attention control group, or an alternative psychological treatment.
- Eligible comparator interventions for pharmacological interventions: placebo, other pharmacological or psychosocial intervention.
- The RCT is not solely a dismantling study.
- Study outcomes include a standardized measure of PTSD symptoms (either clinician-administered or self-report).
- No restriction on the basis of severity of PTSD symptoms or the type of traumatic event.
- Individual, group, and couple interventions.
- No minimum sample size.
- Only studies published in English.
- Unpublished studies eligible.

The inclusion criteria for treatment studies were:

- Any RCT (including cluster and crossover trials) evaluating the efficacy of psychological interventions aimed at reducing symptoms of PTSD.
- For adults, at least 70% of participants required to be diagnosed with PTSD according to DSM or ICD criteria by means of a structured interview or diagnosis by a clinician.
- For children and adolescents, at least 70% diagnosed with partial or full DSM or ICD PTSD by means of a structured interview or diagnosis by a clinician (partial PTSD is defined as at least one symptom per cluster and presence of impairment), or score above a standard cutoff of a validated self-report measure.
- No restrictions on the basis of comorbidity, but PTSD required to be the primary diagnosis.
- Eligible comparator interventions for psychosocial interventions: waitlist, treatment as usual, symptom monitoring, repeated assessment, other minimal-attention control group, or an alternative psychological treatment.
- Eligible comparator interventions for pharmacological interventions: placebo, other pharmacological or psychosocial intervention.

- The RCT is not solely a dismantling study.
- Duration of PTSD symptoms required to be 3 months or more.
- No restriction on the basis of severity of PTSD symptoms or the type of traumatic event.
- Individual, group, and couple interventions.
- No minimum sample size.
- Only studies published in English.
- Unpublished studies eligible.

A total of 361 RCTs fulfilled the criteria for inclusion in the meta-analyses undertaken. Studies that fulfilled the inclusion criteria were further scrutinized to determine if data were available to use in the meta-analyses, and to assess risk of bias according to the Cochrane Collaboration criteria. If sufficient data were not available, requests were made to authors for data that could be used. A total of 327 (91%) of the included RCTs provided data that were included in the meta-analyses. The classification and grouping of the interventions included are described. The final meta-analyses and reference lists of all eligible studies can be found on the ISTSS website (*www. istss.org/getattachment/Treating-Trauma/New-ISTSS-Prevention-and-Treatment-Guidelines/ISTSS_PreventionTreatmentGuidelines_FNL.pdf.aspx*).

Definition of Clinical Importance

To generate recommendations from the results of the meta-analyses, the following definition of clinical importance was developed and agreed upon:

- PTSD symptom change was the primary outcome measure and other outcomes (e.g., diagnosis, functioning, other symptom change, tolerability) were considered as secondary outcome measures.
- The clinically important definition was based on both magnitude of change and strength/quality of evidence.
- Informed by previous work in this area (e.g., NICE, 2005) to be rated clinically important, an intervention delivered 3 or more months after the traumatic event had to demonstrate an effect size, calculated as the standardized mean difference (SMD), for continuous outcomes of >0.8 (<0.65 relative risk for binary outcomes) for wait-list control comparisons, >0.5 for attention control comparisons (no meaningful treatment, but same dosage of time/same number of sessions with a therapist), >0.4 for placebo control comparisons, and >0.2 for active treatment control comparisons.
- To be rated clinically important, an early intervention started within 3 months of the traumatic event had to demonstrate an effect size for continuous outcomes of >0.5 for wait-list control comparisons (<0.8 relative risk for binary outcomes).

- If there was only one RCT, an intervention was not normally recommended as clinically important. Noninferiority RCT evidence alone was not enough to recommend an intervention as clinically important.
- Unless there was a GRADE quality of evidence rating of high or moderate, consideration was given to downgrading the strength of recommendation made with respect to clinical importance.
- The primary analysis for a particular question included data from all included studies. When available, this was clinician rated; when not, self-report was included. In addition, an analysis was also considered of only studies with clinician-rated data. The combination of these two analyses was considered along with the GRADE ratings and risk of bias ratings to determine the strength of recommendation.
- The 95% confidence interval range had to completely exclude the thresholds for the strongest level of recommendation (e.g., lower confidence interval of >0.8 for wait-list control comparisons of treatments).

Recommendation Setting

An algorithm was developed to allow the systematic and objective agreement of recommendations after scrutiny of the meta-analyses pertaining to individual scoping questions. Consideration was given to magnitude of change, strength/quality of evidence, and any other important factors (e.g., adverse effects).

Five different levels of recommendation were possible. A *Strong* recommendation was made for/against interventions with at least reasonable quality of evidence and the highest certainty of effect. A *Standard* recommendation was made when there was at least reasonable quality of evidence and lower certainty of effect. An *Intervention with Low Effect* recommendation was made for interventions with at least reasonable quality of evidence and high certainty of a low level of effect. An *Intervention with Emerging Evidence* recommendation was made for interventions with lower quality of evidence and/or certainty of effect. An *Insufficient Evidence to Recommend* recommendation was made when there was an absence of evidence of effectiveness or ineffectiveness.

The following criteria had to be met for a *Strong* recommendation:

- *Quality*–GRADE rating better than low or mean less than 3 for red-rated risk of bias criteria for the meta-analysis on which results were based. (If the mean number of high risk of bias criteria is 3 or more, a sensitivity analysis excluding the high-risk studies is undertaken and used as the primary meta-analysis if the effectiveness criterion was met.)

- *Effectiveness*–Results met the clinical importance definition for the primary outcome. Alternatively, results showed strong evidence of equivalence (in head-to-head trials) to an intervention that met the clinical importance definition. If the only results pertained to a single RCT, over 300 participants per arm were required.
- *Other factors*–No other factors identified resulted in the Committee recommending against a strong recommendation.

The following criteria had to be met for a *Standard* recommendation:

- *Quality*–GRADE rating better than low or mean less than 3 for red-rated risk of bias criteria for the meta-analysis on which results were based. (If the mean number of high risk of bias criteria was 3 or more, a sensitivity analysis excluding high-risk studies was undertaken and used as the primary meta-analysis if the effectiveness criterion was met.)
- *Effectiveness*–Results did not meet the clinical importance definition for the primary outcome, but the mean difference/relative risk was greater than the threshold. If the results pertained to a single RCT, over 100 participants per arm were required.
- *Other factors*–No other factors resulted in the Committee recommending against a standard recommendation.

The following criteria had to be met for an *Intervention with Low Effect* recommendation:

- *Quality*–GRADE rating better than low or mean less than 3 for red-rated risk of bias criteria for the meta-analysis on which results were based. (If the mean number of high risk of bias criteria is 3 or more, a sensitivity analysis excluding high-risk studies was undertaken and used as the primary meta-analysis if the effectiveness criterion was met.)
- *Effectiveness*–Results did not meet the clinical importance definition for the primary outcome and the mean difference/relative risk was less than the threshold. If the results pertained to a single RCT, over 300 participants per arm were required.
- *Other factors*–No other factors resulted in the Committee recommending against an intervention with low effect recommendation.

Intervention with Emerging Evidence was used if the quality criteria for a strong, standard, or low effect recommendation were not met, but the results and 95% CIs were better than the control condition. If the results pertained to a single RCT, at least 20 participants per arm were required and there had to be no other factors that resulted in the Committee recommending against an emerging intervention recommendation.

Insufficient Evidence to Recommend was used for all interventions when the primary meta-analysis results did not meet the clinical importance definition for the primary outcome and the 95% CIs overlapped with the point of no difference to the control condition.

An example of a generated recommendation follows:

- Scoping question: "For adults with PTSD, do pharmacological treatments, when compared to placebo, result in a clinically significant reduction of symptoms, improved functioning/quality of life, presence of disorder, or adverse effects?"
- Recommendation: Drug X is recommended for the treatment of adults with posttraumatic stress disorder.
- Strength of recommendation: *Standard.*

ISTSS Member Consultation

ISTSS members were consulted at various points of the process. Initially, they were asked to comment on the scoping questions and methodology. They were also asked to consider reference lists of eligible studies to determine if studies were missing. Finally, they were asked to review the initial draft evidence summaries and recommendations, to check them for any apparent inaccuracies, and to consider the following questions:

1. Have the agreed-upon "rules" been applied consistently and appropriately with respect to the levels of recommendation made?
2. Are any studies missing?
3. Are there any apparent inaccuracies in the position papers?

Key Points to Consider in Interpreting the Recommendations

As a result of resource constraints, the focus was on the prevention and treatment of PTSD rather than other conditions/outcomes. The primary outcome measure for all the scoping questions was a continuous measure of PTSD symptoms.

The scoping questions selected did not cover all questions of relevance to the traumatic stress field and resulted in key elements of the evidence base not being considered. For example, community- and school-based interventions for populations in conflict zones that did not occur within 3 months of a traumatic event were not included and studies focusing on comorbidity were not included, unless PTSD was the primary diagnosis.

Studies that did not meet the strict inclusion criteria were not considered. This included a number of high-quality, innovative studies such as dismantling RCTs and RCTs that focused on different ways of delivering the same intervention (e.g., face-to-face or telemedicine delivery).

The recommendations are primarily based on efficacy as determined by meta-analyses of RCTs. RCT evidence of effect is very important and should strongly influence clinical decision making, but it should not dictate it. It is important to remember the maxim, "Absence of evidence does not mean absence of effect" and that "good health care professionals use both individual clinical expertise and the best available external evidence, and neither alone is enough" (Sackett, Rosenberg, Muir Gray, Haynes, & Richardson, 1996).

The studies included in the meta-analyses cover heterogeneous settings and populations. These and other factors—for example, variation in therapist competence, differences between grouped interventions, and the number of sessions/dosage delivered—mean that care should be taken in interpreting recommendations and determining their implications for clinical practice.

It is possible for pharmacological, psychological, and other forms of intervention to cause adverse effects and to be less tolerated by some individuals than others. Although there was no reason found to downgrade the level of recommendation for any intervention on this basis, it cannot be assumed that they will be appropriate for all PTSD sufferers.

Whatever the recommendation, interventions should only be delivered after a thorough assessment of individuals' needs and, where possible, a discussion between the individual (and/or caregivers) and therapist with clear information about the evidence base, potential benefits and risks to allow informed decision making and the development of a coproduced intervention plan.

Classification and Grouping of Interventions

Various interventions have been studied for the prevention and treatment of PTSD, and it is vital that similar and different interventions are grouped in a meaningful way for appropriate meta-analyses to be undertaken. The ISTSS Guidelines Committee therefore agreed to group interventions into categories that would be widely recognized as separate by the traumatic stress community and allow discrimination between different types of intervention.

Individual meta-analyses were undertaken for all pharmacological treatments identified. Psychological and other interventions for the prevention and treatment of PTSD can be divided into those with a trauma focus and those without a trauma focus, and into those delivered to individuals, couples, or groups, but greater granularity is required to maximize the accuracy and usefulness of prevention and treatment recommendations. When sufficient studies were available, the principle that interventions should be grouped according to their broad theoretical base (e.g., CBT-T, EMDR therapy, psychodynamic therapy) was used. Subgroups were then developed if there was good evidence that a more homogeneous grouping could be created that was based on a specific, well-defined intervention that would be widely recognized as a discrete intervention by individuals working in the field (e.g., prolonged exposure, cognitive processing therapy).

Early Interventions

The following groupings/subgroupings were agreed upon for early interventions:

A. *Interventions with a trauma focus*

1. **Brief eye movement desensitization and reprocessing (EMDR therapy).** EMDR therapy is a standardized, eight-phase, trauma-focused therapy involving the use of bilateral physical stimulation (eye movements, taps, or tones). Targeted traumatic memories are considered in terms of an image, the associated cognition, the associated affect, and body sensation. These four components are then focused on as bilateral physical stimulation occurs. It is hypothesized that EMDR therapy stimulates the individual's own information processing to help integrate the targeted memory as an adaptive contextualized memory. Processing targets involve past events, present triggers, and adaptive future functioning. EMDR therapy at times uses restricted questioning related to cognitive processes paired with bilateral stimulation to unblock processing.

2. **Brief individual trauma processing therapy.** This subgroup consisted of a number of brief therapies—lasting two or more sessions—that were theoretically diverse but shared similar core treatment components. These included psychoeducation and therapist-directed reliving of the index trauma to promote elaboration of the trauma memory and help to contextualize or reframe aspects of the experience.

3. **Cognitive-behavioral therapy with a trauma focus (CBT-T).** CBT-T includes all therapies that aim to help PTSD sufferers and those displaying early traumatic stress symptoms by addressing and changing their thoughts, beliefs, and/or behavior. Typically, CBT-T involves homework and includes psychoeducation, exposure work, cognitive work, and more general relaxation/stress management; the relative contribution of these elements varies between different forms of CBT-T.

4. **Debriefing.** The debriefing interventions are single-session and based on critical incident stress debriefing; individuals are asked to provide detailed facts of what happened, their thoughts, reactions,

and symptoms before being provided with psychoeducation about symptoms and how to deal with them.

5. **Group 512 PM.** Group 512 PM is based on debriefing but supplemented with cohesion training exercises, for example, playing games that require team cooperation.

6. **Internet virtual reality therapy.** This involves CBT-T delivered through a virtual reality therapy room, rather than face-to-face.

7. **Nurse-led intensive care recovery program.** This intervention, based on several models, involved delivery of a nurse-led psychological intervention aimed at developing a narrative about the individual's admission and stay in an intensive care unit.

8. **Stepped/collaborative care (SCC).** SCC involves the provision of flexible and modular interventions based on needs identified through screening and direct assessment. Individuals may be offered a range of different psychological interventions based on identified need. Intervention is normally CBT based, but sometimes based on other psychological approaches (e.g., motivational interviewing) and may include components of case management and prescription of pharmacological intervention.

9. **Structured writing therapy (SWT).** SWT involves individuals undertaking guided homework-based writing assignments about their trauma experience and their thoughts and feelings. SWT does not involve the teaching or practice of cognitive therapy-based techniques.

10. **Telephone-based CBT-T.** CBT-T delivered by telephone, rather than face-to-face.

B. *Interventions without a trauma focus*

1. **Behavioral activation (BA).** BA aims to help the individual learn to manage negative feelings through activity planning. Core features of intervention include psychoeducation, behavioral analysis, activity planning, goal identification, troubleshooting, homework, and relapse prevention.

2. **Brief dyadic therapy.** This subgroup consisted of brief CBT-based therapies delivered dyadically with the aim of improving communication and fostering a shared approach to addressing psychological and practical difficulties.

3. **Brief interpersonal psychotherapy (IPT).** IPT focuses on individuals' social and interpersonal functioning and helps patients develop skills in social interactions and social support mobilization. The focus is on current interpersonal encounters rather than past trauma.

4. **Brief parenting intervention.** This intervention is delivered following premature birth primarily focused on supporting the interaction between the neonate and mother.

5. **Cognitive therapy.** This includes a variety of non-trauma-focused techniques commonly used in generic CBT, including, but not limited to, stress management, emotional stabilization, relaxation training, breathing retraining, positive thinking and self-talk, assertiveness training, thought stopping, and stress inoculation training. Cognitive therapy does not involve exposure to trauma memories with the aim of undertaking reprocessing.

6. **Communication facilitator in an intensive care setting.** This approach involves intervention aimed at trying to understand the needs of patients and their families in an intensive care setting and active liaison between clinicians and patients and family members to improve communication and expectations.

7. **Computerized neurobehavioral training.** This intervention aims to teach participants skills to improve neurocognitive functioning through an online program. Participants are encouraged to practice new skills through regular practice.

8. **Computerized visuospatial task.** This involves playing a computer game (e.g., Tetris) to disrupt consolidation of trauma memories.

9. **Intensive care diaries.** This approach is based on the provision of postdischarge daily feedback to patients admitted to intensive care units to help promote an understanding of events that occurred during their admission.

10. **Self-guided Internet-based intervention.** This approach uses Internet-based programs to treat PTSD sufferers using CBT approaches. Use of the intervention is self-directed.

11. **Supportive/nondirective counseling (SC).** SC involves active, empathic listening to the patient who is usually provided with unconditional positive regard. The therapist helps the patient to explore and clarify issues, may provide advice, reflect and confirm appropriate reactions, and introduce problem-solving techniques. SC has been used as a non-trauma-focused control condition in several trials, and focused attention on the index trauma event is usually avoided.

12. **Supported psychoeducational intervention.** This intervention involves the provision of psychoeducational information, normally in booklet or leaflet form, with follow-up guidance, typically by telephone, aimed at reinforcing use of the psychoeducational material.

13. **Telephone-based CBT.** CBT delivered by telephone, rather than face-to-face.

Treatment Interventions

The following groupings/subgroupings were agreed upon for treatment interventions:

A. *Psychological interventions with a trauma focus*

1. **CBT-T.** CBT-T includes all therapies that aim to help PTSD sufferers by addressing and changing their thoughts, beliefs, and/or behavior. Typically, CBT-T involves homework and includes psychoeducation, exposure work, cognitive work, and more general relaxation/stress management; the relative contribution of these elements varies between different forms of CBT-T.

   For children and adolescents, separate meta-analyses were undertaken for CBT-T delivered to child/adolescent only, child/adolescent and caregiver, and caregiver only. TF-CBT is a specific, phase-based model of CBT-T delivered to child/adolescent and caregiver. The first phase includes affect regulation skills and the second phase processing of the trauma narrative. Gradual exposure is incorporated into all components to enhance the child's/adolescent's and caregiver's mastery of trauma reminders. Caregivers are included, when possible, throughout treatment to support the child's/adolescent's practice and mastery of skills and to enhance positive parenting and parental support.

   For adults, the following therapies have been included in meta-analyses as subgroups of CBT-T for individuals or couples (there were not enough RCTs of different types of group therapy to allow meaningful subgroup analyses):

   a. *Brief eclectic psychotherapy for PTSD (BEPP)*. BEPP draws on elements of CBT-T and psychodynamic therapy, including the relationship between the patient and the therapist. It includes exposure to traumatic memories, therapeutic letter writing, and consideration of how the individual has been affected by his or her experience(s). BEPP usually ends with a farewell ritual.

   b. *Cognitive therapy for PTSD (CT-PTSD)*. CT-PTSD focuses on the identification and modification of negative appraisals and behaviors that lead the PTSD sufferer to overestimate current threat (fear). It also involves modification of beliefs related to other aspects of the experience and how the individual interprets his or her behavior during the trauma (e.g., issues concerning guilt and shame).

   c. *Cognitive processing therapy (CPT)*. The main focus of CPT is on the evaluation and modification of problematic thoughts that have developed following the traumatic experience(s). For example, using cognitive techniques to challenge typical thoughts of PTSD, that the individual is to blame for his or her trauma or that the world is now unsafe. An optional component of CPT is the development of a detailed written narrative account of the trauma.

   d. *Internet-based CBT-T*. Internet-based CBT-T uses Internet-based programs to treat PTSD sufferers using CBT-T approaches. A therapist who has less contact with the patient than in traditional face-to-face CBT-T often guides Internet-based CBT-T.

e. *Narrative exposure therapy (NET)*. NET allows PTSD sufferers to describe and develop a coherent, chronological, autobiographical narrative of their life that includes their traumatic experiences (a testimony). The therapist facilitates emotional processing through the use of cognitive-behavioral techniques. A modified version (KidNET) has been developed for children.

f. *Prolonged exposure (PE)*. The primary focus of PE is to help the PTSD sufferer to confront her or his traumatic memories using a verbal narrative technique that involves detailed recounting of the traumatic experience, which is then recorded and listened to on a repeated basis with the goal of habituation. In addition, real-life repeated exposure to avoided and fear-evoking situations, which are now safe but associated with the trauma, is undertaken, again with the aim of habituation.

g. *Reconsolidation of traumatic memories (RTM)*. RTM involves activation of a traumatic memory and a subsequent procedure that includes imagining a black-and-white movie of the event, dissociated from its content, and rewinding it when fully associated over 2 seconds. This is designed to change the perspective from which a memory is recalled.

h. *Virtual reality therapy (VRT)*. VRT involves the PTSD sufferer being exposed to a computer-generated virtual reality that is representative of the individual's traumatic experience(s). A therapist is present and regulates the amount of exposure according to the patient's response. The aim is to achieve habituation.

i. *Written emotional disclosure (WED)*. WED involves the PTSD sufferer writing about his or her traumatic experience(s) based on the belief that suppressed thoughts and emotions maintain PTSD symptoms and accessing, expressing, and processing them will be beneficial.

2. **Dialogical exposure therapy (DET).** DET uses CBT techniques (with and without a trauma focus) and a Gestalt-based exposure method (chair work) in a dialogical framework. Supported by the therapist, the individual enters into a dialogue with aspects of the traumatic experience.

3. **Emotional freedom techniques (EFT).** EFT is a trauma-focused intervention that involves recalling a traumatic event and pairing it with a statement of self-acceptance. This statement is verbally repeated while energy meridians used in acupuncture are stimulated using finger taps rather than needles.

4. **EMDR therapy.** EMDR therapy is a standardized, eight-phase, trauma-focused therapy involving the use of bilateral physical stimulation (eye

movements, taps, or tones). Targeted traumatic memories are considered in terms of an image, the associated cognition, the associated affect, and body sensation. These four components are then focused on as bilateral physical stimulation occurs. It is hypothesized that EMDR therapy stimulates the individual's own information processing to help integrate the targeted memory as an adaptive contextualized memory. Processing targets involve past events, present triggers, and adaptive future functioning. EMDR therapy at times uses restricted questioning related to cognitive processes paired with bilateral stimulation to unblock processing.

5. **Observed and experiential integration (OEI).** OEI involves alternately covering and uncovering the eyes ("switching") and the eyes tracking different locations in the visual field ("glitch-work") while experiencing a disturbing thought, feeling, or memory. It also includes observation of differences between the two eyes' perceptions.

6. **Rapid eye movement desensitization (REM-D).** REM-D initially involves conditioning soothing images with a calming piece of music. Individuals then wear glasses during sleep that detect rapid eye movements (as would occur during dreams) and activate playing of the same piece of music for a period of 30 seconds with the aim of desensitization during nightmares.

B. *Psychological and other interventions without a trauma focus*

1. **Acupuncture.** Acupuncture involves the insertion of fine needles at specific points on the body (acupressure points) to reduce symptoms of PTSD.

2. **Attentional bias modification (ABM).** ABM is a treatment designed for the management of anxiety disorders based on the finding that patients with anxiety disorders selectively attend to threatening information. It involves computer-based training to divert attention away from threatening information.

3. **CBT without a trauma focus.** This includes a heterogeneous group of therapies that use a variety of non-trauma-focused techniques commonly used in generic CBT, including, but not limited to, stress management, emotional stabilization, relaxation training, breathing retraining, positive thinking and self-talk, assertiveness training, thought stopping, and stress inoculation training.

4 **Hypnotherapy.** Hypnotherapy uses hypnosis to induce an altered state of consciousness before undertaking therapeutic work.

5. **IPT.** IPT is an attachment-based treatment that focuses on current interpersonal problems and the resolution of these to improve symptoms.

6. **Mantram repetition.** This involves repeating a holy word(s) or phrase(s).

7. **Metacognitive therapy (MT).** MT involves a focus on metacognition, the aspect of cognition that controls our thinking and conscious experience. MC aims to change unhelpful thinking patterns that may be maintaining symptoms by addressing the metacognitive beliefs that give rise to them.

8. **Mind–body skills.** Mind–body skills include various techniques, including mindfulness, meditation, guided imagery, expressive drawing and writing, self-hypnosis, and biofeedback.

9. **Mindfulness-based stress reduction (MBSR).** MBSR aims to help individuals experience traumatic memories without significant distress by facilitating acceptance of them. MBSR includes meditation practice, mindful awareness practice, and its application to real-life situations.

10. **Neurofeedback.** Neurofeedback involves real-time displays of brain activity that are used to help individuals train (self-regulate) their brain activity.

11. **Parent–child relationship enhancement.** Parent–child relationship enhancement describes therapies that use different techniques, for example, play, with a primary focus to improve parent–child relationships.

12. **Present-centered therapy (PCT).** PCT is designed to target daily challenges that PTSD sufferers encounter as a result of their symptoms. It includes psychoeducation about the impact of PTSD symptoms, the development of effective strategies to deal with day-to-day challenges, and homework to practice newly developed skills.

13. **Psychodynamic therapy.** Psychodynamic therapy uses psychoanalytic theories and practices to help individuals understand and resolve their problems by increasing awareness of their inner world and its influences over current and past relationships.

14. **Psychoeducation.** Psychoeducation provides individuals with information about traumatic stress reactions, PTSD, and how to manage them.

15. **Saikokeishikankyoto.** This is a traditional Japanese herbal medicine.

16. **Somatic experiencing.** This involves a focus on perceived body sensations and to learn how to regulate these with the aim of resolving symptoms.

17. **Stepped-care CBT-T.** This is an intervention developed for children with the introduction of a first step (before therapist-led CBT-T) of parent-led treatment supported by a therapist and Web-based materials. If children require more treatment, they then receive CBT-T.

18. **Supportive/nondirective counseling (SC).** SC involves active, empathic listening to the patient, who is usually provided with unconditional positive regard. The therapist helps the patient to explore

and clarify issues, may provide advice, reflect and confirm appropriate reactions, and introduce problem-solving techniques.

19. **Transcranial magnetic stimulation (TMS).** TMS uses magnetic fields to stimulate nerve cells in targeted areas of the brain. It is usually given in a repetitive manner and is noninvasive.

20. **Yoga.** Yoga is an integrative practice of body postures, breathing, and meditation. It aims to increase present-focused attention and awareness and to facilitate mindfulness and acceptance.

REFERENCES

Australian Centre for Posttraumatic Mental Health. (2007). *Australian guidelines for the treatment of adults with acute stress disorder and posttraumatic stress disorder.* Melbourne, Australia: Author.

Higgins, J. P. T., & Green, S. (Eds.). (2011, March). Cochrane handbook for systematic reviews of interventions, Version 5.1.0. Retrieved from *http://training. cochrane.org/handbook.*

National Institute for Health and Clinical Excellence. (2005). *Post-traumatic stress disorder.* London: Royal College of Psychiatrists & the British Psychological Society.

Sackett, D., Rosenberg, W., Muir Gray, J., Haynes, R., & Richardson, W. (1996). Evidence based medicine: What it is and what it isn't. *British Medical Journal, 312,* 71–72.

World Health Organization. (2013). *Guidelines for the management of conditions specifically related to stress.* Geneva, Switzerland: Author.

APPENDIX 6.1. ISTSS Committee for the Development of the PTSD Prevention and Treatment Guidelines

Lucy Berliner

Jonathan I. Bisson (Chair)

Marylene Cloitre

David Forbes (Vice Chair)

Lutz Goldbeck[1]

Tine Jensen[1]

Catrin Lewis

Candice M. Monson

Miranda Olff

Stephen Pilling

David S. Riggs

Neil P. Roberts

Francine Shapiro[2]

---

[1]Lutz Goldbeck tragically died on October 30, 2017, and Tine Jensen subsequently joined the Committee.

[2]Francine Shapiro tragically died on June 16, 2019, following completion of the guidelines and her contributions to this volume.

APPENDIX 6.2. Scoping Questions

1. For children and adolescents within the first 3 months of a traumatic event, do psychosocial interventions, when compared to intervention as usual, waiting list, or no intervention, result in a clinically important reduction/prevention of symptoms, improved functioning/quality of life, presence of disorder, or adverse effects?

2. For children and adolescents within the first 3 months of a traumatic event, do psychosocial interventions, when compared to other psychosocial interventions, result in a clinically important reduction/prevention of symptoms, improved functioning/quality of life, presence of disorder, or adverse effects?

3. For adults within the first 3 months of a traumatic event, do psychosocial interventions, when compared to intervention as usual, waiting list, or no intervention, result in a clinically important reduction/prevention of symptoms, improved functioning/quality of life, presence of disorder, or adverse effects?

4. For adults within the first 3 months of a traumatic event, do psychosocial interventions, when compared to other psychosocial interventions, result in a clinically important reduction/prevention of symptoms, improved functioning/quality of life, presence of disorder, or adverse effects?

5. For children and adolescents within the first 3 months of a traumatic event, do pharmacological interventions, when compared to placebo, result in a clinically important reduction/prevention of symptoms, improved functioning/quality of life, presence of disorder, or adverse effects?

6. For children and adolescents within the first 3 months of a traumatic event, do pharmacological interventions, when compared to other pharmacological or psychosocial interventions, result in a clinically important reduction/prevention of symptoms, improved functioning/quality of life, presence of disorder, or adverse effects?

7. For adults within the first 3 months of a traumatic event, do pharmacological interventions, when compared to placebo, result in a clinically important reduction/prevention of symptoms, improved functioning/quality of life, presence of disorder, or adverse effects?

8. For adults within the first 3 months of a traumatic event, do pharmacological interventions, when compared to other pharmacological or psychosocial interventions, result in a clinically important reduction/prevention of symptoms, improved functioning/quality of life, presence of disorder, or adverse effects?

9. For children and adolescents with clinically relevant posttraumatic stress symptoms, do psychological treatments, when compared to treatment as usual, waiting list, or no treatment, result in a clinically important reduction of symptoms, improved functioning/quality of life, presence of disorder, or adverse effects?

10. For children and adolescents with clinically relevant posttraumatic stress symptoms, do psychological treatments, when compared to other psychological treatments, result in a clinically important reduction of symptoms, improved functioning/quality of life, presence of disorder, or adverse effects?

11. For adults with PTSD, do psychological treatments, when compared to treatment as usual, waiting list, or no treatment, result in a clinically important reduction of symptoms, improved functioning/quality of life, presence of disorder, or adverse effects?

12. For adults with PTSD, do psychological treatments, when compared to other psychological treatments, result in a clinically important reduction of symptoms, improved functioning/quality of life, presence of disorder, or adverse effects?

13. For children and adolescents with clinically relevant posttraumatic stress symptoms, do pharmacological treatments, when compared to placebo, result in a clinically important reduction of symptoms, improved functioning/quality of life, presence of disorder, or adverse effects?

14. For children and adolescents with clinically relevant posttraumatic stress symptoms, do pharmacological treatments, when compared to other pharmacological or psychosocial interventions, result in a clinically important reduction of symptoms, improved functioning/quality of life, presence of disorder, or adverse effects?

15. For adults with PTSD, do pharmacological treatments, when compared to placebo, result in a clinically important reduction of symptoms, improved functioning/quality of life, presence of disorder, or adverse effects?

16. For adults with PTSD, do pharmacological treatments, when compared to other pharmacological or psychosocial interventions, result in a clinically important reduction of symptoms, improved functioning/quality of life, presence of disorder, or adverse effects?

17. For children and adolescents with clinically relevant posttraumatic stress symptoms, do nonpsychological and nonpharmacological treatments/interventions, when compared to treatment as usual, waiting list, or no treatment, result in a clinically important reduction of symptoms, improved functioning/quality of life, presence of disorder, or adverse effects?

18. For children and adolescents with clinically relevant posttraumatic stress symptoms, do nonpsychological and nonpharmacological treatments/interventions, when compared to other treatments, result in a clinically important reduction of symptoms, improved functioning/quality of life, presence of disorder, or adverse effects?

19. For adults with PTSD, do nonpsychological and nonpharmacological treatments/interventions, when compared to treatment as usual, waiting list, or no treatment, result in a clinically important reduction of symptoms, improved functioning/quality of life, presence of disorder, or adverse effects?

20. For adults with PTSD, do nonpsychological and nonpharmacological treatments/interventions when compared to other treatments, result in a clinically important reduction of symptoms, improved functioning/quality of life, presence of disorder, or adverse effects?

CHAPTER 7

ISTSS PTSD Prevention and Treatment Guidelines

Recommendations

Jonathan I. Bisson, Lucy Berliner, Marylene Cloitre,
David Forbes, Tine Jensen, Catrin Lewis, Candice M. Monson,
Miranda Olff, Stephen Pilling, David S. Riggs, Neil P. Roberts,
and Francine Shapiro

The ISTSS guidelines recommendations should be used with an understanding of the methodology and the key points to consider in their interpretation, as described in the prior chapter. The recommendations for specific early interventions and treatments are listed under summaries of the relevant scoping questions. The recommendations are grouped according to the five different levels of strength of recommendation possible: *Strong, Standard, Low Effect, Intervention with Emerging Evidence,* and *Insufficient Evidence to Recommend.* For an intervention or treatment to be listed, there must have been at least one randomized controlled trial included in at least one of the meta-analyses undertaken to answer the relevant scoping questions. The recommendations were generated with the information available to the ISTSS Guidelines Committee on October 10, 2018; as more knowledge becomes available, it is likely that the level of some of the recommendations will change.

Children and Adolescents

Early Psychosocial Intervention

Summary of relevant scoping questions: "For children and adolescents within the first 3 months of a traumatic event, do psychosocial interventions, when compared to intervention as usual, waiting list, no intervention, or other psychosocial interventions, result in a clinically important reduction/prevention of symptoms, improved functioning/quality of life, presence of disorder, or adverse effects?"

Early Preventative Interventions[1]

Intervention with Emerging Evidence–Self-directed online psychoeducation for caregivers and children and *self-directed online psychoeducation for children* within the first 3 months of a traumatic event have emerging evidence of efficacy for the prevention of clinically relevant posttraumatic stress symptoms in children and adolescents.

Emerging Evidence Not to Recommend–Individual psychological debriefing within the first 3 months of a traumatic event has emerging evidence of increasing the risk of clinically relevant posttraumatic stress symptoms in children and adolescents.

*Insufficient Evidence to Recommend–*There is insufficient evidence to recommend *brief CBT-T* or *self-directed online psychoeducation for caregivers only* within the first 3 months of a traumatic event for the prevention of clinically relevant posttraumatic stress symptoms in children and adolescents.

Early Treatment Interventions[2]

*Insufficient Evidence to Recommend–*There is insufficient evidence to recommend *brief CBT-T, CBT-T,* or *stepped preventative care* within the first 3 months of a traumatic event for the treatment of clinically relevant posttraumatic stress symptoms in children and adolescents.

Early Pharmacological Intervention

Summary of relevant scoping questions: "For children and adolescents within the first 3 months of a traumatic event, do pharmacological interventions, when compared to placebo, other pharmacological, or psychosocial interventions, result in a clinically important reduction/prevention of symptoms, improved functioning/quality of life, presence of disorder, or adverse effects?"

*Insufficient Evidence to Recommend–*There is insufficient evidence to recommend *propranolol* within the first 3 months of a traumatic event as an early pharmacological intervention to prevent clinically relevant posttraumatic stress symptoms in children and adolescents.

Psychological Treatment

Summary of relevant scoping questions: "For children and adolescents with clinically relevant posttraumatic stress symptoms, do psychological treatments, when compared to treatment as usual, waiting list, no treatment, or other psychological treatments, result in a clinically important reduction of symptoms, improved functioning/quality of life, presence of disorder, or adverse effects?"

---

[1]Targeted at unscreened or minimally screened populations.

[2]Provided to individuals with emerging traumatic stress symptoms.

Strong Recommendation–CBT-T (caregiver and child), *CBT-T (child)*, and *EMDR therapy* are recommended for the treatment of children and adolescents with clinically relevant posttraumatic stress symptoms.

Intervention with Emerging Evidence–Group CBT-T (child), *group psychoeducation*, and *parent–child relationship enhancement* have emerging evidence of efficacy for the treatment of children and adolescents with clinically relevant posttraumatic stress symptoms.

*Insufficient Evidence to Recommend–*There is insufficient evidence to recommend *CBT-T (caregiver)*, *family therapy*, *group CBT-T (caregiver and child)*, *KidNET*, *nondirective counseling*, or *stepped-care CBT-T (caregiver and child)* for the treatment of children and adolescents with clinically relevant posttraumatic stress symptoms.

Pharmacological Treatment

Summary of relevant scoping questions: "For children and adolescents with clinically relevant posttraumatic stress symptoms, do pharmacological treatments, when compared to placebo, other pharmacological, or psychosocial interventions, result in a clinically important reduction of symptoms, improved functioning/quality of life, presence of disorder, or adverse effects?"

*Insufficient Evidence to Recommend–*There is insufficient evidence to recommend *sertraline* for the treatment of children and adolescents with clinically relevant posttraumatic stress symptoms.

Nonpsychological and Nonpharmacological Treatment

Summary of relevant scoping questions: "For children and adolescents with clinically relevant posttraumatic stress symptoms, do nonpsychological and nonpharmacological treatments/interventions, when compared to treatment as usual, waiting list, no treatment, or other treatments, result in a clinically important reduction of symptoms, improved functioning/quality of life, presence of disorder, or adverse effects?"

*Insufficient Evidence to Recommend–*There is insufficient evidence to recommend *mind–body skills* or *trauma-focused expressive art therapy* for the treatment of children and adolescents with clinically relevant posttraumatic stress symptoms.

Adults

Early Psychosocial Intervention

Summary of relevant scoping questions: "For adults within the first 3 months of a traumatic event, do psychosocial interventions, when compared to intervention as usual, waiting list, no intervention, or other psychosocial interventions, result in a clinically important reduction/prevention of symptoms, improved functioning/quality of life, presence of disorder, or adverse effects?"

Single-Session Interventions

Intervention with Emerging Evidence—*Group 512 PM* and *single-session EMDR therapy* within the first 3 months of a traumatic event have emerging evidence of efficacy for the prevention and treatment of PTSD symptoms in adults.

Insufficient Evidence to Recommend—*There is insufficient evidence to recommend *group debriefing, group education, group stress management, heart stress counseling, individual debriefing, individual psychoeducation/self-help, reassurance, single-session computerized visuospatial task,* or *trauma-focused counseling* within the first 3 months of a traumatic event for the prevention or treatment of PTSD symptoms in adults.

Multiple-Session Prevention Interventions[3]

Intervention with Emerging Evidence—*Brief dyadic therapy* and *self-guided Internet-based intervention* within the first 3 months of a traumatic event have emerging evidence of efficacy for the prevention of PTSD symptoms in adults.

Insufficient Evidence to Recommend—*There is insufficient evidence to recommend *brief individual trauma processing therapy, brief IPT, brief parenting intervention following premature birth, collaborative care, communication facilitator in an intensive care setting, intensive care diaries in an intensive care context, nurse-led intensive care recovery program, supported psychoeducational intervention,* or *telephone-based CBT* within the first 3 months of a traumatic event for the prevention of PTSD symptoms in adults.

Multiple-Session Early Treatment Interventions[4]

Standard Recommendation—*CBT-T, cognitive therapy,* and *EMDR therapy* within the first 3 months of a traumatic event are recommended for the treatment of PTSD symptoms in adults.

Intervention with Low Effect—*Stepped/collaborative care* within the first 3 months of a traumatic event is recommended as a low effect treatment of PTSD symptoms in adults.

Intervention with Emerging Evidence—*Internet-based guided self-help* and *structured writing intervention* within the first 3 months of a traumatic event

---

[3]Targeted at unscreened or minimally screened populations.

[4]Provided to individuals with emerging traumatic stress symptoms.

have emerging evidence of efficacy for the treatment of PTSD symptoms in adults.

Insufficient Evidence to Recommend–There is insufficient evidence to recommend *behavioral activation, computerized neurobehavioral training, Internet virtual reality therapy, supportive counseling,* or *telephone-based CBT-T* within the first 3 months of a traumatic event for the treatment of PTSD symptoms in adults.

Early Pharmacological Intervention

Summary of relevant scoping questions: "For adults within the first 3 months of a traumatic event, do pharmacological interventions, when compared to placebo, other pharmacological, or psychosocial interventions, result in a clinically important reduction/prevention of symptoms, improved functioning/quality of life, presence of disorder, or adverse effects?"

Intervention with Emerging Evidence–*Hydrocortisone* within the first 3 months of a traumatic event has emerging evidence of efficacy for the prevention of PTSD symptoms in adults.

Insufficient Evidence to Recommend–There is insufficient evidence to recommend *docosahexaenoic acid, escitalopram, gabapentin, oxytocin,* or *propranolol* within the first 3 months of a traumatic event for the prevention or treatment of PTSD symptoms in adults.

Psychological Treatment

Summary of relevant scoping questions: "For adults with PTSD, do psychological treatments, when compared to treatment as usual, waiting list, no treatment, or other psychological treatments, result in a clinically important reduction of symptoms, improved functioning/quality of life, presence of disorder, or adverse effects?"

Strong Recommendation–*Cognitive processing therapy, cognitive therapy, EMDR therapy, individual CBT with a trauma focus (undifferentiated),*[5] and *prolonged exposure* are recommended for the treatment of adults with PTSD.

Standard Recommendation–*CBT without a trauma focus, group CBT with a trauma focus, guided Internet-based CBT with a trauma focus, narrative exposure therapy,* and *present-centered therapy* are recommended for the treatment of adults with PTSD.

Intervention with Emerging Evidence–*Couples CBT with a trauma focus, group and individual CBT with a trauma focus, reconsolidation of traumatic memories, single-session CBT, virtual reality therapy,* and *written exposure therapy*

---

[5] The *individual CBT with a trauma focus (undifferentiated)* recommendation is made from a meta-analysis of all studies meeting the CBT-T definition provided in the prior chapter.

have emerging evidence of efficacy for the treatment of adults with PTSD.

Insufficient Evidence to Recommend–There is insufficient evidence to recommend *brief eclectic psychotherapy for PTSD, dialogical exposure therapy, emotional freedom techniques, group interpersonal therapy, group stabilizing treatment, group supportive counseling, interpersonal psychotherapy, observed and experimental integration, psychodynamic psychotherapy, psychoeducation, relaxation training, REM desensitization,* or *supportive counseling* for the treatment of adults with PTSD.

Pharmacological Treatment

Scoping question: "For adults with PTSD, do pharmacological treatments, when compared to placebo, other pharmacological, or psychosocial interventions, result in a clinically important reduction of symptoms, improved functioning/quality of life, presence of disorder, or adverse effects?"

Intervention with Low Effect–*Fluoxetine, paroxetine, sertraline,* and *venlafaxine* are recommended as low effect treatments for adults with PTSD.

Intervention with Emerging Evidence–*Quetiapine* has emerging evidence of efficacy for the treatment of adults with PTSD.

Insufficient Evidence to Recommend–There is insufficient evidence to recommend *amitriptyline, brofaromine, divalproex, ganaxolone, imipramine, ketamine, lamotrigine, mirtazapine, neurokinin-1 antagonist, olanzapine, phenelzine, tiagabine,* or *topiramate* for the treatment of adults with PTSD.

Nonpsychological and Nonpharmacological Treatment

Summary of relevant scoping questions: "For adults with PTSD, do nonpsychological and nonpharmacological treatments/interventions, when compared to treatment as usual, waiting list, no treatment, or other treatments, result in a clinically important reduction of symptoms, improved functioning/ quality of life, presence of disorder, or adverse effects?"

Intervention with Emerging Evidence–*Acupuncture, neurofeedback, saikokeishikankyoto, somatic experiencing, transcranial magnetic stimulation,* and *yoga* have emerging evidence of efficacy for the treatment of adults with PTSD.

Insufficient Evidence to Recommend–There is insufficient evidence to recommend *attentional bias modification, electroacupuncture, group mindfulness-based stress reduction, group music therapy, hypnotherapy, mantram repetition, mindfulness-based stress reduction, nature adventure therapy,* or *physical exercise* for the treatment of adults with PTSD.

PART II

EARLY INTERVENTION IN ADULTS

CHAPTER 8

Early Intervention for Trauma-Related Psychopathology

Meaghan L. O'Donnell, Belinda J. Pacella, Richard A. Bryant, Miranda Olff, and David Forbes

In many ways, posttraumatic stress disorder (PTSD) and other trauma-related psychopathology are the primary candidates for early intervention because in all instances a discrete event(s) precipitates the disorder. It is seductive to think that if we can identify who has been exposed to the traumatic event, we can identify who would benefit from early intervention. Unfortunately, the process is not quite that easy. Before examining the efficacy and effectiveness of interventions designed to prevent and/or treat the mental health impacts of trauma exposure, it is important to consider how early intervention has been understood from different perspectives.

Background and Context

What Is Early Intervention?

There is no doubt that early intervention is a confusing term, especially in the context of mental health. Often early intervention is described in terms of preventing the prevalence and incidence of disorder (Magruder, Kassam-Adams, Thoresen, & Olff, 2016; Magruder, McLaughlin, & Elmore Borbon, 2017). Primary and secondary prevention are terms frequently used when discussing early intervention in health contexts. Primary prevention aims to prevent a disease before it occurs by preventing exposures to hazards that cause the disease. Secondary prevention aims to reduce the impact of disease that has already occurred by detecting and treating disease as soon as possible. In a trauma context, primary prevention would be activities that decrease the risk of being exposed to traumatic events, such as increasing lighting on campus to prevent sexual assault. Secondary prevention would be all activities designed to decrease the risk of trauma psychopathology developing once exposed to trauma, such as treating acute stress disorder (ASD) to prevent the development of PTSD. Other more complex models have built on the primary/secondary prevention approach, such as a social-ecological model developed by the International Society for Traumatic Stress Studies (ISTSS) that presents a multilevel approach for developing an array of strategies aimed at preventing the occurrence and sequelae of trauma (Magruder et al., 2017).

An alternative categorization of prevention may provide another useful framework. The Institute of Medicine (IOM; Institute of Medicine–Committee on Prevention of Mental Disorders, 1994) presents a continuum of care that provides a more graded approach to early intervention. In this approach, early interventions fall under the prevention rubric of universal, selective, and indicated activities. These categories of services differ according to the level of risk of the target population. From a trauma perspective, universal interventions are those that target the whole population of those exposed to a traumatic event regardless of risk. Like primary prevention, universal interventions would also include interventions designed to prevent exposure to traumatic events. Selective interventions are those that target individuals who risk developing disorder (but who may not yet be symptomatic); indicated interventions are those that target individuals who have minimal but detectable signs of symptoms suggesting disorder. Early treatment is the delivery of an intervention shortly after an individual has developed disorder.

In this chapter, we will look at the effectiveness of early interventions based on the results from the systematic review/meta-analyses that underpinned the ISTSS treatment guidelines. These systematic reviews defined early intervention as that beginning within 3 months of the trauma. Although the guidelines grouped early interventions into a single prevention session, multiple prevention sessions, and early treatment, from a clinical perspective it is useful to consider their effectiveness from the categorization of universal, selective, indicated, and treatment of disorder. This is because not everyone has the same emotional response to a traumatic event over time. In fact, there are a number of distinct trajectories/patterns of PTSD symptoms after trauma exposure, and we will argue that understanding these trajectories is necessary when interpreting the efficacy of early interventions. Before we describe the findings from the systematic reviews, we will take a small detour to the literature that describes symptom trajectories after trauma exposure.

Symptom Trajectory after Trauma

In the last 5–10 years, a number of studies have used statistical methods such as latent growth mixture modeling to examine the trajectories of PTSD symptoms over time (Armour, Shevlin, Elklit, & Mroczek, 2012; Bonanno, 2004; Bonanno, Galea, Bucciarelli, & Vlahov, 2006; Bonanno et al., 2012;

Bryant et al., 2015; deRoon-Cassini, Mancini, Rusch, & Bonanno, 2010; Fink et al., 2017; Galatzer-Levy et al., 2013; Lam et al., 2010; Norris, Tracy, & Galea, 2009; Pietrzak et al., 2014; Santiago et al., 2013; Steenkamp, Dickstein, Salters-Pedneault, Hofmann, & Litz, 2012; Vojvoda, Weine, McGlashan, Becker, & Southwick, 2008). Generally, these studies show that the majority of people exposed to trauma tend to fall into one of four to five archetypical trajectories of long-term outcome. Figure 8.1 is an example of how these trajectories are represented.

The most common outcome is a relatively stable trajectory of low symptomology and healthy functioning across time (often called the resistant or resilient group). When measured from the immediate aftermath of trauma (i.e., within 1 to 6 months), the proportion of people in the resilient class generally ranges from 60 to 85%, and this appears consistent across various types of trauma (Bonanno et al., 2006, 2012; Bryant et al., 2015; deRoon-Cassini et al., 2010; Fink et al., 2017; Lam et al., 2010; Santiago et al., 2013).

These studies also show a second archetypical trajectory known as the chronic class, which consists of people who have a chronic pattern of high symptoms after trauma exposure, with these remaining high across time.

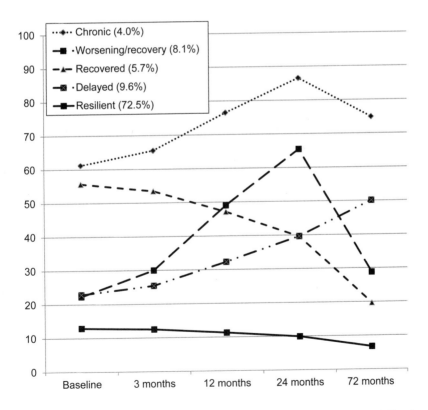

FIGURE 8.1. An example of the different symptom trajectories over time following exposure to a traumatic event. From Bryant et al. (2013).

When measured from the immediate aftermath of trauma, the proportion of people in the chronic class ranges from 2 to 15% (Bryant, O'Donnell, Creamer, McFarlane, & Silove, 2013; Galatzer-Levy et al., 2013; Santiago et al., 2013). However, proportions can reach as high as 20–35% following severe traumatic events, such as physical assault (deRoon-Cassini et al., 2010; Santiago et al., 2013) and sexual assault (Armour et al., 2012).

Studies differ then about the number of remaining class trajectories and what they look like, but generally there is a class with symptoms that start high but then decline over time (often referred to as the recovery class), and there is a class with symptoms that start low but then increase over time (frequently described as delayed onset). Longitudinal studies have found some variability in the proportion of people in the recovery and delayed onset class following different types of trauma. In populations exposed to trauma such as traumatic injury, assault, terrorism, life-threatening medical procedures, natural disaster, and military combat, the proportion of people in the recovery class when measured from the immediate aftermath of trauma ranges from 6 to 15% (Bryant et al., 2015; deRoon-Cassini et al., 2010; Lam et al., 2010), but can range as high as 30–40% in assault (Roy-Byrne et al., 2004) and resettled refugee populations (Vojvoda et al., 2008). Interestingly, in a sample of traumatic injury survivors with a high risk of PTSD, two trajectories of recovery were observed: rapid remitting of symptoms within 5 months and slow remitting of symptoms within 15 months (Galatzer-Levy et al., 2013). However, no delayed onset class was observed. Of the discussed studies, the proportion in the delayed onset class generally ranges from 2 to 14% (Bonanno, 2004; Bryant et al., 2015; deRoon-Cassini et al., 2010; Norris et al., 2009; Pietrzak et al., 2014; Santiago et al., 2013).

Contrary to these overall results that demonstrate resilience to be the modal outcome of trauma exposure, evidence suggests that this theoretical model may not generalize to cases of sexual assault. Rather, chronic and recovery classes are suggested to be a distinct response to sexual assault, with a pattern of high symptoms that decline over time (recovery) being the most modal class. In the aftermath of sexual assault, the proportion in the recovery class appears to range from 65 to 77%, and the proportion in the chronic class ranges from 23 to 35% (Armour et al., 2012; Steenkamp et al., 2012).

Recognizing these PTSD symptom trajectories/patterns (1) helps us interpret the findings from the systematic review/meta-analyses and (2) going forward helps us think about how and when to target interventions. Let us first look at the results from the literature reviews with these trajectories in mind.

Summary and Appraisal of the Evidence

The following tables introduce the findings of the ISTSS guideline recommendations for posttrauma intervention. Table 8.1 presents the findings for a single prevention session, and Table 8.2 gives the outcomes for multiple

TABLE 8.1. ISTSS Recommendations for Single Prevention Session Early Interventions

Intervention with Emerging Evidence–EMDR therapy, Group 512 PM

Insufficient Evidence to Recommend–Computerized visuospatial task, group debriefing: group education, group stress management, heart stress counseling, individual debriefing, psychoeducation/self-help, reassurance, trauma-focused counseling

TABLE 8.2. ISTSS Recommendations for Multiple Prevention Session Early Interventions

Intervention with Emerging Evidence–Brief dyadic therapy, self-guided Internet-based intervention

Insufficient Evidence to Recommend–Brief IPT, brief individual trauma processing therapy, brief parenting intervention following premature birth, collaborative care, communication facilitator in an intensive care setting, guided self-help, intensive care diaries in an intensive care context, self-guided Internet-based intervention, supported psychoeducational intervention, telephone-based CBT

TABLE 8.3. ISTSS Recommendations for Early Treatment

Standard Recommendation–CBT-T, cognitive therapy, EMDR therapy

Intervention with Low Effect–Stepped/collaborative care

Intervention with Emerging Evidence–Internet-based guided self-help, structured writing intervention

Insufficient Evidence to Recommend–Behavioral activation, brief CPT, Internet virtual reality therapy, nurse-led psychological intervention, supportive counseling, telephone-based CBT-T

prevention sessions. Prevention interventions were defined in the guidelines as those interventions that aim to intervene before disorder develops. Table 8.3 presents the early treatment findings defined as those interventions that target disorders such as ASD and early PTSD within the first 3 months of developing.

Although the ISTSS guidelines grouped early interventions into a single prevention session, multiple prevention sessions, and early treatment, from a clinical perspective it is useful to consider their effectiveness from the categorization of universal, selective, indicated, and treatment of disorder.

Universal Interventions

Universal interventions target everyone who has been exposed to traumatic events. As described previously, we know that the majority of trauma survivors have low symptoms over time and will therefore recover on their own. It is therefore difficult to expect that universal intervention would have a significant effect on psychiatric symptoms given that only approximately 25% of survivors will develop moderate to high symptoms.

Single-Session Interventions

Most of the single-session early psychosocial interventions were universal interventions (targeted to the whole population of trauma-exposed survivors), so it is not surprising the studies that fell into this group received a recommendation of *Insufficient Evidence to Recommend*.

An *Insufficient Evidence to Recommend* recommendation was made when there was an absence of evidence of effectiveness or ineffectiveness. Specifically, individual debriefing and group debriefing when delivered as a universal intervention received an *Insufficient Evidence to Recommend* recommendation. This finding is consistent with the 2002 Cochrane review that found there was no evidence debriefing was useful in the prevention of PTSD (Rose, Bisson, Churchill, & Wessely, 2002). This finding is also consistent with the National Institute for Health and Clinical Excellence (NICE), now the National Institute for Health and Care Excellence guidelines for PTSD (National Institute for Health and Clinical Excellence, 2005) that recommend single-session interventions should not be a part of routine practice (although it should be noted that the NICE Triage panel is currently updating this recommendation). Overall, the ISTSS findings are consistent with other guidelines in recommending that single-session psychosocial universal interventions should not be considered a part of routine practice because of the lack of evidence to support their use.

Multiple-Session Interventions

Universal interventions were also not effective when delivered across multiple sessions. Specifically, when delivered as a universal intervention, brief interpersonal counseling therapy (IPT; Holmes et al., 2007), brief individual trauma processing therapy (Brom, Kleber, & Hofman, 1993; Gidron et al., 2001; Rothbaum et al., 2012; Ryding, Wijma, & Wijma, 1998), brief parenting intervention following premature birth (Borghini et al., 2014), intensive care diaries (Jones et al., 2010), and collaborative care (Zatzick et al., 2001) all received an *Insufficient Evidence* rating. This probably represents the fact that the majority of trauma survivors will recover well without the assistance of any intervention. Having said that, we have no current evidence that these interventions would be effective if they were delivered to the minority who would go on to develop PTSD.

Thus, if universal interventions do not seem to demonstrate efficacy in the prevention of PTSD, what should be done after trauma exposure? Should we indeed do anything? Currently, psychological first aid (PFA) is the most frequently endorsed universal approach, having been adopted by the World Health Organization (2011), Red Cross (Australian Red Cross &

Australian Psychological Society, 2013; Gurwitch et al., 2010), and United Nations (Inter-Agency Standing Committee, 2010). PFA represents a set of actions including information provision and advice, emotional and practical support, and monitoring and referral delivered on an as-needed basis, and guided by the aims of promoting safety, calming, self and collectiveness efficacy, connectedness, and hope following trauma exposure. Importantly PFA is not intended as a formal intervention. PFA has been widely applied by lay rescuers in public health settings and workplaces, and during critical and traumatic events. Although PFA has widespread appeal, at least three systematic reviews have consistently reported on the absence of studies that provide rigorous evaluations of PFA interventions (Bisson & Lewis, 2009; Dieltjens, Moonens, Van Praet, De Buck, & Vandekerckhove, 2014; Fox et al., 2012). If PFA is delivered as an intervention rather than an approach, then the need exists to empirically test its efficacy.

Alongside PFA is the approach offered by the European Network for Traumatic Stress (TENTS; *www.tentsproject.eu*). TENTS provides guidelines for offering practical, pragmatic stupport informed by the principles of PFA, but not as an intervention per se. Developed through a consensus approach, these guidelines recommend against the application of formal interventions for all individuals involved in traumatic events. This approach is also consistent with the Australian ASD and PTSD guidelines (Phoenix Australia–Centre for Posttraumatic Mental Health, 2013), which recommend approaches that ensure the survivor's safety and security, provide ongoing practical assistance and information, and encourage the person to use his or her social supports.

Selective/Indicated Interventions

Single-Session Interventions

Interventions that target those with higher symptom levels start to demonstrate more impact on preventing the development of PTSD. In the systematic review/meta-analysis, two single-session interventions were delivered as a selective intervention (eye movement desensitization and reprocessing [EMDR] therapy) or indicated intervention (Group 512 Psychological Intervention Model [PIM]). They both received an *Intervention with Emerging Evidence* recommendation. Group 512 is an intervention that embeds the unique characteristics of Chinese military rescuers within the standard principles of critical-incident stress debriefing (CISD) developed by Mitchell (1983). Group 512 involves four stages—including introduction, discussing the facts, thoughts, reactions, and symptoms related to the trauma, followed by stress management tips—but differs then from standard CISD by including a final stage of cohesion training, where participants play games requiring team cooperation to foster military unit cohesion. This is a critical part of Group 512 PIM, as cohesion is said to have protective effects in preventing stress (Armfield, 1994).

Single-session EMDR therapy also received an *Intervention with Emerging Evidence* recommendation when delivered to trauma survivors with emerging symptoms. Single-session EMDR therapy followed the EMDR Protocol for Recent Critical Incidents (EMDR-PRECI). EMDR-PRECI is a modified version of Shapiro's Recent Traumatic Events Protocol (Shapiro & Laub, 2008), to accommodate memory consolidation that appears to change in the weeks and months following a critical incident (Jarero, Uribe, Artigas, & Givaudan, 2015). EMDR-PRECI involves identifying the worst fragment of the client's trauma memory, followed by the remaining difficult fragments of the memory. Desensitizing occurs by having the client focus on each memory fragment while simultaneously engaging in dual-attention stimulation using eye movements, until all fragments have been processed and the client no longer experiences emotional, cognitive, or somatic distress.

It is important that these two interventions undergo further treatment trials to determine if the evidence associated with them should move both into a higher category of recommendation.

Multiple-Session Interventions

Multiple sessions of a selective intervention, including brief dyadic therapy (Brunet, Des Groseilliers, Cordova, & Ruzek, 2013) and a self-guided Internet intervention (Mouthaan et al., 2013), also received an *Intervention with Emerging Evidence* recommendation. Brief dyadic therapy aims to target the social support process following trauma exposure and involves elements of psychoeducation and motivational interviewing to enhance communication between the patient and his or her significant other. It involves two sessions that aim to promote disclosure of thoughts and emotions relating to the trauma while attempting to reduce social constraints on disclosure and negative interactions between the dyad (Brunet et al., 2013). Trauma TIPS, the Internet-based self-guided intervention, is based on CBT principles of psychoeducation and stress/relaxation techniques in addition to *in vivo* exposure. Trauma TIPS aims to decrease levels of distress and anxiety by providing information on successful coping, instructions, and guidance for *in vivo* exposure in addition to stress management techniques (Mouthaan et al., 2013). *Post hoc* analyses showed a significant decrease in PTSD symptoms in a subgroup of patients with severe initial symptoms, again pointing to the importance of targeting the population at risk with higher symptoms (but note the limitations of *post hoc* analyses). Although these interventions show promise, further evidence is needed to support their efficacy.

Early Treatment

Not surprisingly, the strongest recommendations for early interventions are made in treatments that target disorder. The majority of studies target ASD or early PTSD.

Intervention with *Standard* Recommendations

COGNITIVE-BEHAVIORAL THERAPY WITH A TRAUMA FOCUS

CBT with a trauma focus (CBT-T) received a *Standard* recommendation when delivered as an early intervention to trauma survivors with ASD diagnosis or early PTSD diagnosis. CBT-T is a broad term that encompasses any treatment that employs the standard principles of CBT combined with some form of trauma processing. Generally, CBT-T involves the integration of CBT principles with components of exposure therapy, including imaginal exposure and graded *in vivo* exposure. Across most studies, the typical format of CBT-T included psychoeducation, breathing/relaxation training, imaginal exposure, *in vivo* exposure, and cognitive restructuring (Bisson, Shepherd, Joy, Probert, & Newcombe, 2004; Foa, Zoellner, & Feeny, 2006; Sijbrandij et al., 2007; van Emmerik, Kamphuis, & Emmelkamp, 2008), but one study diverted from this format by excluding the use of *in vivo* exposure (Shaw et al., 2013). The populations within these studies consisted of a fair split of males and females from the United States, United Kingdom, Netherlands, Australia, and Israel, with their mean ages ranging from 33 to 40 years old; these individuals had been exposed to various traumatic experiences, including physical assault, motor vehicle accidents, industrial accidents (Bisson et al., 2004; Bryant et al., 2008; Ehlers et al., 2003; Shalev et al., 2012), sexual assault (Foa et al., 2006; van Emmerik et al., 2008), mixed trauma types (Sijbrandij et al., 2007), and premature births (Shaw et al., 2013).

COGNITIVE THERAPY

Cognitive therapy also received a *Standard* recommendation when delivered as an early intervention to trauma survivors with PTSD symptoms. Cognitive therapy includes identifying and challenging negative automatic thoughts, and modifying underlying cognitive schemas, but involves less potentially distressing exposure to traumatic recollections than other trauma-focused interventions. Populations within these studies ($n = 2$) were comparable, both consisting of a fair split of males and females, with the mean age ranging from 35 to 38 years old, who had been exposed to motor-vehicle accidents, physical injury, or terrorist attacks (Bryant et al., 2008; Shalev et al., 2012).

EMDR THERAPY

Brief EMDR therapy was the final treatment that received a *Standard* recommendation when delivered as an early intervention to survivors with disorder or disorder-level symptoms. Brief EMDR therapy can range from one to two sessions and involves clients focusing on fragments of their trauma memory while simultaneously engaging in dual-attention stimulation using eye movements. When compared to treatment as usual (TAU) or wait-list control, EMDR therapy showed a positive effect on PTSD symptom severity

(n = 4) (Jarero, Artigas, & Luber, 2011; Jarero et al., 2015; Shapiro & Laub, 2015; Shapiro, Laub, & Rosenblat, 2018). Across these studies, the Impact of Event Scale (IES) and the Short PTSD Rating Interview (SPRINT) were used to measure PTSD symptom severity. The populations within these studies mostly included a high proportion of females (44–94%) of Mexican or Israeli descent, with their mean ages ranging from 38 to 42, who had been exposed to an earthquake, manufacturing factory explosion, or fatal missile attack (Jarero et al., 2011, 2015; Shapiro & Laub, 2015; Shapiro et al., 2018).

Intervention with Emerging Evidence Recommendations

Internet-based guided self-help and structured writing intervention received a recommendation of *Intervention with Emerging Evidence.*

INTERNET-BASED GUIDED SELF-HELP

When compared to wait-list control or TAU, a 10-week Internet-based guided self-help program showed a positive effect in reducing PTSD symptoms (measured by the PCL-C) at posttreatment for Swedish parents of children who had been recently diagnosed with cancer. Just over a third of the sample were females, with a mean age of 38, exhibiting a high level of PTSD symptoms. The intervention was based on CBT principles, with a focus on psychoeducation and teaching strategies to cope with psychological distress. Despite experiencing a high dropout rate (62%), the study suggests that CBT-based Internet-guided self-help may have a substantive impact on those who accept Internet-based interventions and report a high level of posttraumatic stress symptoms.

STRUCTURED WRITING

Structured writing is a broad term that encompasses interventions that rely exclusively on writing assignments. Of the two studies that employed structured writing interventions, one study (van Emmerik et al., 2008) adapted its structured writing therapy program from the Interapy program, which is an Internet-based 10-session structured writing intervention (Lange, van de Ven, Schrieken, & Emmelkamp, 2001). Based on the Interapy program, the structured writing intervention followed a three-phase intervention model involving the following phases: (1) self-confrontation, which involves participants writing down detailed accounts of their traumatic experience, paying careful attention to their sensory experiences and most painful trauma-related emotions; (2) cognitive reappraisal, which involves writing an (imaginal) advice letter to a friend who has experienced the same situation and then applying this advice to themselves; and (3) the sharing and farewell phase, which involves writing a letter to a person involved in the situation that describes the letter writer's coping efforts. The other study that employed a structured writing intervention (Bugg, Turpin, Mason, & Scholes, 2009) based its intervention on the Pennebaker writing paradigm, which requires participants to write about the feelings and emotions associated with their traumatic experience once a day for 3 consecutive days (Pennebaker, Kiecolt-Glaser, & Glaser, 1988). The intervention adapted this paradigm slightly by including suggestions to participants to discuss how their experience influenced other areas of their life, including their relationships with loved ones or any other significant issues (Bugg et al., 2009). Across both of these studies, participants were individuals with ASD or PTSD who had sustained a traumatic injury, such as a traffic accident, or sexual or nonsexual assault, with the average age ranging from 37 to 40.

Intervention with Low Effect Recommendations

A number of indicated studies took a *sequencing approach*. These studies reflect an approach that could be (and are) implemented in clinical practice to facilitate early intervention. The collaborative care model devised by Zatzick (Zatzick et al., 2004, 2013, 2015) is a stepped-care model in which injured patients are screened for high PTSD symptoms, and those with risk factors are offered integrated care including pharmacotherapy, motivational interviewing targeting problematic alcohol use, and CBT targeting depression and PTSD symptoms. Elements of the treatment were provided in a stepped fashion such that those with greater ease of delivery, for example, psychoeducation and problem solving, were given initially, followed later by more complex elements like activity scheduling. Patient symptoms were repeatedly measured and higher-intensity care was initiated if the person required it. In a later study, decision making was assisted with a technology-enhanced screening process (Zatzick et al., 2015) that decreased the time required in decision making. Although the studies by Zatzick and colleagues focused on PTSD as the only target outcome, the stepped-care model proposed by O'Donnell and colleagues (O'Donnell et al., 2012) aimed to address a comprehensive range of posttrauma psychopathology. In a two-stage screening process, patients were screened for high-risk symptoms of PTSD, depression, and anxiety, and treated with an evidence-based modular CBT manual that allowed treatment to be tailored to the patient's individual symptom-cluster profiles. The *Intervention with Low Effect* recommendation is a reflection of the small effect sizes associated with these interventions. This was a function of the Zatzick trials including all screened participants in their outcome analyses (not just those who received the intervention). It could be that if the analyses included just those who were allocated into treatment, the effects would have been stronger. These observations are corroborated empirically by recent meta-analyses that systematically assess early intervention overall population impact, an outcome assessment construct that combines both an intervention's treatment effect and breadth of applicability (Giummarra, Lennox, Dali, Costa, & Gabbe, 2018).

Intervention with Insufficient Evidence
to Recommend Recommendations

Of the remaining three treatment modalities, brief cognitive processing therapy (CPT), behavioral activation, and supportive counseling received an *Insufficient Evidence to Recommend* recommendation. Generally, there was only one study of these therapies, and this would have contributed to the classification. Both behavioral activation and supportive counseling contained one study that was compared to a wait-list control or TAU condition, whereas brief CPT contained two studies that were compared to supportive counseling.

Comorbidity

Although PTSD is the main outcome of interest in evaluating early intervention treatments for PTSD, it is also important to consider if, and how, these treatments impacted comorbid psychopathologies. PTSD is more likely to occur as a comorbid disorder than as a sole diagnosis (Bryant et al., 2010; O'Donnell et al., 2016), and anxiety and depression are usually present either as a comorbid diagnosis or at subsyndromal levels. Most studies included measures of anxiety and depression, so the following section reviews the impact of the treatment on anxiety and depression levels.

Of the 18 studies testing CBT-T, 16 included measures of anxiety or depression, while the remaining two studies either did not measure these outcomes (Shalev et al., 2012) or were unpublished (Ost, unpublished). Of the 16 studies that measured depression, three studies found no efficacy for CBT-T in reducing depression at posttreatment and follow-up (Bisson et al., 2004; Bryant, Moulds, Guthrie, & Nixon, 2003, 2005). The majority of studies (*n* = 8) found significant reductions in depression at posttreatment and follow-up (Bryant, Harvey, Dang, Sackville, & Basten, 1998; Bryant, Sackville, Dang, Moulds, & Guthrie, 1999; Ehlers et al., 2003; Nixon, 2012; Nixon et al., 2016; Shaw et al., 2013; van Emmerik et al., 2008; Wu, Li, & Cho, 2014), while a small portion (*n* = 5) found reductions at posttreatment only (Bryant et al., 2008; Echeburúa, de Corral, Sarasua, & Zubizarreta, 1996; Foa et al., 2006; Freyth, Elsesser, Lohrmann, & Sartory, 2010; Sijbrandij et al., 2007). Of the 14 studies that measured anxiety, one study found no efficacy for CBT in reducing anxiety at posttreatment and follow-up (Bisson et al., 2004), while a large portion of these studies (*n* = 6) found reductions in anxiety at posttreatment but not at follow-up (Bryant et al., 1998, 2005, 2008; Bryant, Moulds, Guthrie, & Nixon, 2003; Echeburúa et al., 1996; Sijbrandij et al., 2007). The majority of these studies (*n* = 7) found reductions in anxiety at both posttreatment and follow-up (Bryant et al., 1999; Ehlers et al., 2003; Foa et al., 2006; Freyth et al., 2010; Shaw et al., 2013; van Emmerik et al., 2008; Wu et al., 2014). Of the two studies that evaluated the efficacy of cognitive therapy, only one study included measures of anxiety and depression, and it found reductions in depression and anxiety at 6-month follow-up only (Bryant et al.,

2008). Of the four studies that evaluated brief EMDR therapy, only one brief EMDR study measured comorbid depressive symptoms, and it found a significant reduction in depressive symptoms at 3-month follow-up only (Shapiro & Laub, 2015). The two interventions that received a classification of *Intervention with Emerging Evidence* consisted of a structured writing intervention (*n* = 2; Bugg et al., 2009; van Emmerik et al., 2008) and an Internet-based self-help intervention (*n* = 1; Cernvall, Carlbring, Ljungman, Ljungman, & von Essen, 2015). In general, these interventions were associated with reductions in depressive symptoms at both posttest and follow-up periods (Bugg et al., 2009; van Emmerik et al., 2008), and at posttest when there was no inclusion of follow-up assessments (Cernvall et al., 2015).

Of the 27 studies included in this review, only half showed significant improvements in anxiety and depression symptoms. This is, in part, a function of many studies not measuring anxiety and depression, and other studies not finding a consistent effect on depression and anxiety. This is important for clinicians to consider when treating PTSD in the first few months following trauma exposure. Measuring depression and anxiety in addition to PTSD symptoms as part of the initial assessment and during the course of treatment is important in order to determine if anxiety/depression symptoms are shifting as a consequence of PTSD treatment.

Does "Early" Mean "Brief"?

In the aftermath of trauma, it may appear logical to assume that early intervention requires a reduced treatment dose to target acute symptom presentations, rather than a full treatment dose aimed at targeting enduring disorders. However, a review of the duration of the intervention reveals that this was not always the case. While a small proportion of CBT-T studies (*n* = 3) implemented short treatment lengths of under 4.5 hours (Bisson et al., 2004; Bugg et al., 2009; Freyth et al., 2010), the majority of CBT-T studies ranged between 7.5 and 18 hours (*n* = 12; Bryant et al., 1998, 1999, 2005, 2008; Bryant, Moulds, & Nixon, 2003; Ehlers et al., 2003; Foa et al., 2006; Nixon, 2012; Nixon et al., 2016; Shalev et al., 2012; Sijbrandij et al., 2007; van Emmerik et al., 2008). Cognitive therapy (*n* = 2) ranged from 7 to 12 hours (Ehlers et al., 2003; Shalev et al., 2012). Only EMDR therapy demonstrated what would be considered brief interventions ranging from 45 minutes to 3 hours (*n* = 4; Jarero et al., 2011, 2015; Shapiro & Laub, 2015).

Of those interventions that were recommended as an *Intervention with Emerging Evidence*, Internet-based guided CBT-based self-help required participants to dedicate a total of 10 hours to work through all modules (Cernvall et al., 2015). In comparison, structured writing therapy involved somewhat briefer treatment doses spanning three to five sessions, with total treatment durations as brief as 1 hour (Bugg et al., 2009) or relatively longer at 7.5 hours (van Emmerik et al., 2008).

The idea that early intervention could consist of a reduced dose of treatment does not appear to be supported by the literature. Many of the early treatment interventions administer a similar number of hours of intervention relative to standard treatment protocols. This is because often those individuals presenting for early intervention have a range of complexities that increased their vulnerability to PTSD in the first place (e.g., preexisting anxiety/depression symptoms, negative cognitive style, poor social support, externalizing tendencies). Addressing these factors will likely increase the time taken to achieve successful treatment outcomes.

Future Directions

Since the last treatment guidelines, early intervention has made some progress, but perhaps not as much as expected. The future lies in targeting the different intensity of interventions to different presentations. Here, we can use the trajectory research to help inform our thinking. It may be that the resilience group does not require formal assistance and a universal approach designed to offer general support is all that we should offer. We might consider a low-dose/intensity intervention for those who develop subsyndromal symptoms (on either the delayed onset or recovery trajectory) to speed up their trajectory to recovery or prevent their transition into disorder. And finally, we could consider full treatment for those who develop early disorder.

However, to do this, we need to first be able to identify the level of risk that each trauma survivor presents with (Mouthaan, Sijbrandij, Reitsma, Gersons, & Olff, 2014; Qi et al., 2018; Shalev et al., 2019). Some progress is being made by pooling data from several cohorts of survivors admitted to acute care centers (e.g., as applied in Qi et al., 2018). These studies show us that using early PTSD symptom severity as a predictor produced remarkably accurate estimates of follow-up PTSD (Shalev et al., 2019). However, we are not yet at the place where we can clearly identify which trajectory a trauma survivor will take. It should be noted that trajectory analyses have been able to map the distinct profiles of subgroups within a population, but we still cannot reliably predict in the acute phase how an individual case will fare months later.

Longitudinal studies indicate that the mental health of trauma survivors fluctuates markedly over time, and the main predictors of changing mental health status are factors occurring in the posttrauma environment (Bryant et al., 2013). This poses a major challenge for reliably being able to identify people who most need early intervention. We are best at identifying the resilience class—those who will not develop disorder. That is, most of our screening instruments have high specificity. Screening instruments also do a reasonably good job of identifying who currently has high symptoms, and our trajectory plots show that the high group is likely to be the chronic group. However, our screening instruments are relatively poor at identifying those on other trajectories, so this is something we need to further collaborate on. Identifying the subsyndromal risk profiles will help us design interventions designed to change trajectories and, it is hoped, ultimately help prevent disorder in the long run.

With regard to predicting response to early interventions, some studies indicate that early screening for, for example, severity of acute distress, might predict response to interventions (Frijling, 2017; Mouthaan et al., 2013). Although progess is being made with prediction models, when it comes to identification of risk for disorder or response to treatment, we still have a long way to go. We also need to recognize that early intervention studies have been limited by short-term follow-up assessments. This issue was highlighted in an Israeli study that found although early provision of CBT accelerated the remission of PTSD symptoms, 3 years later the rates of PTSD were not different from those of individuals who did not receive early intervention (Shalev et al., 2016). Furthermore, across early intervention studies, a pattern has emerged that suggests no more than two-thirds of people respond to recommended treatments, which highlights the need for recognition that some people may need additional treatment beyond the recommended early interventions for PTSD. It also highlights that we still require the development of new early interventions so that we can comprehensively address poor recovery in the early aftermath of trauma.

REFERENCES

Armfield, F. (1994). Preventing post-traumatic stress disorder resulting from military operations. *Military Medicine, 159*(12), 739–746.

Armour, C., Shevlin, M., Elklit, A., & Mroczek, D. (2012). A latent growth mixture modeling approach to PTSD symptoms in rape victims. *Traumatology, 18*(1), 20–28.

Australian Red Cross & Australian Psychological Society. (2013). *Psychological first aid: An Australian guide to supporting people affected by disaster.* Victoria, Australia: Authors.

Bisson, J. I., & Lewis, C. (2009). *Systematic review of psychological first aid.* Geneva, Switzerland: World Health Organization.

Bisson, J. I., Shepherd, J. P., Joy, D., Probert, R., & Newcombe, R. G. (2004). Early cognitive–behavioural therapy for post-traumatic stress symptoms after physical injury: Randomised controlled trial. *British Journal of Psychiatry, 184*(1), 63–69.

Bonanno, G. A. (2004). Loss, trauma, and human resilience: Have we underestimated the human capacity to thrive after extremely aversive events? *American Psychologist, 59*(1), 20.

Bonanno, G. A., Galea, S., Bucciarelli, A., & Vlahov, D. (2006). Psychological resilience after disaster: New York City in the aftermath of the September 11th terrorist attack. *Psychological Science, 17*(3), 181–186.

Bonanno, G. A., Mancini, A. D., Horton, J. L., Powell, T. M., LeardMann, C. A.,

Boyko, E. J., et al. (2012). Trajectories of trauma symptoms and resilience in deployed US military service members: Prospective cohort study. *British Journal of Psychiatry, 200*(4), 317–323.

Borghini, A., Habersaat, S., Forcada-Guex, M., Nessi, J., Pierrehumbert, B., Ansermet, F., et al. (2014). Effects of an early intervention on maternal post-traumatic stress symptoms and the quality of mother–infant interaction: The case of pre-term birth. *Infant Behavior and Development, 37*(4), 624–631.

Brom, D., Kleber, R., & Hofman, M. (1993). Victims of traffic accidents: Incidence and prevention of post-traumatic stress disorder. *Journal of Clinical Psychology, 49*(2), 131–140.

Brunet, A., Des Groseilliers, I. B., Cordova, M. J., & Ruzek, J. I. (2013). Randomized controlled trial of a brief dyadic cognitive-behavioral intervention designed to prevent PTSD. *European Journal of Psychotraumatology, 4*(1), 21572.

Bryant, R., Harvey, A., Dang, S., Sackville, T., & Basten, C. (1998). Treatment of acute stress disorder: A comparison of cognitive-behavioral therapy and supportive counseling. *Journal of Consulting and Clinical Psychology, 66*(5), 862–866.

Bryant, R., Mastrodomenico, J., Felmingham, K. L., Hopwood, S., Kenny, L., Kandris, E., et al. (2008). Treatment of acute stress disorder: A randomized controlled trial. *Archives of General Psychiatry, 65*(6), 659–667.

Bryant, R., Moulds, M., Guthrie, R., & Nixon, R. D. (2003). Treating acute stress disorder following mild traumatic brain injury. *American Journal of Psychiatry, 160*(3), 585–587.

Bryant, R., Moulds, M., Guthrie, R. M., & Nixon, R. D. (2005). The additive benefit of hypnosis and cognitive-behavioral therapy in treating acute stress disorder. *Journal of Consulting and Clinical Psychology, 73*(2), 334.

Bryant, R., Moulds, M. L., & Nixon, R. V. (2003). Cognitive behaviour therapy of acute stress disorder: A four-year follow-up. *Behaviour Research and Therapy, 41*(4), 489–494.

Bryant, R., Nickerson, A., Creamer, M., O'Donnell, M., Forbes, D., Galatzer-Levy, I., et al. (2015). Trajectory of post-traumatic stress following traumatic injury: 6-year follow-up. *British Journal of Psychiatry, 206*(5), 417–423.

Bryant, R., O'Donnell, M. L., Creamer, M., McFarlane, A. C., Clark, C. R., & Silove, D. (2010). The psychiatric sequelae of traumatic injury. *American Journal of Psychiatry, 167*(3), 312–320.

Bryant, R., O'Donnell, M. L., Creamer, M., McFarlane, A. C., & Silove, D. (2013). A multisite analysis of the fluctuating course of posttraumatic stress disorder. *JAMA Psychiatry, 70*(8), 839–846.

Bryant, R., Sackville, T., Dang, S. T., Moulds, M., & Guthrie, R. (1999). Treating acute stress disorder: An evaluation of cognitive behavior therapy and supportive counseling techniques. *American Journal of Psychiatry, 156*(11), 1780–1786.

Bugg, A., Turpin, G., Mason, S., & Scholes, C. (2009). A randomised controlled trial of the effectiveness of writing as a self-help intervention for traumatic injury patients at risk of developing post-traumatic stress disorder. *Behaviour Research and Therapy, 47*(1), 6–12.

Cernvall, M., Carlbring, P., Ljungman, L., Ljungman, G., & von Essen, L. (2015). Internet-based guided self-help for parents of children on cancer treatment: A randomized controlled trial. *Psycho-Oncology, 24*(9), 1152–1158.

deRoon-Cassini, T. A., Mancini, A. D., Rusch, M. D., & Bonanno, G. A. (2010).

Psychopathology and resilience following traumatic injury: A latent growth mixture model analysis. *Rehabilitation Psychology, 55*(1), 1.

Dieltjens, T., Moonens, I., Van Praet, K., De Buck, E., & Vandekerckhove, P. (2014). A systematic literature search on psychological first aid: Lack of evidence to develop guidelines. *PLOS ONE, 9*(12), e114714.

Echeburúa, E., de Corral, P., Sarasua, B., & Zubizarreta, I. (1996). Treatment of acute posttraumatic stress disorder in rape victims: An experimental study. *Journal of Anxiety Disorders, 10*(3), 185–199.

Ehlers, A., Clark, D. M., Hackmann, A., McManus, F., Fennell, M., Herbert, C., et al. (2003). A randomized controlled trial of cognitive therapy, a self-help booklet, and repeated assessments as early interventions for posttraumatic stress disorder. *Archives of General Psychiatry, 60*(10), 1024–1032.

Fink, D. S., Lowe, S., Cohen, G. H., Sampson, L. A., Ursano, R. J., Gifford, R. K., et al. (2017). Trajectories of posttraumatic stress symptoms after civilian or deployment traumatic event experiences. *Psychological Trauma: Theory, Research, Practice, and Policy, 9*(2), 138.

Foa, E. B., Zoellner, L. A., & Feeny, N. C. (2006). An evaluation of three brief programs for facilitating recovery after assault. *Journal of Traumatic Stress, 19*(1), 29–43.

Fox, J. H., Burkle, F. M., Bass, J., Pia, F. A., Epstein, J. L., & Markenson, D. (2012). The effectiveness of psychological first aid as a disaster intervention tool: Research analysis of peer-reviewed literature from 1990–2010. *Disaster Medicine and Public Health Preparedness, 6*(3), 247–252.

Freyth, C., Elsesser, K., Lohrmann, T., & Sartory, G. (2010). Effects of additional prolonged exposure to psychoeducation and relaxation in acute stress disorder. *Journal of Anxiety Disorders, 24*(8), 909–917.

Frijling, J. L. (2017). Preventing PTSD with oxytocin: Effects of oxytocin administration on fear neurocircuitry and PTSD symptom development in recently trauma-exposed individuals. *European Journal of Psychotraumatology, 8*(1), Article 1302652.

Galatzer-Levy, I. R., Ankri, Y., Freedman, S., Israeli-Shalev, Y., Roitman, P., Gilad, M., et al. (2013). Early PTSD symptom trajectories: Persistence, recovery, and response to treatment: Results from the Jerusalem Trauma Outreach and Prevention Study (J-TOPS). *PLOS ONE, 8*(8), e70084.

Gidron, Y., Gal, R., Freedman, S., Twiser, I., Lauden, A., Snir, Y., et al. (2001). Translating research findings to PTSD prevention: Results of a randomized-controlled pilot study. *Journal of Traumatic Stress, 14*(4), 773–780.

Giummarra, M. J., Lennox, A., Dali, G., Costa, B., & Gabbe, B. J. (2018). Early psychological interventions for posttraumatic stress, depression and anxiety after traumatic injury: A systematic review and meta-analysis. *Clinical Psychology Review, 62*, 11–36.

Gurwitch, R., Hughes, L., Porter, B., Schreiber, M., Bagwell Kukor, M., Herrmann, J., et al. (2010). *Coping in today's world: Psychological first aid and resilience for families, friends and neighbors: Instructor's manual.* Washington, DC: American Red Cross.

Holmes, A., Hodgins, G., Adey, S., Menzel, S., Danne, P., Kossmann, T., et al. (2007). Trial of interpersonal counselling after major physical trauma. *Australian and New Zealand Journal of Psychiatry, 41*(11), 926–933.

Institute of Medicine—Committee on Prevention of Mental Disorders. (1994). *Reducing risks for mental disorders: Frontiers for preventive intervention reserch.* Washington, DC: National Academy Press.

Inter-Agency Standing Committee. (2010). *IASC guidelines on mental health and psychosocial support in emergency settings.* Geneva, Switzerland: Author.

Jarero, I., Artigas, L., & Luber, M. (2011). The EMDR protocol for recent critical incidents: Application in a disaster mental health continuum of care context. *Journal of EMDR Practice and Research, 5*(3), 82–94.

Jarero, I., Uribe, S., Artigas, L., & Givaudan, M. (2015). EMDR protocol for recent critical incidents: A randomized controlled trial in a technological disaster context. *Journal of EMDR Practice and Research, 9*(4), 166–173.

Jones, C., Bäckman, C., Capuzzo, M., Egerod, I., Flaatten, H., Granja, C., et al. (2010). Intensive care diaries reduce new onset post traumatic stress disorder following critical illness: A randomised, controlled trial. *Critical Care, 14*(5), R168.

Lam, W. W., Bonanno, G. A., Mancini, A. D., Ho, S., Chan, M., Hung, W. K., et al. (2010). Trajectories of psychological distress among Chinese women diagnosed with breast cancer. *Psycho-Oncology, 19*(10), 1044–1051.

Lange, A., van de Ven, J.-P., Schrieken, B., & Emmelkamp, P. M. (2001). Interapy: Treatment of posttraumatic stress through the Internet: A controlled trial. *Journal of Behavior Therapy and Experimental Psychiatry, 32*(2), 73–90.

Magruder, K. M., Kassam-Adams, N., Thoresen, S., & Olff, M. (2016). Prevention and public health approaches to trauma and traumatic stress: A rationale and a call to action. *European Journal of Psychotraumatology, 7*(1), 29715.

Magruder, K. M., McLaughlin, K. A., & Elmore Borbon, D. L. (2017). Trauma is a public health issue. *European Journal of Psychotraumatology, 8*(1), Article 1375338.

Mitchell, J. T. (1983). When disaster strikes: The critical incident stress debriefing process. *Journal of Emergency Medical Services, 8,* 36–39.

Mouthaan, J., Sijbrandij, M., de Vries, G.-J., Reitsma, J. B., van de Schoot, R., Goslings, J. C., et al. (2013). Internet-based early intervention to prevent posttraumatic stress disorder in injury patients: Randomized controlled trial. *Journal of Medical Internet Research, 15*(8).

Mouthaan, J., Sijbrandij, M., Reitsma, J. B., Gersons, B. P., & Olff, M. (2014). Comparing screening instruments to predict posttraumatic stress disorder. *PLOS One, 9*(5), e97183.

National Institute for Health and Clinical Excellence. (2005). *Post-traumatic stress disorder.* London: Royal College of Psychiatrists and the British Psychological Society.

Nixon, R. D. V. (2012). Cognitive processing therapy versus supportive counseling for acute stress disorder following assault: A randomized pilot trial. *Behavior Therapy, 43*(4), 825–836.

Nixon, R. D. V., Best, T., Wilksch, S. R., Angelakis, S., Beatty, L. J., & Weber, N. (2016). Cognitive processing therapy for the treatment of acute stress disorder following sexual assault: A randomised effectiveness study. *Behaviour Change, 33*(4), 232–250.

Norris, F. H., Tracy, M., & Galea, S. (2009). Looking for resilience: Understanding the longitudinal trajectories of responses to stress. *Social Science and Medicine, 68*(12), 2190–2198.

O'Donnell, M. L., Alkemade, N., Creamer, M. C., McFarlane, A. C., Silove, D., Bryant,

R., et al. (2016). The long-term psychiatric sequelae of severe injury: A 6-year follow-up study. *Journal of Clinical Psychiatry, 77*(4), e473–e479.

O'Donnell, M. L., Lau, W., Tipping, S., Holmes, A. C., Ellen, S., Judson, R., et al. (2012). Stepped early psychological intervention for posttraumatic stress disorder, other anxiety disorders, and depression following serious injury. *Journal of Traumatic Stress, 25*(2), 125–133.

Pennebaker, J. W., Kiecolt-Glaser, J. K., & Glaser, R. (1988). Disclosure of traumas and immune function: Health implications for psychotherapy. *Journal of Consulting and Clinical Psychology, 56*(2), 239.

Phoenix Australia—Centre for Posttraumatic Mental Health. (2013). *Australian guidelines for the treatment of acute stress disorder and posttraumatic stress disorder.* Melbourne, Victoria, Australia: Author.

Pietrzak, R., Feder, A., Singh, R., Schechter, C., Bromet, E. J., Katz, C., et al. (2014). Trajectories of PTSD risk and resilience in World Trade Center responders: An 8-year prospective cohort study. *Psychological Medicine, 44*(1), 205–219.

Qi, W., Ratanatharathorn, A., Gevonden, M., Bryant, R., Delahanty, D., Matsuoka, Y., et al. (2018). Application of data pooling to longitudinal studies of early post-traumatic stress disorder (PTSD): The International Consortium to Predict PTSD (ICPP) project. *European Journal of Psychotraumatology, 9*(1), Article 1476442.

Rose, S., Bisson, J., Churchill, R., & Wessely, S. (2002). Psychological debriefing for preventing post traumatic stress disorder (PTSD). *Cochrane Database of Systematic Reviews, 2,* CD000560.

Rothbaum, B., Kearns, M., Price, M., Malcoun, E., Davis, M., Ressler, K., et al. (2012). Early intervention may prevent the development of posttraumatic stress disorder: A randomized pilot civilian study with modified prolonged exposure. *Biological Psychiatry, 72*(11), 957–963.

Roy-Byrne, P. P., Russo, J., Michelson, E., Zatzick, D., Pitman, R. K., & Berliner, L. (2004). Risk factors and outcome in ambulatory assault victims presenting to the acute emergency department setting: Implications for secondary prevention studies in PTSD. *Depression and Anxiety, 19*(2), 77–84.

Ryding, E., Wijma, K., & Wijma, B. (1998). Postpartum counselling after an emergency cesarean. *Clinical Psychology and Psychotherapy, 5*(4), 231–237.

Santiago, P. N., Ursano, R. J., Gray, C. L., Pynoos, R. S., Spiegel, D., Lewis-Fernandez, R., et al. (2013). A systematic review of PTSD prevalence and trajectories in DSM-5 defined trauma exposed populations: Intentional and non-intentional traumatic events. *PLOS ONE, 8*(4), e59236.

Shalev, A., Ankri, Y., Gilad, M., Israeli-Shalev, Y., Adessky, R., Qian, M., et al. (2016). Long-term outcome of early interventions to prevent posttraumatic stress disorder. *Journal of Clinical Psychiatry, 77*(5), e580–e587.

Shalev, A., Ankri, Y., Israeli-Shalev, Y., Peleg, T., Adessky, R., & Freedman, S. (2012). Prevention of posttraumatic stress disorder by early treatment: Results from the Jerusalem trauma outreach and prevention study. *Archives of General Psychiatry, 69*(2), 166–176.

Shalev, A., Gevonden, M., Ratanatharathorn, A., Laska, E., van der Mei, W. F., Qi, W., et al. (2019). Estimating the risk of PTSD in recent trauma survivors: Results of the International Consortium to Predict PTSD (ICPP). *World Psychiatry, 18*(1), 77–87.

Shapiro, E., & Laub, B. (2008). Early EMDR intervention (EEI): A summary, a theoretical model, and the recent traumatic episode protocol (R-TEP). *Journal of EMDR Practice and Research, 2*(2), 79–96.

Shapiro, E., & Laub, B. (2015). Early EMDR intervention following a community critical incident: A randomized clinical trial. *Journal of EMDR Practice and Research, 9*(1), 17–27.

Shapiro, E., Laub, B., & Rosenblat, O. (2018). Early EMDR intervention following intense rocket attacks on a town: A randomised clinical trial. *Clinical Neuropsychiatry: Journal of Treatment Evaluation, 15*(3), 194–205.

Shaw, R. J., St. John, N., Lilo, E. A., Jo, B., Benitz, W., Stevenson, D. K., et al. (2013). Prevention of traumatic stress in mothers with preterm infants: A randomized controlled trial. *Pediatrics, 132*(4), e886–e894.

Sijbrandij, M., Olff, M., Reitsma, J. B., Carlier, I. V., de Vries, M. H., & Gersons, B. P. (2007). Treatment of acute posttraumatic stress disorder with brief cognitive behavioral therapy: A randomized controlled trial. *American Journal of Psychiatry, 164*(1), 82–90.

Steenkamp, M. M., Dickstein, B. D., Salters-Pedneault, K., Hofmann, S. G., & Litz, B. T. (2012). Trajectories of PTSD symptoms following sexual assault: Is resilience the modal outcome? *Journal of Traumatic Stress, 25*(4), 469–474.

van Emmerik, A. A. P., Kamphuis, J., & Emmelkamp, P. M. G. (2008). Treating acute stress disorder and posttraumatic stress disorder with cognitive behavioral therapy or structured writing therapy: A randomized controlled trial. *Psychotherapy and Psychosomatics, 77*(2), 93–100.

Vojvoda, D., Weine, S. M., McGlashan, T., Becker, D. F., & Southwick, S. M. (2008). Posttraumatic stress disorder symptoms in Bosnian refugees 3½ years after resettlement. *Journal of Rehabilitation Research and Development, 45*(3), 421–426.

World Health Organization. (2011). *Psychological first aid: Guide for field workers.* Geneva, Switzerland: War Trauma Foundation and World Vision International.

Wu, K. K., Li, F. W., & Cho, V. W. (2014). A randomized controlled trial of the effectiveness of brief-CBT for patients with symptoms of posttraumatic stress following a motor vehicle crash. *Behavioural and Cognitive Psychotherapy, 42*(1), 31–47.

Zatzick, D., Jurkovich, G., Rivara, F. P., Russo, J., Wagner, A., Wang, J., et al. (2013). A randomized stepped care intervention trial targeting posttraumatic stress disorder for surgically hospitalized injury survivors. *Annals of Surgery, 257*(3), 390–399.

Zatzick, D., O'Connor, S. S., Russo, J., Wang, J., Bush, N., Love, J., et al. (2015). Technology-enhanced stepped collaborative care targeting posttraumatic stress disorder and comorbidity after injury: A randomized controlled trial. *Journal of Traumatic Stress, 28*(5), 391–400.

Zatzick, D., Roy-Byrne, P., Russo, J., Rivara, F., Droesch, R., Wagner, A., et al. (2004). A randomized effectiveness trial of stepped collaborative care for acutely injured trauma survivors. *Archives of General Psychiatry, 61*(5), 498–506.

Zatzick, D., Roy-Byrne, P., Russo, J. E., Rivara, F. P., Koike, A., Jurkovich, G. J., et al. (2001). Collaborative interventions for physically injured trauma survivors: A pilot randomized effectiveness trial. *General Hospital Psychiatry, 23*(3), 114–123.

CHAPTER 9

Early Pharmacological Intervention Following Exposure to Traumatic Events

Jonathan I. Bisson, Laurence Astill Wright, and Marit Sijbrandij

A diagnosis of posttraumatic stress disorder (PTSD) requires a defined external event(s), and this should, in theory, facilitate the development of early interventions to prevent the onset of symptoms and to treat them shortly after they emerge. Unfortunately, despite significant research effort and major developments in our understanding of the learning and memory mechanisms involved in processing traumatic events, we continue to search for effective early interventions. Most early intervention research in humans has focused on psychosocial and behavioral approaches (see O'Donnell, Pacella, Bryant, Olff, & Forbes, Chapter 8, this volume), but there is a growing body of research concerning pharmacological approaches.

This chapter aims to help clinicians interpret the current evidence regarding the prescription of medication in adults within the first 3 months of traumatic events. The chapter provides advice on whether, what, when, and how to prescribe, and discusses key considerations when prescribing medication shortly after traumatic events.

Theoretical Context

Research has provided us with a strong understanding of the involvement of neurotransmitters, neuropeptides, and glucocorticoids in the processing of traumatic memories and the development and maintenance of PTSD. These include catecholamines, opioids, gamma-aminobutyric acid (GABA), gluta-mate, serotonin, oxytocin, and cortisol. There is also considerable evidence that overactivity of the amygdala, driven by overactivity of the noradrenergic system, plays a significant role and that attenuation of this should be benefi-cial in preventing PTSD (Shin, Rauch, & Pitman, 2006).

A key aim of early pharmacological intervention work has been to reduce adrenergic activity, either directly through drugs that work through their effects on adrenergic receptors (e.g., propranolol) or indirectly (e.g., hydrocortisone) to reduce noradrenaline release. Several studies have tried to build on our understanding of the consolidation of traumatic memories by intervening within the so-called golden hours, a time frame up to 6 hours after a traumatic event occurs (Nader, 2003; Zohar et al., 2011).

Although the data from clinical research, specifically with respect to antiadrenergics, have not been as promising as hoped for (Sijbrandij, Klei-boer, Bisson, Barbui, & Cuijpers, 2015), we now have a much better under-standing of the impact of early pharmacological intervention on people at risk of or with PTSD within 3 months of a traumatic event.

Description of Pharmacological Agents

Antiadrenergics. Propranolol, a beta-receptor blocker that was originally developed to treat raised blood pressure, has been tested in a number of randomized controlled trials (RCTs) to prevent PTSD.

Docosahexaenoic acid. Docosahexaenoic acid is an omega-3 fatty acid found in the human body and is present in fish oil. It is widely used as a food supplement and has been tested as an early pharmacological intervention to prevent PTSD.

Gabapentin. Gabapentin was first developed as an antiepileptic drug. Despite its name, it does not act via GABA neurotransmitter receptors and is believed to act through its actions on calcium channels.

Hydrocortisone. The synthetic form of the adrenal-gland-produced hor-mone cortisol has been used to try to bring about homeostasis (stability) to the hypothalamic–pituitary–adrenal axis by inhibiting further release of adrenaline and noradrenaline.

Oxytocin. Interest in this naturally occurring hormone and neuropep-tide was sparked by knowledge of its positive impact on fear responsiveness, stress reactivity, and social–emotional functioning.

Selective serotonin reuptake inhibitors (SSRIs). Members of this class of drugs (fluoxetine, paroxetine, and sertraline) are among those with the strongest evidence of effect for treatment of PTSD present 3 months or more after a traumatic event (see Bisson, Hoskins, & Stein, Chapter 16, this volume). Another SSRI, escitalopram, has been subjected to one RCT as a treatment for acute stress disorder (Suliman et al., 2015) and another for PTSD (Shalev et al., 2012) diagnosed within a month of a traumatic event.

Other pharmacological agents, for example, benzodiazepines and morphine, have been used in an attempt to prevent the development of PTSD, but no studies satisfied the criteria required for inclusion in the evidence summaries prepared for the International Society for Traumatic Stress Studies (ISTSS) guidelines.

Summary and Appraisal of the Evidence

The evidence summaries prepared for the ISTSS guidelines concerned RCTs of pharmacological treatments used within 3 months of a traumatic event that aimed to either prevent or treat symptoms of PTSD. Fifteen includable RCTs were found that considered the six types of drugs described previously. Seven (47%) of the included RCTs had usable data that were included in the primary meta-analyses.

The overall quality of the studies included was low and there was insufficient evidence to recommend all but one of the drugs considered. Only the meta-analysis of the hydrocortisone RCTs showed significant superiority to placebo, leading to it being recommended as an intervention with emerging evidence for the prevention of PTSD in adults.

The RCTs included tended to be conducted within specific populations who were hospital inpatients or outpatients attending the hospital as a result of physical injury or disease. This makes it very difficult to generalize the results to other populations. This is particularly true for hydrocortisone as the majority of participants had septic shock or had undergone major cardiac surgery.

As described by Bisson, Lewis, and Roberts (Chapter 6, this volume), it is very difficult to compare the results of pharmacological treatment trials employing placebo controls and double blinding with psychosocial intervention trials using wait-list or usual-care controls and no blinding of the participant or the treating clinician. In common with other guideline development groups (e.g., National Collaborating Centre for Mental Health, 2005), the ISTSS Guidelines Committee determined a priori rules to allow comparison of different types of treatment, making the threshold required for a *Strong* recommendation for a drug tested through placebo-controlled RCTs 50% less than that for psychological treatments tested through wait-list or usual-care RCTs. Whether the 50% lower threshold accurately reflects the true level is open for debate, but even if the threshold had been lower, this would not have made a difference with respect to the recommendations made for early pharmacological interventions.

The ISTSS guideline recommendations for early pharmacological interventions are shown in Table 9.1.

TABLE 9.1. ISTSS Recommendations for Early Pharmacological Intervention

Intervention with Emerging Evidence—*Hydrocortisone* within the first 3 months of a traumatic event has emerging evidence of efficacy for the prevention of PTSD symptoms in adults.

Insufficient Evidence to Recommend—There is insufficient evidence to recommend *docosahexaenoic acid, escitalopram, gabapentin, oxytocin,* or *propranolol* within the first 3 months of a traumatic event for the prevention or treatment of PTSD symptoms in adults.

Quality of the Evidence

The quality of the pharmacological RCTs, assessed by the Cochrane risk of bias tool (Higgins & Green, 2011) and modified GRADE criteria (see *www.gradeworkinggroup.org*), included in the meta-analyses was low. There were a number of issues that indicated risk of bias in the results, especially with respect to incomplete outcome data and the selective reporting of results. It is also noteworthy that a number of the studies reported significant difficulty in recruiting participants (e.g., Shalev et al., 2012; Stein, Kerridge, Dimsdale, & Hoyt, 2007), with many people refusing to participate as they did not want to take medication.

The studies included in the meta-analyses displayed quite significant clinical heterogeneity, and the majority of the studies were undertaken in higher-income countries. These issues, in addition to the small number of total participants and their physical health and hospital status, raise major questions on the generalizability of these findings. This is particularly pertinent to people exposed to traumatic events who would not have been included in the studies and to individuals living in settings different from those where the research studies were conducted.

Adverse Effects

The participants reported few problematic adverse effects and the drugs considered appeared to be reasonably well tolerated in the included RCTs. That said, an increased rate of dizziness, infection/septic shock, and raised glucose and sodium blood levels were reported in hydrocortisone studies. Although there was no evidence that drugs should not be considered for use because of adverse effects, caution is clearly required, and hydrocortisone, in particular, is associated with problematic adverse effects when taken in higher doses and in the longer term. Hydrocortisone also suppresses the immune system, so it may be contraindicated when there is acute infection risk.

Practical Delivery of the Recommendations

At present, the evidence is not strong enough to recommend the routine use of any medication to prevent or treat PTSD within 3 months of a traumatic event. The *Intervention with Emerging Evidence* recommendation for hydrocortisone suggests the drug is a good candidate for further research in other populations, but, at present, it cannot be argued that hydrocortisone is ready for routine clinical use.

There will, however, be instances when individuals request medication, for example, to help with sleep, refuse evidence-based nonpharmacological approaches, or present with specific troublesome symptoms (e.g., marked insomnia or agitation) following a traumatic event. As with all treatments for PTSD, it is vital that pharmacological treatment only be prescribed after an accurate assessment of an individual's needs that takes into account her or his individual circumstances. Key issues to consider before prescribing medication include primary diagnosis; comorbidity; alternative treatment options; attitude toward medication; previous response to medication; family history of response to medication; expectations of medication; awareness of potential adverse effects; other prescribed drugs and potential interactions; and other substance use and potential interactions. Medication should only be prescribed when a clinician believes the likely benefits outweigh the risks and when the individual is equipped with the knowledge necessary to make a fully informed decision.

Possible Pharmacological Interventions in the First 3 Months

Prevention (Universal Intervention)

No pharmacological intervention can be recommended for routine clinical use to prevent PTSD. Hydrocortisone is the only drug with emerging evidence of benefit and requires further evaluation. In individuals with no contraindications to its prescription, hydrocortisone could be considered as a preventative intervention for people with severe physical illness or injury, shortly after a traumatic event. The doses of hydrocortisone used in the trials varied from 20 mg twice a day orally for 10 days followed by a tapering period where the dose was halved every 2 days (total dose = 400 mg over 10 days), followed by around 70 mg (exact dose not given) over 6 days (Delahanty et al., 2013) to a 100-mg intravenous bolus followed by tapering over 2 days (total dose = 550 mg over 4 days; Weis et al., 2006).

Treatment of Symptoms of PTSD

If an individual with PTSD and her or his treating clinician agree that treatment with medication is indicated and desired, the most logical approach, based on the current evidence base, would be to follow the prescribing algorithm described in Bisson, Hoskins, and Stein (Chapter 16, this volume). It should be acknowledged that no evidence exists for the efficacy of drugs to treat PTSD within 3 months and there is evidence suggesting that escitalopram is no better than placebo in preventing the development of PTSD in individuals with acute stress disorder (ASD) or partial ASD (Suliman et al., 2015) or for the treatment of PTSD diagnosed a month after the traumatic event (Shalev et al., 2012).

Insomnia

Many people find insomnia a particular problem soon after a traumatic event (Hall Brown, Ameenat, & Mellman, 2015) and ask specifically for medication to help them sleep. Although there is no evidence base to support this, if such a scenario occurs, it is recommended that the same approach to the one for pharmacological management of insomnia in PTSD sufferers be taken (see Chapter 16, this volume). A sedative antidepressant should be considered first line, for example, 15 mg of mirtazapine at night (which has the added benefit of RCT evidence supporting its use for PTSD) or 50–100 mg of trazadone at night. Both these drugs are not associated with the addictive potential of drugs such as benzodiazepines or the Z drugs, and there is some evidence of an adverse effect of early temazepam on PTSD symptoms in one RCT that was excluded from the ISTSS evidence syntheses (Mellman, Bustamante, Daniella, & Fins, 2002). An alternative, especially for individuals with significant agitation, is 25 mg of quetiapine at night. It is important to be aware that mirtazapine, trazadone, and quetiapine can cause drowsiness the following day, and other adverse effects such as weight gain, and individuals should be warned about this.

Agitation

Agitation may be present and can be a reason for deciding to treat with medication early on if recommended psychological approaches are not available, have not been effective, or are not wanted. For the majority of people with PTSD, medication for agitation is not necessary, but for some individuals it is likely to be needed and, in addition to reducing agitation, may also enable an individual to tolerate other treatments, for example, psychological treatment for his or her PTSD. Given its adverse effect profile and evidence for use for PTSD, quetiapine is recommended. Some doctors recommend short courses of benzodiazepine for such agitation, but we do not recommend this given the lack of evidence for benzodiazepine use, the risk of dependency, and the risk of increased PTSD symptoms and interference with psychological treatments through their impact on trauma processing by impairing fear extinction (Bouton, Kenney, & Rosengard, 1990; Rothbaum et al., 2014).

Future Developments

There is clearly a need to improve the evidence available for early pharmacological intervention following traumatic events. There is a need to develop and test effective: (1) early universal preventative interventions, (2) indicated interventions to address higher-risk and emerging clinical features of traumatic stress symptomatology, and (3) treatment interventions for diagnosable PTSD by fully exploiting our understanding of the neurobiology of the development and maintenance of PTSD. There are some emerging candidates, but more research is needed to identify novel pharmacological approaches that may help. There is a need for more clinical research with existing drugs, for example, hydrocortisone, in different populations and with a greater focus on dosing and duration of administration.

There is also an urgent need to ensure that our current knowledge with regard to early pharmacological intervention is disseminated and implemented in practice across the world. We need to strive to ensure that people who seek treatment following traumatic events are fully informed about evidence-based pharmacological management so they can make an informed decision on whether to try this approach or not.

Summary

In summary, despite some good candidate drugs, no early pharmacological intervention can be recommended for general use within the first 3 months of a traumatic event. There is emerging evidence that hydrocortisone may prevent the development of PTSD, especially in seriously physically unwell and injured populations. Despite an absence of evidence, some medications can be considered for symptomatic relief within the first 3 months of a traumatic event.

REFERENCES

Bouton, M. E., Kenney, F. A., & Rosengard, C. (1990). State-dependent fear extinction with two benzodiazepine tranquilizers. *Behavioral Neuroscience, 104,* 44–55.

Delahanty, D., Gabert-Quillen, C., Ostrowski, S., Nugent, N., Fischer, B., Morris, A., et al. (2013). The efficacy of initial hydrocortisone administration at preventing posttraumatic distress in adult trauma patients: A randomized trial. *CNS Spectrums, 18,* 103–111.

Hall Brown, T. S., Ameenat, A., & Mellman, T. A. (2015). The role of trauma type in the risk for insomnia. *Journal of Clinical Sleep Medicine, 11,* 735–739.

Higgins, J. P., & Green, S. (Eds.). (2011). Cochrane handbook for systematic reviews of interventions, Version 5.1.0. Retrieved from *training.cochrane.org/handbook.*

Mellman, T. A., Bustamante, V., Daniella, D., & Fins, A. I. (2002). Hypnotic medication in the aftermath of trauma. *Journal of Clinical Psychiatry, 63,* 1183–1184.

Nader, K. (2003). Memory traces unbound. *Trends in Neurosciences, 26,* 65–72.

National Collaborating Centre for Mental Health. (2005). *Post-traumatic stress disorder: The management of PTSD in adults and children in primary and secondary care.* London and Leicester, UK: Gaskell and BPS.

Rothbaum, B. O., Price, M., Jovanovic, T., Norrholm, S. D., Gerardi, M., Dunlop, B., et al. (2014). A randomized, double-blind evaluation of *d*-cycloserine or alprazolam combined with virtual reality exposure therapy for posttraumatic stress disorder in Iraq and Afghanistan war veterans. *American Journal of Psychiatry, 171,* 640–648.

Shalev, A., Ankri, Y., Israeli-Shalev, Y., Peleg, T., Adessky, R., & Freedman, S. (2012). Prevention of posttraumatic stress disorder by early treatment: Results from the Jerusalem Trauma Outreach and Prevention Study. *Archives of General Psychiatry, 69,* 166–176.

Shin, L. M., Rauch, S. L., & Pitman, R. K. (2006). Amygdala, medial prefrontal cortex, and hippocampal function in PTSD. *Annals of the New York Academy of Sciences, 1071,* 67–79.

Sijbrandij, M., Kleiboer, A., Bisson, J. I., Barbui, C., & Cuijpers, P. (2015). Pharmacological prevention of posttraumatic stress disorder and acute stress disorder: A systematic review and meta-analysis. *Lancet Psychiatry, 2,* 413–421.

Stein, M., Kerridge, C., Dimsdale, J., & Hoyt, D. (2007). Pharmacotherapy to prevent PTSD: Results from a randomized controlled proof-of-concept trial in physically injured patients. *Journal of Traumatic Stress, 20,* 923–932.

Suliman, S., Seedat, S., Pingo, J., Sutherland, T., Zohar, J., & Stein, D. (2015). Escitalopram in the prevention of posttraumatic stress disorder: A pilot randomized controlled trial. *BMC Psychiatry, 15*(24).

Weis, F., Kilger, E., Roozendaal, B., de Quervain, D., Lamm, P., Schmidt, M., et al. (2006). Stress doses of hydrocortisone reduce chronic stress symptoms and improve health-related quality of life in high-risk patients after cardiac surgery: A randomized study. *Journal of Thoracic and Cardiovascular Surgery, 131,* 277–282.

Zohar, J., Juven-Wetzler, A., Sonnino, R., Cwikel-Hamzany, S., Balaban, E., & Cohen, H. (2011). New insights into secondary prevention in post-traumatic stress disorder. *Dialogues in Clinical Neuroscience, 13*(3), 301–309.

PART III

EARLY INTERVENTION IN CHILDREN AND ADOLESCENTS

CHAPTER 10

Preventative and Early Interventions

Justin Kenardy, Nancy Kassam-Adams, and Grete Dyb

Preventative and early interventions have the potential to reduce the ongoing impact of trauma exposure. Consistent with public health models, prevention and early intervention to address posttraumatic stress disorder (PTSD) in childhood can be conceptualized as primary prevention (i.e., aiming to prevent the occurrence of a disease/injury), or secondary prevention (i.e., aiming to reduce the impact of a disease/injury early on). PTSD is unusual among mental health problems in that inception is usually clear, and precipitants are included in the definition of the disorder. Having a clear precipitant event or events could mean that early intervention would be more effectively applied. However, identifying children who have experienced trauma is not always straightforward, and trauma-related problems may not be identified for some time. Certain types of trauma and certain settings lend themselves to prevention and early intervention. Natural disasters or war affect populations as a whole; mass violence or a school shooting affect the community or school in which they happen. In medical settings, ill and injured children are populations at risk because they are known to have been exposed to potentially traumatic experiences. Other settings also see children with known recent exposure to trauma, for example, in the United States Child Advocacy Centers (CACs) are a widely used model for service delivery, providing an immediate response to interpersonal traumas such as child abuse, rape, and domestic violence.

Even when a child is identified as being at risk of PTSD following trauma, there is no guarantee that they will receive an appropriate intervention. The evidence base for preventative and early intervention after trauma exposure in children is small and has not been widely disseminated or taken up in clinical practice. In this chapter, we will describe the evidence on prevention and early intervention evaluated by the 2019 treatment guidelines

147

issued by the International Society for Traumatic Stress Studies (ISTSS), as well as practical and clinical implications for applying early interventions in accordance with the current evidence base.

Theoretical Context

Prevention and early intervention for trauma-exposed children have been the focus of a number of theoretical models. Across models, key themes with implications for practice are (1) considering levels of preventive intervention, (2) considering time frame in relation to trauma exposure, and (3) making use of hypothesized predictive factors and etiological mechanisms to select appropriate targets for early intervention.

In the context of both pediatric medical trauma (Kazak, 2006) and children exposed to disaster (Vernberg, 2002), models that frame preventative and early interventions have applied the public health concept of three levels of prevention: universal, targeted, and clinical/treatment. Universal interventions are directed to all children with a trauma exposure. Targeted (sometimes referred to as selective) interventions are delivered to trauma-exposed children with signs of acute distress and/or evident risk factors. Clinical/treatment interventions are for trauma-exposed children who are experiencing clinically significant, persistent, and/or escalating levels of distress and are in need of specialist psychological intervention and support. Both targeted and clinical/treatment interventions require some means of identifying children who need this level of intervention. Screening instruments may be designed to detect those at risk for the development of ongoing problems ("risk screeners") and/or to identify those with current distress warranting clinical attention ("concurrent screeners"). In planning early intervention, this distinction is important, and more research is needed to develop and validate both types of effective screening tools, and to optimize the use of existing screening tools (e.g., timing and presentation; March et al., 2015)

Early intervention models have also delineated the evolving challenges, adaptation, and recovery over time for trauma-exposed children—and the implications of this time frame for intervention. Kazak and colleagues (2006) and Price, Kassam-Adams, Alderfer, Christofferson, and Kazak (2016) described three phases for the trajectory of child and family responses to pediatric medical trauma. In Phase I (the peritrauma period where some aspects of the trauma may still be unfolding), the goal of interventions is to modify the subjective experience of the potentially traumatic event by providing trauma-informed care or services, and to screen for risk. In Phase II (the days to weeks after trauma exposure), intervention goals may include screening for risk, reducing distress from emerging symptoms of traumatic stress, and preventing the development of persistent traumatic stress. In Phase III (months to years after trauma exposure), intervention goals are to identify and treat significant ongoing traumatic stress. Based on work with children exposed to disasters, Vernberg (2002) similarly outlined a framework in which time frame (pre-, peri-, and posttrauma phases) is crucial, and in which the appropriate use of universal, targeted/selected, and clinical/treatment interventions is mapped onto each phase. For example, the purpose of universal interventions would be distinct in each phase, focusing on preparedness in the predisaster phase but on helping children reestablish routines in the early postdisaster phase.

Several models have outlined risk and protective factors for the development and persistence of traumatic stress symptoms. For example, models based on work with children exposed to disasters (La Greca, Silverman, Vernberg, & Prinstein, 1996; Vernberg, 2002) identified the severity and range of exposure to different aspects of the event, individual child characteristics, the environment in which child recovery takes place, and the child's available psychological resources as key risk factors. Biopsychosocial models (Marsac, Kassam-Adams, Delahanty, Widaman, & Barakat, 2014) emphasize processes across pre-, peri-, and posttrauma periods that may contribute to PTSD development. These models point to the importance of considering the interaction of biological factors (genetic and heritable factors, internal physiological processes), psychological factors (memory formation, cognitive state), and social and environmental factors (culture, community support, parent–child interactions). Finally, theoretical models of specific etiological processes provide a strong basis for early interventions that target and interrupt specific mechanisms that drive the development of traumatic stress symptoms. To date, the most fully developed etiological models guiding early interventions are those that highlight the role of cognitive processes in the early development and maintenance of PTSD symptoms (Meiser-Stedman, 2002).

Description of Models and Techniques

There are a few key characteristics of prevention/early interventions that distinguish these from clinical treatments for children who have persisting distress. The models are delivered early on following trauma, and they tend to be briefer than the trauma-focused therapy interventions (generally, one to six sessions). Many models include techniques grounded in CBT approaches, but adapted for the timing and delivery mode of early intervention. Across both early preventative and early treatment interventions, common clinical elements include psychoeducation about responses to trauma, coping skills for trauma-related distress, promotion of facing up to or exposure to nondangerous cues instead of avoidance, promoting helpful cognitions about the trauma, and enhancing parental support. Different models may contain more or less of these common clinical elements.

Models applied in preventative or early treatment interventions are briefly described here, with an emphasis on the core components of each that may be included across specific intervention approaches or studies.

Trauma-Informed Care

Trauma-informed care for prevention and early intervention begins with promoting recognition and awareness of trauma and its impact among professionals across a range of service settings that commonly see children impacted by acute or ongoing trauma, for example, schools, child protection agencies, health care settings, and law enforcement. They are educated that potentially traumatic events are common in children's lives, that there is a range of impacts of trauma exposure for children, and that resilience and recovery are common. The provision of trauma-informed care aims to embed this awareness in the everyday practices of these settings and to minimize new potentially traumatic exposures for children and families (Marsac et al., 2017). Thus, for example, in trauma-informed schools, a change in a student's classroom behavior (becoming withdrawn or disruptive) is understood through a "trauma lens." In trauma-informed medical settings, doctors and nurses work to minimize pain and distress from medical procedures. Trauma-informed care may be appropriate at many points along the posttrauma time frame, from the peritraumatic period onward. In the clinical mental health context where children seek services, the *sine qua non* of trauma-informed care is routine screening for trauma exposure and impact.

Psychological First Aid

Psychological first aid (PFA) techniques, initially developed for postdisaster settings, are applied universally in the very early stages following trauma exposure. The main components are instillation of a sense of safety, promotion of calming through simple skills such as slow breathing and distraction, facilitation of self-efficacy and empowerment, encouragement of personal and community connectedness, and promotion of realistic hope. PFA has been adapted for application with children in a range of settings, through models such as Listen Protect Connect (Ramirez et al., 2013). No studies of PFA were included in the evidence review.

Psychological Debriefing

The primary components of psychological debriefing are the narrative reconstruction of the circumstances of the trauma to improve understanding and change inaccurate interpretations of the circumstances, to promote the referencing of trauma responses to "normalize" reactions, and to provide information about those reactions and possible additional coping resources (Stallard et al., 2006). Psychological debriefing is distinct from other very brief early interventions in its emphasis on a more active psychological processing of the traumatic event. A note of caution is in order, as the review found emerging evidence *not* to recommend individual psychological debriefing as an early preventative intervention.

Information Provision (Self-Help)/Psychoeducation (Self-Directed Online)

Information provision is aimed at promoting more adaptive responses to trauma, thereby reducing the likelihood of the development of long-term psychopathology. The common components of effective information provision are promotion of adaptive appraisals of the potentially traumatic events, reducing excessive and maladaptive early avoidance, and promoting family social support (Kassam-Adams et al., 2016). Information and psychoeducation may involve parents or caretakers as well as children, and may be provided in person, via print materials, or via online/e-health tools. Online interventions offer accessible, self-directed, and initiated interactive information provision where the use and selection of information are within the child's control, possibly with facilitation by a parent, especially with children of a younger age. Many of these interventions have been designed to be engaging and interesting as well as pertinent to the user.

Parent Support and Training

Parent training is a component of many early intervention models, both universal self-directed tools for parents, and in-person interventions (targeted/selective or treatment) that engage parents with or without their child. It commonly includes providing parents with information about trauma and trauma reactions and how they can assist their child in recovery based on trauma-informed care principles, and educating parents as to when their child's reactions may indicate the need to seek further help (Marsac et al., 2013). For example, parents may be taught to help their child return to normal routines as much as possible in the posttrauma period and to interpret behavior changes in the context of trauma responses. Parents are often taught to gently support their child in facing reminders of the trauma so that excessive avoidance does not inadvertently strengthen the development of traumatic stress symptoms. Some early intervention models explicitly include guided practice for parents in applying this new knowledge and set of skills with their child.

School-Based Training for Recovery

Schools provide a unique and well-placed opportunity to deliver preventative care for children following trauma. Schools frequently offer continuity and predictability for children and families, often have well-established relationships with children and their families, and in many cases already deliver universal or targeted/selective interventions for a variety of social-emotional targets. Therefore, schools have been the setting for delivery for many programs following traumatic events: universal programs for parents, children, and teachers in response to a major disaster or ongoing armed conflict to which all children will have been exposed, as well as targeted/selective interventions that are delivered to children with identified distress (Kataoka, Langley, Wong, Baweja, & Stein, 2012). The School-Focused Training for Recovery program is one example (Le Brocque et al., 2017). In this intervention, teachers are provided with in-service training that covers understanding possible responses to trauma, teaching practices that promote recovery, identification of children in need of further assistance, and self-care. Schools have also been the delivery site for early interventions to children exposed to war and violence (Berger, Pat-Horenczyk, & Gelkopf, 2007; Karam et al., 2008; Ramirez et al., 2013; Wolmer et al., 2013).

Active Monitoring

The most likely outcome following exposure to trauma is recovery (Le Brocque, Hendrikz, & Kenardy, 2010). However, the probability of recovery will vary, and it is not always possible to know which children will develop ongoing distress or problems. Therefore, a model of active monitoring (sometimes called "watchful waiting") has been recommended as an approach that does not interrupt natural recovery processes, and effectively utilizes scarce resources (National Institute for Health and Care Excellence, 2018). This approach generally includes universal initial screening for risk, paired with ongoing monitoring for distress or symptoms to determine if targeted/selective or treatment interventions are required.

Stepped Care

Stepped care is not a specific set of techniques, but rather a model that aims to systematically screen or monitor and to deliver the required degree of intervention for each child at the time when needs are identified. Stepped-care models typically begin with less intensive modes of intervention (e.g., psychoeducation, active monitoring) applied universally, and then "step up" to more intensive modes, including treatment for the child or family, if distress does not resolve or if the child's risk level changes (Kazak, 2006). Stepped-care approaches can provide the bridge between universal, targeted/selective, and clinical/treatment levels of early intervention.

Cognitive-Behavioral Therapy with a Trauma Focus

Several variants of traditional cognitive-behavioral therapy with a trauma focus (CBT-T) for children (Cloitre, Karatzias, & Ford, Chapter 20, this volume) have been applied as an early treatment intervention for trauma-exposed children. Compared to treatment of persistent traumatic stress symptoms, CBT-T in early treatment interventions is often briefer, and techniques are frequently adapted for context and setting of delivery (e.g., outside of traditional mental health settings). The KidNET intervention is delivered in six sessions and centers on facilitating the creation of a life narrative, with particular attention to any traumatic experiences (not limited to the recent acute trauma). The aim is construction of a coherent narrative from fragmented reports, and narrative exposure is employed until fear reactions subside. Catani and colleagues (2009) implemented KidNET for war-exposed children in refugee camps soon after a tsunami. Even briefer CBT-T interventions have been employed in the acute posttrauma phase, such as a two-session intervention integrating construction of a trauma narrative, psychoeducation, and coping skills (including exposure) that was implemented in a hospital setting for children postaccident or burn injury (Kramer & Landolt, 2014).

Child and Family Traumatic Stress Intervention

Because parents are likely to be key to successful recovery and early intervention, the Child and Family Traumatic Stress Intervention (CFTSI; Berkowitz, Stover, & Marans, 2011) focuses primarily on enhancing the relationship between a child and parent to promote recovery through psychoeducation, review of results of standard measures, and coping tips. The intervention is delivered over four sessions beginning within 30 days of the trauma and aims to promote communication between child and caregiver/parent about traumatic symptoms and responses, and facilitate the child and parent working together to develop adaptive coping to the traumatic stress responses, including sleep, depressive withdrawal, behavioral problems, and intrusive thoughts and anxiety. Depending on the specific problems of each child, CBT-T elements are incorporated to a greater or lesser extent.

Summary of Evidence

Scoping question: "For children within the first 3 months of a traumatic event, do psychosocial interventions, *when compared to intervention as usual, waiting list, or no intervention*, result in a clinically important reduction/prevention of symptoms, improved functioning/quality of life, presence of disorder, or adverse effects?"

As defined here, early *preventative interventions* target unscreened or minimally screened populations (i.e., any trauma-exposed child) and aim to reduce acute symptoms, prevent development of PTSD, and restore children to everyday functioning. *Early treatment interventions* are provided to children and their families with emerging traumatic stress symptoms and aim to reduce the symptom levels in children with emerging PTSD symptoms or clinical levels of posttraumatic stress. In this review, evidence for efficacy of the studies interventions was defined as clinically important improvements documented in trauma-exposed children and adolescents.

Recommendations

Preventative Interventions

Intervention with Emerging Evidence—Self-directed online psychoeducation for caregivers and children.

Emerging Evidence Not to Recommend—Individual psychological debriefing.

Insufficient Evidence to Recommend—Self-directed online psychoeducation for caregivers only; brief CBT-T.

Early Treatment Interventions

Intervention with Emerging Evidence—Self-directed online psychoeducation for children.

Insufficient Evidence to Recommend—Stepped preventive care; brief CBT-T; CBT-T.

Appraisal of the Evidence

There are several important caveats in appraising the current evidence on early interventions for children and adolescents. These conclusions are based on a relatively small number of studies. Much of the evidence is provided from school-age children and adolescents, identified in hospital settings, who had been exposed to single events, limiting the generalizability of the findings to other ages, settings, and types of trauma exposure. Follow-up assessments were conducted up to 6 months after intervention so that the longer-term impact of early interventions is not yet known.

There is a gap between fairly well-developed theoretical models of what children may need help with after trauma exposure and our current empirical evidence about what works for whom, and how that should be delivered. With regard to delivery, it is notable that the empirical studies included in this review often identified children outside of traditional mental health service systems or online. However, the current empirically supported interventions have not been implemented widely in clinical practice or in response to population-level trauma (i.e., postdisaster outreach programs), so we do not know yet how these interventions would work in broad everyday practice.

Despite these caveats, these studies do provide a useful starting point to inform early preventative and treatment interventions. In most of these studies, child participants had been highly exposed to life threat, had sustained physical injuries, and were at risk of developing or had emerging PTSD symptoms. The studies vary in the manner in which parents were engaged or included, and encompass a range of delivery methods and intervention settings, thus providing useful information about feasibility and practical implementation of early intervention approaches.

Early Preventative Interventions

Self-Directed Online Psychoeducation: *Intervention with Emerging Evidence*

Online psychoeducation for children and their parents was evaluated in a single study of injured children ages 7–16, identified in a hospital setting in Australia (Cox, Kenardy, & Hendrikz, 2010). Self-help tools for relaxation, coping, problem solving, pleasant events, identifying personal strengths, and reflection on the event were provided to children and parents via a website. The study showed promising results in helping families cope in the early aftermath of acute trauma, perhaps being most helpful for children with higher levels of distress (Kenardy, Cox, & Brown, 2015). As noted previously, self-directed online interventions warrant further evaluation in larger samples and across trauma types.

Individual Psychological Debriefing: *Emerging Evidence Not to Recommend*

Two studies evaluated psychological debriefing in children exposed to road traffic accidents and identified in hospital settings in the United Kingdom and Switzerland. Stallard and colleagues (2006) compared debriefing to a neutral discussion. Zehnder, Meuli, and Landolt (2010) compared debriefing with usual care in a hospital. Although intervention and control groups in each study showed a reduction in PTSD symptoms over time, the ISTSS review found that in both studies the debriefing group experienced a smaller reduction in PTSD symptoms at follow-up. Psychological debriefing has been widely used internationally. These results indicate the need for professionals to acknowledge that we should not implement popular methods in clinical practice when there is evidence suggesting they may be ineffective or even slow recovery.

Psychoeducation and Brief CBT-T: *Insufficient Evidence to Recommend*

Two randomized controlled studies evaluated psychoeducation as an early preventative intervention for children. These two small studies evaluated children ages 7–15 exposed to acute injuries in a hospital setting (Kenardy, Thompson, Le Brocque, & Olsson, 2008) and siblings of children diagnosed with cancer (Prchal, Graf, Bergstraesser, & Landolt, 2012). Both used psychoeducation (information about common responses to trauma, common course of symptoms, and coping skills to minimize reactions) via print booklets (Kenardy et al., 2008) or psychoeducation provided in short-term interactions (Prchal et al., 2012). Neither study found evidence for prevention of PTSD symptoms. Similarly, a Web-based intervention (Marsac et al., 2013) for parents of acutely injured children that provided psychoeducation on promoting their children's recovery and reducing child traumatic stress was not effective in preventing child PTSD symptoms. The intervention did enhance parental knowledge about child traumatic stress reactions and adaptive coping.

Early Treatment Interventions

Self-Directed Online Psychoeducation Interventions: *Intervention with Emerging Evidence*

Even though more and more children are very active users of online and social media platforms, very few online early interventions have been evaluated. One exception is the Coping Coach intervention (Kassam-Adams et al., 2016) in which children interact with game characters at three different levels to identify reactions and feelings, explore cognitive appraisals, and reduce avoidance. The ISTSS review found emerging evidence that this technique may reduce PTSD symptoms in recently trauma-exposed children. Caveats are clear—this was a single study with 72 children ages 8–12 facing acute medical events who had some initial distress or risk factors, recruited in a single U.S. hospital. Effectiveness of self-directed online psychoeducation must be explored further in larger samples and with long-term follow-up.

CBT-T and Brief CBT-T: *Insufficient Evidence to Recommend*

CBT-T approaches do not yet have sufficient evidence overall for their effectiveness as early interventions for emerging or clinical symptoms in children. To date, very few early treatment interventions incorporating CBT-T elements have been studied in trials that met inclusion criteria for the ISTSS review. Two interventions delivered over four to six sessions, Narrative Exposure Therapy for Children (KidNET; Catani et al., 2009) and the Child and Family Traumatic Stress Intervention (CFTSI; Berkowitz et al., 2011), showed reduction in PTSD symptoms. A briefer (two-session) intervention (Kramer & Landolt, 2014) was not effective in reducing PTSD symptoms in young children and had some but not sufficient effect for school-aged children.

These interventions each included CBT-T elements and were tailored to target well-known predictors for further development of PTSD and revictimization. But they vary greatly in content, training of providers (schoolteachers, trained mental health professionals), intervention setting (psychiatric clinic, refugee camp, medical hospital), nature of traumatic event, level of PTSD risk or symptoms required for inclusion, and the timing and duration of treatment. This heterogeneity demonstrates the flexibility needed in adapting core CBT elements for early intervention. The intervention studies have demonstrated the feasibility of delivering CBT-T elements in diverse settings and to diverse age groups (young children through adolescents). However, the heterogeneity also creates challenges in taking this evidence to practice. It is important that these and other early intervention approaches that incorporate CBT-T elements go on to be evaluated in additional studies and in different settings. As the current evidence is from studies in only two countries, interventions may need to be tailored to cultural aspects to have the same potential for helping children globally.

Stepped Preventative Care: *Insufficient Evidence to Recommend*

A single study has evaluated a stepped preventative care intervention in a hospital setting in the United States, for injured children ages 8–17 (Kassam-Adams et al., 2011). The intervention did not reduce PTSD compared to usual care. The study's documentation of the feasibility of stepped care delivered by nurses and social workers in a hospital setting can inform ongoing development of early interventions integrated in paediatric health care.

Practical Delivery of the Recommendations

For interventions in the early aftermath of acute trauma exposure, practical considerations are paramount. The type of event and the recovery context help to determine what is needed and what is feasible. Intervention models that aim to prevent PTSD or treat early PTSD symptoms in children must consider how, when, and where to identify children and deliver interventions, the role of parents and caregivers, the roles of mental health and other professionals, as well as developmental and cultural considerations.

Type of Event and Context of Recovery

Acute traumatic events that impact children include those (such as disasters or mass violence) that capture public attention because these events affect whole communities or groups of children and families at one time. Such events may result in disruption of community and family resources that would usually be part of a child's support system. In addition, many millions of children each year experience a potentially traumatic event that primarily affects that child and his or her family (such as a motor-vehicle crash, residential fire, street violence, or a sudden medical event). The context for children's recovery is affected by the extent to which the child's family and community are themselves experiencing distress or disruption and the extent to which they are able to provide support. For children in rural or remote areas, specialized preventative services may be geographically inaccessible.

Where and How Are Preventative and Early Interventions Delivered to Children?

Mental health service settings, designed for treatment-seeking children/families once persistent psychosocial difficulties are present, are unlikely to be the first-line context for early psychosocial interventions. Whether the event impacts one child and family or an entire community, in the early aftermath it is not likely that children will show up to request mental health services, or to be screened for their mental health needs. Whereas clinical/treatment interventions require a trained mental health professional, universal and targeted/selective interventions can often be most feasibly delivered in other settings and by other professionals. There is a key role for professionals who work in service systems (e.g., schools, health care, community-based social services) that routinely see children during and immediately after acute traumatic events.

Mental health professionals can play an important role as consultants for providers in other service settings. It is often useful to establish collaborative agreements with other systems (e.g., Red Cross/Crescent, schools, law enforcement, health care). Forging mutually respectful partnerships allows mental health professionals and other service providers to learn from each other's expertise regarding trauma-exposed children's adaptation and recovery across different contexts (i.e., learning and academics, physical health, and mental health). The studies included in the evidence review reflect this reality—children were identified in health care settings and refugee camps in addition to mental health agencies, and interventions were delivered by mental health therapists or other professionals (teachers and hospital-based nurses and social workers), or were self-directed by children and parents/caretakers.

Mental Health Settings

Trained mental health professionals are needed to provide early treatment interventions to address significant psychological distress after acute trauma. In the studies reviewed here, CBT-T as well as psychoeducation and individual psychological debriefing were delivered by mental health professionals. Mental health providers integrated within settings such as schools and health care facilities are well placed to respond to the needs of recently trauma-exposed children. But mental health professionals without such formal roles can build strong relationships with these and other community settings so they are able to respond quickly when child needs are identified.

Child Advocacy Centers

Widely available in the United States, CACs are multidisciplinary settings that are either stand-alone or embedded in other settings (the hospital, a prosecutors' office). They coordinate early investigative, health, and therapeutic responses for children and families affected by child abuse, sexual assault, and domestic violence. To be accredited, CACs must offer (onsite or through standing agreements) access to both early interventions and trauma-specific treatment services.

Schools

Second only to parents, teachers are likely the adults with the most regular and sustained contact with children following exposure to trauma. Teachers can often have insight into changes in a child's behavior and mood because of their history and ongoing interactions with the child. Thus, teachers can help to facilitate resilience and recovery, and can assist in identifying children with substantial distress who are in need of targeted early intervention. Many schools have behavioral health providers on staff or onsite. Schools can be a venue for preventative intervention (Le Brocque et al., 2017). Although it has been challenging to conduct RCTs, several non-RCT studies have evaluated school-based interventions for children recently exposed to war or disaster, often using pre–post evaluations (Berger et al., 2007; Karam et al., 2008; Ramirez et al., 2013; Wolmer et al., 2013). These interventions were delivered by classroom teachers with additional training or by school nurses or counselors.

Health Care Settings

Primary care and general practitioners have a key trusted role for many families, emergency and hospital settings are among the first to see children after many types of traumatic events, and medical events themselves are potentially traumatic. Many of the existing early preventative interventions were developed in health care settings, likely because these settings provide the opportunity to identify children soon after an exposure to trauma. Studies included in the ISTSS evidence review commonly used health care settings as the venue to identify trauma-exposed children, whether the interventions were eventually delivered by mental health professionals (Berkowitz et al., 2011; Kramer & Landolt, 2014; Prchal et al., 2012; Stallard et al., 2006; Zehnder et al., 2010), hospital-based staff (Kassam-Adams et al., 2011), or as self-directed online materials (Cox et al., 2010; Kassam-Adams et al., 2016; Kenardy et al., 2015; Marsac et al., 2013).

Interventions Delivered Remotely or Online

Practical considerations, combined with the large number of children exposed to acute traumatic events, have driven the development of self-guided interventions that are delivered via print materials or online. Several of the studies in the review exemplify this strategy (Cox et al., 2010; Marsac et al., 2013).

When Should Preventative and Early Interventions Be Delivered?

One of the most debated issues in the prevention of child PTSD is the optimal time frame to provide early intervention. As noted earlier, several key theoretical models have suggested different goals for screening and intervention at different times across the posttrauma recovery period.

There are several challenges to determining the optimal timing for screening and intervention. The best (most feasible) opportunity to screen children can be immediately following the event, when they are in the presence of health care professionals or other first responders. However, it appears that currently available screening tools are more reliable when they are completed at least 1 month after the event (to allow for natural recovery). Some intervention approaches (i.e., watchful waiting, stepped care) suggest that children be initially screened at a time close to the event, and then selectively followed up and rescreened (e.g., >1 month posttrauma; March et al., 2015). Studies included in the ISTSS evidence review initiated preventative or treatment interventions as early as several days posttrauma, and in all but one study interventions were initiated within 1 month posttrauma. Whatever their results regarding effectiveness, many of these studies shed light on the feasibility and practical implications of early screening and intervention with children exposed to acute trauma.

Developmental Considerations in Preventative and Early Interventions

The importance of early and preventative intervention is magnified when viewed through a developmental lens. When trauma is experienced in childhood, changes in psychosocial functioning can have a long-lasting and deeper impact on social, cognitive, and neurological development. Across childhood, from infancy to adolescence, developmental changes and growth add a level of complexity to the design and delivery of preventative and early intervention. Interventions must take into account children's differing and changing needs, as well as age-related mediating and moderating factors that impact responses to trauma. This evidence review points out the relatively small number of studies with children to date and highlights the need for more evaluation of early preventative interventions for the youngest children. Interventions that have been demonstrated to be effective with adults may not necessarily work with children, and interventions that are effective for school-aged children may not be appropriate for preschool children or adolescents. Furthermore, any intervention targeted for children must consider the potential inclusion of parents or caregivers, and the potential need to directly address caregiver needs.

The Role of Parents

Parents and caregivers often play a key role in facilitating resilience and recovery following traumatic events. They do so in a number of ways. Parents act to buffer their child, especially young children, from the impact of stressors. They may achieve this by deflecting the impact of the stressor, helping to reduce or eliminate the child's direct exposure to the event, assisting the child in responding in adaptive ways, and/or modeling more adaptive responses to stressors. Parents' own distress can directly or indirectly affect their child by reducing the parents' capacity to buffer their child's distress and model adaptive responses, and through changes to parenting behaviors that lead to less adaptive and resilient behavior in their child. It is therefore important to consider and potentially address the health of a parent or caregiver when delivering any preventative or early intervention for their child. Finally, parents are often key gatekeepers for appropriate and timely professional assistance for their child. While this is true at any age, parents of younger children are essential for child access to services, and therefore it is crucial to effectively engage parents in the process of intervention.

The interventions included in the ISTSS guidelines review varied in the nature and extent of their engagement of parents, from provision of information (Cox et al., 2010; Kenardy et al., 2008; Marsac et al., 2013) to direct involvement of parents in the intervention as key drivers of child recovery (Berkowitz et al., 2011). Across studies, it appears that interventions provided solely to parents were not as effective.

Ethical Considerations

Across service settings, children with recent exposure to trauma are vulnerable to being retraumatized when the impact of these experiences is not recognized. Thus, the provision of trauma-informed care can be seen as a minimal standard for providing ethical care and services (Kassam-Adams & Butler, 2017). Early interventions raise a number of ethical questions for consideration; several of these are delineated next.

* *Who will recover without intervention and how do we ensure that we do not inadvertently interfere in natural recovery processes for a trauma-exposed child? What is the appropriate role for professional assistance versus promotion of "natural" helping processes in the family and community?* It may go against our natural desire to provide help after trauma, but practitioners should consider whether active early intervention is the best course of action, that is, sometimes "less is more." Respecting and supporting the capacity of a child's natural support systems may be the most important first step. It is especially important that universal interventions delivered soon after trauma "do no harm." Practitioners have a responsibility to consider the potential for harm when deciding whether and how to intervene. Other ethical considerations come into play when families actively request early intervention for a child, for example, after serious interpersonal traumas such as sexual assault or exposure to extreme violence or homicide. In these cases, being responsive to family concerns by offering brief supportive psychoeducational anticipatory guidance can be a way of keeping families engaged and open to other forms of assistance should those be needed later.

* *Do we have evidence to support the optimal method and timing of screening for this child in this setting? Is there evidence to support how screening results will guide subsequent action (i.e., immediate services vs. active monitoring vs. no further follow-up)?* Ethical screening requires a linked pathway of care including resourced intervention options. If screening occurs without these pathways being available, then the process of screening will potentially contribute to distress in the child and family without having any means to address this.

Future Developments

Future development in the area of early intervention requires attention to the practical realities of implementation, the promise of online tools, and the challenges of intervening after acute trauma for children already exposed to chronic trauma. Advances in early interventions will benefit from evaluation conducted in multiple settings by clinicians and front-line programs, and may require adaptation of traditional randomized controlled trial designs.

It is important that interventions developed through a relatively rigorous empirical process be broadly applicable in practical real-world situations. That might be in a mental health setting, but for children it is more likely to be in a school, community, or hospital setting. The field needs to think beyond the mental health setting when considering not just the generalizability of an intervention but also its usability and sustainability. From the outset of the development process, we should consider participatory and user-centered design, and end user input and validation. In the case of children, this entails enlisting feedback not only from children but also from parents and likely providers of the intervention.

Another aspect of practical delivery of early interventions is the opportunity for wider reach provided by online and e-health tools. Children and adolescents are prominent users of digital tools and social media. The ISTSS evidence review points to the promise of these tools for early prevention and treatment. Given the emerging evidence to recommend online interventions, we need continued efforts to assess Web-based interventions for children, both self-directed online interventions and online tools that may complement face-to-face interventions.

The complexity of exposure to traumatic events is also a challenge when choosing early interventions for children. Some children are exposed to multiple types of traumatic events several times and are at higher risk of developing psychopathology. Future development should clarify to what degree children with chronic trauma benefit from early psychosocial interventions after an acute event.

The ISTSS review makes it clear that there is a paucity of evidence from randomized controlled trials about which preventative and early interventions work for children posttrauma. Additional key sources of information and evidence about possible interventions include practitioners and organizations operating in this space. More clinical evaluation needs to be done as part of care, and these findings need to be available to inform development of future interventions. Evaluations may need to think outside of traditional RCT designs to be feasible in applied settings. However, it remains crucial that evaluations of early interventions take into account the confounding effects of natural remission. Finally, as our knowledge of etiological mechanisms grows, this can inform both development and evaluation of new and more effective interventions.

Summary

The two most notable findings of the ISTSS review are the emerging evidence for the effectiveness of self-directed online psychoeducation interventions as early prevention or treatment, and the caution about individual psychological debriefing for children based on emerging evidence. Several cross-cutting themes emerge from this review. The current evidence suggests that early preventative or treatment interventions should include children themselves, not only engaging parents as conduits to support their children. Interventions evaluated in this review demonstrate the need, and the feasibility, of moving beyond the mental health setting to reach children after trauma. Online interventions may have a key role in the "toolkit" of early interventions for children because of their potential global reach, accessibility, and user engagement. Finally, the ISTSS review shows that we still lack sufficient evidence to strongly recommend specific effective early intervention approaches for trauma-exposed children. Given the many millions of children exposed to acute trauma each year, these findings point to the need for clinicians and researchers to work together to develop effective, practical, and sustainable early intervention approaches.

REFERENCES

Berger, R., Pat-Horenczyk, R., & Gelkopf, M. (2007). School-based intervention for prevention and treatment of elementary-students' terror-related distress in Israel: A quasi-randomized controlled trial. *Journal of Traumatic Stress, 20,* 541–551.

Berkowitz, S., Stover, C. S., & Marans, S. R. (2011). The child and family traumatic stress intervention: Secondary prevention for youth at risk of developing PTSD. *Journal of Child Psychology and Psychiatry, 52*(6), 676–685.

Catani, C., Kohiladevy, M., Ruf, M., Schauer, E., Elbert, T., & Neuner, F. (2009). Treating children traumatized by war and tsunami: A comparison between exposure therapy and meditation-relaxation in North-East Sri Lanka. *BMC Psychiatry, 9*(1), 22.

Cox, C., Kenardy, J., & Hendrikz, J. K. (2010). A randomised controlled trial of a web-based early intervention for children and their parents following accidental injury. *Journal of Pediatric Psychology, 35,* 581–592.

Karam, E. G., Fayyad, J., Karam, A. N., Tabet, C. C., Melhem, N., Mneimneh, Z., et al. (2008). Effectiveness and specificity of a classroom-based group intervention in children and adolescents exposed to war in Lebanon. *World Psychiatry: Official Journal of the World Psychiatric Association, 7* (2), 103–109.

Kassam-Adams, N., & Butler, L. (2017). What do clinicians caring for children need to know about pediatric medical traumatic stress and the ethics of trauma-informed approaches? *AMA Journal of Ethics, 19*(8), 793.

Kassam-Adams, N., Garcia-Espana, J. F., Marsac, M. L., Kohser, K. L., Baxt, C., Nance, M., et al. (2011). A pilot randomized controlled trial assessing secondary prevention of traumatic stress integrated into pediatric trauma care. *Journal of Traumatic Stress, 24,* 252–259.

Kassam-Adams, N., Marsac, M. L., Kohser, K. L., Kenardy, J., March, S., & Winston, F. K. (2016). Pilot randomized controlled trial of a novel web-based intervention to prevent posttraumatic stress in children following medical events. *Journal of Pediatric Psychology, 41*(1), 138–148.

Kataoka, S., Langley, A. K., Wong, M., Baweja, S., & Stein, B. D. (2012). Responding to students with PTSD in schools. *Child and Adolescent Psychiatric Clinics of North America, 21*(1), 119–133.

Kazak, A. E. (2006). Pediatric psychosocial preventative health model (PPPHM): Research, practice, and collaboration in pediatric family systems medicine. *Family Systems Health, 24*(4), 381–395.

Kazak, A. E., Kassam-Adams, N., Schneider, S., Zelikovsky, N., Alderfer, M. A., & Rourke, M. (2006). An integrative model of pediatric medical traumatic stress. *Journal of Pediatric Psychology, 31*(4), 343–355.

Kenardy, J., Cox, C. M., & Brown, F. L. (2015). A web-based early intervention can prevent long-term post-traumatic stress reactions in children with high initial distress following accidental injury: A treatment moderator analysis. *Journal of Traumatic Stress, 28,* 366–369.

Kenardy, J., Thompson, K., Le Brocque, R., & Olsson, K. (2008). Information provision intervention for children and their parents following paediatric accidental injury. *European Child and Adolescent Psychiatry, 17,* 316–325.

Kramer, D. N., & Landolt, M. A. (2014). Early psychological intervention in accidentally injured children ages 2–16: A randomized controlled trial. *European Journal of Psychotraumatology, 5*(1), 24402.

La Greca, A. M., Silverman, W. K., Vernberg, E. M., & Prinstein, M. J. (1996). Symptoms of posttraumatic stress in children after Hurricane Andrew: A prospective study. *Journal of Consulting Clinical Psychology, 64*(4), 712–723.

Le Brocque, R., De Young, A., Montague, G., Pocock, S., March, S., & Kenardy, J. (2017). Schools and natural disaster recovery: The unique and vital role that teachers and education professionals play in ensuring the mental health of students following natural disasters. *Journal of Psychologists and Counsellors in Schools, 27,* 1–23.

Le Brocque, R., Hendrikz, J., & Kenardy, J. (2010). The course of post-traumatic stress in children: Examination of recovery trajectories following traumatic injury. *Journal of Pediatric Psychology, 35,* 637–645.

March, S., Kenardy, J., Cobham, V. E., Nixon, R. D. V., McDermott, B., & De Young, A. (2015). Feasibility of a screening program for at-risk children following accidental injury. *Journal of Traumatic Stress, 28,* 34–40.

Marsac, M. L., Hildenbrand, A. K., Kohser, K. L., Winston, F. K., Li, Y., & Kassam-Adams, N. (2013). Preventing posttraumatic stress following pediatric injury: A randomized controlled trial of a web-based psycho-educational intervention for parents. *Journal of Pediatric Psychology, 38*(10), 1101–1111.

Marsac, M. L., Kassam-Adams, N., Delahanty, D. L., Ciesla, J., Weiss, D., Widaman, K. F., et al. (2017). An initial application of a biopsychosocial framework to predict posttraumatic stress following pediatric injury. *Health Psychology, 36*(8), 787–796.

Marsac, M. L., Kassam-Adams, N., Delahanty, D. L., Widaman, K. F., & Barakat, L. P. (2014). Posttraumatic stress following acute medical trauma in children: A proposed model of bio-psycho-social processes during the peri-trauma period. *Clinical Child and Family Psychology Review, 17*(4), 399–411.

Meiser-Stedman, R. (2002). Towards a cognitive–behavioural model of PTSD in children and adolescents. *Clinical Child and Family Psychology Review, 5*(4), 217–232.

National Institute for Health and Care Excellence. (2018). Post-traumatic stress disorder (PTSD): The management of PTSD in adults and children in primary and secondary care (NICE Clinical Guideline 116). Retrieved from *https://www.nice.org.uk/guidance/ng116.*

Prchal, A., Graf, A., Bergstraesser, E., & Landolt, M. A. (2012). A two-session psychological intervention for siblings of pediatric cancer patients: A randomized controlled pilot trial. *Child and Adolescent Psychiatry and Mental Health, 6*(1), 3.

Price, J., Kassam-Adams, N., Alderfer, M. A., Christofferson, J., & Kazak, A. E. (2016). Systematic review: A reevaluation and update of the integrative (trajectory) model of pediatric medical traumatic stress. *Journal of Pediatric Psychology, 41*(1), 86–97.

Ramirez, M., Harland, K., Frederick, M., Shepherd, R., Wong, M., & Cavanaugh, J. E. (2013). Listen protect connect for traumatized schoolchildren: A pilot study of psychological first aid. *BMC Psychology, 1*(1), 26.

Stallard, P., Velleman, R., Salter, E., Howse, I., Yule, W., & Taylor, G. (2006). A randomised controlled trial to determine the effectiveness of an early psychological intervention with children involved in road traffic accidents. *Journal of Child Psychology and Psychiatry, 47*(2), 127–134.

Vernberg, E. M. (2002). Intervention approaches following disasters. In A. M. L. Greca, W. K. Silverman, E. M. Vernberg, & M. C. Roberts (Eds.), *Helping children cope with disasters and terrorism.* Washington, DC: American Psychological Association.

Wolmer, L., Hamiel, D., Slone, M., Faians, M., Picker, M., Adiv, T., et al. (2013). Post-traumatic reaction of Israeli Jewish and Arab children exposed to rocket attacks before and after teacher-delivered intervention. *Israel Journal of Psychiatry and Related Sciences, 50*(3), 165–173.

Zehnder, D., Meuli, M., & Landolt, M. A. (2010). Effectiveness of a single-session early psychological intervention for children after road traffic accidents: A randomised controlled trial. *Child and Adolescent Psychiatry and Mental Health, 4,* Article 7.

PART IV

TREATMENTS FOR ADULTS

CHAPTER 11

Psychological Treatments
Core and Common Elements of Effectiveness

Miranda Olff, Candice M. Monson, David S. Riggs,
Christopher Lee, Anke Ehlers, and David Forbes

A core component of the recent International Society for Traumatic Stress Studies (ISTSS) guidelines for the prevention and treatment of PTSD is a systematic review of the evidence for the psychological treatment of adults with PTSD.

As outlined in Table 11.1, this evidence review resulted in four specific psychological treatments receiving a *Strong* recommendation. These treatments, all trauma-focused, were cognitive processing therapy (CPT), cognitive therapy for PTSD (CT-PTSD), eye movement desensitization and reprocessing (EMDR) therapy, and prolonged exposure (PE). Each of these treatments has not only established a strong evidence base in its own right but also generally demonstrated comparable outcomes in head-to-head studies with each other. As such, these treatments represent the first-line interventions in the psychological treatment of adults with PTSD. In addition to these four specified interventions, "general undifferentiated individual CBT with a trauma focus" also received a *Strong* recommendation.

The ISTSS systematic review also identified a range of other psychological interventions for which the evidence base resulted in a *Standard* recommendation, as well as those for which there is now emerging evidence (see Table 11.1). Brief descriptions of all those treatments can be found in Bisson, Lewis, and Roberts (Chapter 6, this volume), and the relevant research data are summarized in the evidence reviews, evidence statements, and forest plots on the ISTSS website (*www.istss.org/treating-trauma/new-istss-prevention-and-treatment-guidelines.aspx*). Several of those interventions are also briefly described in other chapters of this volume. For example, guided

TABLE 11.1. Recommendation Levels from ISTSS Guidelines for the Prevention and Treatment of PTSD

Strong **Recommendation**—*Cognitive processing therapy, cognitive therapy, EMDR therapy, individual CBT with a trauma focus (undifferentiated),* and *prolonged exposure* are recommended for the treatment of adults with PTSD.

Standard **Recommendation**—*CBT without a trauma focus, group CBT with a trauma focus, guided Internet-based CBT with a trauma focus, narrative exposure therapy,* and *present-centered therapy* are recommended for the treatment of adults with PTSD.

Intervention with Emerging Evidence **Recommendation**—*Couples CBT with a trauma focus, group and individual CBT with a trauma focus, reconsolidation of traumatic memories, single-session CBT, virtual reality therapy,* and *written exposure therapy* have emerging evidence of efficacy for the treatment of adults with PTSD.

Insufficient Evidence to Recommend—There is insufficient evidence to recommend *brief eclectic psychotherapy for PTSD, dialogical exposure therapy, emotional freedom techniques, group interpersonal therapy, group stabilizing treatment, group supportive counseling, individual psychoeducation/self-help, interpersonal psychotherapy, observed and experimental integration, psychodynamic psychotherapy, psychoeducation, reassurance, relaxation training, REM desensitization, supportive counseling,* and *trauma-focused counseling* for the treatment of adults with PTSD.

Internet-based trauma-focused CBT and virtual reality therapy are discussed by Lewis and Olff (Chapter 18, this volume, on e-mental health), while narrative exposure therapy (NET) is described by Cloitre, Cohen, and Schnyder (Chapter 23, this volume) in the context of adaptation of trauma-focused interventions across cultures and populations. It is noteworthy that all of the eleven treatments assigned a *Standard* recommendation or *Intervention with Emerging Evidence* recommendation are also trauma focused, with the exceptions of CBT without a trauma focus and present-centered therapy (PCT).

The final category outlined in Table 11.1 relates to interventions for which there was *Insufficient Evidence to Recommend*. To clarify, this means that a sufficient evidence base has not been established to meet the classifications mentioned previously. It does not necessarily imply that the interventions listed are ineffective, but simply that a suitably robust evidence base does not yet exist. This is, for instance, the case for brief eclectic psychotherapy for PTSD (BEPP). Acceptance and commitment therapy (ACT), although widely used and shown to be superior to control conditions for a range of mental health problems (e.g., A-Tjak et al., 2015; Kelson, Rollin, Ridout, & Campbell, 2019), was not included in any of the recommendation categories as no RCTs of ACT were identified that met the inclusion criteria for the evidence review. The RCT of ACT by Lang and colleagues (2017), while a strong study, was excluded as it did not meet the evidence review requirement for 70% of participants to meet criteria for a diagnosis of PTSD.

This chapter seeks to offer an overview of the four strongly recommended specific treatments, reflecting on the core ingredients of each (also see Figure 11.1 for a brief overview of core ingredients), whether what they have in common may account for their treatment effectiveness, and how these factors may also be reflected in other interventions with (at this point) a weaker evidence base. In addition, the chapter will consider where even the strongly recommended interventions may struggle to achieve optimal outcomes, highlighting future areas that still require investigation. The following four chapters of this volume will address each of these treatments in turn and in detail, outlining a summary and appraisal of the evidence base for each one, detailed guidance on the delivery of each intervention, and

---

CPT
Psychoeducation[e]
Socratic dialogue[a,b,c]
Cognitive worksheets[a,b,c]
Giving and receiving compliments[d]
Addressing cognitive avoidance[c]
Noncontingent nice things for oneself[d]

CT-PTSD
Individualized case formulation[a,e]
Reclaiming/rebuilding your life assignments[a,b,c,d]
Guided discovery[a,c]
Behavioral experiments[a,c]
Updating trauma memories[a,b]
Discrimination training with triggers of reexperiencing[d]
A site visit[a,b,c]
A blueprint[e]

EMDR Therapy
Affect regulation skills[e]
Obtaining a suitable target[b] (perceptual elements, negative meaning,[a] emotional response, body sensation)
Positive belief[a]
Desensitization (e.g., eye movements)[a,b,d]
Body scan[a,b]
Future processing[a,e]

PE
Psychoeducation[e]
Calm breathing[e]
In vivo exposure[a,b,c]
Imaginal exposure[a,b,c]
Postexposure processing[a]

FIGURE 11.1. Core ingredients (techniques) of effective treatments. Superscript letters denote mostly addressing/targeting (a) trauma-related cognitions; (b) engaging with, and activation of, the trauma memory; (c) experiential avoidance; (d) other; (e) general.

issues for consideration by clinicians in managing presentations where initial attempts at delivering the treatment have resulted in suboptimal outcomes.

Core Ingredients of the Four Strongly Recommended Effective Treatments

Cognitive Processing Therapy

The core ingredients that comprise CPT follow from the social-cognitive theory on which it is grounded (Resick, Monson, & Chard, 2017). This theory holds that PTSD symptoms result from cognitions about traumatic events not being incorporated into existing beliefs (i.e., running contrary to preexisting beliefs) or seemingly confirming preexisting negative beliefs. In addition, traumatic events cause significant shifts in beliefs about present and future events. Based on this theory, creating more balanced, adaptive, multifaceted trauma appraisals and beliefs (both looking back on the traumatic experience and in the present) is the primary goal of treatment. "Psychoeducation" at the start of the intervention helps the patient to understand the rationale of the therapy.

There is a predominant focus on cognitive interventions. The two major types of cognitive interventions employed are "Socratic dialogue" and "cognitive worksheets." Socratic dialogue is a cornerstone practice of CPT. It is used to help patients arrive at a different way of thinking about the past, present, and future. It also models curiosity and critical thinking, and encourages patients to actively engage in creating a new narrative for understanding their trauma and its impact. As treatment progresses, patients utilize a series of cognitive worksheets to help them learn how to challenge their unhelpful thoughts.

An additional mechanism of purported action in CPT is "identifying avoidance of trauma memories and reminders," motivating patients to engage in the cognitive interventions designed to challenge their trauma-related thoughts and replace them with something more adaptive. As such, behavioral avoidance is conceptualized as a therapy-interfering behavior that needs to be overcome to profit from the cognitive interventions, rather than a specific target of the intervention per se.

Finally, two brief behavioral interventions are assigned toward the end of the therapy: "giving and receiving compliments on a daily basis" and daily "doing nice things for oneself." Both of these activities are designed to further challenge underlying trauma-related cognitions relating to self-worth and to help with relapse prevention regarding depression.

Cognitive Therapy for PTSD

CT-PTSD comprises eight core components, the first of which is an "individualized case formulation." The therapist and patient collaboratively develop an individualized version of Ehlers and Clark's (2000) model of PTSD, which serves as the framework for therapy. This model suggests that excessively negative appraisals of the trauma and/or its sequelae and disjointed memories, which lead to easy triggering of reexperiencing by matching sensory cues, lead to a sense of current internal or external threat in PTSD. The problem is maintained by behavioral and cognitive strategies that are intended to control the symptoms and perceived threat. Specific treatment procedures are then tailored to this individualized formulation.

"Reclaiming/rebuilding your life assignments" are introduced from the first session onward, designed to address the patient's perceptions that they have been permanently changed as a result of the trauma. These assignments involve helping the patient to reclaim or rebuild previously enjoyed and meaningful activities and social contacts.

"Changing problematic appraisals" of the trauma and its sequelae involves guided discovery and behavioral experiments throughout treatment and is closely integrated with the component of updating the memories. "Updating trauma memories" is a three-step procedure that includes: (1) accessing memories of the worst moments during the traumatic events and their currently threatening meanings, (2) identifying information that updates these meanings (either information from the course of events during the trauma or from guided discovery and testing of predictions), and (3) linking the new meanings to the worst moments in memory.

"Discrimination training with triggers of reexperiencing" involves systematically spotting idiosyncratic triggers (often subtle sensory cues) and learning to discriminate between "now" (cues in a new safe context) and "then" (cue in the traumatic event). A "site visit" completes the memory updating and trigger discrimination. Patient and therapist visit the site of the trauma, in person or virtually (e.g., Google Streetview, recent videos or photos) to discover how the site now looks different from the trauma and to uncover new information that helps update the meaning and memory of the trauma.

"Dropping unhelpful behaviors and cognitive processes" commonly includes discussing their advantages and disadvantages, as well as use of behavioral experiments in which the patient experiments with reducing unhelpful strategies such as rumination, hypervigilance for threat, thought suppression, and excessive precautions (safety behaviors).

Finally, an individualized "blueprint" summarizes what the patient has learned in treatment and includes plans for any setbacks.

EMDR Therapy

EMDR therapy includes several key ingredients. It begins with taking a history, providing psychoeducation, and preparing the patient for EMDR memory processing. Taking a history includes assessing the principal symptoms, such as problematic behaviors, thoughts, and feelings, as well as identifying the patient's existing positive resources. "Affect regulation skills" may be taught at this stage if needed (e.g., safe place imagery).

The next stage involves collaborative case conceptualization and "obtaining a suitable target" for the EMDR therapy. Attention is paid to the key perceptual elements of the memory (usually, an image), the negative meaning the patient associates with this event, and the emotional response, which includes both affect and the corresponding bodily sensation. The patient also identifies a "positive belief," the opposite of the negative meaning. The choice of negative and positive meanings associated with the experience is influenced by the patient's history. Also, congruence needs to exist between the meaning theme and the patient's presenting symptoms. For example, a patient who following a traumatic event avoids situations that might be associated with danger is encouraged to consider a negative meaning such as "I am not safe," while another patient who after sexual abuse has a history of entering into relationships where she is abused might have a theme such as "I am bad/defective."

The next stage of EMDR therapy focuses on "desensitization" in which the target memory is paired with a bilateral task (typically, eye movements). During this phase, the therapist encourages the patient to simply notice what occurs. He or she is not continually redirected to the originally targeted material but, rather, makes his or her own associative responses during each set of bilateral movements. The continued focus on the target or associated material continues until the memories become less vivid and emotional. At this time, adaptive experiences or ideas emerge. Once the target is desensitized (which is defined as a score of 0 or 1 on the Subjective Units of Distress Scale [SUDS]), the therapist then directs patients to think about the original incident and their identified positive belief, and to focus on that positive belief while eye movements are continued. The aim of this is to increase and strengthen positive associations to the original traumatic material. During the "body scan," the patient recalls the event and the desired positive belief and focuses on any somatic sensations. Negative feelings are desensitized and positive feelings are strengthened.

A final phase of the treatment is to prepare the patient for "future processing" with the aim of protecting against relapse. Potentially difficult future situations are identified and the therapist addresses any skill deficits or anticipatory anxiety associated with engaging in those events. Eye movements are used to desensitize such anxiety and create mastery for future engagement.

Prolonged Exposure

PE includes several key components: psychoeducation, *in vivo* exposure, imaginal exposure, and postexposure processing. Psychoeducation about trauma, PTSD, and recovery provides foundational knowledge that helps the patient understand the treatment and engage more fully in treatment activities. Topics include common reactions to trauma, how symptoms develop after trauma and are maintained over time, and how PE reduces PTSD symptoms.

In vivo exposure targets behavioral avoidance of situations, activities, objects, or people that are objectively low risk but are avoided, because they trigger memories and distressing emotions related to the trauma (e.g., fear, shame, guilt). *In vivo* exercises are collaboratively identified by provider and patient and are completed as homework, beginning with a moderately challenging item (one that produces some distress but the patient believes can be completed). Assignments increase to more challenging items in successive sessions as patients develop skill and confidence in the treatment and their ability to manage distress. *In vivo* exposure reduces the intense emotion associated with triggers and provides an opportunity to introduce and process corrective information about safety and tolerability that, in turn, leads to improved functioning.

Imaginal exposure blocks cognitive avoidance and facilitates processing of the trauma memory. In imaginal exposure, the patient revisits a specific trauma memory (typically, the trauma that the patient identifies as the most upsetting, although in some limited instances a progressive hierarchy may also be used here) in imagination while describing the event aloud in detail. During imaginal exposure, the therapist actively listens to, and observes, the patient while limiting his or her own comments to queries of subjective distress, brief words of encouragement, or probing questions to encourage engagement with the memory. After completion of the imaginal exposure exercise, during the postexposure processing stage, the provider and patient examine and process the details of the event and the emotions and thoughts that were experienced during the trauma and during the imaginal exposure session. In addition, the postimaginal processing discussion provides an opportunity to restate and summarize the trauma memory. The provider and patient may discuss new details or perspectives that arose, differentiate the traumatic experience from other life experiences, and consider the meaning of the traumatic event in the context of the patient's current life. Revisiting the event in this way promotes processing of the trauma memory by activating the thoughts and emotions associated with the trauma in a safe context. As such, it helps patients to realize that they can cope with the distress associated with the memory. The imaginal exposure narrative is recorded and the patient is instructed to listen to the recording daily between sessions to maximize its therapeutic value.

It is worth noting that calm (controlled) breathing is also often introduced in the first session as a simple means of managing distressing emotions by slowing the breathing rate. It is not considered a critical part of the protocol by most PE experts; however, because many patients find it useful, it is typically included in the treatment. Importantly, patients are instructed not to engage in controlled breathing while completing an exposure exercise.

Common Elements across These Strongly Recommended Treatments

To summarize our understanding of which elements may be responsible for treatment success based on the four treatments with the strongest evidence, the core elements appear to be (1) addressing trauma-related cognitions; (2) engaging with, and activation of, the trauma memory; and (3) addressing experiential avoidance. Although all three elements are present in each of the four strongly recommended treatments, the manner in which each of the treatments addresses these core elements varies in emphasis, depth, and technique.

Addressing Trauma-Related Cognitions

It is clear from the brief descriptions outlined previously that there is significant overlap in the focus on trauma-related cognitions in CT-PTSD, CPT, and EMDR therapy. It is also a key component of PE, most clearly in the postexposure processing phase that encourages cognitive change, but cognitive change also occurs through experiential learning during the exposure exercises. The cognitive methods and techniques used to modify cognitions might be slightly different, and the emphasis on these interventions varies, but they all share the goal of achieving changes in trauma-related cognitions. It could be argued that all components of these treatments either directly or indirectly serve to modify cognitions, but this section will focus on those components designed to target the cognitions directly.

In CPT, the systematic use of Socratic dialogue to address problematic trauma appraisals and a set of core themes related to current and future beliefs, as well as more structured approaches to cognitive change, are cornerstones of the approach. They are used to directly help patients arrive at a different way of thinking about the past, present, and future. These components model curiosity and critical thinking, encouraging patients to actively engage in creating a new narrative for understanding their trauma and its impact.

In CT-PTSD, the individual case formulation provides a preliminary opportunity to modify trauma-related interpretations, while the updating trauma memories procedure, guided discovery and behavioral experiments, and reclaiming your life assignments serve to change excessively negative meanings that induce a sense of current threat. Guided by the individual case formulation, key appraisals of the trauma and its sequelae are identified and modified collaboratively. The particular cognitive techniques depend on the formulation and type of appraisals. For example, for patients who feel ashamed about the trauma, a survey is helpful to test their predictions of what other people would think about their reactions during the trauma.

In EMDR therapy, a core element of the intervention includes the identification of key negative themes and cognitions associated with the traumatic experience, as well as corresponding opposite positive views of the self or the world. As the negative memories become less vivid and emotional, the patient often spontaneously recalls other life experiences that have a positive sense of self or the world. These are routinely tracked as they evolve over the course of treatment. In the final stage of treatment, the patient is directed to think of potential relapse situations and a positive sense of self, and the therapist enhances this association.

In PE, while exposure is the core element, a second element necessary for recovery is the introduction of information that disconfirms the expectations of negative outcome associated with trauma memories. In PE, this information is introduced experientially through the exposure exercises themselves (e.g., experiencing distress and not "falling apart" or entering a store and not having something bad happen). Imaginal exposure—retelling the trauma narrative in great detail—also provides an opportunity for new appraisals and interpretations of what happened (e.g., around perceived self-blame). These alternative perceptions are discussed and consolidated in the processing that occurs following the imaginal exposure. This postexposure processing tends to be less structured and more reflective than other cognitive approaches. Nevertheless, it encourages change in cognitions and is therefore similar to more formal cognitive interventions.

A final point worthy of mention in a discussion of changing trauma-related conditions relates to the potential role played by psychoeducation. It is important to emphasize that psychoeducation, despite being routinely used in clinical practice, does not have a strong evidence base to support its use in isolation. In conjunction with other active ingredients, however, it may still have a role to play in helping to modify the traumatic memory. For example, education may directly change cognitions and appraisals regarding the symptomatic sequelae of trauma (e.g., "I'm losing my mind; I'm the only person who reacts like this") by providing a better understanding of why the symptoms develop, their evolutionary function, and a positive prognosis for treatment.

In summary, a core component common to all four strongly recommended treatments is that of modifying trauma-related cognitions whether by assisting the patient to reevaluate and reappraise unhelpful thoughts and beliefs through presenting alternative ideas, providing new experiences, or reconnecting with other experiences from the past.

Engagement with and Activation of the Traumatic Memory

All four strongly recommended treatments require and include engagement with, and activation of, the avoided traumatic memory at some level (and, in doing so, recognize the importance of addressing experiential avoidance).

In PE, the emphasis is clearly and primarily on repeated and prolonged exposure to the cognitive, emotional, and physiological elements of the trauma memory (imaginal exposure) and to external cues for the memory (*in vivo* exposure). The theoretical foundation for PE, emotional processing theory, posits that activation of the traumatic memory with all its constituent elements is essential for recovery (Foa, Cahill, Smelser, & Bates, 2001). The other three interventions all include some form of engagement with, and activation of, the traumatic memory, although the degree of depth, duration, and repetition of this engagement varies.

In CT-PTSD, there is some imaginal reliving or narrative writing to access hot spots in memory and update them, but these are not used as repeated exposures. Nevertheless, it is a "trauma-focused" approach and, as such, requires activation of the traumatic memories to access and change the meanings associated with the hot spots. Hence, CT-PTSD uses cognitive change as a means to achieve emotional change. Similarly, CPT utilizes trauma-focused cognitive interventions, with any discussion about the traumatic event and the associated interpretations and beliefs necessarily constituting some form of engagement with, and activation of, the avoided memory. More obviously, the form of CPT that includes written narratives of the trauma account might be interpreted as an exposure paradigm even if that is not the primary goal. A core component of EMDR therapy requires the patient to focus on the key elements of the trauma experience, including perceptual elements, key thoughts, and bodily sensations.

In summary, all four strongly recommended approaches are "trauma focused" and all include direct or indirect activation of, and engagement with, the traumatic memories.

Addressing Experiential Avoidance

The trauma-focused work described in the previous section highlights the issue of changing experiential avoidance of the trauma memory. However, attention to broader experiential avoidance, including behavioral avoidance, is also a core theme. The four strongly recommended interventions differ in approach, but all aim to address the experiential avoidance that is so central to the PTSD clinical picture. In PE, the *in vivo* exposure protocol directly targets behavioral avoidance of situations, activities, objects, or people that are objectively low risk, but are avoided because they trigger memories and distressing emotions related to the trauma (e.g., fear, shame, guilt). In CPT, avoidance of trauma reminders is explicitly identified and patients are encouraged through cognitive interventions to engage in avoided activities. As noted previously, in CPT the behavioral avoidance is conceptualized as a therapy-interfering behavior that attenuates potential gains from the cognitive interventions, rather than a specific target of intervention as in *in vivo* exposure, but the end result is the same. In CT-PTSD, behavioral avoidance is addressed in several ways such as guiding patients through reclaiming or rebuilding activities and social contacts, behavioral experiments, identifying triggers and learning to discriminate between "now" and "then" cues, and finally through the site visit. In EMDR therapy, the experiential avoidance is addressed in the "future processing" phase by imagining future events that might give rise to distress, and targeting the reduction of the associated arousal and then picturing more adaptive behaviors and ideas.

In sum, although the four treatments vary in how they target experiential avoidance, including behavioral avoidance, all include strategies designed to identify and modify this avoidance.

Putative Mechanisms

Having identified the core components that are common to the four strongly recommended treatments, it is worth giving brief consideration to the underlying mechanisms: Do they work in different ways or are all three fundamentally addressing the same process? A full discussion of this complex issue is beyond the scope of this chapter, and only brief consideration will be paid to this question here.

One theme that stands out across the core shared components is that of activating and modifying the traumatic memory. This is achieved in different ways—behavioral, affective, cognitive and somatic/physiological—but it could be argued that all three components involve first activating (engaging with) the trauma memories and, second, incorporating new information that is inconsistent with that contained in the existing memory. Unhelpful, distorted appraisals and beliefs about the self, other people, and the world are challenged and replaced by more adaptive cognitions. This may occur via changing how the memory is stored and the new associations made through behavioral means (e.g., *in vivo* exposure, behavioral experiments, social reengagement), through affective means (e.g., *imaginal* exposure and habituation, reconnecting with positive life experiences), or through direct attempts at changing cognitions. Essentially, all fall under an "information-processing" paradigm, a theoretical approach that has long been used to explain effective treatments for the anxiety disorders in general (e.g., Foa & Kozak, 1986) and PTSD more specifically (e.g., Foa & Rothbaum, 1998). Critically, in addition to introducing new information to the memory system possibly through an underlying information-processing paradigm, all four treatments work to reduce distress associated with the trauma memories.

A related common mechanism appears to be that the treatments change the personal meanings of the trauma so that it becomes less threatening to patients' view of themselves, the world, and their future. Empirical studies have supported the hypothesis that cognitive change drives symptom change across a range of evidence-based treatments for PTSD (Brown, Belli, Asnaani, & Foa, 2019).

Applicability of These Core Elements to the Other Recommended Treatments

While CPT, CT-PTSD, EMDR therapy, and PE are the four specific treatments receiving a *Strong* recommendation in these guidelines, *undifferentiated CBT with a trauma focus* also received a *Strong* recommendation. Importantly, these undifferentiated approaches to trauma-focused CBT routinely include all three of the elements described previously (e.g., Bryant, Moulds, Guthrie, Dang, & Nixon, 2003; Forbes et al., 2007). Given the central place of those three elements in the four strongly recommended interventions, it is not surprising that other approaches incorporating those components would also demonstrate high effectiveness.

Similarly, the trauma-focused treatments that received a *Standard* recommendation in the guidelines (i.e., a good evidence base but insufficiently robust to justify a *Strong* recommendation) also tend to include these elements. Interventions such as *group CBT with a trauma focus, guided Internet-based CBT with a trauma focus*, and *narrative exposure therapy* all require engagement with the traumatic memory, opportunities for cognitive change, and (to varying degrees) encouragement to reduce avoidance. This argument can be extended to many of the newer interventions (for which fewer data are currently available) that are classified here as emerging interventions with promise. These include interventions such as *couples CBT with a trauma focus, group and individual CBT with a trauma focus, reconsolidation of traumatic memories, virtual reality therapy*, and *written exposure therapy*. Thus, a large proportion of treatments for PTSD, particularly those demonstrating high effectiveness, utilize most or all of these three factors, applying them in different formats, for different populations, and in different contexts.

In this context, it is worth noting that there have been previous attempts to identify common elements in a broader range of effective interventions that included, in addition to the four strongly recommended treatments in the current guidelines, interventions such as Skills Training in Affective and Interpersonal Regulation (STAIR; Cloitre, Cohen, & Koenen, 2006) outlined in more detail by Cloitre, Karatzias, and Ford (Chapter 20, this volume) for the treatment of complex PTSD. The common elements identified by those authors included psychoeducation; emotion regulation and coping skills; imaginal exposure; and cognitive processing, restructuring, and/or meaning making (Schnyder et al., 2015). In short, it is a very similar list to the core elements identified previously.

It is important to emphasize that there is also a *Standard* recommendation for non-trauma-focused psychological interventions such as present-centered therapy and group CBT without a trauma focus. It would therefore be wrong to suggest that gains cannot be made without all of these core elements (though it is worth noting that those other approaches each include one or more of them). Rather, the available data suggest that addressing each of these core elements to at least some degree may be central to maximizing the benefits of treatment.

Factors That Account for Treatments Not Being Effective

The evidence is clear that, even with the most effective and strongly recommended treatments, a considerable number of people with PTSD do not respond optimally. Some show little or no demonstrable response, while others may continue to experience significant residual symptoms and may retain a PTSD diagnosis, even after making substantial gains. There clearly is a need to improve this partial response or nonresponse to treatment, and several common areas have been identified in which all four strongly recommended treatments—and, indeed, all psychological treatments—struggle.

Certain populations do not seem to respond as well to any of our established treatments, with often-cited examples being military/veterans or refugees (Foa et al., 2018; Monson et al., 2006; Resick, Wachen, et al., 2017; Sonne et al., 2016) and adults with childhood onset PTSD (Karatzias et al., 2019). The nature and breadth of comorbid conditions such as serious depression, anger, or dissociative disorders (which are often seen in the populations mentioned previously) may also complicate delivery of these interventions. Anger deserves special mention, since the evidence suggests that high levels of anger adversely affect symptom maintenance and treatment outcome by preventing effective engagement with the traumatic memory—and if the memory is not activated, it is not available for modification (Forbes et al., 2008; Gluck, Knefel, & Lueger-Schuster, 2017; Lloyd et al., 2014). The presence of significant comorbidity and associated behaviors sometimes leads to clinically motivated exclusions of patients who, for example, are currently actively suicidal (intent with concrete plans), have an alcohol or drug dependence that dominates everyday life, or are experiencing an acute psychosis. The issue of comorbidity is addressed in more detail by Roberts, Back, Mueser, and Murray (Chapter 22, this volume).

Another issue for consideration is that the patient's primary concern may change, highlighting the importance of collaboratively negotiating treatment goals at the outset and regularly reviewing those goals—just because a person meets criteria for a PTSD diagnosis does not necessarily mean those symptoms are the primary concern. It may emerge in the course of therapy that PTSD is currently not the patient's main problem, and comorbid conditions (e.g., depression, obsessive compulsive disorder, borderline personality disorder, substance use disorder, physical illness), social problems (e.g., debts, no stable housing, illness in the family, family distress), legal problems (e.g., custody issues, asylum), or a new negative life event (e.g., death of a significant other) are his or her main current concern.

Importantly for clinicians, although a patient's primary concern may shift during treatment, it is also possible (particularly in the context of the avoidance features of PTSD) that patients may endeavor to avoid trauma work by bringing up new or ongoing issues. Here, we note the importance of clinicians not being too quick to leave the trauma work and thereby joining with the patients' avoidance. However, with attention to the potential for this shift in patient concern to represent avoidance noted and addressed, continuing to doggedly pursue the chosen treatment in such cases where this persists is likely to prove ineffective. While other life issues are dominating, the person is unlikely to be able to sufficiently engage in a trauma-focused treatment. This may be a function not only of limited cognitive and affective resources to devote to treatment, but also of practical difficulties. People with other significant life concerns may find they are unable to attend sessions regularly due to practical reasons or have little time or privacy to work on their homework assignments (e.g., no stable home). Engagement in treatment may also be adversely affected if patients have doubts that the treatment is right for them (e.g., cultural reasons) or they are worried about the negative consequences of others finding out about the treatment (e.g., fear of retribution from others if they disclose details of trauma or simply the perceived stigma of receiving mental health care). There is also considerable debate and conflicting research evidence as to whether active compensation claims may have the potential to interfere with treatment expectations and efficacy (Belsher, Tiet, Garvert, & Rosen, 2012; Frueh, Grubaugh, Elhai, & Buckley, 2007; Monson et al., 2006). Despite this conflicting research, nevertheless, the impact of active compensation seeking on current needs and treatment expectations and engagement needs to be actively considered.

Other factors that may be implicated in a more attenuated treatment response relate to individual characteristics and circumstances. Lower pretreatment social support has been found to be associated with individual trauma-focused therapy response (Price et al., 2018; Shnaider, Sijercic, Wanklyn, Suvak, & Monson, 2017), and social isolation and negative social interactions are risk factors for the onset and maintenance of PTSD (Olff, 2012; Wagner, Monson, & Hart, 2016). Personality traits such as low levels of openness to new experiences have been demonstrated to reduce the efficacy of TF-CBT (van Emmerik, Kamphuis, Noordhof, & Emmelkamp, 2011). Similarly, low readiness for change has been shown to be predictive of reduced improvements in symptom severity over treatment and follow-up for veterans after PE and CPT (Cook, Simiola, Hamblen, Bernardy, & Schnurr, 2017). These factors offer a potential focus for future research.

A final major challenge of all of these intrapsychic, mostly individually delivered interventions is their variable ability to induce broader psychosocial effects on relationship functioning, work, and quality of life. In routine clinical settings, it is clearly important to go beyond the core, evidence-based treatment for PTSD to assist the patient in addressing these broader issues. A failure to do so, and to address other lifestyle issues such as physical health, is likely to mitigate against treatment gains and to increase the chances of relapse. This issue is further addressed by Forbes, Bisson, Monson, and Berliner (Chapter 26, this volume).

Discussion

The four psychological treatments that have received a *Strong* recommendation in the recent ISTSS systematic reviews (Bisson et al., 2019) were CPT, CT-PTSD, EMDR therapy, and PE. Three core elements were identified that are shared by all of these four effective psychotherapies for PTSD. These comprise addressing trauma-related cognitions, addressing engagement with and activation of the trauma memory, and addressing experiential avoidance. As described, these elements are used in different ways across the treatments but, by focusing on these core elements, clinicians may be better able to remain focused and not be overwhelmed in the context of complex clinical presentations. It is important, however, that the treatment practiced is learned well and delivered with fidelity. Although CPT, CT-PTSD, EMDR therapy, and PE are the four specific treatments receiving a *Strong* recommendation in these guidelines, undifferentiated trauma-focused CBT, which includes all three of the elements described previously, also received a *Strong* recommendation. Other trauma-focused treatments that achieved either a *Standard* or *Intervention with Emerging Evidence* recommendation also utilize most or all of these three factors and apply them in different formats, for different populations, and in different contexts. A greater focus on the common elements across effective PTSD treatments may assist clinicians in delivering the best interventions to their patients and in managing complex cases.

Roberts and colleagues (Chapter 22, this volume) outline approaches to addressing comorbidity in more detail. At this point, it is worth noting the potential for improved outcomes by formalizing (e.g., through manuals, treatment guidelines, and training) how to manage and incorporate comorbid conditions (e.g., substance dependence; personality disorders; self-injury) into the recommended interventions to enhance outcomes. For example, if a person with PTSD is misusing substances in CPT, improvements can be made in training providers on how to target cognitions that are specific to substance use to address misuse that is also conceptually linked to avoidance that maintains PTSD. The broader issues of dissemination, training, and implementation are addressed in more detail by Riggs and colleagues (Chapter 24, this volume).

Four treatments are effective, but there are limitations. Should we provide greater session frequency or more intensive treatment formats? There is some indication of effectiveness here in populations with more chronic or complex PTSD (Ehlers et al., 2014; Mendez, Nijdam, ter Heide, van der Aa, & Olff, 2018; van Woudenberg et al., 2018). Another limitation in our science is to know which people with PTSD benefit more from which particular treatment approach. Personalized medicine is still in its infancy; we still do not know what works for whom. Should we target the ingredients to those that best match the person with PTSD? Should we stick to different interventions but better target the type of intervention to the person with PTSD? Can we tailor the intervention to the needs of different patient groups (e.g., age, sex, culture, comorbidities, type of trauma, illness duration, severity)? These, however, remain open questions and are addressed in more detail by Cloitre and colleagues and Forbes and colleagues (Chapters 23 and 26, respectively, this volume).

As long as we do not have firm evidence for these tailored interventions, the biggest gain will be reached with optimal training in at least one of the four psychotherapies that we know work best. This training should include supervision/consultation in the treatment procedures by someone trained in the therapy protocol, as such consultation has been shown to improve patient-level PTSD outcomes (Monson et al., 2018). Moreover, practicing with fidelity to whichever treatments are offered is important to treatment outcomes (e.g., Farmer, Mitchell, Parker-Guilbert, & Galovski, 2017; Holder, Holliday, Williams, Mullen, & Suris, 2018; Maxfield & Hyer, 2002).

The best-case scenario is for clinicians to learn more than one evidence-based therapy (EBT) to fidelity (i.e., having more than one tool in the toolbox). This will allow a clinician to offer different treatments to different patients based on patient characteristics such as patient preference in the choice of treatment. This is potentially important given data indicating that patient preference is a significant predictor of treatment response in PTSD (Zoellner, Roy-Byrne, Mavissakalian, & Feeny, 2019) and other mental health conditions (see Swift & Callahan, 2009, for meta-analysis).

Each of these treatments, as outlined earlier, while sharing common elements and possibly a core unifying underlying mechanism of action, varies in its focus, depth, and technique. As such, being able to offer different treatment options for consideration will benefit the patient—particularly when one approach has not resulted in optimal outcomes. The option to consider another variant approach that may better suit the patient has the potential to enhance outcomes, with empirical studies needed to test the added effects of offering a second intervention. Future research on individualized effective ingredients in combination with clinicians' experience with different types of treatment will ultimately bring the best treatment to the patient. The issues of future directions in treatment and personalized medicine are addressed in more detail by Cloitre and colleagues and Forbes and colleagues (Chapters 23 and 26, respectively, this volume).

REFERENCES

A-Tjak, J. G., Davis, M. L., Morina, N., Powers, M. B., Smits, J. A., & Emmelkamp, P. M. (2015). A meta-analysis of the efficacy of acceptance and commitment therapy for clinically relevant mental and physical health problems. *Psychotherapy and Psychosomatics, 84*(1), 30–36.

Belsher, B. E., Tiet, Q. Q., Garvert, D. W., & Rosen, C. S. (2012). Compensation and treatment: Disability benefits and outcomes of U.S. veterans receiving residential PTSD treatment. *Journal of Traumatic Stress, 25,* 494–502.

Bisson, J. I., Berliner, L., Cloitre, M., Forbes, D., Jensen, T. K., Lewis, C., et al. (2019). The International Society for Traumatic Stress Studies new guidelines for the prevention and treatment of PTSD: Methodology and development process. *Journal of Traumatic Stress, 32*(7).

Brown, L. A., Belli, G. M., Asnaani, A., & Foa, E. B. (2019). A review of the role of negative cognitions about oneself, others, and the world in the treatment of PTSD. *Cognitive Therapy and Research, 43,* 143–173.

Bryant, R. A., Moulds, M. L., Guthrie, R. M., Dang, S. T., & Nixon, R. D. V. (2003). Imaginal exposure alone and imaginal exposure with cognitive restructuring in treatment of posttraumatic stress disorder. *Journal of Consulting and Clinical Psychology, 71*(4), 706–712.

Cloitre, M., Cohen, L., & Koenen, K. (2006). *Treating survivors of childhood abuse: Psychotherapy for the interrupted life.* New York: Guilford Press.

Cook, J. M., Simiola, V., Hamblen, J. L., Bernardy, N., & Schnurr, P. P. (2017). The influence of patient readiness on implementation of evidence-based PTSD treatments in Veterans Affairs residential programs. *Psychological Trauma, 9*(Suppl. 1), 51–58.

Ehlers, A., & Clark, D. M. (2000). A cognitive model of posttraumatic stress disorder. *Behaviour Research and Therapy, 38,* 319–345.

Ehlers, A., Hackmann, A., Grey, N., Wild, J., Liness, S., Albert, I., et al. (2014). A randomized controlled trial of 7-day intensive and standard weekly cognitive therapy for PTSD and emotion-focused supportive therapy. *American Journal of Psychiatry, 171*(3), 294–304.

Farmer, C. C., Mitchell, K. S., Parker-Guilbert, K., & Galovski, T. E. (2017). Fidelity to the cognitive processing therapy protocol: Evaluation of critical elements. *Behavior Therapy, 48,* 195–206.

Foa, E. B., Cahill, S. P., Smelser, N. L., & Bates, P. B. (2001). Psychological therapies: Emotional processing. In *International encyclopedia of the social and behavioral sciences* (pp. 12363–12369). Oxford, UK: Elsevier.

Foa, E. B., & Kozak, M. J. (1986). Emotional processing of fear: Exposure to corrective information. *Psychological Bulletin, 99*(1), 20–35.

Foa, E. B., McLean, C. P., Zang, Y., Rosenfield, D., Yadin, E., Yarvis, J. S., et al. (2018). Effect of prolonged exposure therapy delivered over 2 weeks vs 8 weeks vs present-centered therapy on PTSD symptom severity in military personnel: A randomized clinical trial. *Journal of the American Medical Association, 319,* 354–365.

Foa, E. B., & Rothbaum, B. O. (1998). *Treating the trauma of rape: Cognitive-behavioral therapy for PTSD.* New York: Guilford Press.

Forbes, D., Creamer, M., Phelps, A., Couineau, A., Cooper, J., Bryant, R., et al. (2007). Treating adults with acute stress disorder and posttraumatic stress disorder in general practice: A clinical update. *Medical Journal of Australia, 187,* 120–123.

Forbes, D., Parslow, R., Creamer, M., Allen, N., McHugh, T., & Hopwood, M. (2008). Mechanisms of anger and treatment outcome in combat veterans with posttraumatic stress disorder. *Journal of Traumatic Stress, 21*(2), 142–149.

Frueh, B., Grubaugh, A., Elhai, J., & Buckley, T. (2007). U.S. Department of Veterans Affairs disability policies for posttraumatic stress disorder: Administrative trends and implications for treatment, rehabilitation, and research. *American Journal of Public Health, 97,* 2143–2145.

Gluck, T. M., Knefel, M., & Lueger-Schuster, B. (2017). A network analysis of anger, shame, proposed ICD-11 post-traumatic stress disorder, and different types of childhood trauma in foster care settings in a sample of adult survivors. *European Journal of Psychotraumatology, 8.*

Holder, N., Holliday, R., Williams, R., Mullen, K., & Surís, A. (2018). A preliminary examination of the role of psychotherapist fidelity on outcomes of cognitive processing therapy during an RCT for military sexual trauma-related PTSD. *Cognitive Behaviour Therapy, 47*(1), 76–89.

Karatzias, T., Murphy, P., Cloitre, M., Bisson, J., Roberts, N., Shevlin, M., et al. (2019). Psychological interventions for ICD-11 complex PTSD symptoms: Systematic review and meta-analysis. *Psychological Medicine, 49*(11), 1761–1775.

Kelson, J., Rollin, A., Ridout, B., & Campbell, A. (2019). Internet-delivered acceptance and commitment therapy for anxiety treatment: Systematic review. *Journal of Medical Internet Research, 21*(1), e12530.

Lang, A. J., Schnurr, P. P., Jain, S., He, F., Walser, R. D., Bolton, E., et al. (2017). Randomized controlled trial of acceptance and commitment therapy for distress and impairment in OEF/OIF/OND veterans. *Psychological Trauma, 9*(Suppl. 1), 74–84.

Lloyd, D., Nixon, R., Varker, T., Elliott, P., Perry, D., Bryant, R. A., et al. (2014). Comorbidity in the prediction of cognitive processing therapy treatment outcomes for combat-related posttraumatic stress disorder. *Journal of Anxiety Disorders, 28,* 237–240.

Maxfield, L., & Hyer, L. (2002). The relationship between efficacy and methodology in studies investigating EMDR treatment of PTSD. *Journal of Clinical Psychology, 58*(1), 23–41.

Mendez, M. Z., Nijdam, M. J., ter Heide, F. J. J., van der Aa, N., & Olff, M. (2018). A five-day inpatient EMDR treatment programme for PTSD: Pilot study. *European Journal of Psychotraumatology, 9*(1).

Monson, C. M., Schnurr, P. P., Resick, P. A., Friedman, M. J., Young-Xu, Y., & Stevens, S. P. (2006). Cognitive processing therapy for veterans with military-related posttraumatic stress disorder. *Journal of Consulting and Clinical Psychology, 74,* 898–907.

Monson, C. M., Shields, N., Suvak, M. K., Lane, J. E. M., Shnaider, P., Landy, M. S. H., et al. (2018). A randomized controlled effectiveness trial of training strategies in cognitive processing therapy for posttraumatic stress disorder: Impact on patient outcomes. *Behaviour Research and Therapy, 110,* 31–40.

Olff, M. (2012). Bonding after trauma: On the role of social support and the oxytocin system in traumatic stress. *European Journal of Psychotraumatology, 3.*

Price, M., Lancaster, C. L., Gros, D. F., Legrand, A. C., van Stolk-Cooke, K., & Acierno, R. (2018). An examination of social support and PTSD treatment response during prolonged exposure. *Psychiatry, 81*(3), 258–270.

Resick, P. A., Monson, C. M., & Chard, K. M. (2017). *Cognitive processing therapy for PTSD: A comprehensive manual.* New York: Guilford Press.

Schnyder, U., Ehlers, A., Elbert, T., Foa, E. B., Gersons, B. P. R., Resick, P. A., et al.

(2015). Psychotherapies for PTSD: What do they have in common? *European Journal of Psychotraumatology, 6,* 28186.

Shnaider, P., Sijercic, I., Wanklyn, S. G., Suvak, M. K., & Monson, C. M. (2017). The role of social support in cognitive-behavioral conjoint therapy for post-traumatic stress disorder. *Behavior Therapy, 48*(3), 285–294.

Sonne, C., Carlsson, J., Bech, P., Vindbjerg, E., Mortensen, E. L., & Elklit, A. (2016). Psychosocial predictors of treatment outcome for trauma-affected refugees. *European Journal of Psychotraumatology, 7.*

Swift, J. K., & Callahan, J. L. (2009). The impact of patient treatment preferences on outcome: A meta-analysis. *Journal of Clinical Psychology, 65*(4), 368–381.

van Emmerik, A. A., Kamphuis, J. H., Noordhof, A., & Emmelkamp, P. M. (2011). Catch me if you can: Do the five-factor model personality traits moderate drop-out and acute treatment response in post-traumatic stress disorder patients? *Psychotherapy and Psychosomatics, 80*(6), 386–388.

van Woudenberg, C., Voorendonk, E. M., Bongaerts, H., Zoet, H. A., Verhagen, M., Lee, C. W., et al. (2018). Effectiveness of an intensive treatment programme combining prolonged exposure and eye movement desensitization and repro-cessing for severe post-traumatic stress disorder. *European Journal of Psychotrau-matology, 9*(1).

Wagner, A. C., Monson, C. M., & Hart, T. L. (2016). Understanding social factors in the context of trauma: Implications for measurement and intervention. *Journal of Aggression, Maltreatment and Trauma, 25*(8), 831–853.

Zoellner, L. A., Roy-Byrne, P. P., Mavissakalian, M., & Feeny, N. C. (2019). Doubly randomized preference trial of prolonged exposure versus sertraline for treat-ment of PTSD. *American Journal of Psychiatry, 176*(4), 287–296.

CHAPTER 12

Prolonged Exposure

David S. Riggs, Larissa Tate, Kelly Chrestman, and Edna B. Foa

Originally developed by Edna Foa and colleagues (Foa, Hembree, & Rothbaum, 2007; Foa, Rothbaum, Riggs, & Murdock, 1991), prolonged exposure (PE) is a manualized treatment for posttraumatic stress disorder (PTSD) with decades of research supporting its efficacy (for reviews, see Cusack et al., 2016; Kline, Cooper, Rytwinski, & Feeny, 2018; Lenz, Haktanir, & Callender, 2017; Powers, Halpern, Ferenschak, Gillihan, & Foa, 2010; Watts et al., 2013). In the current *Posttraumatic Stress Disorder Prevention and Treatment Guidelines* published by the International Society for Traumatic Stress Studies (ISTSS; *www.istss.org/getattachment/Treating-Trauma/ New-ISTSS-Prevention-and-Treatment-Guidelines/ISTSS_PreventionTreatment- Guidelines_FNL.pdf.aspx*), PE received a *Strong* recommendation for the treatment of PTSD. PE has also received similarly strong recommendations in other recent clinical practice/treatment guidelines (e.g., American Psychological Association, 2017; Department of Veterans Affairs & Department of Defense, 2017; National Institute of Health and Care Excellence, 2018; Phoenix Australia–Centre for Posttraumatic Mental Health, 2013). In the following pages, we describe the theoretical foundations of PE and discuss the specific techniques of this therapy. Additionally, we provide a brief overview of the evidence for the efficacy of PE as part of the ISTSS guidelines review. The balance of the chapter consists of a discussion about practical considerations in the delivery of PE and suggestions for future directions in the refinement of PE.

Theoretical Foundations

The theoretical foundations of PE are rooted in the emotional processing theory of fear first applied to anxiety disorders and their treatment by

Foa and Kozak (1986) and later expanded into a comprehensive theory on the effects of trauma, natural recovery from trauma, and the efficacy of cognitive-behavioral approaches to treating PTSD (e.g., Foa & Cahill, 2001; Foa, Huppert, & Cahill, 2006; Foa & Riggs, 1993). Emotional processing theory proposed that emotions are represented as cognitive-memory structures that include representations of stimuli, responses, and meaning associated with the particular emotion. The original formulation of emotional processing theory focused on the emotion of fear; later discussions, particularly in the context of trauma, extrapolated the model to encompass other emotions that commonly accompany traumatic events, such as horror, disgust, anger, guilt, and shame (Harned, Ruork, Liu, & Tkachuck, 2015; Held, Klassen, Brennan, & Zalta, 2018).

These cognitive-emotion networks become "active" and the emotion is experienced when a sufficient number of stimuli and response representations are activated. Foa and Kozak (1986) suggested that these networks (specifically, the fear network) become pathological when there are erroneous associations among the representations in the network. For example, if the representation of a housecat (or any other typically benign object) is erroneously associated with the meaning "threat," then a person would experience feelings of fear when the "cat" representation is activated by environmental cues. It is also possible for the cognitive-emotion networks to be pathological when the response representations produce extremely high arousal when activated (Foa & Kozak, 1986). For instance, many a person has employed the "5-second rule" to eat a cookie that has fallen to the floor; others have very intense feelings of disgust at just the thought of eating something that has touched the floor, so much so that actually eating the cookie would be practically impossible.

In the case of PTSD, it is thought that the traumatic experience results in a specific cognitive emotional memory structure that incorporates stimuli and the varied emotional responses present at the time of the trauma. It is further proposed that this trauma memory structure includes (1) a large number of stimulus elements associated with the emotion networks such as fear, horror, guilt, or sadness; (2) representations of the physiological/emotional/behavioral responses that engender intense arousal; and (3) associations between response representation and the meaning of self-incompetence (Foa et al., 2007). Modification of the pathological network requires the activation of the trauma memory structure and the introduction of new information that is incompatible with the erroneous information included therein (Foa & Kozak 1986; Foa et al., 2007). Avoidance interferes with this process by limiting activation of the trauma memory structure and the opportunities for corrective information to be introduced. PE accomplishes the conditions needed for modification by actively working to overcome avoidance through having the client systematically confront stimuli that create distress and are avoided despite having a low probability of resulting in harm. These stimuli include situations that the person has been avoiding (e.g., crowds, driving, specific locations) and the memories and images associated with trauma. Confronting these stimuli activates the trauma memory structure (and associated emotional structures), rendering new information about the stimuli (e.g., the feared consequence did not occur) and about one's reactions (e.g., I did not "go crazy") that can be incorporated into the network.

Description of Techniques

As suggested by its name, PE promotes the confrontation of distressing stimuli through intentional exposure to these stimuli (Foa et al., 2007). Individuals with PTSD tend to avoid two broad classes of stimuli: external (i.e., objects, places, situations) and internal (i.e., memories, images, emotions, physiological arousal). Therefore, PE utilizes two forms of exposure exercises, including *in vivo* exposures to the external stimuli and imaginal exposure to encourage the activation and processing of the traumatic memory. These techniques, along with other components of PE, are described previously. This discussion highlights the exposure components of PE; it should be noted that other elements of the protocol (i.e., psychoeducation and relaxed breathing) are introduced earlier in the protocol (i.e., in Sessions 1 and 2) than are the exposure exercises, which are initiated after Session 2 (*in vivo*) and in Session 3 (imaginal).

Components of PE

PE is a manualized protocol that includes several key components, all of which are introduced relatively early in treatment.

In vivo Exposure

In vivo exposure targets behavioral avoidance of situations, activities, objects, or people that are objectively low risk, but are avoided because they trigger memories and distressing emotions related to the trauma (e.g., fear, shame, guilt). Specific *in vivo* activities are collaboratively identified by the provider and client and ranked from least to most distressing. Activities are assigned systematically throughout the rest of treatment, starting with less distressing situations and gradually taking on more difficult situations as the individual develops skill and confidence in the treatment, and in his or her own ability to manage distress. *In vivo* assignments are typically completed by the client as homework assignments between sessions and are repeated over several days or weeks until they no longer trigger excessive distress and avoidance. *In vivo* exercises generally begin with a moderately challenging item (one that produces some distress but the patient believes can be completed) and then "steps" up to more challenging items in successive sessions. As part of each session, the *in vivo* exposure homework from the preceding session is reviewed and new assignments are selected. *In vivo* exposures reduce intense emotion associated with triggers and introduce corrective information about safety and tolerability that leads to improved functioning.

Imaginal Exposure

Imaginal exposure blocks cognitive avoidance and facilitates processing of the trauma memory. In imaginal exposure, the client repeatedly revisits a specific trauma memory (the standard is to use the memory of the trauma that the client identifies as the most upsetting) in imagination while describing the event aloud in detail. The narrative of the memory is typically repeated for approximately 40–45 minutes. During the imaginal exposure session, the therapist is actively engaged in listening to and observing the client. The clinician does not engage in conversation or discussion of the traumatic memory, but rather limits his or her comments to queries of subjective distress, brief words of encouragement, or probe questions designed to encourage engagement with the memory. After the completion of the imaginal exposure exercise, the provider and client review and process the details of the event and the emotions and thoughts that were experienced during the trauma and during the imaginal exposure session. Revisiting the event in this way promotes processing of the trauma memory by activating the thoughts and emotions associated with the trauma in a safe context. Imaginal exposure also helps clients realize they can cope with the distress associated with the memory. The imaginal exposure narrative is recorded, and the client is instructed to listen to the recording daily between sessions to maximize its therapeutic value.

The postimaginal exposure processing discussion may in some ways appear similar to more formal cognitive interventions; in contrast, it is generally informal, supportive, and reflective. The discussion follows the experiences reported by the client and serves to restate and summarize both the trauma memory and the thoughts and emotions that arose during exposure. During processing, the provider and client may discuss additional details or new perspectives that arose, differentiate the traumatic experience from other life experiences that may trigger similar emotions but are not dangerous in the way the trauma was, and consider the meaning of the traumatic event in the context of the client's current life and future goals. Although formal cognitive interventions are not standard in PE processing, it has not been found to hinder the therapeutic outcome when used in conjunction with imaginal exposure (Foa et al., 2005). It has been suggested that some clients, principally those who lack basic emotion regulation skills, may benefit from a more structured approach, such as the addition of emotion regulation skills training that is included in dialectical behavior therapy (M. Harned, personal communication, May 22, 2019). Generally, however, the added effort on the part of client and provider has not been shown to result in additional therapeutic gain in most PTSD clients.

Psychoeducation

Psychoeducation about trauma, PTSD, and recovery provides foundational knowledge that helps the patient understand the treatment and engage more fully in treatment activities. Most of the educational material in PE is delivered in the first three sessions, but topics may be revisited throughout treatment, as needed, to reinforce learning. Topics include common reactions to trauma, how symptoms develop after trauma and are maintained over time through processes such as avoidance and cognitive errors, and how the treatment reduces PTSD symptoms by targeting these maintaining factors.

Relaxed Breathing

Relaxed breathing is an optional component of PE and is typically introduced in the first session as a simple means of managing distressing emotions by slowing the breathing rate. It is not considered a critical part of the protocol by most PE experts; however, many clients have found it useful and so relaxed breathing is typically included in the treatment. Importantly, clients should be instructed not to engage in controlled breathing while completing an exposure exercise. Although adverse reactions to relaxed breathing are not noted in the literature, in our clinical experience there are some clients for whom the controlled breathing can serve as a trauma reminder. For example, medics and corpsmen are often taught to control their breathing when treating a wounded service member on the battlefield. In some cases, this controlled breathing can become associated with the trauma of the injury (or death) of the service member and similar breathing may cue the trauma memory. In these cases, omitting the relaxed breathing training from PE is recommended. However, it may be useful to include such breathing on the list of *in vivo* exposure exercises.

Summary and Appraisal of the Evidence

The ISTSS Guidelines Revision Committee conducted meta-analyses of PTSD symptoms posttreatment, answering various scoping questions posed a priori (as outlined by Bisson, Lewis, & Roberts, Chapter 6, this volume). The Committee included PE in these analyses and specifically reported on how PE compared to wait list or treatment as usual (TAU), interpersonal psychotherapy (IPT; Markowitz et al., 2015), and metacognitive therapy (MCT; Wells, Walton, Lovell, & Proctor, 2015). Overall, the results prompted the Committee to make a strong recommendation for PE in the treatment of PTSD in adults. Specifically, PE was found to be more effective in reducing PTSD symptoms than no treatment with consistently large effect sizes.

Research has demonstrated the effectiveness of PE across a variety of populations (Cahill, Rothbaum, Resick, & Follette, 2009), including military veterans (e.g., Cooper & Clum, 1989; Goodson, Lefkowitz, Helstrom, & Gawrysiak, 2013; Schnurr et al., 2007; Tuerk et al., 2011) and active duty populations (e.g., Blount, Cigrang, Foa, Ford, & Peterson, 2014; Foa, McLean, et al., 2018). PE has also been shown to be effective in the treatment of PTSD in victims of physical and sexual assault (e.g., Foa et al., 1999, 2005; Resick, Nishith, Weaver, Astin, & Feuer, 2002; Resick, Williams, Suvak, Monson, & Gradus, 2012), motor vehicle accidents (e.g., Blanchard et al., 2003), and mixed traumas (e.g., Bryant et al., 2008). Importantly, evidence supporting the effectiveness of PE for PTSD has emerged from research centers around the world.

PE versus Wait List or TAU

In the review conducted by the ISTSS Guidelines Revision Committee, a total of 12 studies were included that examined the effectiveness of PE in reducing PTSD symptoms versus a wait-list or TAU control group. Overall, PE showed a positive effect when compared to these groups and was more effective in treating PTSD than wait list or TAU. These results were demonstrated across a variety of populations, including sexual assault victims (e.g., Foa et al., 1991, 1999; Resick et al., 2002; Rothbaum, Astin, & Marsteller, 2005), other assault or abuse victims (e.g., Foa et al., 2005), non-Western patients (e.g., Asukai, Saito, Tsuruta, Kisimoto, & Nshikawa, 2010), veterans (e.g., Nacasch et al., 2011), and active duty service members (e.g., Foa, McLean, et al., 2018; Reger et al., 2016).

Limitations

Several limitations to these studies should be discussed. First, a few of these studies had relatively small sample sizes (e.g., Asukai et al., 2010; Foa et al., 1991; Nacasch et al., 2011; Wells et al., 2015), which makes it difficult to generalize the findings to the larger population of patients with PTSD. Second, some additional potential biases must be noted, as highlighted by the meta-analyses conducted by the ISTSS Guidelines Revision Committee. For example, there was a high risk of bias due to incomplete outcome data or attrition (e.g., Foa et al., 1991; Rothbaum et al., 2005; Wells et al., 2015), lack of blinding of outcome assessment or detection bias (e.g., Wells et al., 2015), and other reasons (e.g., Asukai et al., 2010; Foa et al., 1991, 1999; Nacasch et al., 2011; Resick et al., 2002; Wells et al., 2015). Additionally, there was an unclear risk for bias in regard to random sequence generation (e.g., Foa et al., 1991, 1999; Resick et al., 2002; Rothbaum et al., 2005), allocation concealment (e.g., Foa et al., 1991, 1999; Fonzo et al., 2017; Nacasch et al., 2011; Pacella et al., 2012; Resick et al., 2002; Rothbaum et al., 2005), blinding of outcome assessment or detection bias (e.g., Fonzo et al., 2017), and selective reporting bias (e.g., Asukai et al., 2010; Foa et al., 1991, 1999, 2005; Pacella et al., 2012; Reger et al., 2016; Resick et al., 2002; Rothbaum et al., 2005; Wells et al., 2015).

PE versus IPT

To date, only one RCT has been conducted examining the efficacy of PE compared with IPT (Markowitz et al., 2015). The researchers also included relaxation therapy (RT) as an active control condition. At random, 110 eligible participants were assigned to one of the three conditions. All three groups showed improvement in clinician-rated PTSD symptoms, and the PE and IPT groups did not differ in the amount of symptom improvement. However, only the PE group showed a reduction in PTSD symptoms significantly greater than the RT group.

Limitations

One of the major limitations of determining the efficacy of IPT in treating PTSD versus PE is that only one empirical study has been conducted comparing the two treatments. Additionally, meta-analyses determined a high risk for other biases in the Markowitz and colleagues (2015) study. Currently, PE cannot be determined to be a superior treatment to IPT.

PE versus MCT

Only one RCT has been conducted comparing the efficacy of PE to MCT. MCT is a therapy that focuses on changing how one responds to negative thoughts and beliefs, rather than changing thought content. In the previously mentioned study by Wells and colleagues (2015), MCT showed a superior effect in self-reported PTSD symptoms compared with PE, and MCT resulted in these improvements more rapidly than PE.

Limitations

Although the results of the aforementioned study demonstrated the success of MCT, there has only been one study conducted examining the comparison of this therapy to PE. Additionally, the sample size was relatively small and the study contained several potential risks for biases, including a high risk for incomplete outcome data or attrition, high risk for blinding of outcome assessment or detection bias, high risk for other biases, and an unclear risk for selective reporting or reporting bias.

Practical Delivery of PE

In its standard form, PE is delivered in a series of 90-minute outpatient sessions typically held once or twice per week. Studies included in the review that formed the foundation of the ISTSS treatment guidelines revision recommendation provided 9–12 sessions of PE. Practically, though, clients may demonstrate significant improvement in fewer than nine sessions and others may require more than 12 sessions. We currently recommend that clinicians plan to provide 8–15 sessions of PE for their clients with PTSD. Each PE session is structured much as other cognitive-behavioral treatment sessions are, beginning with a review of homework (after the first session), continuing through specified exercises, and ending with the assignment of homework exercises to be completed prior to the next session.

PE is a fairly structured treatment, with aspects of the protocol introduced sequentially across the first several sessions. The first session is largely dedicated to psychoeducation around issues related to trauma, the development and maintenance of PTSD, and an overview of PE procedures. The second session continues psychoeducation, with a focus on conveying the common reactions to trauma and their relation to PTSD symptoms. This session also includes introduction of *in vivo* exposure and development of a hierarchy to guide the *in vivo* exposure exercises. The initial *in vivo* exposure exercises are assigned as homework at the end of this session. In Session 3, the procedures for imaginal exposure are introduced and the initial imaginal exposure exercise is completed. The imaginal exposure exercise in this and all ensuing sessions is audiorecorded to allow the client to review it daily between sessions as homework. The balance of sessions introduce more challenging *in vivo* homework exercises and continue the imaginal exposure exercises in session. In the final session, the therapist and client review the progress made through treatment, develop a plan to prevent relapse, and explore the patient's feelings related to the end of treatment.

Although the basic structure of many of the PE sessions is similar, clinicians will likely find that each session takes on different characteristics. For example, in early sessions, therapists are likely to find themselves in the role of "coach," encouraging clients to try to overcome their tendency to avoid upsetting memories or emotions. Portions of these early sessions may also be devoted to discussing resistance to homework exercises or troubleshooting exercises that have not been successful. In later sessions, as clients begin to gain confidence and overcome anxiety, therapists may find themselves largely serving as "consultants," providing guidance as clients select and plan the exercises to be completed that week. Clinicians will also likely notice that the trauma narrative changes as sessions proceed, one reason that it is important to record each imaginal exposure session. Clients will add or drop specific details from the narrative, often with each repetition, but the nature of the narrative may also change. Our clinical experience suggests that the narrative tends to gain a greater coherence and temporal order with repetitions. Such changes in content and structure may serve as discussion points in the processing of the imaginal exposure exercises.

Despite the overall structure of the PE protocol, there is a great deal of flexibility that allows clinicians to individualize the treatment to address the needs of specific clients. Some of this is built into the protocol itself. Thus, the specific items included on the *in vivo* hierarchy will reflect the avoidance behavior of each individual client. Similarly, each client will relate the events of his or her own trauma during imaginal exposure exercises. Beyond this, though, clinicians will work with each client to plan which *in vivo* items to use for exercises and how rapidly to proceed through the exercises. Imaginal exposure, too, can be modulated to meet clients' needs. These and other modifications to the PE protocol are discussed below.

Challenges to Delivery of PE

There can be a number of challenges to the delivery of PE, including very practical issues pertaining to the delivery of sessions, resistance from clients, and reticence on the part of clinicians. The practical barriers to PE delivery that we most commonly encounter include having to schedule 90-minute sessions, logistic barriers to holding regular weekly sessions, and the requirements to record sessions for use in homework assignments. Some clients are resistant to engaging in PE because it requires them to confront memories and situations that are distressing. Clinicians, too, can be resistant to engaging in PE because we do not want our clients to be upset, or exacerbate the patient's symptoms, or because we do not want to become upset ourselves as we listen to clients describe their traumas. Clinicians may also be reticent to engage a client in PE because this approach to therapy is different from treatment with which they are more familiar. Fortunately, the many years of experience using PE in a variety of settings, as well as a number of recent research efforts, provide guidance on how to address these challenges.

Modifications of PE and Strategies to Address Logistical Challenges

One key barrier to the adoption of PE is the requirement to schedule 90-minute treatment sessions. As a result, clinicians sometimes shorten sessions to 60 minutes in duration. Clinical experience suggests that this can often be accomplished with little or no detriment in outcome, particularly with later sessions where the imaginal exposure exercise may take only 30 minutes to complete (Foa et al., 2007). In addition, in the U.S. Veterans Affairs health care system, for example, the second session is commonly divided into two separate sessions: one focused on education about common reactions and another introducing *in vivo* exposure. Some recent research also supports the efficacy of PE delivered in 60-minute sessions. Nacasch and colleagues (2015) found that 60-minute PE sessions that included at least 20 minutes of imaginal exposure were noninferior to the standard 90-minute sessions that include 40 minutes of imaginal exposure. Similar results were found by van Minnen and Foa (2006) in an uncontrolled trial. A third study (Foa, Zandberg, et al., 2018) is currently under way to replicate these findings with U.S. military personnel and a sample large enough to provide adequate power to test the noninferiority between 60- and 90-minute sessions.

There are sometimes logistical issues related to recording sessions for use in imaginal homework exercises. One solution to this is the development of smartphone applications such as the PE Coach app developed by the U.S. Departments of Veterans Affairs and Defense. This application is installed on the client's smartphone and includes a range of capabilities to support PE, including the ability to record sessions for later playback. In addition, PE Coach includes the ability to construct the *in vivo* hierarchy, track homework completion, and monitor symptom severity over time (Reger et al., 2013). Initial studies demonstrate client and therapist interest in using smartphone applications as part of therapy for PTSD (e.g., Erbes et al., 2014; Reger, Skopp, Edwards-Stewart, & Lemus, 2017).

Another logistical challenge that may arise is clients finding it difficult to attend weekly (or biweekly) therapy sessions. Recent advances in the use of tele-health offer a method for addressing these logistical challenges in PE delivery. Tuerk, Yoder, Ruggerio, Gros, and Acierno (2010) conducted an uncontrolled study in which 12 veterans with combat-related PTSD were treated with PE delivered via telephone therapy sessions. These veterans experienced statistically significant decreases in PTSD symptoms, with effect sizes on a par with those veterans that receive standard in-person PE. Additional controlled studies support the efficacy of PE delivered via tele-health. In one study, participants in both a home-based tele-health group and an in-person PE group experienced significant reductions in clinician-rated symptoms of PTSD, depression, and anxiety (Yuen et al., 2015). Furthermore, tele-health PE was found noninferior to the in-person PE at the end of treatment. Another RCT found home-based tele-health PE noninferior to in-person PE with regard to reducing PTSD. Reductions in PTSD in both groups were maintained at 3- and 6-month follow-ups (Acierno et al., 2017).

Clinician Concerns about Using PE

Despite years of research supporting PE's effectiveness in treating PTSD, many clinicians still do not utilize it. One most often-cited reason by clinicians is concern the treatment could cause patient decompensation (Becker, Zayfert, & Anderson, 2004; van Minnen, Hendriks, & Olff, 2010), despite research demonstrating that this is an extremely unlikely outcome with PE (Jayawickreme et al., 2014). Ruzek and colleagues (2016) surveyed nearly 1,300 U.S. mental health clinicians serving veterans enrolled in a national Veterans Affairs PE training program. Prior to training, these clinicians were interested in and had positive expectations about PE, but were concerned the treatment might increase patient distress and worsen symptoms.

The studies reviewed for the ISTSS guidelines revision indicated that PE is both effective and safe for treating PTSD. Despite the fact that PE is a safe procedure, it is possible that some clients will become so distressed during exposure exercises, particularly imaginal exposure exercises, that they are unable to integrate new information into the trauma memory network.

Indeed, the protocol recognizes this and builds in strategies for what is termed patient overengagement with the trauma memory (Foa et al., 2007). It is important to note that overengagement does not mean the client has become emotional or upset. Rather, overengagement is defined by a level of emotional distress that precludes learning or processing exposure exercise (Foa et al., 2007). The PE protocol anticipates this possibility and provides therapists with strategies that allow treatment to continue, while helping to manage the client's extreme distress. Although a full explication of these strategies is beyond the present chapter, clinicians would be well served to remember that the standard PE instructions for imaginal exposure (e.g., closing one's eyes, using the present tense) are designed to maximize client engagement with the imaginal exposure because clients tend to try to avoid it. Therefore, when faced with the challenge of an overengaged client, the clinician can reverse some of these standard instructions (e.g., ask the client to complete the exercise with his or her eyes open or relate the traumatic event in the past tense). Additional approaches that, in our clinical experience, have been used with success include having the client write a trauma narrative and read it to the therapist, or having the client relate the events of the trauma through a question-and-answer-type conversation with the therapist. For a more detailed description of these strategies, the reader is referred to the PE treatment manual (Foa et al., 2007).

The PE manual also indicates that PE may not be the treatment of choice for clients with severe comorbid conditions, such as imminent threat of suicide or homicide, severe and recent self-injurious behavior, and psychosis (Foa et al., 2007). However, clinicians appear to think PE is more generally contraindicated for PTSD patients with comorbid symptoms or disorders. For example, in a study by Becker and colleagues (2004), clinicians considered imaginal exposure contraindicated for patients with comorbid psychotic disorder (85%), suicidality (85%), dissociation (51%), any comorbid diagnosis (37%), or a comorbid anxiety disorder (32%). Similarly, van Minnen and colleagues (2010) found that clinicians believed depression was a contraindication for PE, especially for patients with multiple childhood traumas. These beliefs persist, despite evidence that PE can be used effectively with clients who have comorbid conditions (McLean & Foa, 2014; van Minnen, Harned, Zoellner, & Mills, 2012).

In one of the most thorough examinations of PE in the context of comorbid conditions, van Minnen and colleagues (2012) reviewed the literature on PE, including randomized controlled trials, open-label trials, and pilot studies to determine the impact of several potential comorbidities on PE's effectiveness. The conditions they examined included dissociation, borderline personality disorder (BPD), psychosis, suicidal and nonsuicidal self-injury, substance use, and depression. These researchers concluded that PE can be used effectively with clients experiencing each of these comorbid issues (van Minnen et al., 2012). Importantly, however, when comorbid conditions are severe, it may be best to treat the comorbid condition concurrently, or prior to, implementing PE for the PTSD. For example, in the few studies that have examined PE in the presence of comorbid psychosis, all patients were maintained on their treatment regimen for the psychosis when they completed PE (van Minnen et al., 2012). Similarly, efforts to utilize PE with clients suffering from severe BPD have been provided prior to or concurrent with treatment for BPD (e.g., dialectical behavior therapy; Harned et al., 2015), and sometimes the basic PE protocol is modified, such as by adding skills training sessions prior to initiating exposure (see van Minnen et al., 2012, for a more thorough discussion).

PE is efficacious in reducing PTSD symptoms among patients with comorbid depression (e.g., Foa et al., 2005). In another study, PTSD patients with current major depression, past major depression, and no history of major depression experienced similar reductions in PTSD with PE treatment (Hagenaars, van Minnen, & Hoogduin, 2010). Although comorbid depression has not been found to contraindicate PE, it is recommended that therapists consider alternative treatment or crisis management prior to PE when major depression is the primary disorder or when clients are at high risk of suicide (McLean & Foa, 2014).

Traumatic brain injury (TBI) and PTSD commonly co-occur in military combat veterans (Hoge et al., 2008). TBI has also been suggested as a contraindication for PE. However, research indicates that PE is efficacious in clients with TBI. For example, Sripada and colleagues (2013) found no difference between veterans with and without a history of mild TBI in the degree to which PTSD symptoms were reduced by PE treatment. Similar results emerged from a study of active duty service members and veterans (Wolf et al., 2015). Another recent study found no differences between veterans with and without TBI on a number of PE treatment processes, including fear activation, length and number of exposure sessions, within-session habituation, and extinction rate (Ragsdale et al., 2018).

Clinicians sometimes express concern about using PE when PTSD is accompanied by dissociative symptoms. However, research indicates that dissociative symptoms are not related to improvement or dropout from PE. In one study, individuals with high levels of dissociation experienced similar reductions of PTSD symptoms as did patients with low levels of dissociation (Merrill & Strauman, 2004). Wolf, Lunney, and Schnurr (2016) found that outcomes of PE were no different between groups of individuals with the dissociative subtype of PTSD and those without dissociation. Burton, Feeny, Connell, and Zoellner (2018) found similar results, suggesting that PTSD patients with dissociation respond well to exposure-based treatments.

When using PE with patients who have a high tendency to dissociate, it is important to remember that the success of PE is premised on the client being able to incorporate new information into the cognitive-emotion network associated with the trauma. This requires the client to process "new" information while the trauma memory is activated; metaphorically, the client must keep one foot in the present while the other revisits the past. Highly dissociative clients may find this difficult. Therefore, it might be necessary to modify imaginal exposure instructions to help the client process new information. This can be done by having the client complete the imaginal exposure exercise with his or her eyes open (as with an overengager). The client may also use simple grounding techniques (e.g., visual focusing on an object, gripping the arms of a chair) as a means of maintaining connection to the present. Similarly, therapists may increase their verbalizations during the exercise (e.g., offering words of encouragement, reminders that they are present) to help ground their clients.

Questions about using PE with PTSD clients who have substance use disorder (SUD) persist, primarily because most prior studies of PE excluded participants with comorbid substance dependence (although they typically included those with substance abuse diagnoses). Traditionally, clients presenting with comorbid PTSD and substance dependence were treated sequentially beginning with the substance use problems. Once they achieved a period of abstinence from substance use (the exact period of time varied), treatment for PTSD was introduced. To date, there are no studies of sequential treatment for PTSD and SUD in which the PTSD is treated first. Our clinical experience suggests that this approach can be quite challenging, and it is not recommended. However, several recent studies have found PE to be efficacious when used in combination, or concurrently, with treatment for SUD. It has been suggested that PE may be effective not only in reducing PTSD, but may also help maintain reductions in substance use (McLean & Foa, 2014). Some of these studies have focused on one particular substance such as alcohol dependence (Foa, McLean, Capaldi, & Rosenfield, 2013) or cocaine dependence (Brady, Dansky, Back, Foa, & Carroll, 2001), whereas others have included participants who were dependent on a variety of substances (Mills et al., 2012). A manual for combined PE and SUD treatment has been developed (Back et al., 2015).

The results described previously indicate that patients with PTSD and co-occurring disorders or symptoms can be successfully and safely treated with PE. Perhaps of equal importance is the finding that PE often improves comorbid symptomatology. Studies that examined change in depression found that PE leads to a reduction in depression (e.g., Aderka, Gillihan, McLean, & Foa, 2013; Asukai et al., 2010; Foa et al., 1999; Foa & Rauch, 2004; Gilboa-Schechtman et al., 2010; Moser, Cahill, & Foa, 2010; Schnurr et al., 2007) and in suicidal and self-injurious urges and behaviors (Harned, Korslund, & Linehan, 2014). PE also has demonstrated effectiveness in reducing trauma-related guilt (Pacella et al., 2012; Resick et al., 2002), anger (Cahill, Rauch, Hembree, & Foa, 2003), and general anxiety (Foa et al., 2005; Nacasch et al., 2011). In addition, PE can significantly improve social adjustment and functioning (Foa et al., 2005; Foa, Yusko, et al., 2013; Shemesh et al., 2011) and decrease physical health complaints (Rauch et al., 2009). Thus, not only is PE effective in the face of comorbid problems, but researchers have demonstrated its ability to broadly impact the lives of individuals with

PTSD by fostering improvement in PTSD, as well as associated symptoms, and by improving general functioning and quality of life.

New Advances and Future Directions for PE

Recent years have seen significant advances in the application of PE in the treatment of PTSD. Several studies have examined variations in the delivery modality, timing, and setting of PE with promising results. Although these studies maintain the basic content and structure of the PE protocol, they incorporate fairly major modifications that could alter the processes or outcomes of the treatment. These changes include the use of virtual reality technology (Maples-Keller, Bunnell, Kim, & Rothbaum, 2017; Reger et al., 2016), the use of daily PE sessions (e.g., Blount et al., 2014; Foa, McLean, et al., 2018), and the delivery of PE in primary care settings (Cigrang et al., 2015, 2017).

Virtual-Reality-Augmented PE

Reger and colleagues (2016) compared virtual reality exposure (VRE) to standard PE, hypothesizing that the added multisensory virtual reality component would increase emotional engagement during exposure, resulting in superior outcomes relative to exposure delivered in the standard manner. In this study with military personnel who had combat-related PTSD, VRE followed the standard PE treatment protocol (Foa et al., 2007) with two exceptions. First, in Session 2 of VRE, the patient was briefly introduced to the VR equipment and instructed in its use while immersed in a calm virtual environment. Beginning in Session 3 of VRE, the therapist placed the patient in a relevant VR environment and patients confronted their memory with their eyes open, wearing a virtual reality headset. As the patient articulated his or her memory, the therapist customized the scene and associated stimuli to match the memory in relevant respects. Although VRE was efficacious in reducing PTSD symptoms posttreatment, improvements were not significantly different from those achieved with standard PE. In addition, *post hoc* analyses showed greater improvement in the standard PE group at 3- and 6-month follow-up.

Massed PE

Blount and colleagues (2014) presented the case study of a U.S. military service member treated in an intensive outpatient protocol (IOP) that delivered PE every day for 2 weeks. At the end of the 2 weeks, the client exhibited clinically meaningful reductions in PTSD, depression, and anxiety, and also no longer met the diagnostic criteria for PTSD. These gains were maintained at 6-month follow-up. Foa, McLean, and colleagues (2018) conducted a randomized trial comparing "massed PE" (daily sessions for 2 weeks) to the standard PE protocol (weekly sessions for 10 weeks). Massed PE was found to be noninferior to standard PE. Furthermore, massed PE had a lower dropout rate (Foa, McLean, et al., 2018).

PE in Primary Care Settings

Cigrang and colleagues (2015) examined the initial efficacy of a brief version of PE for primary care (PE-PC) protocol. In this study, PE-PC was delivered in four 30-minute appointments over 4–6 weeks. Patients who received PE-PC experienced significant improvements in PTSD, depression, and general mental health that were maintained at 6- and 12-month follow-ups. A subsequent RCT comparing PE-PC to a minimal contact control condition found similar results (Cigrang et al., 2017) that were generally maintained at 6-month follow-up, indicating that PE-PC delivered in integrated primary care may be effective for the treatment of PTSD.

Conclusions

PE has been used and studied for more than 30 years, and the empirical literature that supports its efficacy in treating PTSD is among the most extensive of any PTSD treatment. PE has been found effective in treating PTSD following a variety of different traumatic events, and in different countries and settings. PE is effective in treating PTSD in the presence of significant comorbidities and, importantly, improves these other conditions as well. Despite this evidence, some clinicians are reticent to put PE into practice. A number of reasons for this hesitancy were described in this chapter, along with several modifications or adjustments that can be made to the PE protocol to address such concerns or challenges. Many of these procedural adjustments are actually reflective of the flexibility built into the PE protocol, which appears not to be well understood by clinicians. Other adjustments to the protocol represent substantial changes, and several of these alterations have been the subject of empirical study (e.g., massed sessions, tele-health delivery, virtual reality exposure). The positive effects of PE appear robust enough to persist, even with the variations in procedure.

Despite the strength of the research underlying and supporting PE, there are a number of questions that remain, and additional research is needed to provide guidance to clinicians as they incorporate this treatment into their repertoire. For example, not all clients benefit from PE; research is needed to help determine how to best help those clients who do not respond to PE in its current format. Should PE be modified to treat these clients, or would they be more effectively treated with another approach? Similarly, the techniques of PE appear quite robust to modifications in delivery, including massed sessions, tele-health, and the use of virtual reality. However, research is needed to provide guidance on whether and how such modifications impact the effectiveness of PE for particular patients. Another area in need of research is implementation. What tools, techniques, processes, and policies are needed to support clinicians as they begin to use PE to treat PTSD?

Beyond the practical questions outlined previously, a number of theoretical questions and issues related to PE require additional research. There have been some initial attempts at identifying and understanding the mechanisms that underlie the changes observed with PE, but additional work is needed. PE is sometimes conceptualized as a treatment that focuses on the habituation of fear to achieve its gains. However, we recognize that PTSD is associated with many emotions beyond fear, including guilt, shame, horror, and disgust. The success of PE with clients whose traumatic memories likely include many of these feelings other than fear suggests that the treatment does not work solely through habituation of fear. A better delineation of the mechanisms of change may offer the opportunity to improve the efficiency of PE and to better identify clients who are most likely to benefit from the treatment.

In sum, PE is a treatment with an extensive record of research supporting its use to treat PTSD arising from a variety of traumas. That being said, not all clients benefit from PE and dropout rates can be high, although no higher than in other treatments for PTSD (Imel, Laska, Jakupcak, & Simpson, 2013). The protocol appears robust to modifications in delivery parameters and useful in the context of a number of conditions that commonly co-occur with PTSD. Despite the strengths of PE, clinicians have been slow to adopt the protocol into their practices. Future work should examine barriers to implementation and identify procedures to encourage the use of this effective treatment.

REFERENCES

Acierno, R., Knapp, R., Tuerk, P., Gilmore, A. K., Lejuez, C., Ruggiero, K., et al. (2017). A non-inferiority trial of prolonged exposure for posttraumatic stress disorder: In person versus home-based telehealth. *Behaviour Research and Therapy, 89,* 57–65.

Aderka, I. M., Gillihan, S. J., McLean, C. P., & Foa, E. B. (2013). The relationship between posttraumatic and depressive symptoms during prolonged exposure with and without cognitive restructuring for the treatment of posttraumatic stress disorder. *Journal of Consulting and Clinical Psychology, 81*(3), 375–382.

American Psychological Association. (2017). Clinical practice guideline for the treatment of PTSD for adults. Retrieved from *www.apa.org/ptsd-guideline/ptsd.pdf.*

Asukai, N., Saito, A., Tsuruta, N., Kisimoto, J., & Nshikawa, T. (2010). Efficacy of exposure therapy for Japanese patients with posttraumatic stress disorder due to mixed traumatic events: A randomized controlled study. *Journal of Traumatic Stress, 23*(6), 744–750.

Back, S. E., Foa, E. B., Killeen, T. K., Mills, K. L., Teesson, M., Cotton, B. D., et al.

(2015). *Concurrent treatment of PTSD and substance use disorders using prolonged exposure (COPE)*. New York: Oxford University Press.

Becker, C. B., Zayfert, C., & Anderson, E. (2004). A survey of psychologists' attitudes towards and utilization of exposure therapy for PTSD. *Behaviour Research and Therapy, 42*(3), 277–292.

Blanchard, E. B., Hickling, E. B., Devineni, T., Veazey, C. H., Galovski, T. E., Mundy, E., et al. (2003). A controlled evaluation of cognitive behavioral therapy for posttraumatic stress in motor vehicle accident survivors. *Behaviour Research and Therapy, 41*(1), 79–96.

Blount, T. B., Cigrang, J. A., Foa, E. B., Ford, H. L., & Peterson, A. L. (2014). Intensive outpatient prolonged exposure for combat-related PTSD: A case study. *Cognitive and Behavioral Practice, 21*, 89–96.

Brady, K. T., Dansky, B. S., Back, S. E., Foa, E. B., & Carroll, K. M. (2001). Exposure therapy in the treatment of PTSD cocaine dependent individuals: Preliminary findings. *Journal of Substance Abuse Treatment, 21*(1), 47–54.

Bryant, R. A., Moulds, M. L., Guthrie, R. M., Dang, S. T., Mastrodomenico, J., Nixon, R. D., et al. (2008). A randomized controlled trial of exposure therapy and cognitive restructuring for posttraumatic stress disorder. *Journal of Consulting and Clinical Psychology, 76*(4), 695–703.

Burton, M. S., Feeny, N. C., Connell, A. M., & Zoellner, L. A. (2018). Exploring evidence of a dissociative subtype in PTSD: Baseline symptom structure, etiology, and treatment efficacy for those who dissociate. *Journal of Consulting and Clinical Psychology, 86*(5), 439–451.

Cahill, S. P., Rauch, S. A. M., Hembree, E. A., & Foa, E. B. (2003). Effect of cognitive–behavioral treatments for PTSD on anger. *Journal of Cognitive Psychotherapy, 17*(2), 113–131.

Cahill, S. P., Rothbaum, B., Resick, P. A., & Follette, V. M. (2009). Cognitive–behavioral therapy for adults. In E. B. Foa, T. M. Keane, M. J. Friedman, & J. A. Cohen (Eds.), *Effective treatments for PTSD: Practice guidelines from the International Society for Traumatic Stress Studies* (2nd ed., pp. 139–222). New York: Guilford Press.

Cigrang, J. A., Rauch, S. A., Mintz, J., Brundige, A., Avila, L. L. Bryan, C. J., et al. (2015). Treatment of active duty military with PTSD in primary care: A follow-up report. *Journal of Anxiety Disorders, 36*, 110–114.

Cigrang, J. A., Rauch, S. A., Mintz, J., Mitchell, J. A., Najera, E., Litz, B. T., et al. (2017). Moving effective treatment for posttraumatic stress disorder to primary care: A randomized controlled trial with active duty military. *Family, Systems, and Health, 35*(4), 450–462.

Cooper, N. A., & Clum, G. A. (1989). Imaginal flooding as a supplementary treatment for PTSD in combat veterans: A controlled study. *Behavior Therapy, 20*(3), 381–391.

Cusack, K., Jonas, D. E., Forneris, C. A., Wines, C., Sonis, J., Middleton, J. C., et al. (2016). Psychological treatments for adults with posttraumatic stress disorder: A systematic review and meta-analysis. *Clinical Psychology Review, 43*, 128–141.

Department of Veterans Affairs & Department of Defense. (2017). VA/DoD clinical practice guideline for the management of posttraumatic stress disorder and acute stress disorder. Retrieved from *www.healthquality.va.gov/guidelines/MH/ptsd/VADoDPTSDCPGFinal.pdf*.

Erbes, C. R., Stinson, R., Kuhn, E., Polusny, M., Urban, J., Hoffman, J., et al. (2014). Access, utilization, and interest in mHealth applications among veterans receiving outpatient care for PTSD. *Military Medicine, 179*(11), 1218–1222.

Foa, E. B., & Cahill, S. P. (2001). Psychological therapies: Emotional processing. In N. J. Smelser & B. Bates (Eds.), *International encyclopedia of the social and behavioral sciences* (Vol. 12, pp. 12363–12369). Oxford, UK: Elsevier Science.

Foa, E. B., Dancu, C. V., Hembree, E. A., Jaycox, L. H., Meadows, E. A., & Street, G. P. (1999). A comparison of exposure therapy, stress inoculation training, and their combination for reducing posttraumatic stress disorder in female assault victims. *Journal of Consulting and Clinical Psychology, 67*(2), 194–200.

Foa, E. B., Hembree, E. A., Cahill, S. P., Rauch, S. A., Riggs, D. S., Feeny, N. C., et al. (2005). Randomized trial of prolonged exposure for posttraumatic stress disorder with and without cognitive restructuring: Outcome at academic and community clinics. *Journal of Consulting and Clinical Psychology, 73*(5), 953–964.

Foa, E. B., Hembree, E. A., & Rothbaum, B. O. (2007). *Prolonged exposure therapy for PTSD: Emotional processing of traumatic experiences: Therapist guide.* New York: Oxford University Press.

Foa, E. B., Huppert, J. D., & Cahill, S. P. (2006). Emotional processiong theory: An update. In B. O. Rothbaum (Ed.), *Pathological anxiety: Emotional processing in etiology and treatment* (pp. 3–24). New York: Guilford Press.

Foa, E. B., & Kozak, M. J. (1986). Emotional processing of fear: Exposure to corrective information. *Psychological Bulletin, 99*(1), 20–35.

Foa, E. B., McLean, C. P., Capaldi, S., & Rosenfield, D. (2013). Prolonged exposure vs supportive counseling for sexual abuse-related PTSD in adolescent girls: A randomized clinical trial. *Journal of the American Medical Association, 310*(24), 2650–2657.

Foa, E. B., McLean, C. P., Zang, Y., Rosenfield, D., Yadin, E., Yarvid, J. S., et al. (2018). Effect of prolonged exposure therapy delivered over 2 weeks vs 8 weeks vs present centered therapy on PTSD symptom severity in military personnel: A randomized clinical trial. *Journal of the American Medical Association, 319*(4), 354–364.

Foa, E. B., & Rauch S. A. (2004). Cognitive changes during prolonged exposure versus prolonged exposure plus cognitive restructuring in female assault survivors with posttraumatic stress disorder. *Journal of Consulting and Clinical Psychology, 72*(5), 879–884.

Foa, E. B., & Riggs, D. S. (1993). Post-traumatic stress disorder in rape victims. In J. Oldham, M. B. Riba, & A. Tasman (Eds.), *American Psychiatric Press review of psychiatry* (Vol. 12, pp. 273–303). Washington, DC: American Psychiatric Press.

Foa, E. B., Rothbaum, B. O., Riggs, D. S., & Murdock, T. B. (1991). Treatment of post-traumatic stress disorder in rape victims: A comparison between cognitive-behavioral procedures and counseling. *Journal of Consulting Clinical Psychology, 59*(5), 715–723.

Foa, E. B., Yusko, D. A., McLean, C. P., Suvak, M. K., Bux, D. A., Oslin, D., et al. (2013). Concurrent naltrexone and prolonged exposure therapy for patients with co-morbid alcohol dependence and posttraumatic stress disorder: A randomized control trial. *Journal of the American Medical Association, 310*(5), 488–495.

Foa, E. B., Zandberg, L. J., McLean, C. P., Rosenfield, D., Fitzgerald, H., Tuerk, P. W., et al. (2018). The efficacy of 90-minute versus 60-minute sessions of prolonged exposure for posttraumatic stress disorder: Design of a randomized controlled trial in active duty military personnel. *Psychological Trauma: Theory, Research, Practice, and Policy, 11*(3), 307–313.

Fonzo, G. A., Goodkind, M. S., Oathes, D. J., Zaiko, Y. V., Harvey, M., Peng, K. K., et al. (2017). PTSD psychotherapy outcome predicted by brain activation during emotional activity and regulation. *American Journal of Psychiatry, 174*(12), 1163–1174.

Gilboa-Schechtman, E., Foa, E. B., Shafran, N., Aderka, I., Powers, M. B., Rachamim, L., et al. (2010). Prolonged exposure versus dynamic therapy for adolescent PTSD: A pilot randomized controlled trial. *Journal of the American Academy of Child and Adolescent Psychiatry, 49*(10), 1034–1042.

Goodson, J. T., Lefkowitz, C. M., Helstrom, A. W., & Gawrysiak, M. J. (2013). Outcomes of prolonged exposure therapy for veterans with posttraumatic stress disorder. *Journal of Traumatic Stress, 26*(4), 419–425.

Hagenaars, M. A., van Minnen, A., & Hoogduin, K. A. (2010). The impact of dissociation and depression on the efficacy of prolonged exposure treatment for PTSD. *Behaviour Research and Therapy, 48*(1), 19–27.

Harned, M. S., Korslund, K. E., & Linehan, M. M. (2014). A pilot randomized controlled trial of dialectical behavior therapy with and without the dialectical behavior therapy prolonged exposure protocol for suicidal and self-injuring women with borderline personality disorder and PTSD. *Behaviour Research and Therapy, 55,* 7–17.

Harned, M. S., Ruork, A. K., Liu, J., & Tkachuck, M. A. (2015). Emotional activation and habituation during imaginal exposure for PTSD among women with borderline personality disorder. *Journal of Traumatic Stress, 28,* 253–257.

Held, P., Klassen, B. J., Brennan, M. B., & Zalta, A. K. (2018). Using prolonged exposure and cognitive processing therapy to treat veterans with moral injury-based PTSD: Two case examples. *Cognitive and Behavioral Practice, 25,* 377–390.

Hoge, C. W., McGurk, D., Thomas, J. L., Cox, A. L., Engel, C. C., & Castro, C. A. (2008). Mild traumatic brain injury in U.S. soldiers returning from Iraq. *New England Journal of Medicine, 358*(5), 453–463.

Imel, Z. E., Laska, K., Jakupcak, M., & Simpson, T. L. (2013). Meta-analysis of dropout in treatments for posttraumatic stress disorder. *Journal of Consulting and Clinical Psychology, 81,* 394–404.

Jayawickreme, N., Cahill, S. P., Riggs, D. S., Rauch, S. A., Resick, P. A., Rothbaum, B. O., et al. (2014). Primum non nocere (first do no harm): Symptom worsening and improvement in female assault victims after prolonged exposure for PTSD. *Depression and Anxiety, 31*(5), 412–419.

Kline, A. C., Cooper, A. A., Rytwinski, N. K., & Feeny, N. C. (2018). Long-term efficacy of psychotherapy for posttraumatic stress disorder: A meta-analysis of randomized controlled trials. *Clinical Psychology Review, 59,* 30–40.

Lenz, A. S., Haktanir, A., & Callender, K. (2017). Meta-analysis of trauma-focused therapies for treating symptoms of posttraumatic stress disorder. *Journal of Counseling and Development, 95,* 339–353.

Maples-Keller, J. L., Bunnell, B. E., Kim, S. J., & Rothbaum, B. O. (2017). The use of virtual reality technology in the treatment of anxiety and other psychiatric disorders. *Harvard Review of Psychiatry, 25*(3), 103–113.

Markowitz, J. C., Petkova, E., Neria, Y., Van Meter, P. E., Zhao, Y., Hembree, E., et al. (2015). Is exposure necessary?: A randomized clinical trial of interpersonal psychotherapy for PTSD. *American Journal of Psychiatry, 172*(5), 430–440.

McLean, C. P., & Foa, E. B. (2014). The use of prolonged exposure therapy to help patients with posttraumatic stress disorder. *Clinical Practice, 11*(2), 233–241.

Merrill, K. M., & Strauman, T. J. (2004). The role of personality in cognitive-behavioral therapies. *Behavior Therapy, 35*(1), 131–146.

Mills, K. L., Teesson, M., Back, S. E., Brady, K. T., Baker, A. L., Hopwood, S., et al. (2012). Integrated exposure-based therapy for co-occurring posttraumatic stress disorder and substance dependence: A randomized controlled trial. *Journal of the American Medical Association, 308*(7), 690–699.

Moser, J. S., Cahill, S. P., & Foa, E. B. (2010). Evidence for poorer outcome in patients with severe negative trauma-related cognitions receiving prolonged exposure plus cognitive restructuring: Implications for treatment matching in posttraumatic stress disorder. *Journal of Nervous and Mental Disease, 198*(1), 72–75.

Nacasch, N., Foa, E. B., Huppert, J. D., Tzur, D., Fostick, L., Dinstein, Y., et al. (2011). Prolonged exposure therapy for combat- and terror-related posttraumatic stress disorder: A randomized control comparison with treatment as usual. *Journal of Clinical Psychiatry, 72*(9), 1174–1180.

Nacasch, N., Huppert, J. D., Su, Y. J., Kivity, Y., Dinshtein, Y., Yeh, R., et al. (2015). Are 60-minute prolonged exposure sessions with 20-minute imaginal exposure to traumatic memories sufficient to successfully treat PTSD?: A randomized noninferiority clinical trial. *Behavior Therapy, 46*(3), 328–341.

National Institute of Health and Care Excellence. (2018). Post-traumatic stress disorder. Retrieved from *www.nice.org.uk/guidance/ng116/resources/posttraumatic-stress-disorder-pdf-66141601777861.*

Pacella, M. L., Armelie, A., Boarts, J., Wagner, G., Jones, T., Feeny, N., et al. (2012). The impact of prolonged exposure on PTSD symptoms and associated psychopathology in people living with HIV: A randomized test of concept. *AIDS and Behavior, 16*(5), 1327–1340.

Phoenix Australia—Centre for Posttraumatic Mental Health. (2013). Australian guidelines for the treatment of acute stress disorder and posttraumatic stress disorder. Retrieved from *https://phoenixaustralia.org/wp-content/uploads/2015/03/Phoenix-ASD-PTSD-Guidelines.pdf.*

Powers, M. B., Halpern, J. M., Ferenschak, M. P., Gillihan, S. J., & Foa, E. B. (2010). A meta-analytic review of prolonged exposure for posttraumatic stress disorder. *Clinical Psychology Review, 30,* 635–641.

Ragsdale, K. A., Gramlich, M. A., Beidel, D. C., Neer, S. M., Kitsmiller, E. G., & Morrison, K. I. (2018). Does traumatic brain injury attenuate the exposure therapy process? *Behavior Therapy, 49*(4), 617–630.

Rauch, S. A., Grunfeld, T. E., Yadin, E., Cahill, S. P., Hembree, E., & Foa, E. B. (2009). Changes in reported physical health symptoms and social function with prolonged exposure therapy for chronic posttraumatic stress disorder. *Depression and Anxiety, 26*(8), 732–738.

Reger, G. M., Hoffman, J., Riggs, D. S., Rothbaum, B. O., Ruzek, J., Holloway, K. M., et al. (2013). The "PE Coach" smartphone application: An innovative approach to improving implementation, fidelity, and homework adherence during prolonged exposure. *Psychological Services, 10*(3), 342–349.

Reger, G. M., Koenen-Woods, P., Zetocha, K., Smolenski, D. J., Holloway, K. M., Rothbaum, B. O., et al. (2016). Randomized controlled trial of prolonged exposure using imaginal exposure vs. virtual reality exposure in active duty soldiers with deployment-related posttraumatic stress disorder (PTSD). *Journal of Consulting and Clinical Psychology, 84*(11), 946–959.

Reger, G. M., Skopp, N. A., Edwards-Stewart, A., & Lemus, E. L. (2017). Comparison of PE Coach to treatment as usual: A case series with two active duty soldiers. *Military Psychology, 27*(5), 287–296.

Resick, P. A., Nishith, P., Weaver, T. L., Astin, M. C., & Feuer, C. A. (2002). A comparison of cognitive processing therapy with prolonged exposure and a waiting condition for the treatment of chronic posttraumatic stress disorder in female rape victims. *Journal of Consulting and Clinical Psychology, 70*(4), 867–879.

Resick, P. A., Williams, L. F., Suvak, M. K., Monson, C. M., & Gradus, J. L. (2012). Long-term outcomes of cognitive-behavioral treatments for posttraumatic stress disorder among female rape survivors. *Journal of Consulting and Clinical Psychology, 80*(2), 201–210.

Rothbaum, B. O., Astin, M. C., & Marsteller, F. (2005). Prolonged exposure versus eye movement desensitization and reprocessing (EMDR) for PTSD rape victims. *Journal of Traumatic Stress, 18*(6), 607–616.

Ruzek, J. I., Eftekhari, A., Rosen, C. S., Crowley, J. J., Kuhn, E., Foa, E. B., et al. (2016). Effects of a comprehensive training program on clinician beliefs about and intention to use prolonged exposure therapy for PTSD. *Psychological Trauma, 8*(3), 348–355.

Schnurr, P. P., Friedman, M. J., Engel, C. C., Foa, E. B., Shea, M. T., Chow, B. K., et al. (2007). Cognitive behavioral therapy for posttraumatic stress disorder in women: A randomized controlled trial. *Journal of the American Medical Association, 297*(8), 820–830.

Shemesh, E., Annunziato, R. A., Weatherley, B. D., Cotter, G., Feaganes, J. R., Santra, M., et al. (2011). A randomized controlled trial of the safety and promise of cognitive-behavioral therapy using imaginal exposure in patients with posttraumatic stress disorder resulting from cardiovascular illness. *Journal of Clinical Psychiatry, 72*(2), 168–174.

Sripada, R. K., Rauch, S. A., Tuerk, P. W., Smith, E., Defever, A. M., Mayer, R. A., et al. (2013). Mild traumatic brain injury and treatment response in prolonged exposure for PTSD. *Journal of Traumatic Stress, 26*(3), 369–375.

Tuerk, P. W., Yoder, M., Grubaugh, A., Myrick, H., Hammer, M., & Acierno, R. (2011). Prolonged exposure therapy for combat-related posttraumatic disorder: An examination of treatment effectiveness for veterans of the wars in Afghanistan and Iraq. *Journal of Anxiety Disorders, 25*(3), 397–403.

Tuerk, P. W., Yoder, M., Ruggiero, K. J., Gros, D. F., & Acierno, R. (2010). A pilot study of prolonged exposure therapy for posttraumatic stress disorder delivered via telehealth technology. *Journal of Traumatic Stress, 23*(1), 116–123.

van Minnen, A., & Foa, E. B. (2006). The effect of imaginal exposure length on outcome of treatment for PTSD. *Journal of Traumatic Stress, 19*(4), 427–438.

van Minnen, A., Harned, M. S., Zoellner, L., & Mills, K. (2012). Examining potential contraindications for prolonged exposure therapy for PTSD. *European Journal of Psychotraumatology, 3*, 1–14.

van Minnen, A., Hendriks, M., & Olff, M. (2010). When do trauma experts choose exposure therapy for PTSD patients?: A controlled study of therapist and patient factors. *Behaviour Research and Therapy, 48*(4), 312–320.

Watts, B. V., Schnurr, P. P., Mayo, L., Yinong, Y., Weeks, W. B., & Friedman, M. J. (2013). Meta-analysis of the efficacy of treatments for posttraumatic stress disorder. *Journal of Clinical Psychiatry, 74,* e541–e550.

Wells, A., Walton, D., Lovell, K., & Proctor, D. (2015). Metacognitive therapy versus prolonged exposure in adults with chronic post-traumatic stress disorder: A parallel randomized controlled trial. *Cognitive Therapy and Research, 39*(1), 70–80.

Wolf, E. J., Lunney, C. A., & Schnurr, P. P. (2016). The influence of the dissociative subtype of posttraumatic stress disorder on treatment efficacy in female veterans and active duty service members. *Journal of Consulting and Clinical Psychology, 84*(1), 95–100.

Wolf, G. K., Kretzmer, T., Crawford, E., Thors, C., Wagner, H. R., Strom, T. Q., et al. (2015). Prolonged exposure therapy with veterans and active duty personnel diagnosed with PTSD and traumatic brain injury. *Journal of Traumatic Stress, 28*(4), 339–347.

Yuen, E. K., Gros, D. F., Price, M., Zeigler, S., Tuerk, P. W., Foa, E. B., et al. (2015). Randomized controlled trial of home-based telehealth versus in-person prolonged exposure for combat-related PTSD in veterans: Preliminary results. *Journal of Clinical Psychology, 71*(6), 500–512.

CHAPTER 13

Cognitive Processing Therapy

Kathleen M. Chard, Debra L. Kaysen, Tara E. Galovski,
Reginald D. V. Nixon, and Candice M. Monson

Our goal in this chapter is to provide a review of information critical to understanding cognitive processing therapy (CPT) (Resick, Monson, & Chard, 2017), its origins, and its uses as a treatment for posttraumatic stress disorder (PTSD). The chapter begins with a description of the theoretical underpinnings of CPT and the techniques that comprise each CPT session. The evidence supporting CPT as a recommended PTSD treatment is summarized, including a detailed appraisal of the data regarding generalizability and gaps in the literature. The chapter concludes with recommendations for conducting CPT with special populations and areas for future development from clinical and research perspectives.

Theoretical Context

CPT is based on a sociocognitive or constructivist model to explain failure to recover following trauma, and the resulting PTSD (for details, see Resick, Monson, & Chard, 2014, 2017; Resick & Schnicke, 1993). Although informed by information-processing theories of fear and PTSD, in addition to traditional cognitive theory (e.g., Beck, Rush, Shaw, & Emery, 1979; Foa, Steketee, & Rothbaum, 1989; Inhelder & Piaget, 1958; Lang, 1977), the role and importance of cognitions and emotions in CPT differ somewhat compared with these and other theoretical accounts of PTSD (e.g., Brewin, 2001; Ehlers & Clark, 2000). According to CPT theory, when traumas occur, the brain attempts to reconcile the meaning of the event in relation to prior existing cognitive structures, or schemas. It is posited that recovery from traumatization through natural processes or with intervention occurs because of *accommodation* of the traumatic information with existing schema. In other words, preexisting belief structures are modified enough to be consonant with realistic appraisals about the trauma. PTSD is thought to occur when there is dissonance between pretrauma schemas and posttraumatic appraisals of the event (see Resick, Monson, & Chard, 2017, for a detailed discussion). In making sense of traumatic experiences, those with PTSD attempt to maintain their preexisting positive beliefs and alter their appraisals of the trauma to be consistent with them. Or, if there are preexisting negative schemas, they incorporate this information to confirm those prior negative beliefs. In both cases, assimilation of the traumatic information takes place because individuals attempt to incorporate traumatic information without changing existing schemas. Symptoms are also maintained if clients radically modify their pretrauma beliefs following trauma, a process labeled as *overaccommodation*. For example, they may go from believing that the world is generally safe to believing that they are in constant threat of harm. Assimilated beliefs are targeted first in the course of CPT based on the notion that correcting historical trauma appraisals has cascading effects on here-and-now and future-oriented cognitions that represent problematic overaccommodated beliefs. Thus, the goal of CPT is to have clients develop realistic appraisals about the trauma and adapt their schema in a balanced manner to account for the traumatic information, and then correct overaccommodated beliefs that emanate from traumatic experiences. This cognitive processing is core to successful CPT and accounts for the title of the therapy.

A critical component of the model underpinning CPT is its position on emotions. CPT differentiates between what are considered instinctual, hardwired emotions (i.e., natural emotions), such as fear in the face of real danger or sadness that might follow a loss, versus "manufactured" emotions that are posited to be driven by effortful cognition. CPT encourages the expression of natural emotions that have been suppressed or avoided, with the view that they will dissipate with time. Resolution of maladaptive manufactured emotions occurs by modifying underlying unhelpful beliefs through cognitive intervention.

In summary, CPT operates from a sociocognitive framework that has a particular emphasis on addressing the meaning and interpretations clients make of themselves, others, and the world more generally following trauma. It encourages emotional expression while addressing unhelpful or erroneous thinking that leads to the problematic symptoms seen in PTSD. The techniques and processes of CPT are detailed next.

Description of Techniques

As elaborated in a later section, CPT can be delivered in a number of formats, including individual and group sessions, across various delivery formats (e.g., face-to-face, tele-health), and for varying duration, typically an average of 12 sessions on an outpatient basis. Each session follows a similar framework: an agenda is set for the session, practice assignments given in the previous session are reviewed and discussed, a new skill or therapy component is introduced, practice assignments around that new component given, and potential challenges in undertaking the new skills problem-solved. CPT has the same characteristics of good cognitive-behavioral approaches, balancing structure, a collaborative, nonjudgmental therapeutic relationship, and sometimes requiring, as discussed later, a gentle "push" by therapists to address the avoidance that maintains PTSD and can interfere with optimal therapeutic outcomes.

CPT can be viewed as having three phases, with the first occurring in the early sessions (Sessions 1–3). This phase includes psychoeducation about PTSD as a disorder of nonrecovery, socializing clients to the sociocognitive model, and introducing the relationship between beliefs and emotions in PTSD. This phase also includes a focus on identifying "stuck points," or unhelpful beliefs that are interfering with recovery. The first session of CPT provides an opportune time to discuss the role that avoidance plays in maintaining PTSD and for clinicians to get a sense of stuck points that might interfere with optimal engagement of therapy (e.g., "If I think about my trauma, it will make me worse"). Socratic dialogue is a key element of CPT, and in this early phase it is particularly helpful in identifying these types of beliefs. In this phase of therapy, gentle questioning and alternative perspectives are explored, with a focus on assimilation-type stuck points (e.g., self-blame). Practice assignments are established after each session, with the first being an impact statement. Here, a client writes a statement, approximately one page long, explaining why she thinks the trauma happened and how it has impacted her beliefs in the domains highlighted earlier (i.e., safety, trust, power/control, esteem, and intimacy). In this phase, a client also completes a worksheet, allowing her to learn about the relationship between events, thoughts, and feelings. One format of CPT can involve the use of a written trauma account (CPT + A). If clinicians use this format, clients are asked to write a detailed account of their traumatic event at the end of Session 3.

The second phase of CPT (Sessions 4 and 5) comprises further processing of the traumatic event(s), with more formal cognitive intervention. Socratic dialogue remains a key element of therapy and, through it, clients are helped to question and challenge their stuck points. Clients are also introduced to ways to identify their idiosyncratic thinking styles that frequently reinforce these stuck points. For example, clients learn to recognize if their thoughts typically could be categorized as catastrophizing. A client might therefore come to understand that his initial interpretation of an incident in which a driver honked at him was an overreaction. That is, rather than viewing what happened as a dangerous situation that the client perceived he was lucky to escape without being attacked, he instead recognizes his habit of catastrophizing around certain incidents (and in this instance, despite no evidence that physical confrontation was ever a likely outcome). Assimilated beliefs continue to be a focus, with self-blame and hindsight bias (the idea that one could have predicted a traumatic event or should have done something to prevent it) targeted in particular. Clients might also minimize or distort the nature of the trauma in an attempt to make it fit with pretrauma schemas. Thus, therapy involves labeling the event for what it was (e.g., a rape) and addressing stuck points around accepting the traumatic event, as it occurred. If clients are doing CPT-A, this phase also involves reading their description of the most traumatic account in session and writing it up again as a practice assignment, with a focus on incorporating current thoughts and feelings.

In the final phase of CPT, clinicians assist clients to become more independent in their challenging of stuck points and developing healthier, more balanced beliefs. A goal here is to help clients become their own therapists, and it is accompanied by worksheets that incorporate questions to challenge stuck points, identifying how a point might represent a problematic pattern of thinking, and most importantly, documenting an alternative and more helpful belief. Throughout CPT, emotions are attended to and sometimes amplified, with clients encouraged to express and feel natural emotions, and to identify stuck points that might maintain unhelpful manufactured emotions. Although residual assimilated beliefs are still worked on in this phase, the majority of time is spent on overaccommodated beliefs largely in the domains of safety, trust, power/control, esteem, and intimacy. Clients identify how stuck points in these domains can be both self- and other-focused. For example, most clients readily relate to the concept of poor self-esteem; however, their esteem of others (e.g., people from other cultures, people associated with particular organizations) can also be negatively impacted by trauma (e.g., "All people who are [insert race] are dangerous"). In this phase, clients work through these domains with the help of handouts that describe how stuck points in these areas maintain PTSD, and that give examples of common types of stuck points and possible resolution statements. If the client has stuck points regarding other areas, for example, religion, grief, or moral injury, those are also addressed during this phase of therapy.

CPT usually ends when the entire protocol has been worked through, a client's PTSD symptoms have significantly lessened, and client and clinician are in agreement that it is appropriate to terminate therapy. The CPT manual provides directions for how to lengthen or shorten the protocol, while still covering all of the recommended material, depending on how quickly clients achieve the criterion outcomes. Clients are asked to write a new impact statement that focuses on their *current* beliefs and thoughts about the trauma. This is read to the therapist in the final session. It represents another indicator of PTSD recovery, with significant changes in beliefs typically observed. The new impact statement is also helpful in identifying any residual stuck points on which clients might need to continue to work after therapy has ended. As with most therapeutic approaches, a review of therapy skills is conducted, relapse prevention and plans for the future are discussed, and the importance of continued practice of skills is emphasized. A routine review 1–3 months after therapy has ceased is recommended to assist in identifying any unresolved stuck points and to encourage ongoing practice of the skills.

Appraisal of the Evidence

Evidence from Randomized Controlled Clinical Trials

To date, there have been over twenty published randomized controlled trials (RCTs) evaluating the efficacy of CPT. On the weight of this body of evidence, CPT has received a *Strong* recommendation in the International Society for Traumatic Stress Studies (ISTSS; 2018) guidelines for the prevention and treatment of PTSD. This body of evidence for CPT was originally developed and tested in an open trial designed to treat PTSD in civilian female victims of sexual assault and rape. Given the initial evidence that emerged from this study supporting the effectiveness of CPT, Resick and colleagues (2002) conducted the first RCT of CPT using a direct comparison design and evaluated the efficacy of CPT as compared to the gold standard treatment at the time, prolonged exposure (PE; Foa, Hembree, & Rothbaum, 2007), and to a minimal attention (MA) condition. This initial RCT was conducted with female rape survivors, most of whom (85.8%) described a history of multiple traumatic events across their lifespan, including childhood sexual assault (41%). The results of this first trial were strong, with participants in both CPT and PE demonstrating significant improvements in PTSD and depression and improvements in both active conditions being significantly greater than those observed in the MA group. In perhaps the most extensive long-term follow-up study in the PTSD literature to date, Resick, Williams, Suvak, Monson, and Gradus (2012) assessed the maintenance of treatment gains 5–10 years after the completion of treatment in this trial and found that gains were well maintained for participants who received both CPT and PE.

Over the course of the next decade, several additional RCTs were designed and conducted with the goal of building on Resick and colleagues' (2002) foundational trial and advancing the understanding of the mechanisms of action, as well as exploring flexible approaches to delivering treatment and optimizing outcomes. First, to better understand the relative contribution of the different theorized therapeutic elements of CPT, Resick, Nishith, Weaver, Astin, and Feuer (2008) conducted a dismantling trial comparing the treatment protocol with the account to the treatment protocol without the account, to a condition that focused *only* on writing the account of the trauma and then processing the associated emotions. Participants in all three conditions improved significantly on PTSD, depression, anger, guilt, anxiety, and shame; however, those who received CPT without the account improved faster and had significantly less dropout from treatment. These study results suggest that change in trauma-related beliefs is a critical mechanism of action in CPT. This study has important clinical implications, because it gives both therapists and patients demonstrably equally effective choices in delivering and receiving versions of CPT, thereby optimizing patient agency and increasing the likelihood of engagement and retention.

Galovski, Blain, Mott, Elwood, and Houle (2012) then explored the benefit of modifying the length of therapy such that therapy's end be determined by patient progress versus by a prescribed number of sessions. Flexibly administering the protocol yielded higher response rates; by the end of the study, 92% of the participants no longer had a diagnosis of PTSD. As a result of this study, CPT is now administered over a variable number of sessions, depending on patient needs. This study further assessed the impact of inserting non-trauma-focused crisis sessions into the protocol (in the case of midprotocol major psychosocial stressors or non-trauma-related patient crises) and found that CPT was able to easily accommodate intentional and thoughtful divergence from the protocol. Importantly, dropout rates were relatively low in this trial (i.e., 25%), suggesting that variable lengths of treatment (i.e., allowing patients to be done when they are improved and remain in therapy longer if they need additional assistance) and specific attention to major life stressors (with forethought as to how to return to the protocol as expediently as possible) may increase patient engagement and retention.

Consideration of the potentially more profound impact of early exposures to trauma in treating PTSD, particularly childhood sexual abuse, has long been an empirical and clinical concern. Clinicians and researchers alike have noted challenges with chronic abuse that occurs during important developmental years and wondered as to whether brief, protocol-driven therapies are adequate in cases of complex trauma histories. Chard (2005) expanded the CPT protocol to 17 sessions and compared this treatment to an MA wait-list condition. Adult study participants had all experienced childhood sexual abuse and the majority reported chronic abuse histories (57% recalled over 100 incidents of abuse). CPT participants showed significantly greater improvement than MA participants, with large effect size differences on PTSD and depression outcomes. This trial provides support for the effectiveness of CPT in cases of chronic PTSD stemming from trauma exposures during patients' formative years. Ahrens and Rexford (2002) also tested the CPT protocol with adolescents with a history of child interpersonal trauma. Their study included 38 incarcerated male adolescents who had typically experienced multiple traumas, largely interpersonal violence in nature. Eight sessions of CPT were compared to a wait-list control, and patients in the CPT condition reported, on average, a 50% reduction in PTSD symptoms via a self-report measure.

In an effort to assess the generalizability of CPT to noncivilian populations, several RCTs were conducted with both veteran and active duty military samples. The generalizability to military populations is particularly important, given the smaller effects of trauma-focused treatment in this population as compared to those observed in civilians (Steenkamp, Litz,

Hoge, & Marmar, 2015). The first CPT study conducted with a veteran sample included primarily male veterans (93% male; 80% from the Vietnam era; 78% with combat-related trauma) and compared the 12-session CPT protocol with a 10-week wait list (Monson et al., 2006). CPT participants demonstrated greater improvements in PTSD than the wait-list controls, with large effect size differences. Suris, Link-Malcolm, Chard, Ahn, and North (2013) also conducted a CPT trial with U.S. veterans. This study specifically included veterans who had suffered military sexual trauma (MST), and the sample was 85% female. CPT was compared to an active treatment condition, present-centered therapy (PCT), and CPT demonstrated a large effect for PTSD, with PCT having slightly less significant improvements. Finally, Sloan, Marx, Lee, and Resick (2018) recently compared CPT to written exposure therapy (WET) in a sample of civilian and veterans (52% male) who had been diagnosed with PTSD secondary to different types of trauma. CPT and WET were largely equivalent in effectively treating PTSD. CPT has also been tested in veterans outside the United States. Forbes and colleagues (2012) compared CPT to an active largely CBT-focused treatment as usual (TAU) condition in a sample of Australian veterans (97% male and 67% from the Vietnam era) attending for care at a veterans' counseling service. Study results indicated that veterans who participated in CPT improved significantly more in PTSD symptoms than those in TAU, with a large effect size reported. Resick and colleagues (2015) first tested CPT in an active duty military sample and compared CPT to PCT. Both treatments showed significant improvement over time, with CPT resulting in a slightly larger effect, although not significantly different from PCT. These comparison trials continue to demonstrate strong evidence supporting the efficacy of CPT in military and active duty populations. However, they also indicate substantial room for improvement in terms of overall outcomes and retention.

CPT has been tested in a range of different contexts and with diverse populations. The efficacy of CPT has been demonstrated in randomized controlled clinical trials internationally, including in the Democratic Republic of Congo, Iraq, Australia, and Germany (Bass et al., 2013; Bolton et al., 2014; Butollo, Karl, Konig, & Rosner, 2016; Nixon, 2012; Weiss et al., 2015). The therapy has been tested as well across diverse populations within the United States, including Bosnian war refugees (Schulz, Resick, Huber, & Griffin, 2006), African American clients (Lester, Artz, Resick, & Young-Xu, 2010), Latinos (Marques et al., 2016; Valentine et al., 2017), and Native Americans (Pearson, Kaysen, Huh, & Bedard-Gilligan, 2019). CPT has been translated into 12 different languages (Resick, Monson, & Chard, 2017) and has been shown to be effective when delivered through an interpreter (Schulz et al., 2006).

CPT continues to evolve, with the overarching goal of developing the therapy to enhance reach, access, and treatment for more diverse groups of trauma survivors. Toward this end, several RCTs have utilized augmentation designs or directly compared different versions of the protocol or methods of administration of CPT. Augmentation studies have sought to address sleep impairment prior to commencing trauma-focused treatment and found that sleep impairment could be significantly improved, and that the improved sleep augmented recovery from depression, but not from PTSD (Galovski et al., 2016). In a second augmentation study, Kozel and colleagues (2018) added transcranial magnetic stimulation (TMS) to CPT to improve outcomes in veterans with PTSD and showed a significantly greater effect on PTSD in the TMS + CPT condition, as compared to a sham TMS + CPT control. A series of studies were also conducted comparing the method of treatment delivery of CPT. For example, several noninferiority trials found that delivering CPT via tele-videoconferencing was noninferior to delivering the therapy in person for primarily male veterans (Morland et al., 2014), for civilian and veteran women (Morland et al., 2015), and in post-9/11 veterans (Maieritsch et al., 2016). Importantly, the groups did not differ with respect to therapeutic alliance, treatment compliance, and treatment satisfaction (Morland et al., 2014), suggesting that treatment via tele-videoconferencing is a feasible, palatable, and engaging modality of care.

Finally, although CPT was originally developed as a group therapy, the intervention has primarily been tested as an individual therapy. Resick, Wachen, and colleagues (2017) sought to evaluate the relative efficacy of group- versus individually administered CPT with active duty service members and found that participants improved significantly in PTSD and depression in both treatment conditions, but improvements in PTSD were significantly greater when the therapy was administered individually.

Evidence from Clinical Effectiveness Studies

PTSD rarely occurs in isolation, and treatment trials have assessed the effects of the intervention on a host of clinically complex patient populations. A number of studies assessing the effects of treatment on secondary outcomes and the effects of the decreases of PTSD and depression on comorbid disorders and conditions have been published. To date, studies have shown CPT to be effective in individuals who are also diagnosed with one or more personality disorders (Clarke, Rizvi, & Resick, 2008; Farmer, Mitchell, Parker-Guilbert, & Galovski, 2017; Walter, Bolte, Owens, & Chard, 2012). Kaysen and colleagues (2014) found that participants with current or past histories of alcohol use disorders recovered as well from PTSD as compared to participants without this comorbidity. In a later study with Native American women with PTSD, substance use, and HIV risk behavior, CPT was associated with significant reductions in PTSD severity, high-risk sexual behavior, and frequency of alcohol use (Pearson et al., 2019).

Traumatic brain injury (TBI) is a signature wound of American combat veterans who served post-9/11 and has high rates of comorbidity with PTSD (Hoge et al., 2008). Treating PTSD with CPT as part of a larger 8-week residential VA treatment program for comorbid PTSD and TBI was found to be beneficial, including for individuals with moderate to severe TBIs (Chard, Schumm, McIlvain, Bailey, & Parkinson, 2011; Walter et al., 2012; Walter, Varkovitzky, Owens, Lewis, & Chard, 2014). In addition, Jak and colleagues (2019) found that CPT with or without added cognitive rehabilitation training was effective in treating veterans with PTSD and a history of TBI in a randomized trial. CPT has been successfully implemented in an urban community mental health clinic as the trauma recovery portion of a larger program designed to provide mental health services to individuals diagnosed with severe mental illness, having unstable housing, and recently diverted from jail (Feingold, Fox-Galalis, & Galovski, 2018).

Additional treatment gains on impairment in functioning, comorbid symptoms, and clinical correlates of PTSD have been reported across RCTs and effectiveness studies, including improvements in depression, suicidal ideation, health-related concerns and sleep, sexual functioning, physiological reactivity, dissociation, occupational performance, and functioning across other important life domains (Galovski, Monson, Bruce, & Resick, 2009; Galovski, Sobel, Phipps, & Resick, 2005; Gradus, Suvak, Wisco, Marx, & Resick, 2013; Griffin, Resick, & Galovski, 2012; Mesa, Dickstein, Wooten, & Chard, 2017; Monson et al., 2012; Resick, Williams, et al., 2012; Speicher, Walter, & Chard, 2014; Wells et al., 2018). CPT is a relatively robust treatment that has been utilized in a variety of contexts, with research and implementation studies that have evaluated aspects of optimal delivery of the intervention. Also of note, in separate dissemination initiatives with U.S. and Australian veterans, very large effect sizes were found in naturalistic data collection of therapists' first cases using CPT—thus showing that even in the consultation process, therapists from different professions and with various levels of clinical expertise can facilitate significant positive changes for their clients (Chard, Ricksecker, Healy, Karlin, & Resick, 2012; Lloyd et al., 2015). Taken together, these studies showed that CPT is robust with demonstrable effect when administered in variable lengths, with added crisis sessions, with or without a trauma account, when delivered through videoconferencing, and in group, individual, or combined formats. It should be noted that in all of these trials, the actual protocol content was preserved with careful attention to fidelity. The richness of this clinical effectiveness and implementation literature helps inform the guidelines for providers in delivery of CPT across varying clinical contexts.

Practical Delivery of the Recommendations

Setting the Stage for CPT Delivery

Prior to starting CPT, it is essential to ensure that the clinical setting will allow for CPT to be delivered in a way that it is likely to be effective. As noted previously, CPT has been delivered in a variety of settings, including outpatient clinics, intensive day programs, low resource areas, and residential treatment programs (Bass et al., 2013; Walter et al., 2014). When offering the various formats of CPT to a client, we recommend relying on client preference when at all possible. Although many clients want to tell their trauma account to a therapist, we have found that just as many do not want to focus on the details of the event and would prefer moving to the cognitive challenging phase sooner. Thus, we find it helpful to discuss the treatment options with each client prior to starting CPT and allowing them to make an informed choice. Individual CPT is recommended to be delivered in 60-minute psychotherapy sessions, typically delivered weekly or biweekly. Group CPT consists of 90- to 120-minute group sessions, delivered weekly or biweekly. There is new, promising research that has examined more frequent sessions, such as three times per week or even daily sessions, which suggests that this type of spacing for sessions does not reduce efficacy and may reduce dropout (Bryan et al., 2018; Zalta et al., 2018). However, at the present time, the findings on more frequent dosing of treatment than twice weekly are based on open trials or single case studies. This has great promise for clients whose work, school, family demands or geographical limitations necessitate they receive treatment in a short period of time, or for clinical contexts such as inpatient settings, where more frequent sessions are necessary due to the length of stay. In these studies, clients are asked to complete all practice assignments prior to each session. In contrast, spacing out CPT more than once weekly may increase dropout and may also reduce the therapy's effectiveness (Gutner, Suvak, Sloan, & Resick, 2016). This can be a challenge in clinical settings with high caseloads or with a treatment model of monthly sessions. Thus, it is important when working with both clients and clinic administrators to ensure that at least weekly sessions are feasible.

CPT relies on the concept of "treat to target," which means that treatment plans are oriented toward achieving a well-defined, clinically relevant end-target. The assumption with this model is that the treatment plan will be both dynamic and responsive and will adjust the intervention based on measurement of clinical response. In the case of CPT, this means that clinicians should be using standardized measures to monitor the client's response to treatment (i.e., change in PTSD symptom severity), ideally weekly. By tracking PTSD symptom improvements frequently and reliably over the course of CPT, clinicians can help to ensure that the treatment is addressing core symptoms effectively and can help to identify times when CPT has gone awry early enough to correct the course. The PTSD checklist (PCL; Blevins, Weathers, Davis, Witte, & Domino, 2015) is a common tool used for this purpose, as it is both free and standardized. Clinicians should also use standardized instruments to track other symptoms that may be of clinical importance, such as depression, substance use, panic attacks, or suicidal ideation/self-injury. Monitoring changes in symptoms weekly accomplishes several goals. It allows both client and therapist to observe CPT progress. For therapists, this is an active process and allows CPT clinicians to notice whether symptoms are improving and, if they are not, to address these barriers. It also can provide a helpful point of discussion for both client and therapist around practice compliance and practice engagement. It can be helpful if the clinical setting is one in which clients can fill in the outcome measures in the waiting room or prior to beginning each session and where these measures can be tracked over time.

Who Is Appropriate for CPT?

In selecting clients for CPT, the existing clinical trials literature is used as a guideline. In general, these trials have had relatively minimal exclusion criteria, which often mirror the realities of most clinical settings. Exclusion criteria for CPT have generally been based on issues around clinical safety (suicidal/homicidal ideation with active intent, active psychosis or mania, substance dependence, active and severe nonsuicidal self-injury) or around ensuring that treatment effects can be attributed to the intervention (i.e., stability on psychiatric medications, typically for 1–2 months). Based on the literature, reviewed previously, individuals have been included in trials for CPT with personality disorders and other psychiatric disorders (e.g., depression, obsessive compulsive disorder, atttention-deficit/hyperactivity disorder, panic disorder, traumatic brain injury), as well as with both childhood and adult traumatic events, and with both single-incident and chronic trauma experiences. Thus, in general, CPT is a flexible intervention that can be applied to a broad array of individuals with PTSD, or subthreshold PTSD (Dickstein, Walter, Schumm, & Chard, 2013).

In determining whether CPT is a good fit for a particular client, there are various factors to consider. First of all, it is essential to determine that a client has PTSD. This may seem self-evident, but for the most part, CPT has been tested for individuals presenting with a clinical diagnosis of PTSD. Many individuals who have experienced traumatic events may present for treatment with other disorders and may not have PTSD. In these cases, it is more appropriate to use an evidence-based intervention for the presenting complaint. In cases where an individual may have subthreshold PTSD, CPT may be an appropriate intervention should it seem as if the trauma-related symptoms are what is driving client distress and another intervention does not make more sense in terms of one's case conceptualization.

Other factors to consider are safety-related concerns, such as suicidality, homicidality, and nonsuicidal self-injury. In these cases, it is essential that clinicians obtain a comprehensive history of the behavior. Factors such as the recency, frequency, and severity of the behavior, whether it is acute or chronic, the client's overall level of impulsivity, his or her level of supports and coping skills, and the degree/frequency with which he or she is using drugs and alcohol should be considered. For individuals whose suicidal behavior or nonsuicidal self-injurious behavior are likely to lead to CPT needing to be interrupted, interventions like the collaborative assessment and management of suicidality (CAMS) or dialectical behavior therapy may be helpful prior to, or concurrent with, the start of CPT to assist with stabilization, although this has never been directly examined in a CPT trial (Harned, Korslund, Foa, & Linehan, 2012; Jobes et al., 2017; van Minnen, Harned, Zoellner, & Mills, 2012). It is also helpful to examine how PTSD symptoms may fit in with these behaviors. In many cases, treating PTSD is an efficacious way of reducing suicidal ideation, as long as the client can engage in CPT (Gradus et al., 2013).

For substance use, individuals were included in earlier CPT research trials if they met criteria for mild to moderate substance abuse disorders (i.e., the fourth edition of the *Diagnostic and Statistical Manual of Mental Disorders* [DSM-IV]; American Psychiatric Association, 1994) and if they agreed to not use before, during, or after homework assignments or sessions. Individuals were excluded on the basis of severe substance use disorders (DSM-IV dependence). This exclusion criterion was established due to unexplored concerns about CPT leading to increased risk of substance relapse. However, more recent research has failed to demonstrate that trauma-focused therapies lead to substance relapse more than substance-use-focused therapies or relaxation treatment (Killeen et al., 2008; Roberts, Roberts, Jones, & Bisson, 2015; Simpson, Lehavot, & Petrakis, 2017). Moreover, unremitted PTSD increases the risk of substance use relapse (Ouimette, Coolhart, Funderburk, Wade, & Brown, 2007; Ouimette, Moos, & Finney, 2003; Read, Brown, & Kahler, 2004). Recent studies have only excluded individuals who were in need of current detoxification procedures, and typically, these individuals start the studies right after detoxification is complete (Resick, Monson, & Chard, 2017). Thus, the decision for the clinician is whether CPT is more likely to lead to harm than just treating the substance use alone or engaging in concurrent treatment. Similar to safety-related behaviors, factors such as the recency, frequency, quantity, and severity of use; chronicity; and the length of time the client has been able to maintain sobriety must be considered. Some clinicians may not be comfortable assessing substance use, although there are brief screening measures that may be helpful in this regard (Hays, Merz, & Nicholas, 1995; Tiet, Finney, & Moos, 2008). In addition, it is critical to assess whether the client has physiological dependence, as acute withdrawal from some substances such as alcohol can require medical attention. During treatment, it is important that clinicians monitor quantity and frequency of use during treatment and monitor urges to use. It is not yet known to what extent substance use over the course of CPT may impact clinical outcomes. Thus, prior to starting CPT, it can be helpful to create a contract around use and set up guidelines for how much and when the patient is using substances. For example, it is common to establish limits making clear that clients will not be seen if they are intoxicated or high. Clinicians may also wish to set up guidelines requiring clients to limit their use before or after practice completion, or to use CPT cognitive skills prior to deciding to use. Some of these limits may also depend on where a client is in terms of his or her own substance use treatment goals and the severity of current use and presence/absence of a substance use disorder.

A common concern for clinicians is what to do with clients when the traumatic event occurred long ago or whether CPT is appropriate for clients who have extensive trauma histories, especially with chronic traumatic events. Despite these concerns, the evidence suggests that CPT appears to work well even with clients having extensive and complex trauma histories. There may be challenges with selecting an index trauma. However, empirical evidence indicates that multiple trauma exposures or a history of childhood trauma does not appear to interfere with CPT treatment outcomes (Chard, 2005).

In terms of other factors that might influence the delivery of CPT, such as issues surrounding literacy, or working with clients who have experienced a TBI, clients with physical disabilities that may interfere with writing or reading, or clients with learning disabilities, CPT is still possible to implement, but may require some modifications. Modifications can include using simplified worksheets or worksheets formatted in ways that make them easier for clients to complete (i.e., a more linear presentation of material, simplified language, larger text). Clients who cannot write can voice-record their responses. In international contexts with very low levels of literacy, CPT materials have been simplified and clients have even memorized the materials. The key point is that there still will be regular practice working on the core skills of CPT: cognitive processing, identification of stuck points and maladaptive emotions, learning to challenge those stuck points, and moving toward creation of more balanced beliefs.

Trials in low-resource settings have, by necessity, utilized pioneering and less traditional rigorous methodology to achieve study aims in challenging circumstances (such as lack of normed instruments available in local languages, lack of trained mental health professionals for assessments or treatment delivery, armed conflict) and locales (such as lack of electricity, Internet access and technical support, physical infrastructure). The challenges to conducting an RCT in the Democratic Republic of Congo, for example, include working with study assessors and therapists with minimal training in mental health, which necessitates increasing training time, removing jargon from the treatment manual and training materials, training in the provision of clinical supervision, conducting training sessions using more hands-on practice, and providing more training in basic psychotherapy or assessment skills. Additional challenges working in the Democratic Republic of Congo and in Northern and Southern Iraq include delivering the therapy and assessments, and training, in multiple languages; creating materials to help promote basic buy-in around talk therapy; managing extensive travel distances for clients, providers, and supervisors given poor structural infrastructure; and addressing the delivery of a trauma-focused therapy in an active conflict setting where, in some cases, supervisors are not able to travel to sites to observe sessions and clients and counselors may need to sleep outside their homes due to concerns about safety in their communities.

Common Pitfalls in CPT Delivery

Throughout the course of CPT, one of the common pitfalls in delivery occurs when therapists themselves avoid or when they reinforce client avoidance. Therapist avoidance can manifest itself in adding extra sessions prior to starting CPT without a strong clinical rationale. It can also manifest itself as repeating sessions during the early and middle phases of CPT, either out of a concern that the client "masters" the skill or in response to incomplete practice. At times, therapist avoidance may be prompted by a therapist's own stuck points about the treatment process (i.e., "I'll make them worse," "My client won't be able to tolerate this," or "I am hurting my client"). It is extremely helpful when good supervision or peer consultation is available, both to identify therapist avoidance and to challenge therapist stuck points.

Therapists reinforcing client avoidance can happen in a variety of ways. For example, therapists may try to reassure clients with regard to out-of-session practice noncompliance ("That's OK that you did not do the assignment"), may fail to reassign practice assignments as recommended in the manual, or may avoid talking about the index trauma or asking for details about it. They may inadvertently shut down emotions rather than letting a client sit with his or her natural emotions or they may allow the client to avoid talking about the traumatic events during the session.

Therapists also may fail to notice and respond appropriately to client-level avoidance, inadvertently reinforcing these behaviors. As client avoidance is conceptualized in CPT as any behavior that serves to escape trauma-related cues, emotions, and reminders, it can manifest in multiple ways and can, at times, be difficult to identify. In general, with avoidance behavior in CPT, the optimal response is to identify the behavior, motivate the client to make a change (i.e., not avoiding), and address stuck points around the avoidance. With regard to practice noncompliance, this would include completing the assignment in session, followed by reassignment of the missed practice and assignment of the new practice.

Another common pitfall in CPT is the failure to identify and address assimilation-related stuck points, especially in the early sessions (Sessions 2–5). Often overaccommodation stuck points are easier for clinicians and clients to hear and identify. For clients, these frequently are easier beliefs to discuss, because they are more distal from the traumatic event itself. Assimilation stuck points such as those reflecting self-blame, undoing, and hindsight bias may be more subtle. Also, as these stuck points may be linked to intense emotions about the event itself, they may contribute more to client-related avoidance. However, the failure to address and challenge these assimilated stuck points is likely to leave PTSD symptoms untouched and also makes it more difficult to gain traction on the overaccommodated stuck points.

Another challenge in CPT can be helping the client pick the "index trauma." An index trauma in CPT refers to the trauma that the client defines as his or her most traumatic event. For some clients, identifying a "most distressing traumatic event" can be a challenge, especially for clients with more extensive trauma histories. To determine the index trauma, it can be helpful to question which trauma is interfering with a client's functioning the most and/or which one is most associated with PTSD symptoms (e.g., "Which one do you want to avoid talking about the most?" "Which event shows up more than others in intrusive memories or nightmares?"). At times, clinicians may recognize the need to focus on a different traumatic event, either because the client did not disclose the most distressing trauma in Session 1 or because, as symptoms from the initial trauma resolved, it became clear that another traumatic event was actually fueling symptoms and stuck points. In these cases, it is important to include the new traumatic event and continue working on relevant stuck points. It is acceptable in CPT to work on stuck points from multiple traumatic events.

Over and above all the pitfalls mentioned, the biggest area where CPT therapists struggle is in the execution of Socratic dialogue. Socratic dialogue is the bedrock of CPT and is the art of asking curious questions to guide new learning. This includes learning how to identify what we are saying to ourselves, to question the accuracy of those beliefs, and to generate new, more balanced thoughts. Therapists may be tempted to tell clients the answer or to assume that they already know what the answer is. At times, it can even seem more expedient to try to jump ahead in the process, rather than to pursue questions as a way of guiding the therapeutic process. However, what is most important in guiding change is the process of discovery for the client and the ability to learn to make these discoveries on one's own that tends to enhance perceived self-efficacy and to create new learning. In addition, in other therapies, when changed beliefs are uttered by the client rather than the therapist, they are more predictive of behavioral change (Amrhein, Miller, Yahne, Palmer, & Fulcher, 2003; Moyers et al., 2007), although this has not been tested in CPT directly. The process of Socratic dialogue should be one that is collaborative and warm; this creates a safe environment within which to look, together, at some of the most difficult parts of the traumatic event. As such, if the therapist finds that he or she is trying to win an argument or to convince the client of a certain perspective or point of view, then the therapist has exited the realm of Socratic dialogue. Defensiveness on the part of the client is conceptualized as a behavioral indicator that the therapist is too change-oriented or has moved out of Socratic dialogue and should return to a mode of curious exploration.

Training and Support in the Delivery of CPT

For therapists who are not trained in CBT, delivery of manualized treatments, or cognitive interventions, moving to CPT treatment delivery may represent a shift and they may need more training and consultation in making those changes. There are online trainings in CPT (*https://cpt.musc.edu* or *https://*

deploymentpsych.org/online-courses/cpt) that can help interested providers gain a foundation in core CPT skills prior to training, or strengthen their skills after attending a training session. Attending an in-person CPT workshop is strongly recommended and required to become an approved CPT provider, and to gain a better sense of how to deliver the treatment with fidelity. These trainings involve didactic content, role plays, and video of the therapy being conducted with various types of clients. This is also a helpful medium within which to see how different therapists maintain their voice as clinicians while still delivering CPT that is true to the model. Following attendance at a CPT workshop, it is recommended that clinicians attend supervision or case consultation with an approved CPT trainer/consultant. The type of case oversight depends on the clinicians' setting and whether experienced CPT clinicians are on-site; it also depends on the therapists' prior level of related training and expertise. The current recommendation is that a therapist complete 20 group consultation sessions or complete 7.5 hours of individual supervision to become an approved CPT provider. It is also recommended that they start at least four cases or two groups, so they can complete at least two individual cases or two groups. This is to ensure they experience enough of the therapy while they have the support of consultation or supervision. This allows for a place to discuss issues, such as those touched on in this chapter: who is an appropriate client for CPT, how to deliver CPT with fidelity to real-world clients, and what to do when one encounters challenges along the road.

Future Developments

Although the efficacy and effectiveness research that has accumulated on CPT is compelling, there is room for further developments to ultimately improve the health and well-being of those with PTSD. While a great majority of clients receiving CPT show dramatic improvement in their symptoms, we know that some clients have little to no improvement in their symptoms during CPT. There is little consistent data across studies predicting who does not do as well in CPT based on client variables, but two common themes that have emerged are lack of therapist fidelity to the protocol and problems with homework compliance (Farmer et al., 2017; Wiltsey Stirman et al., 2018). Currently, the CPT manual recommends that avoidance and lack of homework completion be addressed very early in treatment through brainstorming about types of avoidance that may emerge and completing A-B-C sheets in session on the thoughts that may be reinforcing the avoidance behavior. If the client continues to be largely noncompliant, the CPT manual recommends considering termination around Sessions 5 and 6 as there is little evidence to suggest that the client will get better when not actively participating in all aspects of the treatment protocol. In other situations, the client may be compliant with the therapy, but still show minimal improvement in his or her PCL assessment scores. This may be the result of an undiscussed trauma that needs to be identified with its resulting stuck points, but the lack of improvement can also be caused by internal or external factors that motivate the client to remain symptomatic. We encourage the therapist to help the client identify the reasons why and, when possible, look for the stuck points that may be inhibiting change. If a client continues to show minimal improvement in CPT, it may become necessary to discuss available alternative treatment strategies that the client might find more effective. Future studies are examining which of the evidence-based treatments are more effective for which type of client, and this may help to improve client outcomes in the future (Schnurr et al., 2015).

With research showing that various components of CPT work (Resick et al., 2008), the next generation of CPT research should aim to determine treatment matching based on client characteristics, their social milieu, and treatment context. Relatively few client characteristics have been elucidated predicting treatment response to CPT. One factor found to predict a differential response to different versions of CPT is level of dissociation, with those higher in dissociation responding better to CPT + A versus CPT or written accounts only (Resick, Suvak, Johnides, Mitchell, & Iverson, 2012). Galovski and colleagues' (2012) CPT variable-length study revealed that those with more depressive symptoms required more sessions of CPT. Increasing client age (Rizvi, Vogt, & Resick, 2009), lower social functioning (Lord et al., 2019), and higher levels of anger (Lloyd et al., 2014) have also been found to predict poorer outcomes. Most of these factors have only been found in single studies and in certain samples, and thus require replication. More studies testing potential treatment moderators will help provide guidance to clinicians and their patients with regard to the best match and dose of treatment for a given client. In the meantime, client preference for treatment has been found to predict PTSD treatment outcomes in the broader PTSD field (Zoellner, Roy-Byrne, Mavissakalian, & Feeny, 2018) and should guide selection of the version of CPT delivered. Moreover, there are certain low-resource contexts in which different components of CPT might be offered. Although more research on CPT and CPT + A is ongoing, it is important to remember that the written-accounts-only version was not significantly different from the other conditions at posttreatment and follow-up in the one dismantling trial with female interpersonal violence victims conducted to date (Resick et al., 2008). Future research on this treatment component may help facilitate access to treatment in certain contexts with few clinicians or limited training.

The next generation of CPT research will extend to address other essential health care delivery questions and adjunctive interventions to optimize CPT outcomes. As reviewed previously, there have been creative efforts to address such questions, including the examination of CPT dosing, delivery via video technology, delivery in low-resource areas, and delivery in residential settings. Efforts are afoot to test the massed dosing of CPT (i.e., sequential days of delivery; Wachen, 2019) and via therapist-assisted online delivery (Monson, Fitzpatrick, & Wagner, 2017) to facilitate more efficient outcomes and access to treatment, respectively. With regard to optimizing CPT with adjunctive interventions, there is at least one study beginning to test the addition of 3,4-methylenedioxy-methamphetamine (MDMA; Wagner & Monson, 2018) to potentiate the effects of CPT, especially in cases of refractory PTSD.

Another avenue of potential research is how much CPT might be simplified or "degraded" and still maintain its efficacy. This is a natural extension of determining the active ingredients of CPT from the essential ones. As concrete examples: Do clients need to learn both challenging questions and patterns of problematic thinking? Would a focus on altering assimilated thoughts only yield the same outcomes? Are the behavioral assignments in Sessions 10 and 11 essential? Do clients need to progress through a series of worksheets designed to challenge cognitions? This vein of research aimed at developing as parsimonious a treatment as possible has important implications to client uptake, retention, ease of delivery, and training clinicians in CPT.

Related to training clinicians in CPT, there is room to improve access to CPT by understanding the best methods to train clinicians in the model. Monson and colleagues (2018) found significantly better patient engagement and symptom outcomes when clinicians learning the therapy received expert postworkshop consultation in the model. More implementation research needs to be conducted to determine not only how to bring clinicians up to fidelity in CPT, but also how to sustain such practices over time and with efficient use of resources. On the latter point, some health care settings with PTSD clients most in need do not have the resources to train clinicians or experience significant staff turnover, making travel to in-person workshops offered at set times a barrier to learning and delivering CPT. Implementation studies that assess the noninferiority of other methods to train clinicians (e.g., on-demand online workshop training) and determine fidelity to the treatment (e.g., self-assessment) are needed to identify the most efficient methods in clinician training.

In summary, the past 25 years have yielded a significant number of RCTs and clinical effectiveness studies that not only demonstrate the efficacy of CPT in creating lasting changes in PTSD symptoms, but also show how effective CPT is in treating a broad spectrum of comorbid conditions that are often considered complex presentations by clinicians. Studies have borne out the utility of CPT's various forms (e.g., with and without accounts, modified worksheets) and flexible treatment options (e.g., group, individual, combined) in helping clients suffering from the aftermath of a variety of traumatic events in many parts of the world. We anticipate that current and future research efforts will lead to further refinement of CPT, which ultimately will translate to better outcomes for our clients.

REFERENCES

Ahrens, J., & Rexford, L. (2002). Cognitive processing therapy for incarcerated adolescents with PTSD. *Journal of Aggression, Maltreatment and Trauma, 6*, 201–221.

American Psychiatric Association. (1994). *Diagnostic and statistical manual of mental disorders* (4th ed.). Washington, DC: Author.

Amrhein, P. C., Miller, W. R., Yahne, C. E., Palmer, M., & Fulcher, L. (2003). Client commitment language during motivational interviewing predicts drug use outcomes. *Journal of Consulting and Clinical Psychology, 71*, 862–876.

Bass, J. K., Annan, J., McIvor Murray, S., Kaysen, D., Griffiths, S., Cetinoglu, T., et al. (2013). Controlled trial of psychotherapy for Congolese survivors of sexual violence. *New England Journal of Medicine, 368*(23), 2182–2191.

Beck, A. T., Rush, A. J., Shaw, B. F., & Emery, G. (1979). *Cognitive therapy of depression.* New York: Guilford Press.

Blevins, C. A., Weathers, F. W., Davis, M. T., Witte, T. K., & Domino, J. L. (2015). The posttraumatic stress disorder checklist for DSM-5 (PCL-5): Development and initial psychometric evaluation. *Journal of Traumatic Stress, 28*, 489–498.

Bolton, P., Bass, J. K., Zangana, G. A. S., Kamal, T., Murray, S. M., Kaysen, D., et al. (2014). A randomized controlled trial of mental health interventions for survivors of systematic violence in Kurdistan, Northern Iraq. *BMC Psychiatry, 14*(1), 360.

Brewin, C. R. (2001). A cognitive neuroscience account of posttraumatic stress disorder and its treatment. *Behaviour Research and Therapy, 39*, 373–393.

Bryan, C. J., Leifker, F. R., Rozek, D. C., Bryan, A. O., Reynolds, M. L., Oakey, D. N., et al. (2018). Examining the effectiveness of an intensive, 2 week treatment program for military personnel and veterans with PTSD: Results of a pilot, open-label, prospective cohort trial. *Journal of Clinical Psychology, 74*, 2070–2081.

Butollo, W., Karl, R., Konig, J., & Rosner, R. (2016). A randomized controlled clinical trial of dialogical exposure therapy versus cognitive processing therapy for adult outpatients suffering from PTSD after type I trauma in adulthood. *Psychotherapy Psychosomatics, 85*, 16–26.

Chard, K. M. (2005). An evaluation of cognitive processing therapy for the treatment of posttraumatic stress disorder related to childhood sexual abuse. *Journal of Consulting and Clinical Psychology, 73*(5), 965–971.

Chard, K. M., Ricksecker, E. G., Healy, E. T., Karlin, B. E., & Resick, P. A. (2012). Dissemination and experience with cognitive processing therapy. *Journal of Rehabilitation Research and Development, 49*, 667–678.

Chard, K. M., Schumm, J. A., McIlvain, S. M., Bailey, G. W., & Parkinson, R. B. (2011). Exploring the efficacy of a residential treatment program incorporating cognitive processing therapy-cognitive for veterans with PTSD and traumatic brain injury. *Journal of Traumatic Stress, 24*(3), 347–351.

Clarke, S. B., Rizvi, S. L., & Resick, P. A. (2008). Borderline personality characteristics and treatment outcome in cognitive-behavioral treatments for PTSD in female rape victims. *Behavior Therapy, 39*(1), 72–78.

Dickstein, B. D., Walter, K. H., Schumm, J. A., & Chard, K. M. (2013). Comparing response to cognitive processing therapy in military veterans with subthreshold and threshold posttraumatic stress disorder. *Journal of Traumatic Stress, 26*, 1–7.

Ehlers, A., & Clark, D. M. (2000). A cognitive model of posttraumatic stress disorder. *Behaviour Research and Therapy, 38*, 319–345.

Farmer, C. C., Mitchell, K. S., Parker-Guilbert, K., & Galovski, T. E. (2017). Fidelity to the cognitive processing therapy protocol: Evaluation of critical elements. *Behavior Therapy, 48*(2), 195–206.

Feingold, Z. R., Fox-Galalis, A. B., & Galovski, T. E. (2018). Effectiveness of evidence-based psychotherapy for posttraumatic distress within a jail diversion program. *Psychological Services, 15*(4), 409.

Foa, E. B., Hembree, E. A., & Rothbaum, B. O. (2007). *Prolonged exposure therapy for PTSD: Emotional processing of traumatic experiences.* London: Oxford University Press.

Foa, E. B., Steketee, G., & Rothbaum, B. O. (1989). Behavioral/cognitive conceptualizations of post-traumatic stress disorder. *Behavior Therapy, 20,* 155–176.

Forbes, D., Lloyd, D., Nixon, R. D., Elliott, P., Varker, T., Perry, D., et al. (2012). A multisite randomized controlled effectiveness trial of cognitive processing therapy for military-related posttraumatic stress disorder. *Journal of Anxiety Disorders, 26*(3), 442–452.

Galovski, T. E., Blain, L. M., Mott, J. M., Elwood, L., & Houle, T. (2012). Manualized therapy for PTSD: Flexing the structure of cognitive processing therapy. *Journal of Consulting and Clinical Psychology, 80,* 968–981.

Galovski, T. E., Harik, J. M., Blain, L. M., Elwood, L., Gloth, C., & Fletcher, T. D. (2016). Augmenting cognitive processing therapy to improve sleep impairment in PTSD: A randomized controlled trial. *Journal of Consulting and Clinical Psychology, 84,* 167–177.

Galovski, T. E., Monson, C., Bruce, S. E., & Resick, P. A. (2009). Does cognitive-behavioral therapy for PTSD improve perceived health and sleep impairment? *Journal of Traumatic Stress, 22*(3), 197–204.

Galovski, T. E., Sobel, A. A., Phipps, K. A., & Resick, P. A. (2005). Trauma recovery: Beyond posttraumatic stress disorder and other axis I symptom severity. In T. A. Corales (Ed.), *Trends in posttraumatic stress disorder research* (pp. 207–227). Hauppauge, NY: Nova Science.

Gradus, J. L., Suvak, M. K., Wisco, B. E., Marx, B. P., & Resick, P. A. (2013). Treatment of posttraumatic stress disorder reduces suicidal ideation. *Depression and Anxiety, 30*(10), 1046–1053.

Griffin, M. G., Resick, P. A., & Galovski, T. E. (2012). Does physiologic response to loud tones change following cognitive–behavioral treatment for posttraumatic stress disorder? *Journal of Traumatic Stress, 25*(1), 25–32.

Gutner, C. A., Suvak, M., Sloan, D. M., & Resick, P. A. (2016). Does timing matter?: Examining the impact of session timing on outcome. *Journal of Consulting and Clinical Psychology, 84*(12).

Harned, M. S., Korslund, K. E., Foa, E. B., & Linehan, M. M. (2012). Treating PTSD in suicidal and self-injuring women with borderline personality disorder: Development and preliminary evaluation of a dialectical behavior therapy prolonged exposure protocol. *Behaviour Research Therapy, 50,* 381–386.

Hays, R. D., Merz, J. F., & Nicholas, R. (1995). Response burden, reliability, and validity of the CAGE, Short MAST, and AUDIT alcohol screening measures. *Behavior Research Methods, Instruments, and Computers, 27,* 277–280.

Hoge, C. W., McGurk, D., Thomas, J. L., Cox, A. L., Engel, C. C., & Castro, C. A. (2008). Mild traumatic brain injury in US soldiers returning from Iraq. *New England Journal of Medicine, 358*(5), 453–463.

Inhelder, B., & Piaget, J. (1958). *The growth of logical thinking from childhood to adolescence: An essay on the construction of formal operational structures.* London: Routledge.

International Society for Traumatic Stress Studies. (2018). *ISTSS PTSD guidelines: Methodology and recommendations.* Chicago: Author.

Jak, A. J., Jurick, A., Crocker, L. D., Sanderson-Cimino, M., Aupperle, R., Rodgers, C. S., et al. (2019). SMART-CPT for veterans with comorbid posttraumatic stress disorder and history of traumatic brain injury: A randomized controlled trial. *Journal of Neurology, Neurosurgery, and Psychiatry, 90*(3), 333–341.

Jobes, D. A., Comtois, K. A., Gutierrez, P. M., Brenner, L. A., Huh, D., Chalker, G., et al. (2017). A randomized controlled trial of the collaborative assessment and management of suicidality versus enhanced care as usual with suicidal soldiers. *Psychiatry, 80,* 339–356.

Kaysen, D., Schumm, J., Pedersen, E. R., Seim, R. W., Bedard-Gilligan, M., & Chard, K. (2014). Cognitive processing therapy for veterans with comorbid PTSD and alcohol use disorders. *Addictive Behaviors, 39,* 420–427.

Killeen, T., Hien, D., Campbell, A., Brown, C., Hansen, C., & Jiang, H. (2008). Adverse events in an integrated trauma-focused intervention for women in community substance abuse treatment. *Journal of Substance Abuse Treatment, 35,* 304–311.

Kozel, F. A., Motes, M. A., Didehbani, N., DeLaRosa, B., Bass, C., Schraufnagel, C. D., et al. (2018). Repetitive TMS to augment cognitive processing therapy in combat veterans of recent conflicts with PTSD: A randomized clinical trial. *Journal of Affective Disorders, 229,* 506–514.

Lang, P. J. (1977). Imagery in therapy: An information processing analysis of fear. *Behavior Therapy, 8,* 862–886.

Lester, K., Artz, C., Resick, P. A., & Young-Xu, Y. (2010). Impact of race on early treatment termination and outcomes in posttraumatic stress disorder treatment. *Journal of Consulting and Clinical Psychology, 78*(4), 480.

Lloyd, D., Couineau, A. L., Hawkins, K., Kartal, D., Nixon, R., Perry, D., et al. (2015). Preliminary outcomes of implementing cognitive processing therapy for posttraumatic stress disorder across a national veterans' treatment service. *Journal of Clinical Psychiatry, 76*(11), e1405–e1409.

Lloyd, D., Nixon, R., Varker, T., Elliott, P., Perry, D., Bryant, R. A., et al. (2014). Comorbidity in the prediction of cognitive processing therapy treatment outcomes for combat-related posttraumatic stress disorder. *Journal of Anxiety Disorders, 28,* 237–240.

Lord, K. A., Suvak, M. K., Holmes, S., Shields, N., Lane, J., Sijercic, I., et al. (2019). Bidirectional relationships between posttraumatic stress disorder and social functioning during cognitive processing therapy. *Behavior Therapy.* [Epub ahead of print]

Maieritsch, K. P., Smith, T. L., Hessinger, J. D., Ahearn, E. P., Eickhoff, J. C., & Zhao, Q. (2016). Randomized controlled equivalence trial comparing videoconference and in person delivery of cognitive processing therapy for PTSD. *Journal of Telemedicine and Telecare, 22,* 238–243.

Marques, L., Eustis, E. H., Dixon, L., Valentine, S. E., Borba, C. P., Simon, N., et al. (2016). Delivering cognitive processing therapy in a community health setting: The influence of Latino culture and community violence on posttraumatic cognitions. *Psychological Trauma: Theory, Research, Practice, and Policy, 8*(1), 98.

Mesa, F., Dickstein, B. D., Wooten, V. D., & Chard, K. M. (2017). Response to cognitive processing therapy in veterans with and without obstructive sleep apnea. *Journal of Traumatic Stress, 30*(6), 646–655.

Monson, C. M., Fitzpatrick, S., & Wagner, A. (2017). *Therapist-assisted cognitive therapy for posttraumatic stress disorder.* Toronto, ON: Beacon Digital Therapy.

Monson, C. M., Macdonald, A., Vorstenbosch, V., Shnaider, P., Goldstein, E., Ferrier-Auerbach, A. G., et al. (2012). Changes in social adjustement with cognitive processing therapy: Effects of treatment and association with PTSD symptom change. *Journal of Traumatic Stress, 25,* 519–526.

Monson, C. M., Schnurr, P. P., Resick, P. A., Friedman, M. J., Young-Xu, Y., & Stevens, S. P. (2006). Cognitive processing therapy for veterans with military-related posttraumatic stress disorder. *Journal of Consulting and Clinical Psychology, 74*(5), 898–907.

Monson, C. M., Shields, N., Suvak, M. K., Lane, J. E., Shnaider, P., Landy, M., et al. (2018). A randomized controlled effectiveness trial of training strategies in cognitive processing therapy for posttraumatic stress disorder: Impact on patient outcomes. *Behaviour Research and Therapy, 110,* 31–40.

Morland, L. A., Mackintosh, M. A., Greene, C. J., Rosen, C., Chard, K., Resick, P., et al. (2014). Cognitive processing therapy for posttraumatic stress disorder delivered to rural veterans via telemental health: A randomized noninferiority clinical trial. *Journal of Clinical Psychiatry, 75*(5), 470–476.

Morland, L. A., Mackintosh, M., Rosen, C. S., Willis, E., Resick, P., Chard, K., et al. (2015). Telemedicine versus in-person delivery of cognitive processing therapy for women with posttraumatic stress disorder: A randomized non-inferiority trial. *Depression and Anxiety, 32*(11), 811–820.

Moyers, T. B., Martin, T., Christopher, P. J., Houck, J. M., Tonigan, S. J., & Amrhein, P. C. (2007). Client language as a mediator of motivational interviewing efficacy: Where is the evidence? *Alcoholism: Clinical and Experimental Research, 31,* 40–47.

Nixon, R. D. (2012). Cognitive processing therapy versus supportive counseling for acute stress disorder following assault: A randomized pilot trial. *Behavior Therapy, 43*(4), 825–836.

Ouimette, P., Coolhart, D., Funderburk, J. S., Wade, M., & Brown, P. J. (2007). Precipitants of first substance use in recently abstinent substance use disorder patients with PTSD. *Addiction Behavior, 32,* 1719–1727.

Ouimette, P., Moos, R. H., & Finney, J. W. (2003). PTSD treatment and 5-year remission among patients with substance use and posttraumatic stress disorders. *Journal of Consulting and Clinical Psychology, 71,* 410–414.

Pearson, C. R., Kaysen, D., Huh, D., & Bedard-Gilligan, M. (2019). Randomized control trial of culturally adapted cognitive processing therapy for PTSD substance misuse and HIV sexual risk behavior for Native American women. *AIDS and Behavior, 23*(3), 695–706.

Read, J. P., Brown, P. J., & Kahler, C. W. (2004). Substance use and posttraumatic stress disorders: Symptom interplay and effects on outcome. *Addiction Behavior, 29,* 1665–1672.

Resick, P. A., Galovski, T. E., Uhlmansiek, M. O., Scher, C. D., Clum, G. A., & Young-Xu, Y. (2008). A randomized clinical trial to dismantle components of cognitive processing therapy for posttraumatic stress disorder in female victims of interpersonal violence. *Journal of Consulting and Clinical Psychology, 76,* 243–258.

Resick, P. A., Monson, C. M., & Chard, K. M. (2014). *Cognitive processing therapy:*

Veteran/military version: Therapist's manual. Washington, DC: Department of Veterans Affairs.

Resick, P. A., Monson, C. M., & Chard, K. M. (2017). *Cognitive processing therapy for PTSD: A comprehensive manual.* New York: Guilford Press.

Resick, P. A., Nishith, P., Weaver, T. L., Astin, M. C., & Feuer, C. A. (2002). A comparison of cognitive processing therapy, prolonged exposure and a waiting condition for the treatment of posttraumatic stress disorder in female rape victims. *Journal of Consulting and Clinical Psychology, 70,* 867–879.

Resick, P. A., & Schnicke, M. K. (1993). *Cognitive processing therapy for rape victims: A treatment manual.* Newbury Park, CA: SAGE.

Resick, P. A., Suvak, M. K., Johnides, B. D., Mitchell, K. S., & Iverson, K. M. (2012). The impact of dissociation on PTSD treatment with cognitive processing therapy. *Depression and Anxiety, 29,* 718–730.

Resick, P. A., Wachen, J. S., Dondanville, K. A., Pruiksma, K. E., Yarvis, J. S., Peterson, A. L. et al. (2017). Effect of group versus individual cognitive processing therapy in active-duty military seeking treatment for posttraumatic stress disorder: A randomized clinical trial. *JAMA Psychiatry, 74,* 28–36.

Resick, P. A., Wachen, J. S., Mintz, J., Young-McCaughan, S., Roache, J. D., Borah, A. M., et al. (2015). A randomized clinical trial of group cognitive processing therapy compared with group present-centered therapy for PTSD among active duty military personnel. *Journal of Consulting and Clinical Psychology, 83,* 1058–1068.

Resick, P. A., Williams, L. F., Suvak, M. K., Monson, C. M., & Gradus, J. L. (2012). Long-term outcomes of cognitive–behavioral treatments for posttraumatic stress disorder among female rape survivors. *Journal of Consulting and Clinical Psychology, 80*(2), 201–210.

Rizvi, S. L., Vogt, D. S., & Resick, P. A. (2009). Cognitive and affective predictors of treatment outcome in cognitive processing therapy and prolonged exposure for posttraumatic stress disorder. *Behaviour Research and Therapy, 47,* 737–743.

Roberts, N. P., Roberts, P. A., Jones, N., & Bisson, J. I. (2015). Psychological interventions for post-traumatic stress disorder and comorbid substance use disorder: A systematic review and meta-analysis. *Clinical Pyschology Review, 38,* 25–38.

Schnurr, P. P., Chard, K. M., Ruzek, J. I., Chow, B. K., Shih, M., Resick, P. A., et al. (2015). Design of a VA cooperative study #591: CERV-PTSD, comparative effectiveness research in veterans with PTSD. *Contemporary Clinical Trials, 41,* 75–84.

Schulz, P. M., Resick, P. A., Huber, L. C., & Griffin, M. G. (2006). The effectiveness of cognitive processing therapy for PTSD with refugees in a community setting. *Cognitive and Behavioral Practice, 13*(4), 322–331.

Simpson, T. L., Lehavot, K., & Petrakis, I. L. (2017). No wrong doors: Findings from a critical review of behavioral randomized clinical trails for individuals with co-occurring alcohol/drug problems and posttraumatic stress disorder. *Alcoholism: Clinical and Experimental Research, 41,* 681–702.

Sloan, D. M., Marx, B. P., Lee, D. J., & Resick, P. A. (2018). A brief exposure-based treatment vs cognitive processing therapy for posttraumatic stress disorder: A randomized noninferiority clinical trial. *JAMA Psychiatry, 75*(3), 233–239.

Speicher, S. M., Walter, K. H., & Chard, K. M. (2014). Interdisciplinary residential treatment of posttraumatic stress disorder and traumatic brain injury: Effects on symptom severity and occupational performance and satisfaction. *American Journal of Occupational Therapy, 68*(4), 412–421.

Steenkamp, M. M., Litz, B. T., Hoge, C. W., & Marmar, C. R. (2015). Psychotherapy for military-related PTSD: A review of randomized clinical trials. *Journal of the American Medical Association, 314,* 489–500.

Suris, A., Link-Malcolm, J., Chard, K., Ahn, C., & North, C. (2013). A randomized clinical trial of cognitive processing therapy for veterans with PTSD related to military sexual trauma. *Journal of Traumatic Stress, 26*(1), 28–37.

Tiet, Q. Q., Finney, J. W., & Moos, R. H. (2008). Screening psychiatric patients for illicit drug use disorders and problems. *Clinical Psychology Review, 28*(4), 578–591.

Valentine, S. E., Borba, C. P., Dixon, L., Vaewsorn, A. S., Guajardo, J. G., Resick, P. A., et al. (2017). Cognitive processing therapy for Spanish-speaking Latinos: A formative study of a model-driven cultural adaptation of the manual to enhance implementation in a usual care setting. *Journal of Clinical Psychology, 73*(3), 239–256.

van Minnen, A., Harned, M. S., Zoellner, L., & Mills, K. (2012). Examining the potential contraindications for prolonged exposure therapy for PTSD. *European Journal of Psychotraumatology, 3.*

Wachen, J. (2019). *Massed cognitive processing therapy for combat-related PTSD.* Washington, DC: National Institutes of Health, U.S. National Library of Medicine. Retrieved from *https://clinicaltrials.gov/ct2/show/NCT03808727.*

Wagner, A., & Monson, C. M. (2018). *An initial test of MDMA-facilitated cognitive processing therapy for posttraumatic stress disorder.* Study funded by the Multidisciplinary Association for Psychedelic Studies.

Walter, K. H., Bolte, T. A., Owens, G. P., & Chard, K. M. (2012). The impact of personality disorders on treatment outcome for veterans in a posttraumatic stress disorder residential treatment program. *Cognitive Therapy and Research, 36*(5), 576–584.

Walter, K. H., Varkovitzky, R. L., Owens, G. P., Lewis, J., & Chard, K. M. (2014). Cognitive processing therapy for veterans with posttraumatic stress disorder: A cross-sectional and longitudinal comparison between outpatient and residential PTSD treatment. *Journal of Consulting and Clinical Psychology, 82,* 551–561.

Weiss, W. M., Murray, L. K., Zangana, G. A. S., Mahmooth, Z., Kaysen, D., Dorsey, S., et al. (2015). Community-based mental health treatments for survivors of torture and militant attacks in Southern Iraq: A randomized control trial. *BMC Psychiatry, 15*(1), 249–275.

Wells, S. Y., Glassman, L. H., Talkovsky, A. M., Chatfield, M. A., Sohn, M. J., Morland, L. A., et al. (2018). Examining changes in sexual functioning after cognitive processing therapy in a sample of women trauma survivors. *Women's Health Issues, 29,* 72–79.

Wiltsey Stirman, S., Gutner, C. A., Suvak, M. K., Adler, A., Calloway, A., & Resick, P. (2018). Homework completion, patient characteristics, and symptom change in cognitive processing therapy for PTSD. *Behavior Therapy, 49,* 741–755.

Zalta, A. K., Held, P., Smith, D. L., Klassen, B. J., Lofgreen, A. M., Normand, P., et al. (2018). Evaluating patterns and predictors of symptom change during a three-week intensive outpatient treatment for veterans with PTSD. *BMC Psychiatry, 18,* 242–245.

Zoellner, L. A., Roy-Byrne, P. P., Mavissakalian, M., & Feeny, N. C. (2018). Doubly randomized preference trial of prolonged exposure versus sertraline for treatment of PTSD. *American Journal of Psychiatry, 176,* 287–296.

CHAPTER 14

Eye Movement Desensitization and Reprocessing Therapy

Francine Shapiro, Mark C. Russell, Christopher Lee, and Sarah J. Schubert

Eye movement desensitization and reprocessing (EMDR) therapy is an integrative, client-centered psychotherapy (Shapiro, 1989, 2018) that emphasizes the brain's information-processing system and memories of disturbing events as the bases of psychopathology. EMDR therapy focuses on experiences contributing to both pathology and resilience. Randomized controlled trials (RCTs) have established the efficacy of EMDR therapy and resulted in its recognition as an evidence-based treatment (EBT) for posttraumatic stress disorder (PTSD). In this chapter, we review the theory underlying EMDR therapy and the evidence base supporting it. The practical aspects and challenges of implementing EMDR therapy in clinical practice are then discussed.

Theoretical Context

The adaptive information processing (AIP) model guides the therapeutic application of EMDR therapy (Shapiro, 2018). This model emphasizes that learning occurs as we assimilate new experiences into existing neurophysiological memory networks. Pathology arises when memories of negative life experiences are inadequately processed. Unprocessed memories are dysfunctionally stored and contain images, thoughts, emotions, and sensations

---

In memory of Francine Shapiro—a brilliant clinician with theoretical foresight, who dedicated her life to healing human suffering.

that were experienced at the time of the adverse event. When triggered, the unprocessed memories negatively influence perception, attitudes, and behavior in the present. Recovery from PTSD with EMDR therapy occurs through accessing dysfunctionally stored memories and the initiation of an accelerated learning state via focused processing that integrates them into adaptive memory networks. Understanding how memory processing occurs in EMDR therapy largely stems from research that has examined the eye movements (EMs) used during EMDR memory processing. Presently, more than 30 RCTs and a meta-analysis (Lee & Cuijpers, 2013) have demonstrated that the EMs in EMDR therapy significantly add to its beneficial treatment effects. Current explanations of mechanisms underlying EMDR therapy include theories related to working memory, the orienting response, and REM.

Working memory theory holds that components of working memory have limited capacity (Baddeley, 2012). In EMDR therapy, engaging in EMs or other dual-attention stimuli such as bilateral taps or tones while focusing on trauma-related memories simultaneously taxes working memory, impairing the ability to hold a visual image in awareness, which causes image quality to deteriorate and the memory to be integrated in a less vivid and therefore less emotional form (van den Hout et al., 2012). Orienting response theory posits that EMs or other dual-attention stimuli elicit an orienting response with associated decreases in physiological arousal (i.e., de-arousal) that aids memory processing (Landin-Romero et al., 2013). An orienting response is an autonomic, attentional reaction evoked by a new stimulus that is assessed for threat (Bradley, 2009). Repeated presentation of nonthreatening stimuli leads to the orienting response quickly habituating and to physiological de-arousal. Investigations of physiological correlates of the EMs in EMDR therapy demonstrate the presence of orienting responses (Schubert et al., 2016), de-arousal via increased parasympathetic tone during EM sets (Sack, Hofmann, Wizelman, & Lempa, 2008), and physiological changes characteristic of a REM-like state (Elofsson, von Scheele, Theorell, & Sondergaard, 2008). A third explanation of the underlying mechanism of EMDR therapy derives from REM research and posits that EMs induce slow wave sleep and REM-like neurobiological mechanisms, which facilitate integration and consolidation of episodic traumatic memories into semantic networks (Pagani et al., 2007; Stickgold, 2002).

A comprehensive understanding of EMDR therapy requires consideration of all three theories and how the mechanisms proposed may simultaneously contribute to the information processing seen in effective PTSD treatment. Currently, these mechanisms appear consistent with neurobiological theories of memory reconsolidation (Suzuki et al., 2004), which propose that a recalled memory is labile and can be linked to new and existing adaptive information and then restored in an altered form. Recent research has found that memory reconsolidation may be disrupted by a distractor stimulus presented during reactivation (Crestani et al., 2015).

In addition to theoretical accounts of how EMDR therapy processes memory, there is evidence from neurophysiological research suggesting that effective EMDR therapy results in repair of the structure and functioning of areas within the brain that facilitate information processing and memory integration (Landin-Romero et al., 2013). For example, after the effective EMDR treatment of patients diagnosed with PTSD, there have been reports of increased hippocampal volume (Bossini et al., 2017), left amygdala volumetric increase (Laugharne et al., 2016), increased prefrontal cortex gray matter (Boukezzi et al., 2017), and functional normalization in limbic structures implicated in PTSD (Lansing, Amen, Hanks, & Rudy, 2005; Oh & Choi, 2004; Pagani et al., 2007, 2012). Using functional magnetic resonance imaging (fMRI) techniques, EMDR therapy has been found to be associated with increased activity in the left hippocampus and left amygdala (Rousseau et al., 2019). Recent investigation into the neural circuits underlying EMDR therapy has demonstrated, through animal research, that alternate bilateral visual stimulation suppresses fear (Baek et al., 2019). Baek and colleagues (2019) found evidence that lasting fear reduction occurred via a neuronal pathway driven by the superior colliculus and supporting activity in the mediodorsal thalamus and prefrontal cortex to compete with emotional amygdala activity. This effect was not found for auditory or other types of visual stimulation. Overall, continued research is needed to fully understand the theory underlying EMDR therapy and the interrelationships among different psychological, physiological, and neurological mechanisms in EMDR treatment of PTSD.

Description of Techniques

EMDR therapy employs an eight-phase approach to address the full range of clinical symptoms caused or exacerbated by past adverse experiences. The phases include history taking; preparation; four reprocessing phases (assessment, desensitization, installation, body scan); closure; and reevaluation.

EMDR therapy emphasizes working with imagery, cognitions, emotions, somatic sensations, and behavior linked to the disturbing memory, as well as attending to past, current, and future-oriented experiential contributors. The following is an overview of the main goals and procedural objectives of the eight phases of EMDR therapy.

Phase I: Client History

Phase I comprises standard history taking, rapport building, and informed consent. The clinician obtains background information and determines client suitability for EMDR therapy. If treatment goals are PTSD symptom reduction, the clinician identifies *target memories* that are not only "Criterion A" trauma experiences related to emergence of the client's major diagnostic presentation (DSM-5; American Psychiatric Association, 2013), but also other associated memories of adverse life experiences that are hypothesized to be driving and maintaining current trauma and associated symptoms. Comprehensive EMDR treatment involves evaluation and remediation of the client's entire clinical picture, including emotional dysregulation, addressing fears, anxieties and avoidance, negative self-beliefs, problematic behaviors, and attachment issues (Shapiro, 2018). The clinician identifies current problems and uses direct questioning and several techniques (e.g., "floatback," also known as "affect bridge") to focus on current somatic and/or cognitive responses in order to associate them with and identify unprocessed memories that are the foundation of the symptoms. For example, in an affect bridge, the clinician instructs the client to "hold the experience in mind, notice the emotions you're having right now and notice what you're feeling in your body. Now let your mind scan back to an earlier time when you may have felt this way before and just notice what comes to mind."

Phase II: Client Preparation

The goal during this phase is to establish client readiness for EMDR therapy by enhancing client trust and rapport, describing the therapy procedures, explaining the theory, testing the eye movements or other type of bilateral stimulation (BLS), teaching affect regulation techniques such as the "safe/calm place," which links a positive emotional state to a word or image, or other methods for building affect tolerance and stability. An affect regulation technique utilized in EMDR therapy preparation is resource development and installation (RDI; Korn & Leeds, 2002). The aim is to identify and enhance the client's awareness of his or her strengths, qualities, and capacities, with the aim of increasing that individual's ability to cope with overwhelming specific daily situations and memory processing itself. For PTSD resulting from a single traumatic event, which research has demonstrated can be treated within three 90-minute sessions (Rothbaum, 1997; Wilson, Becker, & Tinker, 1997), the history taking and preparation phases can be completed in the first session. For multiple or childhood trauma histories, the course of treatment may need to be 12, 90-minute sessions (Boterhoven de Hann et al., 2017).

Phase III: Assessment

EMDR therapy does not require detailed self-disclosure about traumatic events. For example, those debilitated by shame or guilt, such as sexual abuse survivors or combat veterans with a moral injury (i.e., Russell & Figley, 2013), can simply provide a general report of what occurred (e.g., "My stepfather molested me"). In this phase, the clinician asks the client to bring the trauma to awareness, then select a representative image and present-related negative cognition (NC; e.g., "I'm dirty"), emotion(s), physical sensation(s), and body location. The clinician obtains a baseline Subjective Units of Distress Scale (SUDS) rating (Wolpe & Abrams, 1991), from 0, "no distress," to 10, "worst possible." The clinician also elicits a preferred belief or positive cognition (PC)—an adaptive desired self-statement related to the target memory—and a baseline rating for the desired PC on the Validity of Cognitions (VoC) Scale, with 1 indicating "completely untrue" and 7 "completely true." Over the course of treatment, each target memory is assessed for key memory components (e.g., the image, cognition and meaning, and emotion and body sensation). Thus, the therapist asks in each case for a representative picture associated with the traumatic event, what the event means to the person, and his or her emotions as reflected in feelings and body sensations. Following desensitization of all trauma-related memories, anticipated future challenges are also assessed in this manner.

Phase IV: Desensitization

The goal of the desensitization phase is to process the maladaptively stored memory and facilitate its full integration within adaptive memory networks. To initiate EMDR therapy processing, a state of "dual-focused attention" is created by the therapist instructing clients to be aware of the target memory and its representative components (e.g., "Bring up that memory of the motor vehicle accident," the negative cognition, emotion, and physical sensations), while simultaneously directing clients to engage in approximately 24 rhythmic sets of BLS (e.g., eye movements, tapping, auditory tones). It is highly recommended that clinicians initially utilize eye movements for BLS whenever possible (Shapiro, 2018), because over 30 trials have documented the significant positive effects of eye movements in decreasing arousal and memory vividness and/or negative affect (see Lee & Cuijpers, 2013, for a review), increased recognition of true information (Parker, Buckley, & Dagnall, 2009), retrieval of episodic memory (Christman, Garvey, Propper, & Phaneuf, 2003), and attentional flexibility (Kuiken, Bears, Miall, & Smith, 2002). During BLS, the therapist may encourage the client, making statements like "Just let whatever happens, happen" and "Simply notice what occurs." The amount of therapist verbal interaction during EMDR therapy processing is dependent on the client's need for support (e.g., "It's in the past, just notice it"). At the end of each set of BLS, clients are asked, "What do you notice now?" If the client indicates progress in memory processing (e.g., "It's fading," "It switched to another memory"), the therapist initiates further BLS with simple prompts, for instance, "Just stay with that."

In contrast to exposure-based models, the client describing a new negative memory during EMDR therapy is generally considered an example of associated experiences with the targeted event rather than an avoidance of trauma processing. Research demonstrates that in EMDR therapy, responses indicating distancing from the memory, as opposed to reliving responses, are an indication of effective EMDR memory processing (Lee, Taylor, &

Drummond, 2006). It is important for clinicians to trust the innate adaptive information processing and avoid detailed questioning between BLS sets. In effect, EMDR therapy processing involves following the client's spontaneous associations, coupled with BLS sets until no further change in self-report or desensitization occurs (e.g., SUDS ratings of 0–1). If the client is unable to utilize EMs during BLS, then clinicians should offer either tapping or auditory tones and evaluate their effectiveness.

If processing appears to be "blocked," suggested by no cognitive or somatic changes after two sets of BLS, therapists use various brief interventions, such as a change in direction of eye movements (e.g., vertical vs. diagonal), alternating speed of BLS (faster vs. slower), or directing attention to a specific aspect of the trauma experience (e.g., "Notice the tightness in your jaw"), followed immediately by a BLS set (Shapiro, 2018). On occasion, when a client becomes "stuck" (e.g., fails to report a change in SUDS or cognition after two or more consecutive BLS sets, even after the aforementioned adjustment), the therapist may inject a "cognitive interweave," which is a succinct statement or question aimed at eliciting a new adaptive perspective, thought, action, or image (e.g., "Who was responsible for what happened?"). The clinician instructs clients to notice what happens next (e.g., in terms of images, thoughts, feelings, and body sensations) while they focus on their response to the interweave and the therapist initiates another set of BLS. Use of cognitive interweaves or other additions from the standard EMDR therapy protocol should be minimal. Such interventions are viewed as disrupting memory processing by imposing therapist-driven solutions to the issues that might otherwise be achieved by allowing the client's own idiosyncratic, innate adaptive processing to occur.

Processing generally entails simultaneous shifts in affective, cognitive, and somatic components of the memory, and shifts to alternative but associated memory networks. Clinical effects during this phase are measured using SUDS ratings of the target memory. Typically, as SUDS ratings decrease, the content of client self-reports increasingly and spontaneously includes more positive or adaptive information. When the SUDS rating reaches 0 or 1 on a target memory, the desensitization phase is concluded. Commonly, other associated memories have been activated during processing and may also have desensitized to some extent. However, this is not always the case. In simpler cases, the clinician moves to the installation phase after desensitization. For clients with multiple traumas, the clinician may instead reassess the degree of distress associated with other related memories and, if they have not desensitized, target these first before attempting integration.

Phase V: Installation

After desensitization appears complete, the adaptive PC associated with the target memory is paired with BLS sets until a VoC of 6–7 is achieved. Additional processing in this phase addresses any residual disturbances, strengthens the connection with currently existing positive memory networks, and facilitates generalization effects. It should be noted that the target SUDS and VoC numbers are guidelines and that other clinical indicators of progress, such as the elicitation of insights (e.g., the trauma is over, they survived, they can see themselves as safe, supported, and able to manage in the future), are also employed (Shapiro, 2018).

Phase VI: Body Scan

The client focuses on the target memory and searches for negative physical sensations that, if present, are processed with BLS sets until absent. This provides a check for aspects of the traumatic memory that were not fully processed.

Phase VII: Closure

When processing is incomplete, the therapist may utilize relaxation techniques like safe/calm place to stabilize the client if necessary. When processing appears complete, there can be more extensive therapeutic discussion—for example, discussion on the insights that arose during processing and the effect processing may have on current symptoms, particularly those of an avoidance and intrusive nature. Clients are educated about what to expect following desensitization and asked to briefly indicate any between-session disturbance in a "TICES" log, which contains columns to note the trigger, image, cognition, emotion, and physical sensation/SUDS (Shapiro, 2018). They are also instructed to utilize self-calming procedures taught during Phase II.

Phase VIII: Reevaluation

Multiple phases can be completed within a single session. However, at the beginning of the next session, the clinician reevaluates the target memory and TICES log. If the past memories are adequately processed, the clinician can proceed to present triggers, then future templates. Present triggers are typically recent events that triggered distress since the last session. If such an event has occurred, the client is asked to focus on this recent incident (e.g., "I saw a guy in a red sweatsuit similar to the one worn by the person who assaulted me") and associated negative cognition and feelings. The therapist next engages the client in processing using Phases IV–VII. The future template involves imagining future events that might give rise to distress, targeting the reduction of the associated arousal, and then in the imagination, rehearsing more adaptive behaviors and associated ideas.

Additional reevaluation sessions can be scheduled at staggered intervals if clinically indicated or practical, to determine the stability of symptom change over a longer period of time. To complete the standard EMDR therapy protocol, clinicians must complete the three-pronged protocol, which includes reprocessing memories of the past adverse events, processing current triggers, and incorporating "future templates."

Summary and Appraisal of the Evidence

In the 30 years since Shapiro (1989) first described EMDR therapy, there have been over 30 RCTs testing the treatment's efficacy with adults with PTSD, nine RCTs testing its efficacy in treating children with full or partial PTSD, and seven RCTs assessing its efficacy for people recently exposed to a traumatic experience. The cumulative evidence from RCTs led the International Society for Traumatic Stress Studies (ISTSS) guidelines to give EMDR therapy a *Strong* recommendation for the treatment of adults and children with PTSD. This is consistent with other treatment guidelines, such as those published by the World Health Organization (2018) and the Australian Centre for Posttraumatic Mental Health (2013). In this chapter, we provide a summary of the evidence for adults with PTSD. The evidence with respect to treating children is covered by Olff and colleagues and Jensen, Cohen, Jaycox, and Rosner (Chapters 11 and 21, respectively, this volume) and in Chen and colleagues' review (2018), and the evidence of effectiveness for treating recent trauma survivors is described by O'Donnell, Pacella, Bryant, Olff, and Forbes (Chapter 8, this volume).

In reviewing the evidence on the treatment of adults, the ISTSS guidelines identified 11 RCTs where EMDR therapy was compared to a wait-list or treatment as usual (TAU) control. In the meta-analyses, EMDR therapy was found to have a significant positive effect compared with these conditions, and this effect size was large (standardized mean difference [SMD] = 1.24). Once two studies with subclinical dosages were removed, the effect size was even larger (SMD = 1.40).

In addition, a larger number of trials (17) were identified that compared EMDR therapy to another active treatment. The comparisons included cognitive-behavioral therapies (CBT) (Capezzani et al., 2013; Devilly & Spence, 1999; Devilly, Spence, & Rapee, 1999; Ironson, Freud, Strauss, & Williams, 2002; Laugharne et al., 2016; Lee, Gavriel, Drummond, Richards, & Greenwald, 2002; Nijdam, Gersons, Reitsma, de Jongh, & Olff, 2012; Power et al., 2002; Rothbam, Astin, & Marsteller, 2005; Taylor, 2003; Vaughan et al., 1994), supportive counseling (Scheck, Schaeffer, & Gillette, 1998), and relaxation (Carletto et al., 2016; Carlson, Chemtob, Rusnack, Hedlund, & Muraoka, 1998; Taylor, 2003; Vaughan et al., 1994). There are other relevant RCTs that did not meet the ISTSS inclusion criteria, such as the comparison of EMDR therapy to CBT and a wait-list control for patients with a dual diagnosis of PTSD and psychosis (van den Berg et al., 2015), and when EMDR therapy was compared to a placebo control and fluoxetine (van der Kolk et al., 2007).

These RCTs investigated the effects of EMDR therapy on a variety of different trauma exposures, including refugees from war zones (Acarturk et al., 2016; Ter Heide, Mooren, van de Schoot, de Jongh, & Kleber, 2016), motor-vehicle accidents (Aldahadha, Harthy, & Sulaiman, 2012), diagnosis of a life-threatening condition (Capezzani et al., 2013; Carletto et al., 2016), military veterans (Carlson et al., 1998; Himmerich et al., 2016; Jensen, 1994), childhood sexual abuse (Edmond, Rubin, & Wambach, 1999), mixed trauma populations (Laugharne et al., 2016; Lee et al., 2002; Taylor, 2003; van der Kolk et al., 2007), sexual or physical assault (Nijdam et al., 2012), sexual assault (Rothbam et al., 2005), and childhood physical or emotional abuse (Scheck et al., 1998). Thus, the ISTSS guidelines' *Strong* recommendation for the use of EMDR therapy is based on robust findings indicating that EMDR therapy is applicable to a wide range of trauma populations, and its effectiveness is generalizable across contexts and cultures.

Treatment gains following EMDR therapy are substantial and stable. Loss of PTSD diagnosis ranges from 48% (Vaughan et al., 1994) to 94–95% (Capezzani et al., 2013; Nijdam et al., 2012). Moreover, gains in symptom reduction for trauma-related symptoms, depression, and anxiety at posttreatment have been found to be sustained at 18-month follow-up for survivors of childhood sexual abuse treated with EMDR therapy (Edmond & Rubin, 2004). Similarly, trauma-related symptom reduction and improvements in secondary measures after treatment were maintained at 35 months follow-up for a group of Swedish transport workers with chronic PTSD (Högberg et al., 2008).

EMDR therapy is also effective when there are comorbid symptoms. In a meta-analysis of PTSD treatment studies (Chen et al., 2014), EMDR therapy was found to lead to large reductions ($g = 0.64$) for both depression and anxiety compared with inactive and active controls. Subgroup analyses indicated that the duration of the treatment sessions affected these outcomes, such that sessions longer than 60 minutes led to larger reductions in depression and anxiety. Another meta-analysis investigating the effectiveness of EMDR therapy compared to trauma-focused CBT on depressive symptoms when comorbid with a PTSD presentation found a similar large ($g = 0.63$) effect size (Ho & Lee, 2012).

EMDR therapy has been identified as an efficient and effective treatment for adults who experienced childhood sexual trauma and adult-onset sexual assault, beginning with an RCT indicating 90% elimination of PTSD in rape victims after three 90-minute sessions (Rothbaum, 1997). Rothbaum and colleagues (2005) also conducted a head-to-head comparison between EMDR therapy and prolonged exposure with adult sexual assault survivors. Although both treatments resulted in significant improvements compared to a wait-list control, there were no differences between the treatments. However, "an interesting potential clinical implication is that EMDR seemed to do equally well in the main despite less exposure and no homework" (p. 614).

An encouraging finding from RCTs examining EMDR therapy to date is that it can relieve trauma-related symptoms in populations of severe interpersonal trauma and in treatment settings other than a traditional office. For example, therapists working inside a refugee camp with people who had fled a military conflict were able to achieve significant improvements compared to a wait-list control, and treatment gains were maintained at follow-up despite participants living in ongoing unstable conditions (Acarturk et al., 2016). Similar effect sizes were reported when treating survivors of the Timorese war (Schubert et al., 2016). After a mean of four sessions, 95% no longer met PTSD criteria. Also, women with acting-out behaviors and referred mainly from forensic settings did significantly better after receiving only two sessions of EMDR therapy compared to active listening on measures of trauma symptomology and depression, bringing scores within 1 standard deviation of the norm (Scheck et al., 1998).

Practical Delivery Recommendations

Optimal Delivery of EMDR Therapy

A review of the efficacy research on EMDR therapy indicates that optimal delivery is over approximately 4.5 hours of treatment in sessions of 60–90 minutes for comprehensive treatment of PTSD resulting from a single trauma (e.g., Marcus, Marquis, & Sakai, 1997, 2004; Rothbaum, 1997; Wilson, Becker, & Tinker, 1995; Wilson et al., 1997). PTSD resulting from multiple traumas may require longer treatment. For example, 12, 90-minute sessions in the case of combat veterans (Carlson et al., 1998) and for adults with PTSD from childhood experiences may be needed (Boterhoven de Haan et al., 2017). As indicated in the World Health Organization's (2018) practice guidelines, EMDR does not involve: "(a) detailed descriptions of the traumatic event(s), (b) direct challenging of beliefs, (c) extended exposure, or (d) homework" (p. 1).

The standard EMDR therapy protocol is optimal when unimpeded processing occurs. However, when processing gets stuck, as may happen in the case of excessive shame, survivor guilt, or moral injury, then cognitive interweaves can be used by instructing clients to contemplate some missing adaptive information (e.g., "What would you think if it had happened to your son?" or "Did you do what you were trained to do?") while paired with BLS ("Just think of that and follow my hand"). Targets for processing also include flashback scenes and nightmares, which generally rapidly remit, often revealing and resolving the underlying cause.

Special Populations

Complex Traumatic Events

For those who have suffered severe, chronic exposure to adverse childhood events, clinicians should ensure that clients have sufficient capacity to access past traumatic memories, while remaining stabilized in the present.

Consequently, it is considered best to extend the preparation phase to ensure a client's ability to safely tolerate the emotional distress associated with accessing traumatic experiences. This can be accomplished by stabilization interventions such as resource developmental and installation (RDI; Korn & Leeds, 2002), which increases the client's access to positive emotional states (e.g., confidence). For those with multiple, complex trauma histories, the EMDR therapy protocol, which engages the client in unrestricted memory processing, can be adjusted to the initially developed EMD (Shapiro, 1989), which minimizes client associations by focusing on present disturbance or triggers. When containing memory processing in this way, the therapist plans with the client to focus on a defined memory target and restrict associated processing. When adequately prepared (i.e., the client is able to remain present without dissociating or experiencing incapacitating distress), EMDR processing should address the full range of adverse life experiences, including childhood events. During processing, clinicians are advised to (1) target the client's somatic and verbal responses with BLS, (2) frequently assess for hyper- and hypo-arousal, especially dissociation, and (3) be prepared to utilize EMDR strategies like the cognitive interweave for blocked processing, while (4) regularly reassuring clients, "It's old stuff, you are in control and I'm here with you." Current research is investigating the possibility that clients with such traumatic experiences can, in fact, benefit from EMDR therapy without stabilization (Boterhoven de Hann et al., 2017). However, multiple rigorous RCTs providing sufficient treatment time are needed to adequately address this issue.

Another clinical feature of EMDR therapy is the possibility of processing trauma material without the need for detailed information. Clinicians can focus on processing the emotional, cognitive, and somatic (e.g., pain) representations of the traumatic experiences when minimal perceptual details of the event are recalled. For some clients, this has an advantage as he or she can process the trauma without having to disclose details of events.

Children

EMDR therapy has been used with children as young as 1 year old, with limited cognitive capacities or developmental delays, who may find extended exposure overwhelming; live in complex, chaotic family systems; and are unable to engage in therapeutic homework tasks. Contraindications for use of EMDR therapy with children include situations where they are actively being abused or exposed to ongoing threats to their safety. The full eight phases and three-pronged protocol are employed. However, significant variations are introduced to hold the attention of young children, such as the therapist using glove puppets in each hand and focusing each child's attention on these to facilitate bilateral eye movements (Adler-Tapia & Settle, 2017). Adaptations to the EMDR therapy protocol include ensuring developmentally appropriate language is used throughout all phases of treatment.

For example, in taking a history, clients are helped to tell their story and identify target memories in developmentally appropriate ways (e.g., maps, timelines, storybooks). In the target assessment phase, the positive and negative beliefs associated with trauma experiences may be event-specific, rooted in the present tense, and use feeling-based words. Child-friendly adaptations of the VoC and SUD scales (e.g., pictures) are also used. During processing, various BLS tasks are employed to maintain attention (e.g., tapping, drumming). For children with complex trauma presentations and attachment issues, EMDR therapy is effective with appropriate protocol modifications (e.g., Gomez, 2013; Wesselmann, Schweitzer, & Armstrong, 2014).

When EMDR therapy is utilized in creative, flexible, and playful ways, children, even those with multiple trauma histories and complex trauma presentations, are able to fully engage in processing sessions. For example, the EMDR clinician adjusts communication and language to match a child's developmental level. The clinician may vary methods of BLS and keep things playful so the child remains engaged in the therapy. Children may require shorter sets and may need more breaks in reprocessing. Children may be encouraged to express themselves through play and artwork during the assessment phases. The inclusion of parents may be critical to understanding the child's history, and parents might help provide emotional support as needed during the desensitization phases. The integration of family therapy may interrupt negative dynamics in the home and create a more positive and supportive atmosphere for the child's recovery.

Military Veterans

Although EMDR research has demonstrated its usefulness across a variety of military clinical and operational settings (Carlson et al., 1998; Hurley, 2018), the clinician needs to consider therapy targets with flexibility to a client's issues. The possible foci of the therapy include traumatic grief, moral injury, posttraumatic anger, survivor guilt, medically unexplained physical symptoms, phantom limb pain (PLP), and intense betrayal resulting from military sexual trauma (see Russell & Figley, 2013). Moral injury is a construct that describes extreme and unprecedented life experiences, including the harmful aftermath of exposure to such events. Events are considered morally injurious if they transgress deeply held moral beliefs and expectations (Litz et al., 2009).

In each scenario, the client's self-reports of anger, betrayal, guilt, shame, grief, somatic symptoms, or PLP are paired with BLS, along with associated cognitions, memories, emotions, and physical sensations. When processing becomes stuck, then brief therapist-induced interventions like cognitive interweaves are introduced.

Complicating issues can arise with military populations who may experience blocked processing due to deep-seated fears that positive therapeutic change may deprive them of remembering their fallen comrades, or because they view their suffering as just punishment for their perceived or actual moral failings (e.g., participating in an atrocity). In some cases, veterans will directly state their ambivalence toward change. In others, the therapist may have to probe for underlying beliefs that block processing, and/or interject cognitive interweaves (e.g., "What would your buddy say?"). Once uncovered, the client's expressed fears or concerns and related associations are processed with BLS.

Comprehensive trauma-focused treatment of military personnel often goes beyond PTSD diagnosis to include physical symptoms, such as chronic pain including, but not limited to, PLP, which has generally been viewed as an intractable condition. However, EMDR therapy holds that the pain is caused by the unprocessed memory of the injury that, as indicated in the AIP model, contains the somatic sensations and emotions experienced at the time of the event. Successful EMDR treatment of PLP has been reported over the past decade subsequent to processing pivotal memories (e.g., Russell, 2008; Schneider, Hofmann, Rost, & Shapiro, 2008). Recently, an RCT (Rostaminejad, Behnammoghadam, Rostaminejad, Behnammoghadam, & Bashti, 2017) found that EMDR therapy significantly reduced PLP and related psychological symptoms through processing the disturbing memories. All participants reported pain reduction, with 47% claiming to be pain-free. Treatment gains were maintained at 2-year follow-up.

Disaster Survivors

EMDR therapy has been recognized by the international community as a front-line recommended treatment for disaster-related PTSD (e.g., World Health Organization, 2018). Several recent protocols have been developed to help survivors at the time of the event, within 2–3 months, and within 6 months, even while being continuously exposed to trauma (see Shapiro, 2018). Randomized trials have demonstrated the effectiveness of natural and man-made postdisaster protocols in adults (e.g., Acarturk et al., 2016) and children (e.g., Chemtob, Nakashima, & Carlson, 2002; de Roos et al., 2011). In a postdisaster context, clinical and practical concerns lead to EMDR therapy being delivered daily or biweekly, as opposed to weekly (Acarturk et al., 2016; Schubert et al., 2016). Also, in large-scale postdisaster contexts where clinical resources may be limited, an integrative group EMDR therapy protocol can be utilized to process memories of trauma experiences and identify those who may require further individualized EMDR therapy (Jarero, Artigas, & Hartung, 2006).

Limitations of EMDR Therapy

Clients with a seizure disorder, acute traumatic brain injury, or complicated pregnancy are not suitable for EMDR therapy until appropriate safety concerns are cleared. Moreover, although no two clients are identical in their response to EMDR therapy, changes in perceptual detail, cognitions, physiological and emotional responses to traumatic experiences are common (e.g., Shapiro, 2018). Therefore, clinicians should be wary of using EMDR therapy in legal cases without prior consultation with an attorney if the preservation of unaltered, vivid recollections of witnesses is essential.

In addition, trauma survivors may be averse to the potential of recalling earlier traumatic or adverse events warranting appropriate informed consent that EMDR therapy effects may generalize beyond the present incident (see Shapiro, 2018). However, another significant challenge in utilizing EMDR therapy lies within the therapist. Specifically, clinicians experienced in providing mainstream psychotherapies that involve a great deal of therapist probing, reframing, and interpretation may experience some difficulty shifting gears to properly apply EMDR therapy. That said, clients who enter therapy expecting extensive dialogue from a probing therapist, and/or who desire detailed discussion of their traumatic memories and the processing thereof, can become irritated with the EMDR clinician's repeated refrain: "Just think of that . . . and follow my hand" or whatever BLS is utilized. Therapists should be aware of this possibility and be able to adjust accordingly. Additional challenges in utilizing EMDR therapy include securing client buy-in due to its unorthodox procedural framework (i.e., EM and other BLS). In short, EMDR therapy is not a panacea and will not be a good fit for every client and/or therapist.

An issue in treating more complex trauma presentations is that once the trauma memories have been desensitized, the person may indeed no longer have PTSD symptoms but retain disturbances in interpersonal relationships. EMDR therapy on its own cannot fix the skills deficits that a lifetime of trauma or trauma activation has had on a person's functioning. Once the person no longer exhibits PTSD symptoms, therapy for this population needs to focus on providing skills and coaching in behaviors to be better equipped to facilitate growth.

Finally, personality variables may affect how EMDR therapy is received. The treatment requires clients to focus on just noticing what occurs, without judging their experience. However, this might be difficult for clients who score low on traits such as openness to new experience, which research has demonstrated reduces the efficacy of other trauma treatments (van Emmerik, Kamphuis, Noordhof, & Emmelkamp, 2011).

Future Developments

Rigorous research is needed to further our understanding of the crucial processes in EMDR therapy and to test adaptations of the standard protocol and how EMDR therapy can be extended to special populations. An interesting format issue includes frequency of sessions. Is EMDR therapy best delivered every day, twice a week, or once a fortnight? In addition, preliminary findings suggest EMDR therapy can be provided in a group format for those who have acutely suffered trauma, but will such treatment protocols prove effective in other studies? To what extent does cultural context impact treatment effectiveness? Culture may affect how a trauma-focused treatment is received, and trauma may impact culture. The ability of people plagued by ethnopolitical violence to reconcile with each other is often thwarted by unprocessed traumatic memories. One reason for this is the presence of a negative attentional bias that can occur in individuals with PTSD (e.g., Pineles, Shipherd, Mostoufi, Abramovitz, & Yovel, 2009) and hamper their ability to disengage from threatening cues. This can inhibit the ability of historically feuding people, the very sight of whom may cause intractable resistance, to forge agreement. Fortunately, preliminary research suggests that disruptive attentional biases can be ameliorated by EMDR therapy (El Khoury-Malhame et al., 2011). More research is needed to confirm this observation, especially studies that focus on ways to facilitate mediation and reconciliation.

Given the recent inclusion of complex PTSD in the *International Classification of Diseases*, 11th revision (ICD-11; World Health Organization, 2018), RCTs examining efficacy and effectiveness are needed for this population group. Ongoing research is required to understand the optimal stabilization required for effective trauma memory processing in complex PTSD populations, and how to most efficiently attain stability prior to memory processing, and to effectively maintain it during and between processing sessions. Further efforts are also required to understand the tolerability of treatment and dropout rates observed in complex PTSD populations (Boterhoven de Haan et al., 2017). In addition, there are a host of other empirical studies yet to be undertaken with EMDR therapy, including the combined effects of using multiple types of BLS simultaneously, and the effectiveness of EMDR therapy in treating co-occurring conditions, such as moral injury, complicated grief, chronic mild traumatic brain injury, substance abuse, and pain disorders.

In summary, EMDR therapy was introduced three decades ago (Shapiro, 1989). The accumulated literature provides evidence that EMDR therapy is an effective treatment for PTSD and trauma-related conditions arising from different types of traumas, in different contexts and cultures. Encouragingly, the evidence supports its use in interpersonal and simple traumas, for both adults and children, and for chronic and recent trauma events. Further understanding the underlying mechanisms and its limitations requires additional research. Research into the mechanisms of EMDR therapy has to date challenged existing contemporary theories of PTSD and has advanced our understanding of the development and recovery from PTSD. However, there is still much to learn in terms of understanding what constitutes best practice for individuals with complex PTSD and comorbid presentations.

REFERENCES

Acarturk, C., Konuk, E., Cetinkaya, M., Senay, I., Sijbrandij, M., Gulen, B., et al. (2016). The efficacy of eye movement desensitization and reprocessing for post-traumatic stress disorder and depression among Syrian refugees: Results of a randomized controlled trial. *Psychological Medicine, 46*(12), 2583–2593.

Adler-Tapia, R., & Settle, C. (2017). *EMDR and the art of psychotherapy with children: Treatment manual and text* (2nd ed.). New York: Springer.

Aldahadha, B., Harthy, H. A., & Sulaiman, S. (2012). The efficacy of eye movement desensitization reprocessing in resolving the trauma caused by the road accidents in the Sultanate of Oman. *Journal of Instructional Psychology, 39,* 146–158.

American Psychiatric Association. (2013). *Diagnostic and statistical manual of mental disorders* (5th ed.). Arlington, VA: Author.

Australian Centre for Posttraumatic Mental Health. (2013). *Australian guidelines for the treatment of acute stress disorder and posttraumatic stress disorder.* Melbourne: Author.

Baddeley, A. (2012). Working memory: Theories, models, and controversies. *Annual Review of Psychology, 63,* 1–29.

Baek, J., Lee, S., Cho, T., Kim, S. W., Kim, M., Yoon, Y., et al. (2019). Neural circuits underlying a psychotherapeutic regimen for fear disorders. *Nature, 556,* 339–343.

Bossini, L., Santarnecchi, E., Casolaro, I., Koukouna, D., Caterini, C., Cecchini, F., et al. (2017). Morphovolumetric changes after EMDR treatment in drug-naïve PTSD patients. *Rivista di Psichiatria, 52(1),* 24–31.

Boterhoven de Haan, K. L., Lee, C. W., Fassbinder, E., Voncken, M. J., Meewisse, M., Van Es, S. M., et al. (2017). Imagery rescripting and eye movement desensitisation and reprocessing for treatment of adults with childhood trauma-related post-traumatic stress disorder: IREM study design. *BMC Psychiatry, 17*(1), 165.

Boukezzi, S., El Khoury-Malhame, M., Auzias, G., Reynaud, E., Rousseau, P. F., Richard, E., et al. (2017). Grey matter density changes of structures involved in post-traumatic stress disorder (PTSD) after recovery following eye movement desensitization and reprocessing (EMDR) therapy. *Psychiatry Research: Neuroimaging, 266,* 146–152.

Bradley, M. M. (2009). Natural selective attention: Orienting and emotion. *Psychophysiology, 46,* 1–11.

Capezzani, L., Ostacoli, L., Cavallo, M., Carletto, S., Fernandez, I., Solomon, R., et al. (2013). EMDR and CBT for cancer patients: Comparative study of effects on PTSD, anxiety, and depression. *Journal of EMDR Practice and Research, 7,* 134–143.

Carletto, S., Borghi, M., Bertino, G., Oliva, F., Cavallo, M., Hofmann, A., et al. (2016). Treating post-traumatic stress disorder in patients with multiple sclerosis: A randomized controlled trial comparing the efficacy of eye movement desensitization and reprocessing and relaxation therapy. *Frontiers in Psychology 7,* 526.

Carlson, J. G., Chemtob, C. M., Rusnack, K., Hedlund, N. L., & Muraoka, M. Y. (1998). Eye movement desensitization and reprocessing (EMDR) treatment for combat-related posttraumatic stress disorder. *Journal of Traumatic Stress, 11,* 3–24.

Chemtob, C. M., Nakashima, J., & Carlson, J. G. (2002). Brief-treatment for elementary school children with disaster-related PTSD: A field study. *Journal of Clinical Psychology, 58,* 99–112.

Chen, R., Gillespie, A., Zhao, Y., Xi, Y., Ren, Y., & McLean, L. (2018). The efficacy of eye movement desensitization and reprocessing in children and adults who have experienced complex childhood trauma: A systematic review or randomized controlled trials. *Frontiers in Psychology, 9,* 534.

Chen, Y. R., Hung, K. W., Tsai, J. C., Chu, H., Chung, M. H., Chen, S. R., et al. (2014). Efficacy of eye-movement desensitization and reprocessing for patients with posttraumatic-stress disorder: A meta-analysis of randomized controlled trials. *PLOS ONE, 9,* e103676.

Christman, S. D., Garvey, K. J., Propper, R. E., & Phaneuf, K. A. (2003). Bilateral eye movements enhance the retrieval of episodic memories. *Neuropsychology, 17*(2), 221–229.

Crestani, A. P., Zacouteguy Boos, F., Haubrich, J., Ordoñez Sierra, R., Santana, F., Molina, J. M. D., et al. (2015). Memory reconsolidation may be disrupted by a distractor stimulus presented during reactivation. *Scientific Reports, 5,* 13633.

de Roos, C., Greenwald, R., den Hollander-Gijsman, M., Noorthoorn, E., van Buuren, S., & de Jongh, A. (2011). A randomized comparison of cognitive behavioral therapy (CBT) and eye movement desensitization and reprocessing (EMDR) in disaster exposed children. *European Journal of Psychotraumatology, 2,* 5694–5704.

Devilly, G. J., & Spence, S. H. (1999). The relative efficacy and treatment distress of EMDR and a cognitive-behavior trauma treatment protocol in the amelioration of posttraumatic stress disorder. *Journal of Anxiety Disorders, 13,* 131–157.

Devilly, G. J., Spence, S. H., & Rapee, R. M. (1999). Statistical and reliable change with eye movement desensitization and reprocessing: Treating trauma within a veteran population. *Behavior Therapy, 29,* 435–455.

Edmond, T., & Rubin, A. (2004). Assessing the long-term effects of EMDR: Results from an 18-month follow-up study with adult female survivors of CSA. *Journal of Child Sexual Abuse, 13,* 69–86.

Edmond, T., Rubin, A., & Wambach, K. (1999). The effectiveness of EMDR with adult female survivors of childhood sexual abuse. *Social Work Research, 23,* 103–116.

El Khoury-Malhame, M., Lanteaume, L., Beetz, E. M., Roques, J., Reynaud, E., Samuelian, J. C., et al. (2011). Attentional bias in post-traumatic stress disorder diminishes after symptom amelioration. *Behaviour Research and Therapy, 49,* 796–801.

Elofsson, U. O. E., von Scheele, B., Theorell, T., & Sondergaard, H. P. (2008). Physiological correlates of eye movement desensitization and reprocessing. *Journal of Anxiety Disorders, 22,* 622–634.

Gomez, A. (2013). *EMDR therapy and adjunct approaches with children: Complex trauma, attachment, and dissociation.* New York: Springer.

Himmerich, H., Willmund, G. D., Zimmermann, P., Wolf, J. E., Buhler, A. H., Kirkby, K. C., et al. (2016). Serum concentrations of TNF-alpha and its soluble receptors during psychotherapy in German soldiers suffering from combat-related PTSD. *Psychiatria Danubina, 28,* 293–298.

Ho, M. S. K., & Lee, C. W. (2012). Cognitive behaviour therapy versus eye movement desensitization and reprocessing for post-traumatic disorder—Is it all in the homework then? *European Review of Applied Psychology, 62,* 253–260.

Högberg, G., Pagani, M., Sundin, O., Soares, J., Aberg-Wistedt, A., Tarnell, B., et al. (2008). Treatment of post-traumatic stress disorder with eye movement desensitization and reprocessing: Outcome is stable in 35-month follow-up. *Psychiatry Research, 159,* 101–108.

Hurley, E. C. (2018). Effective treatment of veterans with PTSD: Comparison between intensive daily and weekly EMDR approaches. *Frontiers in Psychology, 9,* 1458.

Ironson, G., Freud, B., Strauss, J. L., & Williams, J. (2002). Comparison of two treatments for traumatic stress: A community-based study of EMDR and prolonged exposure. *Journal of Clinical Psychology, 58,* 113–128.

Jarero, I., Artigas, L., & Hartung, J. (2006). EMDR integrative group treatment protocol: A postdisaster trauma intervention for children and adults. *Traumatology, 12*(2), 121–129.

Jensen, J. A. (1994). An investigation of eye movement desensitization and reprocessing (EMD/R) as a treatment for posttraumatic stress disorder (PTSD) symptoms of Vietnam combat veterans. *Behavior Therapy, 25,* 311–326.

Korn, D. L., & Leeds, A. M. (2002). Preliminary evidence of efficacy for EMDR resource development and installation in the stabilization phase of treatment of complex posttraumatic stress disorder. *Journal of Clinical Psychology, 58,* 1465–1487.

Kuiken, D., Bears, M., Miall, D., & Smith, L. (2002). Eye movement desensitization reprocessing facilitates attentional orienting. *Imagination, Cognition and Personality, 21,* 3–20.

Landin-Romero, R., Nova, P., Vicens, V., McKenna, P. J., Santed, A., Pomarol-Clotet, E., et al. (2013). EMDR therapy modulates the default mode network in a subsyndromal, traumatized bipolar patient. *Neuropsychobiology, 67,* 181–184.

Lansing, K., Amen, D. G., Hanks, C., & Rudy, L. (2005). High resolution brain SPECT imaging and EMDR in police officers with PTSD. *Journal of Neuropsychiatry and Clinical Neurosciences, 17,* 526–532.

Laugharne, J., Kullack, C., Lee, C. W., McGuire, T., Brockman, S., Drummond, P. D., et al. (2016). Amygdala volumetric change following psychotherapy for posttraumatic stress disorder. *Journal of Neuropsychiatry and Clinical Neuroscience, 28*(4), 312–318.

Lee, C. W., & Cuijpers, P. (2013). A meta-analysis of the contribution of eye movements in processing emotional memories. *Journal of Behavior Therapy and Experimental Psychiatry, 44,* 231–239.

Lee, C. W., Gavriel, H., Drummond, P. D., Richards, J. & Greenwald, R. (2002). Treatment of PTSD: Stress inoculation training with prolonged exposure compared to EMDR. *Journal of Clinical Psychology, 58,* 1071–1089.

Lee, C. W., Taylor, G., & Drummond, P. D. (2006). The active ingredient in EMDR: Is it traditional exposure or dual focus of attention? *Clinical Psychology and Psychotherapy, 13*(2), 97–107.

Litz, B. T., Stein, N., Delaney, E., Lebowitz, L., Nash, W. P., Silva, C., et al. (2009). Moral injury and moral repair in war veterans: A preliminary model and intervention strategy. *Clinical Psychology Review, 29,* 695–706.

Marcus, S. V., Marquis, P., & Sakai, C. (1997). Controlled study of treatment of PTSD using EMDR in an HMO setting. *Psychotherapy Research Practice and Training, 34,* 307–315.

Marcus, S., Marquis, P., & Sakai, C. (2004). Three- and 6-month follow-up of EMDR treatment of PTSD in an HMO setting. *International Journal of Stress Management, 11,* 195–208.

Nijdam, M. J., Gersons, B. P. R., Reitsma, J. B., de Jongh, A., & Olff, M. (2012). Brief eclectic psychotherapy v. eye movement desensitization and reprocessing therapy for post-traumatic stress disorder: Randomised controlled trial. *British Journal of Psychiatry, 200,* 224–231.

Oh, D.-H., & Choi, J. (2004). Changes in the regional cerebral perfusion after eye movement desensitization and reprocessing: A SPECT study of two cases. *Korean Journal of Biological Psychiatry, 11*(2), 173–180.

Pagani, M., DiLorenzo, G., Verardo, A. R., Nicolais, G., Monaco, L., Lauretti, G., et al. (2012). Neurobiological correlates of EMDR monitoring—An EEG study. *PLOS ONE, 7*(9), e45753.

Pagani, M., Hogberg, G., Salmaso, D., Nardo, D., Sundin, O., Johnson, C., et al. (2007). Effects of EMDR psychotherapy on 99mTc-HMPAO distribution in occupation-related post-traumatic stress disorder. *Nuclear Medicine Communications, 28,* 757–765.

Parker, A., Buckley, S., & Dagnall, N. (2009). Reduced misinformation effects following saccadic bilateral eye movements. *Brain and Cognition, 69,* 89–97.

Pineles, S. L., Shipherd, J. C., Mostoufi, S. M., Abramovitz, S. M., & Yovel, I. (2009). Attentional biases in PTSD: More evidence for interference. *Behaviour Research and Therapy, 47*(12), 1050–1057.

Power, K. G., McGoldrick, T., Brown, K., Buchanan, R., Sharp, D., Swanson, V., et al. (2002). A controlled comparison of eye movement desensitization and reprocessing versus exposure plus cognitive restructuring, versus waiting list in the treatment of posttraumatic stress disorder. *Journal of Clinical Psychology and Psychotherapy, 9,* 299–318.

Rostaminejad, A., Behnammoghadam, M., Rostaminejad, M., Behnammoghadam, Z., & Bashti, S. (2017). Efficacy of eye movement desensitization and reprocessing on the phantom limb pain of patients with amputations within a 24-month follow-up. *International Journal of Rehabilitation Research, 40,* 209–214.

Rothbaum, B. O. (1997). A controlled study of eye movement desensitization and reprocessing in the treatment of posttraumatic stress disordered victims. *Bulletin of the Menninger Clinic, 61,* 317–334.

Rothbaum, B. O., Astin, M. C., & Marsteller, F. (2005). Prolonged exposure versus eye movement desensitization (EMDR) for PTSD rape victims. *Journal of Traumatic Stress, 18,* 607–616.

Rousseau, P.-F., El Khoury-Malhame, M., Reynaud, E., Boukezzi, S., Cancel, A., Zendjidjian, X., et al. (2019). Fear extinction learning improvement in PTSD after EMDR therapy: An fMRI study. *European Journal of Psychotraumatology, 10,* 1–11.

Russell, M. C. (2008). Treating traumatic amputation-related phantom limb pain: A case study utilizing eye movement desensitization and reprocessing (EMDR) within the armed services. *Clinical Case Studies, 7,* 136–153.

Russell, M. C., & Figley, C. R. (2013). *Treating traumatic stress disorders in military personnel: An EMDR practitioner's guide.* New York: Routledge.

Sack, M., Hofmann, A., Wizelman, L., & Lempa, W. (2008). Psychophysiological changes during EMDR and treatment outcome. *Journal of EMDR Practice and Research, 2,* 239–246.

Scheck, M. M., Schaeffer, J. A., & Gillette, C. S. (1998). Brief psychological intervention with traumatized young women: The efficacy of eye movement desensitization and reprocessing. *Journal of Traumatic Stress, 11,* 25–44.

Schneider, J., Hofmann, A., Rost, C., & Shapiro, F. (2008). EMDR in the treatment of chronic phantom limb pain. *Pain Medicine, 9*(1), 76–82.

Schubert, S. J., Lee, C. W., de Araujo, G., Butler, S. R., Taylor, G., & Drummond, P. (2016). The effectiveness of eye movement desensitization and reprocessing (EMDR) therapy to treat symptoms following trauma in Timor Leste. *Journal of Traumatic Stress, 29,* 141–148.

Shapiro, F. (1989). Efficacy of the eye movement desensitization procedure in the treatment of traumatic memories. *Journal of Traumatic Stress, 2,* 199–223.

Shapiro, F. (2018). *Eye movement desensitization and reprocessing: Basic principles, protocols, and procedures* (3rd ed.). New York: Guilford Press.

Stickgold, R. (2002). EMDR: A putative neurobiological mechanism of action. *Journal of Clinical Psychology, 58,* 61–75.

Suzuki, A., Josselyn, S. A., Frankland, P. W., Masushige, S., Silva, A. J., & Kida, S. (2004). Memory reconsolidation and extinction have distinct temporal and biochemical signatures. *Journal of Neuroscience, 24,* 4787–4795.

Taylor, S. (2003). Outcome predictors for three PTSD treatments: Exposure therapy, EMDR, and relaxation training (Special Issue on Posttraumatic Stress Disorder). *Journal of Cognitive Psychotherapy, 17,* 149–162.

Ter Heide, F. J., Mooren, T. M., van de Schoot, R., de Jongh, A., & Kleber, R. J. (2016). Eye movement desensitization and reprocessing therapy v. stabilization as usual for refugees: Randomised controlled trial. *British Journal of Psychiatry, 209,* 311–318.

van den Berg, D. P., de Bont, P. A., van der Vleugel, B. M., de Roos, C., de Jongh, A., van Minnen, A., et al. (2015). Prolonged exposure vs. eye movement desensitization and reprocessing vs. waiting list for posttraumatic stress disorder in patients with a psychotic disorder: A randomized clinical trial. *JAMA Psychiatry, 72,* 259–267.

van den Hout, M. A., Rijkeboer, M. T., Engelhard, I. M., Klugkist, I., Hornsveld, H., Toffolo, M., et al. (2012). Tones inferior to eye movements in the EMDR treatment of PTSD. *Behaviour Research and Therapy, 50,* 275–279.

van der Kolk, B. A., Spinazzola, J., Blaustein, M. E., Hopper, J. W., Hopper, E. K., Korn, D. L., et al. (2007). A randomized clinical trial of eye movement desensitization and reprocessing (EMDR), fluoxetine, and pill placebo in the treatment of posttraumatic stress disorder: Treatment effects and long-term maintenance. *Journal of Clinical Psychiatry, 68,* 37–46.

van Emmerik, A. A., Kamphuis, J. H., Noordhof, A., & Emmelkamp, P. M. (2011). Catch me if you can: Do the five-factor model personality traits moderate dropout and acute treatment response in post-traumatic stress disorder patients? *Psychotherapy and Psychosomatics, 80*(6), 386–388.

Vaughan, K., Armstrong, M., Gold, R., O'Connor, N., Jenneke, W., & Tarrier, N. (1994). A trial of eye movement desensitization compared to image habituation training and applied muscle relaxation in posttraumatic stress disorder. *Journal of Behavior Therapy, 25,* 283–291.

Wesselmann, D., Schweitzer, C., & Armstrong, S. (2014). *Integrative team treatment for attachment trauma in children: Family therapy and EMDR.* New York: Norton.

Wilson, S., Becker, L. A., & Tinker, R. H. (1995). Eye movement desensitization and reprocessing (EMDR): Treatment for psychologically traumatized individuals. *Journal of Consulting and Clinical Psychology, 63,* 928–937.

Wilson, S. A., Becker, L. A., & Tinker, R. H. (1997). Fifteen-month follow-up of eye movement desensitization and reprocessing (EMDR) treatment for posttraumatic stress disorder and psychological trauma. *Journal of Consulting and Clinical Psychology, 65*(6), 1047–1056.

Wolpe, J., & Abrams, J. (1991). Post-traumatic stress disorder overcome by eye movement desensitization: A case report. *Journal of Behavior Therapy and Experimental Psychiatry, 22,* 39–43.

World Health Organization. (2018). *International statistical classification of diseases and related health problems* (11th rev.). Geneva, Switzerland: Author. Retrieved from *https://icd.who.int/browse11/l-m/en.*

CHAPTER 15

Cognitive Therapy

Anke Ehlers

One of the basic ideas of cognitive therapy is that clients' symptoms and behavior make sense if one understands how they perceive themselves and the world, and what they make of these perceptions. To help clients change unhelpful cognitions that contribute to their symptoms and behavior, therapists need to "get into their clients' heads," that is, understand how they perceive and interpret the surrounding world, what they think about themselves, and what beliefs motivate their behavior.

Traumatic events are extremely negative events that everyone would find highly threatening and distressing. Yet what people find *most* distressing about a traumatic event, and what it means to them, varies greatly from person to person, and influences the probability of developing posttraumatic stress disorder (PTSD). Cognitive therapy for PTSD (CT-PTSD) addresses threatening personal meanings of trauma, together with characteristics of trauma memories and unhelpful coping strategies. This chapter describes the treatment procedures used in CT-PTSD and the theory behind them, reviews the evidence collected so far, and discusses the implementation of CT-PTSD in clinical practice, before outlining areas for future development.

Theoretical Background

Ehlers and Clark's (2000) cognitive model of PTSD was developed to explain why some people do not recover from traumatic events and develop chronic PTSD, and to serve as the framework for an individualized formulation of a client's problems and treatment. The model suggests that PTSD develops if individuals process traumatic experiences in a way that produces a sense of a *serious current threat*, which is driven, in turn, by two key processes (see Figure 15.1).

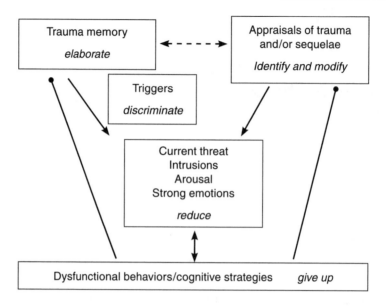

FIGURE 15.1. Treatment goals in cognitive therapy for PTSD (Ehlers & Clark, 2000). Pointed arrow heads indicate "leads to." Round arrow heads indicate "prevents a change in." Dashed arrows indicate "influences." From Ehlers (2013). Copyright © 2013 John Wiley & Sons. Reprinted with permission.

The first source of current threat are *negative appraisals* (personal meanings) of the trauma and/or its sequelae (e.g., reactions of other people, initial PTSD symptoms, physical consequences of the trauma) that go beyond what anyone would find threatening/horrific about the event. The perceived threat can be external or internal, and the type of negative emotion depends on the type of appraisal. Perceived *external* threat can result from appraisals about impending danger (e.g., "I cannot trust anyone"), leading to excessive fear, or appraisals about the unfairness of the trauma or its aftermath (e.g., "I will never be able to accept that the perpetrator got away with it"), leading to persistent anger. Perceived *internal* threat often relates to negative appraisals of one's behavior, emotions, or reactions during the trauma or to the perpetrators' or other people's humiliating or derogatory statements, and may lead to guilt (e.g., "It was my fault") or shame (e.g., "I am a bad person"). A common negative appraisal of consequences of the trauma in PTSD is perceived permanent change of the self or one's life (e.g., "I have permanently changed for the worse"), which can lead to sadness and hopelessness. In the case of multiply traumatized individuals, personal meanings tend to become more generalized (e.g., "I do not matter"; "I deserve bad things happening to me"; "I am worthless"), leading to an enduring sense of degradation, defeat, or low self-worth. The appraisals can become more embedded in a person's belief systems over time. For example, if an early life trauma has led a person to feel that he or she is damaged in some way, or unlucky in life, experiencing further trauma is likely to confirm this belief.

The second source of perceived current threat according to Ehlers and Clark (2000) are *characteristics of trauma memories*. The worst moments of the trauma are poorly elaborated in memory, that is, inadequately integrated into their context (both within the event, and within the context of previous and subsequent experiences/information). The effect of this is that people with PTSD remember the trauma in a disjointed way. When they recall the worst moments, it may be difficult for them to access other information that could correct impressions they had or predictions they made at the time: in other words, the memory for these moments has not been updated with what the individuals know now, and the threat they experienced during these moments is reexperienced as if it were happening right now rather than being a memory from the past.

Ehlers and Clark (2000) also noted that intrusive trauma memories are easily triggered in PTSD by sensory cues that overlap perceptually with those occurring during trauma (e.g., a similar sound, color, smell, shape, movement, or bodily sensation). They suggested that people during trauma mainly process perceptual features of the experience, and that two basic learning mechanisms, perceptual priming and generalized associative learning, lead to a poor discrimination of the stimuli in the current environment from those in the trauma. This means that perceptually similar stimuli are easily spotted and can trigger reexperiencing symptoms.

The problem is maintained by *cognitive strategies and behaviors* that people with PTSD use to reduce the sense of current threat. These strategies (such as effortful suppression of memories, rumination, excessive precautions to prevent future trauma or "safety behaviors," alcohol or drug use) maintain PTSD by preventing change in the appraisals or trauma memory, and/or by increasing symptoms—and thus keep the sense of a current threat going.

Figure 15.1 illustrates the three factors (appraisals, memory characteristics, cognitive/behavioral strategies) that maintain a sense of current threat and PTSD symptoms according to Ehlers and Clark's (2000) model. CT-PTSD targets these three factors. The model suggests three treatment goals:

- To modify excessively negative appraisals (meanings) of the trauma and its sequelae
- To reduce reexperiencing by elaboration of the trauma memories and discrimination of triggers
- To reduce behaviors and cognitive strategies that maintain the sense of current threat

Treatment Approach and Core Techniques

In common with other forms of cognitive therapy, CT-PTSD uses guided discovery as the primary therapeutic style. As the main focus of the intervention is the cognitions that stem from the traumas and induce a sense of current threat, strategies such as Socratic questioning aim to gently guide clients to explore and examine a wider range of evidence by asking questions that help them consider the problem from different perspectives, with the aim of generating a less threatening alternative interpretation. The therapist works from a perspective of curiosity, rather than trying to undermine or prove the client's perspective wrong. A nonthreatening, collaborative style of interaction and establishing a good therapeutic relationship are essential to working with trauma survivors.

Core interventions in CT-PTSD are:

• The therapist and client collaboratively develop an *individualized case formulation* that is an individualized version of Ehlers and Clark's (2000) model of PTSD, which serves as the framework for therapy. Treatment procedures are tailored to the formulation.

• *Reclaiming/rebuilding your life assignments* are designed from the first session onward to address the clients' perceived permanent change after trauma and involve reclaiming or rebuilding activities and social contacts.

• *Changing problematic appraisals* of the traumas and their sequelae (e.g., responses of others, physical consequences, symptoms of PTSD) involves information, guided discovery, and *behavioral experiments* throughout treatment. For appraisals of the traumas, this is closely integrated with the *updating memories procedure*.

• *Updating trauma memories* is a three-step procedure that includes (1) accessing memories of the worst moments during the traumatic events and their currently threatening meanings, (2) identifying information that updates these meanings (either information from the course of events during the trauma or from guided discovery and testing of predictions), and (3) linking the new meanings to the worst moments in memory (see a more detailed description later).

• *Discrimination training with triggers of reexperiencing* involves systematically spotting idiosyncratic triggers (often subtle sensory cues) and learning to discriminate between "now" (cues in a new safe context) and "then" (cues in the traumatic event) (see a more detailed description later).

• A *site visit* completes the memory updating and trigger discrimination (see Murray, Merritt, & Grey, 2015, for a detailed description).

• *Dropping unhelpful behaviors and cognitive processes* commonly includes discussing their advantages and disadvantages and *behavioral experiments*, whereby the patient experiments with reducing unhelpful strategies such as rumination, hypervigilance for threat, thought suppression, and excessive precautions (safety behaviors).

- A *blueprint* summarizes what the client has learned in treatment and includes plans for any setbacks.

Throughout treatment, the work on appraisals is closely interwoven with memory work and is tailored to the case formulation. The specific cognitive therapy techniques depend on the client's pattern of emotions and underlying cognitive themes: for clients with an overgeneralized sense of risk, *behavioral experiments* that test their predictions of impending harm (e.g., "I will be attacked again") are essential. For clients who are ashamed about what they did or did not do during the trauma, *surveys to discover other people's views* and compare them with the reactions they anticipated (e.g., "People will think I am weak and pathetic") are very helpful. If clients blame themselves for the trauma, treatment involves guided discovery of the contribution of other people and situational factors to the event, which are then summarized in a *pie chart*. For clients who are preoccupied with the injustice of the event, writing a letter (which is usually not sent) expressing the effect the trauma has had on their lives and expressing their anger is helpful, as well as a *cost–benefit analysis* of the advantages and disadvantages of staying angry.

Some of the behavioral and cognitive techniques used in other cognitive-behavioral therapy (CBT) treatments for PTSD are not used in CT-PTSD, such as repeated exposures to promote habituation and exposure hierarchies (the updating memories and trigger discrimination procedures are used instead), anxiety ratings in feared situations (Subjective Units of Distress/Discomfort Scale [SUDS]; the degree of conviction in appraisals and nowness of memories are rated instead), or thought records or rehearsal of rational responses (self-instruction).

Summary and Appraisal of the Evidence

Four cognitive therapy studies with a total of 189 participants were included in the evidence review for the prevention and treatment of PTSD guidelines developed by the International Society for Traumatic Stress Studies (ISTSS) and resulted in cognitive therapy receiving a *Strong* recommendation. These studies compared it with a wait-list/repeated-assessment control group (Duffy, Gillespie, & Clark, 2007; Ehlers, Clark, Hackmann, McManus, & Fennell, 2005; Ehlers et al., 2003, 2014) and with an emotion-focused supportive counseling group (Ehlers et al., 2014). All four of the studies were conducted in the United Kingdom. The results of the meta-analysis indicated that cognitive therapy showed a positive effect when compared with wait list or treatment as usual (TAU) and in comparison with emotion-focused supportive counseling, suggesting specificity of treatment effects. There has not, as yet, been a head-to-head trial of cognitive therapy with any of the other strongly recommended treatments: cognitive processing therapy (CPT), eye movement desensitization and reprocessing (EMDR) therapy, prolonged exposure (PE), or undifferentiated CBT with a trauma focus.

The participants in these studies included the survivors of motor vehicle accidents (Ehlers et al., 2003), a terrorist attack and other civil conflicts in Northern Ireland (Duffy et al., 2007), and a variety of different traumatic events (Ehlers et al., 2005, 2014). The range of chronicity of PTSD in these studies varied to include a duration of up to 20 years. In these trials, CT-PTSD was also found to be highly acceptable to clients, as indicated by very low dropout rates (3%, on average). It led to very large improvements in PTSD symptoms (intent-to-treat pre–post treatment effect sizes of around 2.5 for self-reported PTSD symptoms), disability, depression, anxiety, and quality of life, and over 70% of clients (intent-to-treat) recovered from PTSD. CT-PTSD was also shown to be superior to a self-help CBT booklet (not included in the ISTSS evidence review; Ehlers et al., 2003).

Outreach open trials treating consecutive samples of survivors of the Omagh and London bombings replicated the treatment effects observed in the trials (Brewin et al., 2010; Gillespie, Duffy, Hackmann, & Clark, 2002). It is noteworthy that the percentage of clients whose symptoms deteriorated with treatment was close to zero, and smaller than in clients waiting for treatment (Ehlers et al., 2014).

Three effectiveness studies implemented CT-PTSD in routine clinical services and evaluated outcomes in consecutive cases (Ehlers et al., 2013; Ehlers, Grey, et al., 2020) or a randomized controlled trial (RCT) (Duffy et al., 2007). The samples treated in these studies included a very wide range of clients, including those with complicating factors such as serious social problems, currently living in danger, very severe depression, borderline personality disorder, or multiple traumatic events and losses. Therapists included trainees in addition to experienced therapists. Outcomes remained very good, with large intent-to-treat pre–post treatment effect sizes of 1.25 and higher for PTSD symptoms. Around 60% of the clients who started therapy showed clinically significant change/remitted from PTSD. Dropout rates (around 15%) were somewhat higher than those in the RTCs of CT-PTSD (3%), but still below the average for RCTs of trauma-focused CBT of 23% (Bisson, Roberts, Andrew, Cooper, & Lewis, 2013). Hardly any clients experienced symptom deterioration (1.4% in Ehlers et al., 2013), and it is unclear whether this was related to treatment. These results, together with those of Schnurr and colleagues (2007) and Steenkamp, Litz, Hoge, and Marmar (2015) for PE therapy and CPT, are in line with Stewart and Chambless's (2009) conclusion that there is some loss of effectiveness in clinically representative samples compared to RCTs. The reasons remain unclear and require further investigation. They may include client factors (e.g., chronicity, comorbidity, attitude toward treatment), therapist factors (e.g., level of training, experience with PTSD), quality and consistency of treatment delivery (e.g., extent to which the traumas were addressed in treatment), social factors (e.g., financial problems, stability of living situation, ongoing threat), and organizational factors (e.g., limits to number or length of sessions in the service). It is noteworthy that the clients in the CT-PTSD effectiveness studies did not receive more sessions, on average, than those in the RCTs, despite the complexity of their mental health and social problems. There was also evidence that the treatment for clients with multiple traumas and social problems (who had a somewhat less favorable treatment outcome) was less trauma-focused than for other clients in the same cohort (Ehlers et al., 2013). Thus, the dose of trauma-focused work they received was less than ideal.

The efficacy of an intervention does not necessarily show that the underlying theory of its mechanism is correct. Investigations of the mediators of treatment effects are therefore needed. A study using growth curve modeling in a sample of 268 clients treated with CT-PTSD suggested that, in line with Ehlers and Clark's (2000) model, changes in negative appraisals drive changes in symptoms during treatment and not vice versa (Kleim et al., 2013). Wiedemann and colleagues (2020) replicated this result in a second consecutive cohort of clients treated with CT-PTSD and showed that the results extend to the other factors proposed in Ehlers and Clark's model: disjointedness of memories and maintaining behaviors such as safety behaviors, rumination, and thought suppression. Charquero-Ballester and colleagues (2019) analyzed patterns of brain network activation during a task that involved trauma-related and neutral pictures before and after CT-PTSD. Consistent with Ehlers and Clark's model, before therapy the brains of people with PTSD underutilized two subcomponents of the default mode network that are linked to memory contextualization and to mentalizing about self and others, compared to brains of traumatized and nontraumatized controls. After successful cognitive therapy, these differences in brain activity no longer occurred.

Overall, the evidence suggests that CT-PTSD is a safe and efficacious treatment for adults and children with PTSD following a wide range of traumas. However, the sample sizes were modest, and a need exists for further RCTs of CT-PTSD in some populations, such as survivors of abuse in early childhood or military veterans. RCTs comparing CT-PTSD against non-trauma-focused CBT would also be desirable. The treatment techniques used in CT-PTSD complement each other and are theoretically derived, but there are no dismantling studies so that it is not known whether all components are necessary. Effectiveness studies showed good results, but there was some loss of overall effects, and further studies of moderators of treatment effects are needed to determine whether subgroups of clients may require further adaptation of treatment procedures, especially the minority of about 20% who do not show reliable improvement in symptoms. Further studies of treatment mechanisms would also be desirable. For example, it would be interesting to compare the theory-derived specific mechanisms (reduction of maintaining appraisals, memory characteristics, cognitive strategies and behaviors) with nonspecific mechanisms such as therapeutic alliance.

Practical Delivery[1]

Duration of Treatment

For clients who currently reexperience a small number of traumas, CT-PTSD is usually delivered in up to 12 weekly sessions of 60–90 minutes, and up to three optional monthly booster sessions. The mean number of sessions is approximately 10. Weekly measures of PTSD symptoms, depression, and appraisals (the Post-Traumatic Cognitions Inventory [PTCI]; Foa, Ehlers, Clark, Tolin, & Orsillo, 1999), memory characteristics, rumination, and safety behaviors are helpful in monitoring the effects of the interventions and spotting remaining problems. For clients with multiple traumas that need to be addressed in treatment, more sessions are offered (usually around 20, but more may be required if the client has significant comorbidity or needs help with significant social problems). Note that for sessions including work on the trauma memory, such as imaginal reliving, updating memories, or the site visit, the therapist needs to allow sufficient time for the memory to be processed. Before going home, the client needs adequate time to refocus on current reality and his or her further plans for the day. These sessions would usually last around 90 minutes. Variations of the treatment format are also effective. A 7-day intensive version of the treatment (delivered over 7 consecutive working days, with 2–4 hours of treatment per day, plus a few booster sessions; Ehlers et al., 2014; Murray, El-Leithy, & Billings, 2017) and a self-study assisted brief treatment are similarly effective (Ehlers, Wild, et al., 2020). Regular case supervision is strongly recommended as it helps therapists generate different perspectives on the client's appraisals, provides support, and ensures adherence to protocol.

Assessment

After traumatic events, people may develop a range of psychological problems. Having experienced a trauma therefore does not necessarily mean that a client has PTSD and requires trauma-focused treatment. A careful diagnostic assessment is needed to ascertain that PTSD is one of the client's main problems. Risk to self and others must be assessed, and in some cases risky symptoms and behaviors may need to be an initial priority. Comorbid disorders, their onset and relationship to the trauma should also be assessed.

---

[1]A guide for therapists, video illustrations of treatment procedures, and treatment materials are available free of charge at *https://oxcadatresources.com*.

Other problems that may interfere with treatment (e.g., court cases, housing problems, pending surgery, interpersonal issues, debt, unclear outcome of an asylum application) should also be considered but do not rule out treatment.

How to Do CT-PTSD

A therapist's guide to CT-PTSD is available free of charge at *https://oxcadat-resources.com*. Here, we describe two unique procedures of CT-PTSD and some general points.

How to Achieve Emotional Shift through Cognitive Work

Cognitive therapy changes emotions through changes in cognitions, but it is important to bear in mind that generating an alternative interpretation (insight) is usually not sufficient to generate a large emotional shift. Crucial steps in therapy are to test the client's appraisals in behavioral experiments or surveys, which create experiential new evidence against the client's threatening interpretations. For example, behavioral experiments for clients with an overgeneralized sense of danger aim to modify their appraisals (e.g., "People can spot that I am an easy target") by specific assignments (e.g., going to a local shop to buy bread) that test their predictions (e.g., "I will be attacked again"). During the experiment, clients drop any safety behaviors (e.g., crossing the road when someone approaches) and hypervigilance and apply the "then versus now" discrimination technique (i.e., looking at other people to see how different they look from the perpetrator, paying attention to all the differences between the current situation and the trauma). The latter is important as intrusive memories may otherwise give clients the impression that they are under threat. Similarly, they link the new meanings to the relevant moments during the trauma in memory with the updating memories procedure, that is, by simultaneously holding the moment and the new meanings in mind to facilitate an emotional shift.

Focus on Appraisals That Induce a Sense of External or Internal Current Threat

People with PTSD often have a wide range of problems and of unhelpful cognitions. This can feel overwhelming for clients and therapists, and it is important for therapists and clients to agree that they will prioritize the PTSD work for a limited time and remain trauma-focused for the majority of the sessions, that is, to remain focused on the memories and appraisals that stem from the client's traumas and their aftermath. Our experience in supervision is that when therapists feel stuck, it helps to focus again on the question of which cognitions maintain the sense of internal or external current threat.

Changing Meanings of Trauma by Updating Trauma Memories

CT-PTSD uses a special procedure to access and shift problematic meanings (appraisals) of the trauma called the *updating trauma memories* procedure. This involves three steps, as listed below.

- *Step 1: Accessing and identifying personal meanings of the trauma that lead to a sense of current threat*
    - Access *hot spots* in memory (i.e., the moments during the trauma that create the greatest distress and sense of "nowness" during recall). Useful techniques include imaginal reliving, narrative writing, and questions about the worst moments of the trauma.
    - Discuss the content of *intrusive memories* and determine what moments of the trauma they represent (often omitted when talking about the trauma); then include these moments in imaginal reliving or narrative.
    - Explore the *personal meanings* of these moments.
- *Step 2: Identifying updating information*
    - Identify updating information—information that does not fit with the meanings, either from what happened during the course of the event, information from reliable sources, or by considering a wider range of interpretations in cognitive restructuring.
- *Step 3: Incorporating personal meanings of hot spots in memory*
    - Link the new information with the relevant moments in memory; the client holds the moment in mind while reminding him- or herself of updating information (reminders can be verbal, movement, touch, sounds, smells, tastes, or images).
    - Include updates in the narrative of this event.
    - Discuss how the client can remind him- or herself of the updates.

STEP 1: ACCESSING AND IDENTIFYING THREATENING PERSONAL MEANINGS

The first step involves accessing the worst moments of the trauma and their meaning through careful questioning (e.g., "What was the worst thing about this?"; "What did you think was going to happen?"; "What did this mean to you at the time?"; "What does this mean to you now?"; "What would it mean if what you feared most did happen?"). It is important to ask direct questions about clients' worst expected outcome, including their fears about dying, and to elicit the underlying meanings, as this guides what information is needed to update their trauma memory.

Imaginal reliving and narrative writing each have particular strengths in accessing the worst moments of the traumas (hot spots; Foa & Rothbaum, 1998) and their meanings, and the relative weight given to each in CT-PTSD depends on the client's level of engagement with the trauma memory and the length of the event. Imaginal reliving (Foa & Rothbaum, 1998) is particularly powerful in facilitating emotional engagement with the memory and accessing details of the memory (including emotions and sensory components). CT-PTSD only uses a few relivings (usually two to three) to access the hot spots sufficiently to assess their problematic meanings and move on to the steps of updating the meaning. Note that hot spots are addressed one at a time, and straightforward updates such as "I did not die" may be attempted as soon as the hot spot is identified, which can be as early as Session 1 or 2. Identifying hot spots may take longer if clients suppress their reactions or skip over difficult moments because, for example, they are ashamed about what happened.

Writing a narrative (Resick & Schnicke, 1993) is particularly useful when the traumatic event lasted for an extended period of time, if clients dissociate and lose contact with the present situation or have a very strong physical reaction (e.g., feeling faint, vomiting) when remembering the trauma, or when aspects of what happened or the order of events is unclear. The narrative is useful for considering the event as a whole and for identifying information from different moments that have implications for the problematic meanings of the trauma.

STEP 2: IDENTIFYING UPDATING INFORMATION

Once a hot spot and its meaning are identified, the next step is to identify information that does not fit with the problematic meanings (updating information). Some of the updating information may concern what happened in the trauma or afterward, and can be something that the client is already aware of, but has not yet been linked to the meaning of this particular moment in his or her memory, or something the client only remembers during imaginal reliving or narrative writing. Examples include knowledge that the outcome of the traumatic event was better than expected (e.g., the client did not die, is not paralyzed); information that explained the client's or other people's behavior (e.g., the client complied with the perpetrator's instructions because he had threatened to kill him; other people did not help because they were in shock); the realization that an impression or perception during the trauma was not true (e.g., the perpetrator had a toy gun rather than a real gun). Information and explanations from reliable sources or experts (e.g., cars are built in a way that makes explosions after accidents very unlikely; certain distressing procedures in the hospital were done to save the client's life) can also be very valuable in identifying updating information.

For other appraisals, guided discovery to generate an alternative perspective is necessary—for example, for appraisals such as "I am a bad person"; "It was my fault"; "My actions were disgraceful"; or "I attract disaster"—including cognitive therapy techniques such as Socratic questioning, systematic discussion of evidence for and against the appraisals, behavioral experiments, discussion of hindsight bias, pie charts, or surveys. Imagery techniques can also be helpful in widening the client's awareness of other factors that contributed to the event or in considering the value of alternative actions. For example, assault survivors who blame themselves for not fighting back during the trauma may visualize what would have happened if they had. This usually leads them to realize that had they fought back, this would have escalated the violence further, and the assailant might have injured them more seriously.

STEP 3: ACTIVE INCORPORATION OF THE UPDATING INFORMATION INTO THE HOT SPOTS

Once updating information that the client finds compelling has been identified, it is actively incorporated into the relevant hot spot. This can be done as soon as the updating information has been identified for that particular hot spot, for example, in the same session that the first reliving was done. Clients are asked to bring this hot spot to mind (either through imaginal reliving or reading the corresponding part of the narrative) and to then remind themselves (prompted by the therapist) of the updating information either (1) verbally (e.g., "I know now that . . ."); (2) by imagery (e.g., visualizing how one's wounds have healed, visualizing the perpetrator in prison, looking at a recent photo of the family or of oneself, visualizing the person who died in the trauma in a peaceful place where he or she is not suffering any longer); (3) by performing movements or actions that are incompatible with the original meaning of this moment (e.g., moving about or jumping up and down for hot spots that involved predictions about dying or being paralyzed); or (4) through incompatible sensations (e.g., touching a healed arm). To summarize the updating process, a written narrative is created that includes the new meanings for each hot spot and highlights them in a different font or color (e.g., "I know now that it was not my fault").

Identification and Discrimination of Triggers of Reexperiencing Symptoms

Clients with PTSD often report that intrusive memories and other reexperiencing symptoms occur "out of the blue" in a wide range of situations. Careful detective work done in collaboration with the therapist usually identifies sensory triggers that clients have not been aware of (e.g., particular colors, sounds, smells, tastes, touch, body posture, or movement). To identify these subtle triggers, client and therapist carefully analyze where and when reexperiencing symptoms occur. Systematic observation in the session (by the client and the therapist) and through homework is usually necessary to identify all triggers. Once a trigger has been identified, the next aim is to break the link between the trigger and the trauma memory.

This involves several steps. First, the client learns to distinguish between "then" and "now," that is, to focus on how the present triggers and their context (now) are different from the trauma (then). This leads him or her to realize that there are more differences than similarities and that he or she is responding to a memory, not to current reality.

Second, intrusions are intentionally triggered in therapy so that the client can learn to apply the then-versus-now discrimination. For example, traffic accident survivors may listen to sounds that remind them of the crash, such as brakes screeching, collisions, glass breaking, or sirens while focusing on all the differences between these sounds and their safe context and the trauma. Other examples include the following. People who were attacked with a knife may look at a range of metal objects, and those who were shot may listen to the sounds of gunfire generated on a computer. Survivors of bombings or fires may look at smoke produced by a smoke machine. People who saw a lot of blood during the trauma may look at red fluids. The then-versus-now discrimination can be facilitated by carrying out actions that were not possible during the trauma (e.g., movements that were not possible during the trauma, touching objects or looking at photos that remind them of their present life).

Third, clients apply these strategies in their natural environment. When reexperiencing symptoms occur, they remind themselves that they are responding to a memory and focus their attention on how the present situation is different from the trauma, and may carry out actions that were not possible during the trauma to remind themselves that the trauma is not happening again.

Tailored Intervention

As the CT-PTSD case formulation is tailored to each individual, it can be applied to a wide variety of presentations, traumas, age groups (Smith et al., 2007), and cultural backgrounds and can incorporate comorbid conditions, the effects of multiple traumas, or the multiple challenges faced by refugees (Grey & Young, 2008; Raval & Tribe, 2014). For example, comorbid depression may be related to some of the client's appraisals of the trauma and other life experiences (e.g., "I am worthless") and cognitive strategies (e.g., rumination). Comorbid panic disorder may have developed from interpretations of the reexperiencing symptoms (e.g., reexperiencing difficulty breathing, leading to the thought "I will suffocate"). And comorbid obsessive–compulsive disorder (OCD) may be linked to appraisals such as "I am contaminated" and linked behaviors such as excessive washing. Cultural beliefs may influence an individual's personal meanings of trauma and his or her attempts to come to terms with trauma memories in helpful and unhelpful ways. Treatment is tailored to the individual's beliefs, including cultural beliefs.

CT-PTSD allows for flexibility in the order in which the core treatment procedures are delivered. The memory-updating procedure often has a fast and profound effect on symptoms and is generally started early on. For patients with severe dissociative symptoms, training in trigger discrimination is conducted first, and narrative writing is preferred over imaginal reliving. In addition, for certain cognitive patterns, the memory work is prepared through discussion of the client's appraisals and cognitive processing at the time of the trauma. For example, when a client profoundly believes him- or herself to be at fault for a trauma, and the resultant guilt and/or shame prevents him or her from being able to describe it fully to the therapist, therapy would start with addressing such appraisals. If a client experienced mental defeat (the perceived loss of all autonomy; Ehlers, Maercker, & Boos, 2000) during an interpersonal trauma, therapy would start with discussing the traumatic situation from a wider perspective to raise the client's awareness that the perpetrators intended to control and manipulate his or her feelings and thoughts at the time, but that they no longer are exerting control now. Clients who are preoccupied with the injustice of the trauma may first express their anger in an (unsent) letter to the perpetrator.

When Treatment Does Not Work

A minority of clients do not achieve significant clinical benefit from a course of CT-PTSD, and the question then arises how best to manage the further care of these clients. There is no empirical evidence as of yet on how best to handle this circumstance, but clinical experience suggests a few possibilities. First, it may emerge in the course of therapy that PTSD is currently not the respective client's main problem; comorbid conditions (e.g., depression, OCD, borderline personality disorder, substance use disorder, physical problems), social problems (e.g., debts, no stable housing, illness in the family), legal problems (e.g., custody issues, asylum), or a new negative life event (e.g., death of a significant other) may have become their principal problem, making them unable to sufficiently engage in a trauma-focused treatment at this time. These clients may benefit from treatment for the comorbid conditions first, and support and problem solving in managing their social issues or new life event. Non-trauma-focused CBT such as stress management may be helpful in managing their PTSD symptoms during this time. Another course of CT-PTSD may then be attempted when such a client is ready to work on his or her trauma memories. Second, some clients may not fully engage with treatment for practical reasons (e.g., unable to attend sessions regularly, little time or privacy to work on their homework assignments) or concerns about the treatment (e.g., doubts about its rationale or anticipated/threatened negative reactions from others). These clients may find it easier to switch to an intensive or semi-intensive treatment format. Third, some clients whose traumas happened many years ago and were life-changing, who are socially very isolated, who have many traumas to work on or long-standing negative beliefs about themselves and other people, a longer course of treatment may be indicated. Fourth, some clients may prefer to try a course of medication for PTSD or an alternative treatment such as non-trauma-focused CBT.

Future Developments

Not all clients can attend weekly treatment sessions with a therapist. Novel forms of treatment delivery are of interest to increase client choice and to use the therapist's time efficiently so that more patients can benefit from treatment. Several variations of treatment delivery have been shown to be efficacious for CT-PTSD. Intensive delivery of treatment over 5–7 working days, or settings such as residential therapy units, may be preferable for some clients (Ehlers et al., 2014). Self-study modules that cover some of the content of CT-PTSD save about 50% of the therapist's time without loss of efficacy (Ehlers, Wild, et al., 2020). They may also be useful in therapist training. Therapist-assisted Internet-delivered CT-PTSD has also shown promise in a pilot study (Wild et al., 2016) and is currently being investigated in an RCT. Support is delivered through online messages and weekly phone calls in 20–25% of the time needed in face-to-face therapy.

The best ways to deliver training for CT-PTSD remain to be investigated. Observations of large-scale efforts to disseminate trauma-focused CBT, such as the English National Health Service Improving Access to Psychological Therapies (IAPT) program and the Veterans Administration health care system in the United States (Clark, 2018; Foa, Gillihan, & Bryant, 2013), have shown that alongside workshops and a manual, supervision of training cases and use of weekly measures of symptoms to monitor the effect of interventions are important in training therapists to a sufficient standard. Online training materials that are accessible during training and beyond may help increase therapists' competency and confidence in delivering treatment.

Summary

Overall, the evidence suggests that CT-PTSD is a safe and efficacious treatment for adults and children with PTSD with high acceptability to clients, both in RCTs and routine clinical settings. Studies have included clients with a wide range of traumas, chronicity, and comorbidity. Nevertheless, there is a need for further RCTs of CT-PTSD in populations such as survivors of early childhood abuse or military veterans. New forms of treatment delivery have shown promise and may help increase client choice and access to treatment. There are gaps in knowledge, though, that still need to be addressed in further studies. This includes further studies of moderators and mediators of treatment effects, and of the best way to train therapists in CT-PTSD.

REFERENCES

Bisson, J. I., Roberts, N. P., Andrew, M., Cooper, R., & Lewis, C. (2013). Psychological therapies for chronic post-traumatic stress disorder (PTSD) in adults. *Cochrane Database of Systematic Reviews*, Issue 12, Article No. CD003388.

Brewin, C. R., Fuchkan, N., Huntley, Z., Robertson, M., Scragg, P., d'Ardenne, P., et al. (2010). Outreach and screening following the 2005 London bombings: Usage and outcomes. *Psychological Medicine, 40*, 2049–2057.

Charquero-Ballester, M., Kleim, B., Ruff, C., Williams, S. C. R., Woolrich, M., Vidaurre, D., et al. (2019). Spatiotemporal dynamics underlying successful cognitive therapy for posttraumatic stress disorder. *CNS Abstracts*.

Clark, D. M. (2018). Realizing the mass public benefit of evidence-based psychological therapies: The IAPT program. *Annual Review of Psychology, 14*, 159–183.

Duffy, M., Gillespie, K., & Clark, D. M. (2007). Post-traumatic stress disorder in the context of terrorism and other civil conflict in Northern Ireland: Randomised controlled trial. *British Medical Journal, 334*, 1147.

Ehlers, A., & Clark, D. M. (2000). A cognitive model of posttraumatic stress disorder. *Behaviour Research and Therapy, 38*, 319–345.

Ehlers, A., Clark, D. M., Hackmann, A., McManus, F., & Fennell, M. (2005). Cognitive therapy for post-traumatic stress disorder: Development and evaluation. *Behaviour Research and Therapy, 43*, 413–431.

Ehlers, A., Clark, D. M., Hackmann, A., McManus, F., Fennell, M., Herbert, C., et al. (2003). A randomized controlled trial of cognitive therapy, a self-help booklet, and repeated assessments as early interventions for posttraumatic stress disorder. *Archives of General Psychiatry, 60*, 1024–1032.

Ehlers, A., Grey, N., Warnock-Parkes, W., Wild, J., Stott, R., Cullen, D., et al. (2020). *Effectiveness of cognitive therapy for PTSD in routine clinical care: Second phase implementation.* Manuscript submitted for publication.

Ehlers, A., Grey, N., Wild, J., Stott, R., Liness, S., Deale, A., et al. (2013). Implementation of cognitive therapy in routine clinical care: Effectiveness and moderators of outcome in a consecutive sample. *Behaviour Research and Therapy, 51*, 742–752.

Ehlers, A., Hackmann, A., Grey, N., Wild, J., Liness, S., Albert, I., et al. (2014). A randomized controlled trial of 7-day intensive and standard weekly cognitive therapy for PTSD and emotion-focused supportive therapy. *American Journal of Psychiatry, 171*, 294–304.

Ehlers, A., Maercker, A., & Boos, A. (2000). PTSD following political imprisonment: The role of mental defeat, alienation, and permanent change. *Journal of Abnormal Psychology, 109*, 45–55.

Ehlers, A., Wild, J., Stott, R., Warnock-Parkes, E., Grey, N., & Clark, D. M. (2020). *Efficient use of therapist time in the treatment of posttraumatic stress disorder: A randomized clinical trial of brief self-study assisted and standard weekly cognitive therapy for PTSD.* Manuscript submitted for publication.

Ehring, T., Kleim, B., & Ehlers, A. (2013). Cognition and emotion in posttraumatic stress disorder. In M. D. Robinson, E. Watkins, & E. Harmon-Jones (Eds.), *Handbook of cognition and emotion* (pp. 401–420). New York: Guilford Press.

Foa, E. B., Ehlers, A., Clark, D. M., Tolin, D., & Orsillo, S. (1999). The Post-Traumatic Cognitions Inventory (PTCI): Development and validation. *Psychological Assessment, 11*, 303–314.

Foa, E. B., Gillihan, S. J., & Bryant, R. A. (2013). Challenges and successes of evidence-based treatments for posttraumatic stress: Lessons learned from prolonged exposure therapy for PTSD. *Psychological Science in the Public Interest, 14,* 65–111.

Foa, E. B., & Rothbaum, B. O. (1998). *Treating the trauma of rape: Cognitive-behaviour therapy for PTSD.* New York: Guilford Press.

Gillespie, K., Duffy, M., Hackmann, A., & Clark, D. M. (2002). Community based cognitive therapy in the treatment of post-traumatic stress disorder following the Omagh bomb. *Behaviour Research and Therapy, 40,* 345–357.

Grey, N., & Young, K. (2008). Cognitive behaviour therapy with refugees and asylum seekers experiencing traumatic stress symptoms. *Behavioural and Cognitive Psychotherapy, 36*(1), 3–19.

Kleim, B., Grey, N., Hackmann, A., Nussbeck, F., Wild, J., Stott, R., et al. (2013). Cognitive change predicts symptom reduction with cognitive therapy for posttraumatic stress disorder. *Journal of Consulting and Clinical Psychology, 81,* 383–393.

Murray, H., El-Leithy, S., & Billings, J. (2017). Intensive cognitive therapy for posttraumatic stress disorder in routine clinical practice: A matched comparison audit. *British Journal of Clinical Psychology, 56,* 476–478.

Murray, H., Merritt, C., & Grey, N. (2015). Returning to the scene of the trauma in PTSD treatment–why, how and when? *Cognitive Behaviour Therapist, 8,* e26.

Raval, H., & Tribe, R. (2014). *Working with interpreters in mental health.* London: Routledge.

Resick, P. A., & Schnicke, M. K. (1993). *Cognitive processing therapy for rape victims.* Newbury Park, CA: SAGE.

Schnurr, P. P., Friedman, M. J., Engel, C. C., Foa, E. B., Shea, M. T., Chow, B. K., et al. (2007). Cognitive behavioral therapy for posttraumatic stress disorder in women: A randomized controlled trial. *Journal of the American Medical Association, 297,* 820–830.

Smith, P., Yule, W., Perrin, S., Tranah, T., Dalgleish, T., & Clark, D. M. (2007). Cognitive behavioural therapy for PTSD in children and adolescents: A preliminary randomized controlled trial. *Journal of the American Academy of Child and Adolescent Psychiatry, 46,* 1051–1061.

Steenkamp, M. M., Litz, B. T., Hoge, C. W., & Marmar, C. R. (2015). Psychotherapy for military-related PTSD: A review of randomized clinical trials. *Journal of the American Medical Association, 324,* 489–500.

Stewart, R. E., & Chambless, D. L. (2009). Cognitive–behavioral therapy for adult anxiety disorders in clinical practice: A meta-analysis of effectiveness studies. *Journal of Consulting and Clinical Psychology, 77*(4), 595–606.

Wiedemann, M., Wild, J., Grey, N., Warnock-Parkes, E., Clark, D. M., & Ehlers, A. (2020). *Processes of change in cognitive therapy for PTSD.* Manuscript submitted for publication.

Wild, J., Warnock-Parkes, E., Grey, N., Stott, R., Wiedemann, M., Canvin, L., et al. (2016). Internet-delivered cognitive therapy for PTSD: A development pilot series. *European Journal of Psychotraumatology, 7,* 31019.

CHAPTER 16

Pharmacological and Other Biological Treatments

Jonathan I. Bisson, Matthew D. Hoskins, and Dan J. Stein

The majority of people with posttraumatic stress disorder (PTSD) who present for treatment are prescribed medication, either on its own or in combination with psychological treatment. Given the proven efficacy of several pharmacological treatments, this represents a major opportunity to improve the health and well-being of people with PTSD. Unfortunately, the full potential of pharmacological treatment is not currently realized, not least as a result of prescribing practice not being based on the evidence currently available. This chapter aims to help clinicians interpret the current evidence regarding the prescription of medication for PTSD; provide advice on what, when, and how to prescribe; and discuss key considerations when prescribing medication for PTSD. It also considers other biological treatments of PTSD. Although we will include some discussion of pharmacotherapy augmentation, the use of medication for PTSD prophylaxis, agents specifically used as adjuncts to psychotherapy, and pharmacotherapy in children and adolescents are beyond the scope of this chapter.

Theoretical Context

Given our knowledge of the neurobiology of PTSD, there is good reason to believe that pharmacological treatment approaches should be beneficial. Important advances in understanding the neurocircuitry, neurogenetics, and neurochemistry of PTSD have been made. It is currently hypothesized that a number of different systems are involved in the development and maintenance of PTSD, with various neurotransmitters, neuropeptides, and glucocorticoids being implicated in its neurobiology, including catechol-amines, opioids, gamma aminobutyric acid (GABA), glutamate, serotonin, oxytocin, and cortisol.

Considerable evidence exists, for example, from animal research on fear conditioning, and from clinical research on PTSD to suggest that over-activity of the noradrenergic system is a fundamental element of this disor-der and that attenuation should be beneficial (Southwick et al., 1999). There are various ways to do this, either directly through drugs that work through their effects on adrenergic receptors (e.g., propranolol and prazosin) or indi-rectly (e.g., hydrocortisone to reduce noradrenaline release). This neurobio-logical work has given impetus to a range of clinical trials in PTSD.

Promising data from both preclinical and clinical work have the poten-tial to inform prescribing for PTSD. There is also a view that a better under-standing of the range of neurobiological alterations in PTSD will help lead to personalized interventions for this disorder. At the same time, our under-standing of the neurobiology of PTSD remains partial, and the limited effect of many drugs in clinical trials highlights the need for more research that may lead to the development of more effective pharmacological treatments for PTSD.

Description of Techniques

• *Selective serotonin reuptake inhibitors (SSRIs).* The most common approach to the pharmacological treatment of PTSD is the prescription of an SSRI. This class of drugs, which includes citalopram, fluoxetine, parox-etine, and sertraline, is widely prescribed for depression and anxiety.

• *Serotonin and noradrenaline reuptake inhibitors (SNRIs).* Duloxetine and venlafaxine are the most widely used SNRIs. At lower doses, their effect is similar to that of SSRIs, but at higher doses, some of these agents also inhibit the reuptake of another monoamine, noradrenaline, leading to greater avail-ability of this chemical within synapses.

• *Monoamine reuptake inhibitors (MARIs).* This group of drugs, com-monly known as tricyclic antidepressants, includes amitriptyline, dothiepin, and imipramine. In addition to serotonin and noradrenaline, these agents antagonize histamine H1 receptors, a property sometimes used to help insomnia.

• *Monoamine oxidase inhibitors (MAOIs).* Phenelzine and tranylcypro-mine are probably the best known MAOIs and work by inhibiting the actions of enzymes that break down monoamines, thereby also increasing the amounts of synaptic monoamine. Their association with a hypertensive cri-sis after eating certain foods has discouraged practitioners from prescribing them, although with care they can be relatively safe and well-tolerated drugs.

● *Other antidepressants.* Other antidepressants are widely used to treat PTSD. Mirtazapine exerts its main effects on serotonin, noradrenaline, and histamine through a different mechanism than other antidepressants. Sedation is a common side effect that is sometimes used to treat insomnia in PTSD sufferers. Trazadone primarily affects the serotonin system, with a weaker effect on histamine. Its sedative side effect is also used to treat insomnia so the drug is often prescribed in combination with an SSRI or SNRI to assist sleep rather than as an antidepressant per se.

● *Antipsychotics.* The most commonly used antipsychotics for PTSD are the newer-generation "atypical antipsychotics," for example, olanzapine, quetiapine, and risperidone. Like older antipsychotics, they are anti-dopaminergic but they also affect the serotonergic system. The result is generally a tranquilizing drug without as marked motoric side effects as the "typical antipsychotics," although they do have a number of other adverse effects that can be problematic, including weight gain, oversedation, and the development of a metabolic syndrome that is associated with cardiovascular disease and diabetes.

● *Benzodiazepines.* Despite widespread serious concerns about the risk of dependency and regulatory warnings not to prescribe benzodiazepines for more than a few weeks, these medications are still frequently prescribed to PTSD sufferers. Commonly used drugs in this class include those prescribed for anxiety reduction, for example, diazepam, and those prescribed for sedation, for example, temazepam.

● *Anticonvulsants.* Most anticonvulsants impact the GABA system and calcium and/or sodium channels, reducing glutamate release and preventing the excitability that results in a convulsion. These drugs include carbamazepine, lamotrigine, and valproate and have been used increasingly for mood stabilization and as adjunctive treatments across a range of mental disorders.

● *Other drugs.* Other drugs have been used to treat PTSD, including agents that act on the noradrenergic system (e.g., prazosin and propranolol), or other components of the hypothalamic–pituitary–adrenal axis (e.g., hydrocortisone).

Summary and Appraisal of the Evidence

Monotherapy

The evidence summaries prepared for the guidelines issued by the International Society for Traumatic Stress Studies (ISTSS) concerned randomized controlled trials (RCTs) of pharmacological treatments used as monotherapy for PTSD. Forty-nine includable RCTs were found that considered 16 drugs. Thirty-nine (80%) of the included RCTs had usable data that were included in the meta-analyses. Nineteen (49%) were of the SSRIs fluoxetine, paroxetine, and sertraline, with venlafaxine being the only other drug with more than 500 individuals included in a single meta-analysis.

Fluoxetine, paroxetine, sertraline, and venlafaxine all satisfied the requirement for a *Low Effect* recommendation. This signifies robust evidence of reasonably high quality that these treatments will result in small but clinically significant benefits for people with PTSD who take them. The only other drug with strong enough evidence to recommend was quetiapine, which received an *Intervention with Emerging Evidence* recommendation for the treatment of PTSD in adults.

There was insufficient evidence for the other drugs included to be recommended, but it is interesting to note that four of them (amitriptyline, mirtazapine, a neurokinin-1 antagonist, and phenelzine) were significantly superior to placebo in trials with insufficient participants (<20 per arm) to meet the threshold for recommendation. These drugs are good candidates for further research and may prove to be effective treatments for PTSD.

Most of the RCTs included were of general populations of outpatients with PTSD who had been traumatized by a variety of events, and the results therefore should be generalizable to various populations. That said, it has been proposed that there are differential drug effects across PTSD populations (e.g., ICD-11 [World Health Organization, 2018] includes "complex PTSD" as a new diagnosis, which deserves additional pharmacotherapy research).

It is very difficult to compare the results of pharmacological treatment trials employing placebo controls and double blinding with psychological treatment trials using wait-list or usual-care controls, with neither the participant nor the treating clinician being blinded to treatment. In common with other guideline development groups, the ISTSS Guidelines Committee determined a priori rules to allow comparison of different types of treatment, making the threshold required for a *Strong* recommendation for a drug tested through placebo-controlled RCTs 50% less than that for psychological treatments tested through wait-list or usual-care RCTs. Whether the 50% lower threshold accurately reflects the true level is open for debate, but using this meant that the best-evidenced drug treatments for PTSD were recommended at a lower level of strength than the psychological treatments with the best evidence of treatment for PTSD.

There is a small evidence base that directly compares pharmacotherapy, psychotherapy, or combined treatment. An early meta-analysis of four trials (Hetrick, Purcell, Garner, & Parslow, 2010) found insufficient evidence to determine the relative efficacy of combined treatment, and subsequent trials have been inconsistent (Popiel, Zawadzki, Praglowska, & Teichman, 2015; Schneier et al., 2012; Simon et al., 2008). Nevertheless, in clinical practice, combined treatment is often employed (Marshall & Cloitre, 2000), and there is ongoing research interest in "medication-assisted psychotherapy" (Amoroso & Workman, 2016). In many regions, prescribing a drug with evidence of effect is often the only potentially effective treatment available, given waiting lists for evidence-based psychological treatments, with pharmacotherapy becoming the default treatment and psychotherapy combined at a later date.

The ISTSS guideline recommendations for drugs used as monotherapy for PTSD are shown in Table 16.1.

Augmentation

Although the ISTSS guideline scoping questions did not include queries regarding augmentation of pharmacological treatment with additional pharmacological treatment, a parallel review using the same searches was undertaken concerning this question and will be referred to in this chapter. Sixteen studies were included covering three drugs: prazosin (nine studies, 381 participants), risperidone (five studies, 385 participants), and topiramate (two studies, 97 participants). There was sufficient evidence to issue a *Standard* recommendation for prazosin and risperidone but insufficient evidence to recommend topiramate, which was not statistically superior to placebo.

Quality of the Evidence

The quality of the pharmacological RCTs, assessed by the Cochrane risk of bias tool (Higgins & Green, 2011) and modified GRADE criteria (see *www.gradeworkinggroup.org*), included in the meta-analyses was moderate but, overall, comparable with the highest-quality psychological RCTs included in the meta-analyses that informed the guidelines. There were some issues that indicated risk of bias in the results, especially with respect to the selective reporting of results. Some studies did have more fundamental methodological flaws or lack of clarity around randomization concealment and blinding of posttreatment assessors. The studies included in the meta-analyses displayed quite significant statistical and clinical heterogeneity, both of which impact interpretation of the results to a degree. The majority of participants included in the RCTs had had their PTSD for a number of years

---

TABLE 16.1. ISTSS Guideline Recommendations for Pharmacological Monotherapy

Interventions with Low Effect—Fluoxetine, paroxetine, sertraline, and *venlafaxine* are recommended as low effect treatments for adults with PTSD.

Intervention with Emerging Evidence—Quetiapine has emerging evidence of efficacy for the treatment of adults with PTSD.

*Insufficient Evidence to Recommend—*There is insufficient evidence to recommend *amitriptyline, brofaromine, divalproex, ganaxolone, imipramine, ketamine, lamotrigine, mirtazapine, neurokinin-1 antagonist, olanzapine, phenelzine, tiagabine,* or *topiramate* for the treatment of adults with PTSD.

and exhibited moderate to severe symptoms of PTSD. Most RCTs had broad inclusion criteria for traumatic events, meaning that participants had been exposed to various traumatic events. PTSD had to be the primary condition, but some comorbidity was common. Most studies included depression but excluded potential participants who were suicidal, had psychosis or other major comorbidities such as substance dependence. The vast majority of the studies were undertaken in higher-income countries. All of these factors raise questions around the generalizability of the findings to people with PTSD who would not have been included in the studies and to those living in different settings than where the research studies were conducted.

Dosing

Another important factor to consider, especially with respect to implementation of the evidence, is the doses of medication that were used in the studies. Some studies (e.g., Marshall, Beebe, Oldham, & Zaninelli, 2001; Martenyi, Brown, & Caldwell, 2007) used fixed doses, but most studies followed a prescribing algorithm whereby drug dosage was increased every few weeks if individuals did not recover. The mean doses of the recommended drugs used are shown in Table 16.2; they are well above the standard starting doses. It is clear that a number of individuals needed the maximum level of medication allowed and tolerated during the trial to achieve maximum benefit, indicating that they did not improve sufficiently with lower doses.

The caveat here is that if a longer duration of time had elapsed before increasing a dose in the RCTs, then it is possible more participants would have improved on lower doses. Indeed, it has been argued that improvements can take longer to occur following an increase in medication for PTSD than for depression (National Collaborating Centre for Mental Health, 2005), although the evidence for this claim is not strong. The current evidence certainly suggests that it is inappropriate to keep people with PTSD on lower doses of the recommended drugs if they have not or only partially responded, are tolerating the medication prescribed, and treatment remains indicated.

TABLE 16.2. Mean Trial Doses of Recommended Drugs

Drug	Mean dose
Fluoxetine	41.4 mg
Paroxetine	35.1 mg
Sertraline	136.7 mg
Venlafaxine	223.1 mg
Quetiapine	258.0 mg

Adverse Effects

Due to regulatory requirements, the reporting of adverse effects in pharmacological treatment trials tends to be much better than for psychological treatment trials. Those reported in PTSD treatment trials are very similar to those reported in trials with the same drugs for depression, anxiety, and other disorders. Common adverse effects for paroxetine, fluoxetine, sertraline, and venlafaxine include nausea and sexual dysfunction. Quetiapine can cause sedation and weight gain, and has been associated with cardiac effects, meaning that an electrocardiogram is required before initiating treatment with it. Overall, the recommended drugs appeared to be reasonably well tolerated in the included RCTs and there was no evidence that they should not be considered for use because of adverse effects.

Practical Delivery of the Recommendations

As with all treatments for PTSD, it is vital that pharmacological treatment only be prescribed after an accurate assessment of a client's needs that takes into account her or his individual circumstances. Key issues to consider before prescribing medication (or in weighing whether to prescribe medication, psychotherapy, or combined treatment) include primary diagnosis; comorbidity; alternative treatment options; attitude toward medication; previous response to medication; family history of response to medication; expectations of medication; awareness of potential adverse effects; other prescribed drugs and potential interactions with medication for PTSD and other substance use and potential interactions with medication for PTSD. Medication for PTSD should only be prescribed when a clinician believes the likely benefits outweigh the risks and when the individual is equipped with the knowledge necessary to make a fully informed decision.

Prescribing medication is often suboptimal, and this has led to attempts to formalize prescribing through the development of prescribing algorithms. This is common practice in many disorders and is widely used for mental health disorders (e.g., Taylor, Barnes, & Young, 2018). Research in depression has shown that prescribing according to an algorithm resulted in significantly better outcomes than prescribing based purely on clinician choice (Guo et al., 2015). It seems likely that this finding would apply to PTSD, leading the Cardiff University Traumatic Stress Research Group to develop a prescribing algorithm based on the ISTSS treatment recommendations (Bisson, Baker, Dekker, & Hoskins, 2020). This is being introduced nationally through the All Wales Traumatic Stress Quality Improvement Initiative and will be referred to in this chapter to highlight an example of how the ISTSS pharmacological treatment recommendations are being implemented into practice.

There are a number of principles that underpin the Cardiff algorithm:

1. As a general rule, only one medication should be introduced or changed at once.
2. Patients should be reviewed at least every 4 weeks to consider their progress and tolerance of medication, and to determine if a change to medication is required.
3. Although tied to the evidence base, some flexibility based on other factors is allowed, in line with evidence-based practice (Sackett, Rosenberg, Muir Gray, Haynes, & Richardson, 1996).
4. Regular consideration should be given to the accuracy of the diagnosis and the presence of other factors that need addressing to facilitate the effectiveness of medication (e.g., compliance, social factors, and alcohol misuse).

These principles are pragmatic and reflect good clinical practice, but it is acknowledged that other factors, for example, configuration of local services, and mental and physical comorbidities, may necessitate changes to the algorithm.

Algorithm-Based Pharmacological Treatment for PTSD

Step 1

If an individual with PTSD and her or his treating clinician agree that treatment with medication is indicated and desired, the most logical approach, based on the current evidence base, would be to prescribe one of the three recommended SSRIs (fluoxetine, paroxetine, or sertraline). Unless there are any contraindications, the drugs should be prescribed using the doses suggested in Table 16.3. If, after 4 weeks, the patient continues to experience significant PTSD symptoms and is tolerating the medication, and it is agreed that pharmacological treatment should be continued, the dose ought to be increased by the amount shown in Table 16.3. This procedure would be repeated, resulting in an individual with PTSD who is tolerating medication but continues to exhibit symptoms, reaching the maximum dose of fluoxetine and paroxetine at Week 8 and sertraline at Week 12. A further 4 weeks

TABLE 16.3. Recommended Pharmacological Treatment Doses

Drug	Starting Dose (daily)	Dosing Increment (monthly)	Maximum Dose (daily)
Fluoxetine	20 mg	20 mg	60 mg
Paroxetine	20 mg	20 mg	60 mg
Sertraline	50 mg	50 mg	200 mg
Venlafaxine	75 mg	75 mg	300 mg

should be allowed to determine the response to the maximum dose before making any further changes.

Step 2

If an individual has not responded to the maximum tolerated dose of one of the SSRIs, an alternative medication should be considered. Before doing this, it is important to check that there have been no changes to the clinical presentation and that both the patient and the clinician consider ongoing pharmacological treatment appropriate. The next step involves reducing the existing drug and replacing/cross-tapering it with an alternative. It would be reasonable to try a different SSRI, particularly if an individual has not tolerated one SSRI and may improve with another. If an individual has not shown a significant response to a particular SSRI, it is theoretically unlikely that he or she will do significantly better with an alternative SSRI, and the introduction of venlafaxine is therefore a logical next step. To introduce venlafaxine, the SSRI should be reduced by the incremental dose on a weekly basis and, at the point of stopping, venlafaxine introduced at 37.5 mg twice a day or 75 mg in the morning if the long-acting preparation has been prescribed. The individual should be reviewed monthly with the dose of venlafaxine titrated up by 75 mg at a time to a maximum of 300 mg daily, if needed.

Step 3

In the absence of an adequate response to venlafaxine and subject to it being tolerated, the next step would be to augment it with either prazosin (with particular attention being paid to postural hypotension[1]) or risperidone. (If an individual does not tolerate venlafaxine or responds less well to it than to an SSRI, it is recommended that the SSRI be reinstated in place of venlafaxine and augmented.) Given the side-effect profile of risperidone, the *Intervention with Emerging Evidence* recommendation of quetiapine, and its more favorable side-effect profile, this drug may be used in preference to risperidone. It is, however, acknowledged that the current evidence for quetiapine comes from an RCT in which it was used as a monotherapy and not for augmentation. Quetiapine is initiated at 25 mg a day at night. After 1 week, if tolerated, it is increased to 25 mg twice a day. The dose can be increased by 50 mg a day increments, as indicated, at monthly appointments with a clinician. A maximum of 400 mg a day, based on clinical response and

---

[1]As there is a risk of severe first-dose hypotension, the first and second doses should be taken while sitting on a bed just before lying down. It is important to keep well hydrated while taking prazosin and to get up slowly—initially sitting up on the bed and then slowly standing up. For the first two nights, it is important for men to sit on the toilet to urinate rather than stand up.

tolerability, is recommended in the algorithm, although up to 800 mg daily was used in the trial (Villarreal et al., 2016).

Additional Steps

If people with PTSD do not respond to fluoxetine, paroxetine, sertraline, or venlafaxine on their own or in combination with prazosin, risperidone, or quetiapine, prescribed as described in Steps 1, 2, and 3, they have reached the end of the current evidence-based pharmacological treatment algorithm for PTSD. Unfortunately, this is not an uncommon occurrence, especially in individuals with more complex or severe presentations of PTSD. It is also not uncommon for people with PTSD to be unable to tolerate the maximum dose of one or more drugs. In both these scenarios, alternative steps can be considered but become more evidence-informed than evidence-based. Before embarking on such an approach, it is clearly vital that the patient be fully aware of the situation and able to make a fully informed decision about continuing with pharmacological treatment.

As stated, other pharmacological treatments have been shown to benefit people with PTSD in RCTs but did not meet the requirements to be recommended in the latest ISTSS treatment guidelines. Several of these have been recommended in previous guidelines for the treatment of PTSD, for instance, the National Institute of Health and Care Excellence in the United Kingdom recommended amitriptyline, mirtazapine, and phenelzine based on the same RCT evidence available when the current ISTSS guidelines were developed. A network meta-analysis of drug trials in PTSD also highlighted the potential value of phenelzine (Cipriani et al., 2018). It is therefore reasonable to consider these drugs as alternatives to those recommended by ISTSS if the latter do not work or cannot be tolerated.

Mirtazapine has the advantage of being able to be prescribed in combination with SSRIs and venlafaxine; indeed, some evidence of benefit has been reported for such combinations in depression (Blier et al., 2010), although a large recent pragmatic RCT did not show benefit from the addition of mirtazapine in primary care (Kessler et al., 2018). In general, mirtazapine is started at 30 mg at night, although it can be prescribed at 15 mg that, paradoxically, is more sedative than higher doses, and this dose tends to be favored if the drug is being prescribed primarily to help with sleep.

Amitriptyline and, particularly, phenelzine should not be prescribed in combination with SSRIs or venlafaxine, and a wash-out period of at least a week (or 5 weeks for fluoxetine) is required before starting phenelzine. The prescribing regimen for amitriptyline is to start low (25 mg at night) and gradually build up to a maximum dose of 300 mg, although this is rarely required or tolerated and a more common dose is approximately 150 mg. Phenelzine should be started at 15 mg three times a day. It is important to consider postural hypotension with phenelzine, which is a not uncommon side effect, and warn patients about this.

The other group of drugs that can be considered as an evidence-informed treatment of PTSD are anticonvulsants. There is no strong RCT evidence for any of these medications; indeed, the RCTs have been neutral to date for those tested (valproate, topiramate, lamotrigine) but they are widely used as mood stabilizers, show evidence of effect in other mental disorders, and have been reported to help some people with PTSD (Berlin, 2007). Another anticonvulsant, carbamazepine, has been shown to help with episodic dyscontrol (Lewin & Sumners, 1992), a feature of some presentations of PTSD, and there is non-RCT evidence of benefit in military veterans with PTSD (Lipper et al., 1987).

Other Factors That Influence Prescribing

There are a number of commonly experienced challenges to prescribing medication for PTSD that deserve particular attention and are described next.

Inability to Tolerate Medication Due to Adverse Effects

Although all the commonly prescribed medications are reasonably well tolerated overall, adverse effects are, unfortunately, common. As described previously, it is important for the clinician to discuss possible common adverse effects with the patient as part of the shared decision-making process. The presence of adverse effects should be considered at every review, and a discussion must ensue if they are detected. Key issues to consider before determining how to proceed include the severity of the adverse effect, likelihood of improvement or deterioration, impact on the patient, and balance against any benefits or potential benefits accruing from the medication.

In some instances, it may be that discussion and some reassurance will allow a patient to decide to continue with his or her medication and tolerate an adverse effect as the potential benefits outweigh the potential harms. For example, nausea is relatively common when individuals start taking SSRIs or venlafaxine, but it tends to lessen over a few weeks and can also be reduced by taking the medication with food. It may be that, due to adverse effects, a patient can tolerate a lower dose but not a higher dose of a particular drug. It is then important to discuss the pros and cons of continuing with that drug. For example, paroxetine is more likely to cause agitation than sertraline, and the inability to tolerate paroxetine beyond 20 mg would be a good reason to consider switching to sertraline to determine if it is better tolerated at higher doses before trying a different class of drug.

Insomnia

Many people with PTSD find insomnia to be a particular problem and ask specifically for medication to help them sleep. Individuals who respond well to SSRIs and venlafaxine will generally report improved sleep, but these drugs are not sedatives and can be associated with increased wakefulness (hence the general recommendation to take them in the morning). It is important that patients are aware of this effect. Most will be willing to wait for these drugs to work, but this usually takes several weeks and it is sometimes appropriate to consider prescribing a sedative medication in addition.

When indicated, it is recommended that a sedative antidepressant be considered first line, for example, 15 mg of mirtazapine at night (which has the added benefit of RCT evidence to support its use for PTSD) or 50–100 mg of trazadone at night. Both of these drugs can be safely prescribed with SSRIs and venlafaxine and are not associated with the addictive potential of drugs such as benzodiazepines or the Z drugs. An alternative, especially for individuals with significant agitation (see below) is 25 mg of quetiapine at night. It is important to be aware that mirtazapine, trazadone, and quetiapine can cause drowsiness the following day and to warn patients about this.

Agitation

Agitation is common when individuals present with PTSD and, unfortunately, an unwanted early adverse effect of the SSRIs and venlafaxine is agitation/increased anxiety and even suicidality. For the majority of people with PTSD, adjunctive medication for agitation is not necessary, but for some individuals it is likely to be needed and, in addition to reducing agitation, may also enable a person to tolerate and continue medication likely to help her or his PTSD. Given its profile and evidence for use for PTSD, quetiapine is recommended as an adjunct or even on its own if a patient is very agitated or does not want to take SSRIs or venlafaxine. Some doctors recommend short courses of benzodiazepine for such agitation, but we do not recommend this, given the lack of evidence for benzodiazepine use for PTSD and also the risk of dependency.

Future Developments

There is clearly a need to improve the evidence available for pharmacological approaches to PTSD. There are some emerging candidates, but more research is needed to identify novel pharmacological treatments that may help. This is likely to result from greater neurobiological research; recent larger-scale PTSD genetics research has identified specific genes associated with PTSD (Duncan et al., 2017) that may herald a new, more focused approach to the development of effective pharmacological treatments. There is also a need for more clinical research with existing drugs; for example, we need to develop a greater understanding of the efficacy of drugs for different presentations of PTSD and combination pharmacological and psychological treatment.

An urgent need also exists to ensure that our current knowledge with regard to the pharmacological treatment of PTSD is disseminated and implemented in practice across the world, and that we move to pragmatic trials and the study of treatment algorithms in everyday clinical practice. We must strive to ensure that people with PTSD are fully informed about evidence-based pharmacological treatment so they can make an informed decision on whether to try a particular approach or not. If such a scenario was the norm, many more people with PTSD would be provided with evidence-based pharmacological treatment and experience improved health and well-being as a result.

Other Biological Treatments

Currently, other biological treatments have less evidence to support their use than pharmacological treatments but, in recent years, some promising approaches have emerged. Transcranial magnetic stimulation, neurofeedback, and Saikokeishikankyoto (an herbal preparation) were all recommended by the ISTSS guidelines as having emerging evidence of effect as interventions for the treatment of PTSD. The relatively small number of RCTs and participants involved, and other methodological issues, mean that further work is required before they can be recommended for routine use, but all are good candidates for more research.

Transcranial magnetic stimulation (TMS) uses magnetic fields to stimulate nerve cells in targeted areas of the brain. It is usually administered in a repetitive manner and is noninvasive. TMS is licensed for the treatment of depression, and there has been a significant rise in interest in its potential as a treatment for PTSD in recent years. The four RCTs that have been undertaken to date show signs of early promise in individuals who have not been helped by other approaches. TMS needs to be delivered in a specialist facility and, although it appears to be well tolerated, there is a risk of reduced seizure threshold.

Neurofeedback involves real-time displays of brain activity through EEG or fMRI that train individuals to self-regulate their brain activity and, for example, feel more relaxed. The two included RCTs showed evidence of efficacy, and the treatment was well tolerated. Neurofeedback also needs to take place in a specialist facility.

Saikokeishikankyoto is a traditional Japanese herbal medicine that was shown to be superior to placebo in a small RCT. It is too early to determine if this is an effective treatment or not, but the promising positive results obtained suggest it is a good candidate for future research.

Summary

In summary, there are a number of drugs with strong evidence for the treatment of PTSD as monotherapy or to augment pharmacological treatments.

Fluoxetine, paroxetine, sertraline, and venlafaxine show strong evidence of being effective, albeit low effect, treatments for PTSD, and there is emerging evidence that quetiapine is an effective monotherapy for PTSD. Prazosin and risperidone have good evidence of being effective for the augmentation of other pharmacological treatment. There is an urgent requirement to ensure that people with PTSD are offered optimal pharmacological treatments based on the current evidence. It is also important that further work be undertaken to better understand the neurobiology of PTSD and to use this knowledge to identify better pharmacological treatments in the future.

REFERENCES

Amoroso, T., & Workman, M. (2016). Treating posttraumatic stress disorder with MDMA-assisted psychotherapy: A preliminary meta-analysis and comparison to prolonged exposure therapy. *Journal of Psychopharmacology, 30,* 595–600.

Berlin, H. A. (2007). Antiepileptic drugs for the treatment of post-traumatic stress disorder. *Current Psychiatry Reports, 9,* 291–300.

Bisson, J. I., Baker, A., Dekker, W., & Hoskins, M. D. (2020). Evidence-based prescribing for post-traumatic stress disorder. *British Journal of Psychiatry, 216*(3), 125–126.

Blier, P., Ward, H. E., Tremblay, P., Laberge, L., Hebert, C., & Bergeron, R. (2010). Combination of antidepressant medications from treatment initiation for major depressive disorder: A double-blind randomized study. *American Journal of Psychiatry, 167,* 281–288.

Cipriani, A., Williams, T., Nikolakopoulou, A., Salanti, G., Chaimani, A., Ipser, J., et al. (2018). Comparative efficacy and acceptability of pharmacological treatments for post-traumatic stress disorder in adults: A network meta-analysis. *Psychological Medicine, 48*(12), 1975–1984.

Duncan, L. E., Ratanatharathorn, A., Aiello, A. E., Almli, L. M., Amstadter, A. B., Ashley-Koch, A. E., et al. (2017). Largest GWAS of PTSD (*N* = 20,070) yields genetic overlap with schizophrenia and sex differences in heritability. *Molecular Psychiatry, 23*(3), 666–673.

Guo, T., Xiang, Y., Xiao, L., Hu, C., Chiu, H., Ungvari, G., et al. (2015). Measurement-based care versus standard care for major depression: A randomized controlled trial with blind raters. *American Journal of Psychiatry, 172,* 1004–1013.

Hetrick, S. E., Purcell, R., Garner, B., & Parslow, R. (2010). Combined pharmacotherapy and psychological therapies for posttraumatic stress disorder (PTSD). *Cochrane Database Systematic Reviews,* Issue 7, Article No. CD007316.

Higgins, J. P., & Green, S. (Eds.). (2011). Cochrane handbook for systematic reviews of interventions, Version 5.1.0. Retrieved from *http://training.cochrane.org/handbook.*

Kessler, D. S., MacNeill, S. J., Tallon, D., Lewis, G., Peters, T. J., Hollingworth, W., et al. (2018). Mirtazapine added to SSRIs or SNRIs for treatment resistant depression in primary care: Phase III randomised placebo-controlled trial. *British Medical Journal, 363,* k4218.

Lewin, J., & Sumners, D. (1992). Successful treatment of episodic dyscontrol with carbamazepine. *British Journal of Psychiatry, 161,* 261–262.

Lipper, S., Davidson, J., Grady, T. A., Edinger, J. D., Hammett, E. B., Mahorney, S. L., et al. (1987). Preliminary study of carbamazepine in post-traumatic stress disorder. *Psychosomatics, 27,* 849–854.

Marshall, R. D., Beebe, K. L., Oldham, M., & Zaninelli, R. (2001). Efficacy and safety of paroxetine treatment for chronic PTSD: A fixed-dose, placebo-controlled study. *American Journal of Psychiatry, 158,* 1982–1988.

Marshall, R. D., & Cloitre, M. (2000). Maximizing treatment outcome in post-traumatic stress disorder by combining psychotherapy with pharmacotherapy. *Current Psychiatry Reports, 2,* 335–340.

Martenyi, F., Brown, E. B., & Caldwell, C. D. (2007). Failed efficacy of fluoxetine in the treatment of posttraumatic stress disorder. *Journal of Clinical Psychology, 27,* 166–170.

National Collaborating Centre for Mental Health. (2005). *Post-traumatic stress disorder: The management of PTSD in adults and children in primary and secondary care.* London and Leicester, UK: Gaskell & BPS.

Popiel, A., Zawadzki, B., Pragłowska, E., & Teichman, Y. (2015). Prolonged exposure, paroxetine and the combination in the treatment of PTSD following a motor vehicle accident: A randomized clinical trial—The "TRAKT" study. *Journal of Behavior Therapy and Experimental Psychiatry, 48,* 7–26.

Sackett, D. L., Rosenberg, W. M. C., Muir Gray, J. A., Haynes, R. B., & Richardson, W. S. (1996). Evidence based medicine: What it is and what it isn't. *British Medical Journal, 312,* 71.

Schneier, F. R., Neria, Y., Pavlicova, M., Hembree, E., Suh, E. J., Amsel, L., et al. (2012). Combined prolonged exposure therapy and paroxetine for PTSD related to the World Trade Center attack: A randomized controlled trial. *American Journal of Psychiatry, 169,* 80–88.

Simon, N. M., Connor, K. M., Lang, A. J., Rauch, S., Krulewicz, S., LeBeau, R. T., et al. (2008). Paroxetine CR augmentation for posttraumatic stress disorder refractory to prolonged exposure therapy. *Journal of Clinical Psychiatry, 69,* 400–405.

Southwick, S. M., Bremner, J. D., Rasmusson, A., Morgan, C. A., Amsten, A., & Charney, D. S. (1999). Role of norepinephrine in the pathophysiology and treatment of PTSD. *Biological Psychiatry, 46,* 1192–1204.

Taylor, D. M., Barnes, T. R. E., & Young, A. H. (2018). *The Maudsley prescribing guidelines in psychiatry.* London: Wiley-Blackwell.

Villarreal, G., Hamner, M., Canive, J., Robert, S., Calais, A. L., Durklaski, V., et al. (2016). Efficacy of quetiapine monotherapy in posttraumatic stress disorder: A randomized, placebo-controlled trial. *American Journal of Psychiatry, 173,* 1205–1212.

World Health Organization. (2018). *International classification of diseases and related health problems* (11th rev.). Geneva, Switzerland: Author. Retrieved from *https:// icd.who.int.*

CHAPTER 17

Combined Psychotherapy and Medication Treatment

Mark Burton, Jessica Maples-Keller, Mathew D. Hoskins,
Yilang Tang, Katarzyna Wyka, JoAnn Difede,
and Barbara O. Rothbaum

The literature supports several psychotherapeutic and pharmacological approaches as first- and second-line treatments for posttraumatic stress disorder (PTSD). Meta-analytic reviews consistently demonstrate that trauma-focused psychotherapies outperform wait-list control and placebo-therapy conditions in randomized clinical trials (Cusack et al., 2016; Lee et al., 2016; Watts et al., 2013), with greater reductions in PTSD symptom severity that is maintained after treatment ends (Kline, Cooper, Rytwinski, & Feeny, 2018). Manualized, evidence-based, trauma-focused psychotherapies include prolonged exposure (PE), cognitive processing therapy (CPT), cognitive therapy (CT), and eye movement desensitization and reprocessing (EMDR) therapy. However, some patients will not achieve full response to psychotherapy for PTSD. One strategy to improve outcome is to augment psychotherapy with medication. Several medications demonstrate efficacy as monotherapies for treating PTSD (Hoskins et al., 2015). Medication monotherapy for PTSD is further described by Bisson, Hoskins, and Stein (Chapter 16, this volume).

The most recent U.S. Department of Veterans Affairs and Department of Defense (VA/DoD) *Clinical Practice Guideline for the Management of Posttraumatic Stress Disorder and Acute Stress Disorder* (2017) recommends manualized, trauma-focused psychotherapies, such as PE and CPT, as first-line treatments and pharmacotherapy with sertraline, paroxetine, fluoxetine, or venlafaxine recommended as second-line treatments only for those who do not choose or cannot access trauma-focused therapy. The American Psychological Association (2017) *Clinical Practice Guideline for the Treatment of PTSD* also suggests that the evidence is strong for the recommendation of

287

trauma-focused psychotherapy as monotherapy for PTSD and that the evidence is conditional for the use of sertraline, paroxetine, fluoxetine, and venlafaxine. Likewise, the *Posttraumatic Stress Disorder Prevention and Treatment Guidelines* formulated by the International Society for Traumatic Stress Studies (ISTSS) recommend psychological treatments with a trauma focus more strongly than pharmacotherapy. In terms of combination therapy, the ISTSS guidelines did not include a scoping question to consider this. The VA/DoD guidelines state there is insufficient evidence to suggest the addition of medication for psychotherapy nonresponders, the addition of psychotherapy for medication nonresponders, or the combination of medication and psychotherapy from the start of treatment. Furthermore, they recommend against augmentation of psychotherapy with antipsychotics, benzodiazepines, topiramate, divalproex, baclofen, and pregabalin, due to low-quality evidence, insufficient evidence, and known adverse effects of these treatments. Augmentation of exposure therapy with D-cycloserine (DCS) is recommended for research settings only. The American Psychological Association guidelines do not address combination treatment, citing a lack of comparative effectiveness trials. In general, the literature supports multiple trauma-focused treatments and some medications as monotherapies for PTSD. Although combination approaches are not as well studied, there is a growing body of literature to inform clinical research moving forward.

Description of Techniques

The current chapter examines this literature and discusses research and clinical practice issues related to combined psychotherapy and pharmacotherapy for the treatment of PTSD. The studies reviewed are described in Table 17.1. Our review is divided into two broad categories: (1) evidence for combining psychotherapy with empirically supported medications prescribed daily as monotherapies for PTSD, such as selective serotonin reuptake inhibitors (SSRIs), and (2) evidence for combining psychotherapy with acute-acting medications and interventions prescribed to enhance specific psychotherapeutic processes, such as extinction learning and emotional engagement. Such psychotherapy-specific adjunctive interventions discussed in this chapter include D-cycloserine (DCS), methylene blue, yohimbine, propranolol, dexamethasone, hydrocortisone, and repetitive transcranial magnetic stimulation (rTMS). A novel psychotherapy that utilizes 3,4-methylenedioxymethamphetamine (MDMA) as an adjunct is also discussed.

Summary of the Evidence

The literature for combination treatment is not as well developed as that for monotherapies. However, there are a growing number of randomized

TABLE 17.1. Reviewed Studies

Study and methods	Participants	Outcomes	Interventions	Results	Notes
Conventional medications plus therapy					
Buhmann et al. (2016); Denmark; study type: pragmatic; duration: 6 months	$N = 280$; mean age: 49 years; sex: 41% female; diagnosis: DSM-IV PTSD; predominant trauma type: asylum experience; mean duration of symptoms: 14.7 years	HTQ; HSCL-25; HRSD; HRSA; SCL-90; VAS; SDS; WHO-5	• Group 1: Sertraline (25–200 mg, mean dose 132.1 mg) ± mianserin (10–30 mg, mean dose 20 mg); $n = 71$ • Group 2: Sertraline (25–200 mg, mean dose 132.1 mg) ± mianserin (10–30 mg, mean dose 20 mg) plus therapy; $n = 71$ • Group 3: Therapy (16 sessions CBT over 6 months); $n = 70$ • Group 4: Waiting list; $n = 68$	No significant difference between medication, psychotherapy, or combination on PTSD symptoms.	54% of sessions were translated; 25% in therapy actually received exposure treatment; additionally, 27% of the therapy group received another antidepressant.
Hien et al. (2015); U.S.; study type: RCT; duration: 12 weeks	$N = 69$; mean age: 42.2; sex: 81% female; diagnosis: DSM-IV-TR PTSD and alcohol use disorder; predominant trauma type: CSA (46%); mean duration of symptoms: 14 years	CAPS; SCID-I; TLFB	• Group 1: Sertraline (50–200 mg, mean dose not available) plus 12 weekly sessions of Safety Seeking (SS) therapy; $n = 32$ • Group 2: Placebo plus SS; $n = 37$	Significant improvement in PTSD symptoms in sertraline plus SS group compared to placebo plus SS.	Medication titrated over 2 weeks prior to therapy; patients had PTSD and co-occurring alcohol use disorder.
Popiel et al. (2015); Poland; study type: RCT; duration: 12 weeks	$N = 228$; mean age: 36.9 years; sex: unclear; diagnosis: DSM-IV-TR PTSD; predominant trauma type: motor-vehicle accident (100%); mean duration of symptoms: 17.7 months	SCID-I; PDS; BDI-II	• Group 1: PE × 12 weekly sessions; $n = 114$ • Group 2: Paroxetine 20 mg × 12 weeks; $n = 57$ • Group 3: PE plus paroxetine 20 mg × 12 weeks; $n = 57$	Significant improvement in PTSD symptoms across all groups, with higher remission rates after PE alone compared to paroxetine alone.	Max medication dose was achieved in 3–7 days after starting the trial and reduced within 2 weeks following the 12-week trial.

(continued)

TABLE 17.1. *(continued)*

Study and methods	Participants	Outcomes	Interventions	Results	Notes
Rothbaum et al. (2006); U.S.; study type: RCT; duration: 16 weeks	$N = 65$ (88 completed 10-week open label); mean age: 39.3; sex: 64.6% female; diagnosis: DSM-IV PTSD; predominant trauma type: sexual assault; mean duration of symptoms: 8.1 years	SIP; BDI; STAI-S	• Group 1: Sertraline 50–200 mg × 10 weeks (mean dose 173.1 mg) open label followed by 5 weeks double-blind sertraline plus 10 sessions of twice-weekly PE; $n = 34$ • Group 2: Sertraline 50–200 mg × 10 weeks open label followed by 5 weeks sertraline alone; $n = 31$	Sertraline plus PE was better than sertraline alone for weaker medication responders in *post hoc* analyses.	Flexible dosing schedule was used for Phase I (0–10 weeks). Minor adjustments in dose allowed in weeks 6–10. No further adjustments were permitted in Phase II (Weeks 10–15).
Schmeier et al. (2012); U.S.; study type: RCT; duration: 10 weeks	$N = 37$; mean age: 50.3 years; sex: 54% female; diagnosis: DSM-IV PTSD; predominant trauma type: World Trade Center attacks; mean duration of symptoms: 6.5 years	CAPS; HAMD; QLESQ	• Group 1: Paroxetine (12.5–50 mg, mean dose 32.2 mg) plus 10 weekly sessions of PE; $n = 19$ • Group 2: Placebo plus 10 weekly sessions of PE; $n = 18$	Greater PSTD symptom reduction and higher remission rates in paroxetine plus PE group compared to placebo plus PE at posttreatment; no differences at follow-up.	Paroxetine was dosed at 12.5 mg/day for Week 1, then 25 mg/day for Week 3, then increased dosage up to 50 mg/day as tolerated for remainder of trial. The sample consisted entirely of adult survivors of the World Trade Center attacks.
Simon et al. (2008); U.S.; study type: RCT; duration: 10 weeks	$N = 68$; mean age: 46 years; sex: 56% female; diagnosis: DSM-IV PTSD; predominant trauma type: physical and sexual abuse (78%); mean duration of symptoms: unclear	SPRINT; CGI-S	• Group 1: Paroxetine (12.5–62.5 mg) + PE; $n = 9$ • Group 2: Placebo + PE; $n = 14$	No significant difference between paroxetine plus PE versus placebo plus PE group, with a small trend toward greater symptom reduction in	Therapy course: eight sessions of open-label PE (90–120 minutes); non-responders randomized to treatment arms; five sessions of double-blind PE plus paroxetine/

placebo (90–120 minutes, fortnightly) × 10 weeks.

placebo group.

DCS-assisted therapy

de Kleine et al. (2012); the Netherlands; study type: RCT; duration: 10 weeks	N = 67; mean age: 38.3 years; sex; 80.6% female; diagnosis: DSM-IV PTSD; predominant trauma type: sexual abuse (52%); mean duration of symptoms: unknown	CAPS; BDI; STAI	• Group 1: 50 mg DCS administered orally 1 hour prior to each face-to-face session of manualized PE; n = 33 • Group 2: Administered orally 1 hour prior to each face-to-face session of manualized PE; n = 34	No significant difference between DCS plus exposure and placebo plus exposure, with greater symptom reduction in those with more severe pretreatment PTSD in *post hoc* analyses.	No take-home DCS for homework; concomitant psychotropics were allowed.
Difede et al. (2014); U.S.; study type: RCT; duration: 12 weeks	N = 25; mean age: 45.8 years; sex: 24% female; diagnosis: DSM-IV PTSD; predominant trauma type: World Trade Center attacks; mean duration of symptoms: unclear	CAPS; SCID-MDD; BDI-II; STAXI-2; PCL	• Group 1: 12 weekly sessions of CBT, including PE enhanced by virtual reality (VRE) with 100 mg DCS 90 min before Sessions 2–11; n = 13 • Group 2: 12 weekly sessions of CBT, including PE enhanced by VRE with placebo 90 min before Sessions 2–11; n = 12	Significantly greater remission rates in DCS plus VRE compared to placebo plus VRE.	Pharmacotherapy (on a stable dose for 2 months) allowed during therapy.
Litz et al. (2012); U.S.; study type: RCT; duration: 6 weeks	N = 26; mean age: 32 years; sex: 100% male; diagnosis: DSM-IV PTSD; predominant trauma type: combat; mean duration of symptoms: unclear	CAPS; BDI	• Group 1: 6 weekly exposure sessions with 50 mg DCS given 30 min prior to Sessions 2–5; n = 13 • Group 2: 6 weekly exposure sessions with placebo given 30 min prior to Sessions 2–5; n = 13	Significantly less symptom reduction in DCS plus exposure group compared to placebo plus exposure.	Trial stopped before planned recruitment of 68 was reached.

(continued)

291

TABLE 17.1. (continued)

Study and methods	Participants	Outcomes	Interventions	Results	Notes
Rothbaum et al. (2014); U.S.; study type: RCT; duration: 6 weeks	N = 106; mean age: 34.6 years; sex: 6% female; diagnosis: DSM-IV PTSD; predominant trauma type: combat (100%); mean duration of symptoms: unknown	CAPS; startle response; salivary cortisol	• Group 1: 6 weekly 90- min VRE sessions with DCS 50 mg given 30 min prior to each session; n = 53 • Group 2: 6 weekly 90-min VRE sessions with alprazolam given 30 min prior to each session; n = 50 • Group 3: 6 weekly 90-min VRE sessions with placebo given 30 min prior to each session; n = 53	Significant improvement in PTSD symptoms across all VRE groups, but no significant difference between DCS and placebo; DCS group showed significantly greater improvements on startle and salivary cortisol maintained at follow-up.	56% were on a stable dose of psychotropic medications.
MDMA-assisted therapy					
Mithoefer et al. (2011); U.S.; study type: RCT; duration: 12 weeks	N = 23; mean age: 40.4 years; sex: 85% female; diagnosis: DSM-IV PTSD; predominant trauma type: crime related (95%); mean duration of symptoms: 19 years	CAPS; IES-R; SCL-90-R; RBANS; PASAT; RCFT	• Group 1: 12 therapy sessions with 125 mg MDMA given prior to Sessions 3 and 8; n = 15 • Group 2: 12 therapy sessions with placebo given prior to Sessions 3 and 8; n = 8	Significant improvement in PTSD symptoms and rates of clinical response in MDMA group compared to placebo.	MDMA-assisted therapy model includes male–female therapist dyad; drug-assisted sessions last 6–8 hours, are nondirective, and include music, eye mask, and overnight stay; all participants were deemed to be treatment-resistant.

(continued)

| Mithoefer et al. (2018); U.S.; study type: RCT; duration: 12 weeks | $N = 24$; mean age: 37.2 years; sex: 27% female; diagnosis: DSM-IV PTSD; predominant trauma type: service personnel; mean duration of symptoms: 85.4 months | CAPS-IV; BDI-II; PSQI; PTGI; NEO-PI-R; DES-II; GAF; C-SSRS | • Group 1: 12 therapy sessions with 30 mg (active placebo) MDMA given prior to Sessions 4 and 8; $n = 7$
• Group 2: 12 therapy sessions with 75 mg MDMA given prior to Sessions 4 and 8; $n = 7$
• Group 3: 12 therapy sessions with 125 mg MDMA given prior to Sessions 4 and 8; $n = 12$ | Significant improvement in PTSD symptoms and rates of clinical response in MDMA groups (with 75 mg being greatest) compared to active placebo. | MDMA-assisted therapy model includes male–female therapist dyad; drug-assisted sessions last 6–8 hours, are nondirective, and include music, eye mask, and overnight stay; all participants were deemed to be treatment-resistant. |
| Oehen et al. (2013); Switzerland; study type: RCT; duration: 12 weeks | $N = 14$; mean age: 41.4 years; sex: 83% female; diagnosis: DSM-IV PTSD; predominant trauma type: CSA (50%); mean duration of symptoms: 18.3 years | CAPS; PDS | • Group 1: 12 therapy sessions with 25 mg (active placebo) MDMA given prior to Sessions 3 and 8; $n = 5$
• Group 2: 12 therapy sessions with 125 mg (active placebo) MDMA given prior to Sessions 3 and 8; $n = 9$ | Significant improvement in PTSD symptoms on self-reported but not clinically rated measures in MDMA group compared to placebo. | MDMA-assisted therapy model includes male–female therapist dyad; drug-assisted sessions last 6–8 hours, are nondirective, and include music, eye mask, and overnight stay; all participants were deemed to be treatment-resistant. |

TABLE 17.1. *(continued)*

Study and methods	Participants	Outcomes	Interventions	Results	Notes
Other agents					
Brunet et al. (2018); Canada; study type: RCT; duration: 6 weeks	$N = 61$; mean age: 39.4 years; sex: 58% female; diagnosis: DSM-IV-TR PTSD; predominant trauma type: physical and sexual (57%); mean duration of symptoms: unknown	CAPS; PCL-S	• Group 1: 6 weekly trauma memory reactivation sessions with propranolol (0.67 mg/kg short-acting plus 1 mg/kg long-acting preparations with food); $n = 30$ • Group 2: 6 weekly trauma memory reactivation sessions with placebo; $n = 30$	Significant improvement in PTSD symptoms in propranolol group compared to placebo.	Brief intervention; first session 30 min of written narrative; subsequent sessions 10–20 min.
Tuerk et al. (2018); U.S.; study type: RCT; duration: 15 weeks	$N = 26$; mean age: 32.4 years; sex: 100% male; diagnosis: DSM-IV PTSD; predominant trauma type: combat; mean duration of symptoms: unclear	Trauma-cued heart rate reactivity; PCL-M; BDI-II	• Group 1: Yohimbine 21.6 mg taken 1 hour prior to each PE session; $n = 14$ • Group 2: Placebo taken 1 hour prior to each PE session; $n = 12$	No significant difference in posttreatment PTSD symptom severity or remission.	The sample consisted entirely of male, post-9/11 combat veterans.
Zoellner (2017); U.S.; study type: RCT; duration:	$N = 42$; mean age: 37.5 years; sex: 100% female; diagnosis: DSM-IV-TR PTSD; predominant	PSS-I; CGI; SCID-IV; PSS-SR; QIDS-SR;	• Group 1: 6 sessions of imaginal exposure (IE) plus 260 mg methylene blue (MB) administered post-IE; $n = 15$	Significantly enhanced treatment response and quality of life in MB plus IE	Treatment was modified from the PE manual and included daily imaginal exposures with no *in vivo*

6 weeks	trauma type: physical assault (28.6%); mean duration of symptoms: unclear	PTCI; OSPAN; SF-36 SUDS; MEF	• Group 2: 6 sessions of IE plus placebo administered post-IE; $n = 16$ • Group 3: Waiting list; $n = 11$	compared to placebo group.	exposures.
Kozel et al. (2018); U.S.; study type: RCT; duration: 15 weeks	$N = 103$; mean age: 31 years; sex: 100% male; diagnosis: DSM-IV PTSD; predominant trauma type: combat (100%); mean duration of symptoms: unclear	CAPS; PCL; M-PTSD; QIDS; IPF	• Group 1: Cognitive processing therapy (CPT) plus repetitive transcranial magnetic stimulation (rTMS); $n = 54$ • Group 2: CPT plus sham rTMS; $n = 49$	Greater symptom reduction across both clinician-rated and self-reported PTSD symptoms in CPT plus rTMS compared to sham group.	The sample consisted of male and female post-9/11 combat veterans. The rTMS stimulator coil was positioned over the dorsolateral prefrontal cortex at 110% of motor threshold at 1hz rTMS continuously for 30 minutes for a total of 1,800 pulses immediately prior to CPT session.

Note. BDI, Beck Depression Inventory; CAPS, Clinician-Administered PTSD Scale; CGI-S, Clinical Global Impression Severity; CSS, Crisis Support Scale; C-SSRS, Columbia-Suicide Severity Rating Scale; DES-II, Dissociative Experiences Scale II; GAF, Global Assessment of Functioning; HAMA, Hamilton Rating Scale for Anxiety; HAMD, Hamilton Rating Scale for Depression; HRSA, Hamilton Rating Scale for Anxiety; HRSD, Hamilton Rating Scale for Depression; HSCL-25, Hopkins Symptom Checklist-25; HTQ, Harvard Trauma Questionnaire; IES-R, Impact of Event Scale Revised; IPF, Inventory of Psychosocial Functioning; MEF, Medication Effects Form; M-PTSD, Mississippi Scale for Combat-Related PTSD; NEO-PI-R, Neuroticism–Extroversion–Openness–Personality Inventory–Revised; OSPAN, Automated Operation Span; PASAT, Paced Auditory Serial Addition Task; PCL-M, Posttraumatic Stress Checklist–Military Version; PCL-S, PTSD Checklist-Specific; PDS, Posttraumatic Diagnostic Scale; PSQI, Pittsburgh Sleep Quality Index; PSS-I, PTSD Symptom Scale–Interview Version; PSS-SR, PTSD Symptom Scale–Self-Rated; QLESQ, Quality of Life Enjoyment and Satisfaction Questionnaire; RBANS, Repeatable Battery for the Assessment of Neuropsychological Status; RCFT, Rey–Osterrieth Complex Figure; SAS-SR, Social Adjustment Scale Self-Report; SCID-I, Structured Clinical Interview for DSM-IV-TR Axis I Disorders; SCID-I, Structured Clinical Interview for DSM-IV; SCL-90, Symptom Checklist-90; SDS, Sheehan Disability Scale; SF-36, Short Form Health Survey; SIP, Structured Interview for PTSD; SPRINT, Short PTSD Rating Interview; STAI-S, State–Trait Anxiety Inventory–State Portion; STAXI-2, State–Trait Anger Expression Inventory-2; SUDS, Subjective Units of Distress; TLFB, Timeline Follow-Back; VAS, Visual Analogue Pain Scales; WHO-5, WHO-Five Well-Being Index.

controlled trials (RCTs) examining incremental benefits for medications combined with evidence-based psychotherapy. This chapter will critically review the evidence for combination treatments, specifically focused on randomized clinical trials that compare combination approaches to either medication alone or psychotherapy alone.

Several types of trials have examined the effects of combination treatment. The first type randomizes individuals to evidence-based psychotherapy with either an active medication adjunct or placebo. This method provides a test of the effects of combining medication and psychotherapy from the start of treatment and has been applied to the study of daily-dosed medications like SSRIs and novel psychotherapy augmentation agents. The second type of trial involves maintaining all individuals in a sample on a monotherapeutic medication for a given duration, then randomizing individuals to either receive adjunctive psychotherapy or continue medication only. This method allows for a clinically relevant analysis of the benefits of adding psychotherapy for individuals who already are on a medication. The third type of trial involves providing individuals with a course of psychotherapy, then adding a medication or placebo. The current chapter outlines studies utilizing each of these methodological approaches and discusses their clinical implications.

Combining Efficacious Monotherapies

Several studies have examined combination treatment of evidence-based monotherapeutic medications and psychotherapy for adults with PTSD. The first combination study conducted by Rothbaum and colleagues (2006) examined the benefits of adding evidence-based psychotherapy (PE) to ongoing sertraline treatment for a sample of 88 civilians diagnosed with PTSD mostly related to assault. In Phase I, all participants were started on open-label sertraline treatment for 10 weeks. Medication was titrated up to 200 mg/day or the maximum tolerated dose over the first 6 weeks, with minor adjustments allowed until Week 10 and maintenance of dosage thereafter. Phase II of the study was conducted from Week 10 to Week 15. In this phase, participants with at least a 20% reduction in PTSD severity were randomized to either start PE in conjunction with sertraline ($n = 34$) or continue sertraline only for 5 weeks ($n = 31$). PE was provided in twice-weekly, 90- to 120-minute sessions for a total of 10 sessions. PTSD, depression, and state anxiety severity were measured at Week 0, Week 10 (post–Phase I), and Week 15 (post–Phase II). Results showed that both those who went on to receive sertraline-only in Phase II and those who received sertraline plus PE had equal reductions in PTSD symptoms across Phase I, as expected given that they were both receiving monotherapy with sertraline. During the second phase, PTSD symptom severity continued to decrease for those randomized to combined medication treatment with PE, while it leveled out for those who continued sertraline-only treatment (Week 15 between-group

d = 0.38).[1] For depression and state anxiety, symptom severity reduced from Week 0 to Week 10, but not from Week 10 to 15, with no significant difference found between treatment groups (Week 15 combined within-group d = 1.26 and 1.10, respectively).

Secondary analyses comparing treatment outcomes in high responders to sertraline-only treatment (Phase I) and partial responders showed that high responders continued to see reductions in PTSD symptoms in Phase II of treatment regardless of whether they received additional combination PE or stayed on sertraline only (Week 15 between-group d = -0.18). However, for partial responders in Phase I, further reductions in PTSD severity in Phase II were only found for those who received combination treatment (Week 15 between-group d = 0.90). Taken together, these findings suggest that adding PE to sertraline treatment may be indicated for those who do not fully respond to medication alone. Notably, this study did not include a placebo control condition in Phase I or an evidence-based control therapy in Phase II. As such, findings cannot elucidate specific mechanisms for clinical improvement.

Simon and colleagues (2008) examined the benefits of adding medication to ongoing psychotherapy for PTSD due to mixed trauma. This trial started 44 adult participants on psychotherapy (PE) and then added medication (paroxetine). Specifically, during Phase I, all participants received eight sessions of PE over 4–6 weeks and were then randomized to receive combination treatment with paroxetine (n = 9) or a placebo control (n = 14) in the second phase while continuing to receive PE (five sessions). Only individuals who were designated as nonremitters after Phase I were randomized to Phase II (n = 23). Strong effects were found for PE as a monotherapy in Phase I, with significant mean reductions in PTSD symptom severity. Thirty-eight percent of the sample met full PTSD remission status (<6 on the Short PTSD Rating Interview; Davidson et al., 2001). Twenty-five individuals did not fully remit and were thus randomized to receive either paroxetine or placebo. Paroxetine was initiated at 12.5 mg/day and titrated according to tolerability up to a maximum dose of 62.5 mg/day for 10 weeks. The mean end-point medication dose for paroxetine was 45.8 mg/day (SD = 16.5 mg/day) compared to 44.8 mg/day (SD = 15.5 mg/day) for placebo. Medication was given in combination with PE, which was provided at a lower frequency in Phase II compared to Phase I (every 2 weeks compared to twice per week). Phase II results showed no significant difference in PTSD symptom severity between the paroxetine and placebo groups at the end of treatment (Weeks 14–16 between-group d = 0.35). Remission rates by the end of Phase II for this treatment refractory group were low, with 3/9 (33%) of those receiving

---

[1]Between-group effect sizes were calculated when not provided in the original manuscript using Cohen's d formula, d = mean 1 – mean 2/pooled standard deviation, and are denoted in the text with an asterisk (*). There was insufficient data to calculate within-group effect sizes when they were not reported in the manuscript.

paroxetine and 2/14 (14%) of those receiving placebo demonstrating remission.

These two clinical trials examined benefits of adding a second intervention after an unsuccessful course of monotherapy. Although these studies suggest a benefit for adding PE for low responders to sertraline, methodological limitations, including small sample sizes (e.g., $N = 44$ in Simon et al., 2008) and the lack of placebo controls for therapy and medication, make it difficult to draw broad, clinically applicable conclusions.

In a third trial, Schneier and colleagues (2012) tested the idea that starting combination therapy from the initiation of treatment would be more effective than PE alone for treating PTSD for survivors of the World Trade Center terrorist attacks on September 11, 2001. Thirty-seven participants were randomized to receive 10 weekly sessions of PE with paroxetine ($n = 19$) or placebo ($n = 18$). Paroxetine was initiated at 12.5 mg/day and titrated according to tolerability to a maximum dose of 50 mg/day. Average final dose for the combined group was 32.2 mg/day ($SD = 13.4$) and 36.8 mg/day ($SD = 12.1$) for the paroxetine equivalent in the placebo group. Participants could choose to continue medication (or placebo) after the end of PE for up to 12 weeks. Results showed that those who received paroxetine demonstrated better treatment response compared to those who received placebo, with greater reductions in PTSD symptom severity (Week 10 between-group $d = 1.66*$), higher remission rates (42.1% vs. 16.7%), and greater improvements in quality of life (Week 10 between-group $d = 0.75*$). Depression severity was lower for the combination group (Week 10 between-group $d = 0.82*$), although this difference was not statistically significant. For those who continued on double-blinded medication ($n = 13$) or placebo ($n = 13$) for the maintenance period after PE was discontinued, no additional gains were made, and PTSD symptom severity did not differ between groups after the 12 extra weeks of medication maintenance (Week 22 between-group $d = 0.37$). One individual who was a remitter at Week 10 became a nonaremitter at Week 22, four individuals discontinued before Week 22, and the rest either maintained or gained remitter status in the maintenance phase. Notably, sample size was small and patients were not randomly selected for the second phase, which could have impacted the treatment differences identified. Future research with improved power can determine if this advantage of combined treatment persists over long follow-up time points.

A more recent trial examined the benefits of combined PE and paroxetine treatment in a sample of 228 motor-vehicle crash (MVC) survivors (Popiel, Zawadzki, Praglowska, & Teichman, 2015). MVC survivors diagnosed with PTSD were randomized to receive either PE alone ($n = 144$), paroxetine alone ($n = 57$), or combination treatment ($n = 57$). Treatment was administered over 12 weeks. PE was based on the standard protocol of one 90-minute session per week. The medication-only condition included 45-minute meetings with a psychiatrist every 2 weeks for medication and symptom monitoring and support. Medication was titrated up through Week 7 to a maximum dose of 20 mg/day. Of note, a study limitation included that the dose of paroxetine was a lower maximum than in other combination studies and the authors did not report the mean and standard deviation of dosing for their sample. The combination group received treatment from PE-trained psychiatrists who provided additional 15-minute medication management sessions after PE every 2 weeks. Results of the modified intent to treat analyses (n = 179 participants who started treatment) indicated that PTSD remission rates were significantly higher for the PE group (80.8%) compared to the medication-only group (56.6%), but no significant differences were found for the combination group compared to either of the monotherapy groups (76.9%). Among treatment refusers (n = 49), rates of refusal were higher in the medication-only (47.4%) and combination (31.6%) groups compared to the PE group (3.5%), possibly indicating a preference for starting PE as a monotherapy.

Two additional trials examined the efficacy of combining sertraline and PE from treatment inception. Rauch and colleagues (2019) randomized 223 post-9/11 veterans of the Iraq or Afghanistan wars with combat-related PTSD to combination treatment (PE plus sertraline; n = 75), PE plus placebo (n = 74), or sertraline plus enhanced medication management (n = 74). Participants, recruited across four sites, were randomized to receive treatment over 24 weeks. PE participants received up to 13 standard sessions. Sertraline dosing was adjusted between 50 mg/day and 200 mg/day and titrated upward through Week 10 and then maintained across the 24-week study period. Average dose by the end of treatment for PE plus sertraline, PE plus placebo, and sertraline plus enhanced medication management was 171.6 (SD = 45.0), 197.4 (SD = 11.3), and 170.7 (SD = 46.9), respectively. Enhanced medication management included medical management, psychoeducation, and active listening. Discussion of trauma-related details and guidance on addressing PTSD symptoms were not permitted in medication management sessions. To monitor this, all sessions were taped and 20% were randomly selected for review, with 96.7% of reviewed tapes demonstrating adherence to session protocol. Results indicated that PTSD symptoms reduced significantly, on average, for all study participants with no significant differences found between study conditions (Week 24 between-group d = 0.38 for PE plus placebo vs. sertraline plus enhanced medication management; d = 0.28 for PE plus placebo vs. PE plus sertraline). Notably, the medication management in this protocol was enhanced compared to standard medication management, which may be associated with positive results in this group.

Feeny, Mavissakalian, Roy-Byrne, Bedard-Gilligan, and Zoellner (2020) compared PE plus sertraline to PE alone (without a placebo) in a trial examining the effect of choice (i.e., being allowed to choose your treatment) on treatment outcome for a civilian population. In a doubly randomized preference trial, 150 participants across two sites were first randomized to *choice* or *no-choice* groups. Those in the choice group could choose whether they received PE alone or in combination with sertraline. Those in the no-choice group were randomized to a treatment condition. Standard PE was provided over 10 weekly sessions. Sertraline was dosed as low as 25 mg/day at Week 1 and titrated up to a maximum of 200 mg/day. Analyses are currently being conducted for this recently completed trial. It is expected that the trial will inform clinical recommendations for combining PE and sertraline for the treatment of PTSD, as well as the role of preference and choice in treatment outcome.

Few trials have examined the effects of combination PTSD treatment in which the psychotherapy component was not PE. One study randomized 280 refugees with war-related PTSD to receive an antidepressant medication alone (either sertraline or the tetracyclic antidepressant, mianserin; $n = 71$), psychotherapy alone ($n = 70$), these treatments in combination ($n = 71$), or to remain in a wait-list control condition ($n = 68$) (Buhmann, Nordentoft, Ekstroem, Carlsson, & Mortensen, 2016). The psychotherapy component was described as "flexible," allowing clinicians to choose from multiple CBT components, such as mindfulness and cognitive methods. Only 19% of participants received any exposure component, while 7% received exposure more than three times, which was reportedly related to both patient preference and therapist reluctance. The mean duration of treatment was approximately 6 months for all four groups. No effect on PTSD symptoms or depressive symptoms was demonstrated for any of these treatments (between-group $d < 0.32$). The psychotherapy offered was of moderately short duration, which may have impacted the results. A similar study showed an effect for "flexible" treatment in combination with medication (venlafaxine vs. sertraline) for refugees (Sonne, Carlsson, Bech, Elklit, & Mortensen, 2016). Treatment included a total of 10 sessions with a psychiatrist or medical doctor and 16 sessions with a psychologist and optional individual, as well as group session with social workers (the average number of social work sessions was not included in the original manuscript). No effect on PTSD or depressive symptoms was found between the sertraline and venlafaxine group (between-group $d < 0.22$). Importantly, since the study did not have a monotherapy comparison, the results cannot address the incremental benefits of combination treatment. Additionally, patient and clinical staff were not blind to treatment conditions and there was no placebo control or wait-list group, so it was not possible to compare the effects of pharmacological treatments to a control condition. Finally, Hien and colleagues (2015) examined the effects of adding sertraline ($n = 32$) versus placebo ($n = 37$) for 69 individuals receiving Seeking Safety (SS), a manualized treatment for mixed-trauma PTSD and comorbid alcohol use disorder (Najavitz, 2002). Results showed larger reductions in PTSD symptoms at posttreatment (Week 12 between-group $d = 0.83$) and follow-up (6- and 12-month between-group $d = 0.71$ and $d = 0.65$, respectively) for those receiving sertraline compared to placebo. These findings may be difficult to generalize because not all participants met full diagnostic criteria for PTSD, and the treatment, which lacks robust empirical support, was reduced to half the typical course of sessions.

Thus, the extant literature does not demonstrate compelling evidence for the addition of SSRI medications to psychotherapy based on a limited number of RCTs and mixed study designs. Further research in this area is needed.

Novel Augmentation Strategies

Novel pharmacological and physiological approaches that can catalyze the psychotherapeutic process offer an alternative strategy to traditional additive combination therapies. Currently, multiple approaches are in the early stage of investigation, including DCS, MDMA, methylene blue, yohimbine, propranolol, hydrocortisone, dexamethasone, and rTMS.

D-Cycloserine

D-Cycloserine (DCS) is a partial NMDA receptor agonist. In animal models, DCS has been shown to facilitate the extinction of fear (Davis, Ressler, Rothbaum, & Richardson, 2006), and has thus been studied as an adjunctive medication to improve exposure-based psychotherapy. A 2017 systematic review and meta-analysis of 21 human studies showed a positive DCS augmentation effect on exposure-based cognitive-behavioral therapy (CBT) for anxiety, obsessive–compulsive disorder (OCD), and posttraumatic stress disorder (Mataix-Cols et al., 2017). However, the effect was small ($k = 21$, $n = 1,047$, mean difference = -3.62 [-0.81 to -6.43], $d = -0.25$) and may be highly dependent on the number of DCS doses and timing as well as baseline symptom severity. No differences were found between diagnoses. A subsequent reanalysis showed that DCS effects were optimal when medication was received at least 60 minutes prior to treatment as compared to less than 60 minutes before treatment (Rosenfield et al., 2019). A recent unpublished meta-analysis of four DCS trials for PTSD specifically suggested no significant benefit for DCS over placebo as an augmentation strategy for the treatment of PTSD ($k = 4$, $n = 224$, $SMD = -0.07$ [-0.52, 0.39]; Hoskins et al., 2020).

Findings from individual PTSD studies are mixed. Specifically, the effect of DCS augmentation of exposure-based therapies in PTSD has been evaluated in four published RCTs (de Kleine, Hendriks, Kusters, Broekman, & van Minnen, 2012; Difede et al., 2014; Litz et al., 2012; Rothbaum et al., 2014) and a fifth recently completed, unpublished trial (Difede, Rothbaum, Rizzo, Roy, & Reist, 2019). The study by de Kleine and colleagues (2012) randomized 67 mostly female sexual abuse survivors with PTSD to receive either 50 mg DCS ($n = 33$) or placebo ($n = 34$) 60 minutes prior to prolonged exposure (PE). PE included 8–10 weekly sessions lasting 90 minutes. There was adequate random sequence generation, allocation concealment, and blinding of participants, personnel, and outcome assessors. However, this study allowed the use of concomitant psychotropic medications and there was incomplete outcome data, with data missing from more than 40% of randomized participants.

PTSD symptoms reduced across time for the sample as a whole, but treatment group (DCS vs. placebo) did not have a significant effect on slope of change (Week 10 between-group $d = 0.43*$). However, treatment group was significantly associated with responder status (there was at least a 10-point drop on CAPS), with those receiving DCS more likely to be responders at the end of treatment (63.6%) compared to the placebo group (38.2%). Furthermore, exploratory session analyses indicated that DCS resulted in greater symptom reduction in participants with greater baseline PTSD severity who required more treatment sessions. Dropout rates were 27.3% in the DCS group and 38.2% in the placebo group.

Difede and colleagues (2014) randomized 25 mostly male survivors of the World Trade Center attacks to receive virtual reality exposure (VRE) plus 100 mg DCS ($n = 13$) or placebo ($n = 12$). The manualized VRE intervention included 12 weekly, 90-minute sessions with DCS or placebo administered 90 minutes prior to the session. All dropouts from the study were reported, and all from the placebo group (12% of randomized participants). However, this study allowed the use of concomitant psychotropic medications. Participants, personnel, and outcome assessors were adequately blinded, and there were small sample sizes per arm.

DCS showed a trend for greater symptom reduction at posttreatment (Week 10 between-group $d = 0.68$) and a significant reduction in symptoms at 6-month follow-up (between-group $d = 1.13$) as well as increased PTSD remission rates (Week 10, 46% vs. 8%; 6-month follow-up 69% vs. 17%). There were no DCS dropouts, compared to 25% in the placebo group.

Litz and colleagues (2012) randomized 26 male Iraq and Afghanistan veterans with combat-related PTSD to receive a brief six-session, manualized exposure therapy plus 50 mg DCS ($n = 13$) or placebo ($n = 13$) 30 minutes beforehand. In contrast with previous findings, the DCS group demonstrated less symptom reduction than the placebo group (Week 6 between-group $d = 1.15*$). Remission rates at posttreatment were similar (33.3% vs. 36.4%). Dropout rates were 30.8% in the DCS group and 15.4% in the placebo group. There was adequate random sequence generation and allocation concealment, and outcome assessments were conducted by an independent blind rater. However, the method of blinding participants and personnel was not adequately described. Also, the trial was stopped before the planned recruitment of $n = 68$ was reached, leaving a small sample size per arm. There is some question if adequate extinction of fear occurred in the psychotherapy sessions in the study.

Rothbaum and colleagues (2014) randomized 156 mostly male Iraq and Afghanistan veterans with combat-related PTSD in a three parallel-armed study to compare 50 mg DCS ($n = 53$), 0.25 mg alprazolam ($n = 50$), and placebo prior to VRE ($n = 53$). The manualized VRE intervention included six weekly 90-minute sessions with the experimental medication given 30 minutes beforehand. Concomitant psychotropics were allowed during this study. The random sequence generation and blinding of participants, personnel, and outcome assessors were not adequately described, and there was a high dropout rate, with data missing for more than 40% of randomized participants, with nearly a third being from participants who had dropped out before their first treatment.

PTSD symptom severity significantly decreased for all groups. No significant differences in PTSD symptom severity between the DCS and placebo groups were identified, but the alprazolam group had significantly worse severity of symptoms than the placebo group at posttreatment. Remission rates at posttreatment were similar (21.4% vs. 25.7% vs. 26.5%). The DCS group demonstrated enhanced between-session extinction learning and demonstrated lower cortisol and startle reactivity to virtual trauma cues at posttreatment. Dropout rates were high (DCS 45%, alprazolam 30%, placebo 36%), but occurred generally before the first treatment session (20% of the sample). These findings provide converging evidence that benzodiazepines are not effective medications for PTSD, especially when combined with exposure therapy.

Finally, Difede and colleagues (2019) randomized 192 mostly male combat veterans to 50 mg DCS or placebo combined with VRE or PE treatments for combat-related PTSD. The manualized VRE intervention included nine weekly sessions lasting 90 minutes. Sessions 3–9 included experimental medication given 30 minutes beforehand. All patients in all conditions improved significantly at posttreatment and maintained their gains at follow-up. The main effect of DCS was not significant, suggesting that participants improved at a similar rate regardless of medication. Dropout rates were 26.3% in the DCS group compared to 36.1% in the placebo group.

In summary, although the findings across studies are suggestive of a DCS effect on exposure-based therapy (Mataix-Cols et al., 2017; Rosenfield et al., 2019), single studies of PTSD treatment were likely underpowered to detect such an effect, given that all participants were randomized to receive a known effective treatment. Detecting an effect is likely obscured by differences in trauma type, number of treatment sessions received, and the dosage and timing of DCS. For example, a recent meta-analysis (Hoskins et al., 2020) found that a higher dose of 100 mg DCS was more effective in one RCT (de Kleine et al., 2012). Likewise, when timing is isolated in two RCTs (de Kleine et al., 2012; Difede et al., 2014), giving 50–100 mg DCS 90 minutes before therapy is modestly more effective than placebo (kappa = 2, n = 92, SMD = –0.47 [–0.89, –0.06]). The single positive RCT suggests that further research, in the direction of higher DCS doses given at longer intervals prior to exposure-based therapies, is needed to establish the clinical utility of this augmentation strategy for the treatment of PTSD.

3,4-Methylenedioxy-methamphetamine

3,4-Methylenedioxy-methamphetamine (MDMA) is a ring-substituted phenethylamine with a unique psychopharmacological profile, typically characterized by 2–6 hours of subjective feelings of well-being, sociability, and positive mood. MDMA exerts its effect mainly through both an increased release and reuptake inhibition of presynaptic serotonin and, to a lesser effect, dopamine. MDMA is associated with a robust release of the neuropeptide oxytocin and is associated with prosocial subjective experiences in healthy controls. MDMA stimulates release of cortisol and noradrenaline, which may enhance both emotional engagement and extinction learning (Young et al., 2017). Given its potential to reduce fear responding, enhance fear extinction, and increase prosocial emotional states, MDMA has been proposed as a candidate for assisting psychological therapies in traumatized people. The effects of MDMA-assisted psychotherapy (MDMA-AP) have been evaluated in three published RCTs with small sample sizes (Mithoefer, Wagner, Mithoefer, Jerome, & Doblin, 2011; Mithoefer et al., 2018; Oehen, Traber, Widmer, & Schnyder, 2013) and one long-term follow-up study (Mithoefer et al., 2013).

A novel MDMA-assisted therapeutic approach was developed and manualized by the nonprofit Multidisciplinary Association for Psychedelic Studies (MAPS), which includes a female–male therapist dyad, weekly 90-minute preparation and integration sessions, and two to three 8-hour-long, drug-assisted sessions. During the drug-assisted sessions, the participants are encouraged to focus their attention inward. The sessions are self-directed and unstructured, with participants allowed to think and talk about their trauma spontaneously. However, specific discussion of trauma can be encouraged by the therapist when needed. An initial pilot study of six patients with PTSD due to a sexual assault provided support for the safety and tolerability of this approach (Bouso, Doblin, Farre, Alcazar, & Gomez-Jarabo, 2008). In a small randomized trial of mostly female participants (n = 20) with treatment-resistant PTSD who received 16 weeks of manualized MAPS MDMA-AP with two 8-hour sessions of either 125 mg MDMA (plus a supplemental dose of 62.5 mg after 2 hours; n = 12) or matching inactive placebo (n = 8), the MDMA group demonstrated greater improvement in PTSD symptoms than the placebo group (Mithoefer et al., 2011). There was adequate random sequence generation and allocation concealment, although a high risk of performance bias existed, with participants and personnel likely unblinded by the novel nature of the drug. However, independent blinded outcome assessors were used. The clinical response, defined as more than 30% reduction in CAPS, was achieved in 83.3% of the MDMA group, compared to 25% of the placebo group, indicating that the MDMA-AP benefited this small treatment-resistant population. Clinical gains were largely maintained at 2- to 4-year follow-up (Mithoefer et al., 2013).

As MDMA demonstrates acute effects likely noticeable compared to placebo, maintaining the blind complicates the interpretation of results. As such, a subsequent investigation compared two doses of MDMA. In a randomized trial of 12 mostly female participants with chronic, treatment-resistant PTSD, participants received MDMA-AP via three drug-assisted sessions and either 125 mg MDMA (plus 62.5 supplemental dose; n = 8) or active placebo 25 mg MDMA (plus 12.5 mg supplemental dose; n = 4). A significant difference in PTSD symptoms was identified on self-reported symptoms but not on clinician-rated symptoms (Oehen et al., 2013). Dropout rates were 12.5% and 25% in the 125 mg and active control groups, respectively.

Finally, Mithoefer and colleagues (2018) randomized 24 mostly male service personnel (firefighters, police officers, and veterans) with PTSD to MDMA-assisted psychotherapy with three mediation doses: 125 mg ($n = 12$), 75 mg ($n = 7$), and active placebo 30 mg MDMA ($n = 7$) plus a 50% supplemental dose after 2 hours in all conditions. The 75 mg and 125 mg demonstrated significantly greater reduction in PTSD symptoms compared to the 30 mg group (1 month after the second experimental session between-group $d = 1.1$ for 125 mg vs. active placebo; $d = 2.8$ for 75 mg vs. active placebo). As in the previous Mithoefer study, there was adequate random sequence generation, allocation concealment, and blinding of outcome assessors, and the use of an active placebo dose also ensured adequate blinding of participants and personnel.

While recent meta-analytical findings (Hoskins et al., 2020) demonstrate impressive effects for this novel drug-assisted therapy (kappa = 3, $n = 58$, $SMD = -1.31$ [-1.92, -0.69]), effects for MDMA-AP are difficult to interpret given the sparse literature and methodological issues, including inability to maintain participants blind to the study drug, where an inactive placebo was used, and the use of a novel psychotherapy approach that has not been compared to conventional trauma-focused psychological therapies without drug augmentation. There are currently several ongoing Phase II studies in the United States, Canada, and Israel, with more open-label feasibility studies planned across Europe. In the United States, the Food and Drug Administration has granted a Breakthrough Therapy Designation for MDMA-AP, with Phase III studies commencing soon. Future research will benefit from follow-up studies replicating and extending this work in additional research groups and comparisons with empirically supported psychotherapies.

Other Novel Augmentation Agents

Additional agents that show promise for augmenting PE include methylene-blue and yohimbine. In a sample of 42 patients with chronic PTSD, methylene-blue plus imaginal exposure resulted in more treatment responders (number needed to treat = 7.5) and a higher reported quality of life (3-month follow-up between-group $d = 0.58$) compared to placebo plus imaginal exposure (Zoellner et al., 2017). In a sample of 26 males with combat-related PTSD, yohimbine plus PE was associated with higher objective arousal, indicated by increased heart rate and blood pressure, and subjective arousal, indicated by increased subjective report of distress, during the combined drug and exposure session. Those who received yohimbine showed lower trauma-cued heart rate reactivity during a script-driven imagery task 1 week following this session (between-group difference in heart rate = 3.15 beats per minute, $d = 0.25$; Tuerk et al., 2018). Notably, yohimbine was associated with greater between-session habituation (d = 0.32) and more rapid improvement in depression (d = 0.21) but not PTSD symptoms over the course of treatment.

One recent study examined the effect of propranolol provided 90 minutes before brief (15–25 minutes) memory reactivation sessions for 60 adults diagnosed with PTSD (Brunet et al., 2018). Participants received 0.67 mg/kg of short-acting propranolol, plus 1.0 mg/kg of long-lasting propranolol 90 minutes prior to six weekly sessions, during which participants read their trauma narrative out loud. This study was designed to target reconsolidation of trauma memories specifically. Those randomized to receive propranolol (n = 30) reported significantly lower PTSD symptom severity from clinical interview compared to those who received placebo (n = 31) after six sessions (within-group d = 1.76 and d = 1.25, respectively).

Corticosteroids have also been investigated as augmentation agents for PE with mixed results. Dexamethasone (0.5 mg) or placebo was administered the night before VRE in 27 post-9/11 veterans (n = 13 and n = 14, respectively; Maples-Keller et al., 2019). The dropout rate was significantly higher in the dexamethasone + VRE group (76.9%) compared to the placebo + VRE group (28.5%). Results suggested that the dexamethasone group may have experienced an increase in reexperiencing symptoms at Session 2 following drug administration. In contrast, hydrocortisone administered 20 minutes prior to imaginal exposure sessions in a sample of veterans receiving PTSD treatment (PE) resulted in greater retention in treatment and subsequently greater reductions in PTSD severity compared to placebo (Yehuda et al., 2015).

One additional augmentation strategy of recent interest combines repetitive transcranial magnetic stimulation (rTMS) with trauma-focused treatment. In one study, this approach involved rTMS right over dorsolateral prefrontal cortex compared to sham just prior to weekly cognitive processing therapy (CPT) sessions. One hundred three Iraq and Afghanistan veterans with combat-related PTSD were randomized to receive either rTMS + CPT (n = 54) or Sham + CTP (n = 49). Results showing that the rTMS + CPT group demonstrated greater symptom reduction across both clinician-rated and self-reported PTSD symptoms (Session 5 through 6-month follow-up between-group $d \geq 0.79$; Kozel et al., 2018). Future work should investigate mechanisms of this effect as well as optimal timing and dose.

Practical Delivery of Combined Efficacious Monotherapies

As a general clinical strategy, combination treatment of PTSD has not been well studied. In line with recent clinical recommendations (American Psychological Association, 2017; U.S. Department of Veterans Affairs & Department of Defense, 2017), patients should be offered evidence-based, trauma-focused therapy first. If a patient declines therapy or is unable to participate, medications should be recommended based on several clinical considerations, including patient preference, symptom profile, comorbid diagnosis, and the medication's side effects (Ehlers, Chapter 15, this volume). For patients who have not fully responded to medication alone, the addition of exposure therapy, like PE, may be indicated, in line with findings from Rothbaum and colleagues (2006). However, findings from Simon and colleagues (2008) suggest that nonreponse to exposure therapy does not warrant the addition of medication, at least not the addition of an SSRI after nonresponse to PE. Furthermore, a clear benefit for starting evidence-based psychotherapy and pharmacotherapy simultaneously at the start of treatment has not been found in the literature, with multiple studies showing no added benefit of combinatin therapy over PE alone for PTSD (Popiel et al., 2015; Rauch et al., 2019) or benefits that were not sustained (Schneir et al., 2012). There is a lack of research examining evidence-based psychotherapies other than exposure therapy in combination with medication for the treatment of PTSD. However, there is no reason to expect findings would be different for these other evidence-based approaches. Taken together, these studies suggest that SSRIs do not boost the effects of PE whether administered after nonresponse or throughout therapy. Thus, providers may need to temper expectations regarding combination approaches and look at alternative strategies to make "course corrections" after nonresponse to PE, especially if PE session frequency is low. Maintaining weekly or more frequent PE sessions without adding an SSRI may be a more effective approach. The finding of added benefits from the addition of PE after nonresponse to an SSRI is encouraging given that patients are more likely to present after nonresponse to SSRI monotherapy due to greater access to this treatment compared to evidence-based psychotherapy. Although these studies are informative, research on combining evidence-based pharmacotherapy and psychotherapy is limited. Novel methods are needed to identify additional factors that could inform the prescription of combination therapy. For example, it may be the case that adding an SSRI to PE is beneficial, but only for those with certain preferences or diagnostic profiles. Studies to date have not been able to tease apart these potential prescriptive predictors. Until clear benefits for combination therapy can be identified for specific populations of patients, this approach should not be recommended, consistent with published guidelines.

Practical Delivery of Augmentation Strategies

The literature on psychotherapy-specific augmentation of exposure-based PTSD treatment is young, making strong practical clinical recommendations premature. However, the studies outlined in this chapter can inform recommendations for future research. It is theorized that augmentation strategies for exposure-based treatments work by enhancing extinction learning and consolidation processes both during and after exposure sessions (see Singewald, Schmuckermair, Whittle, Holmes, & Ressler, 2015), suggesting a window of optimal combination effect that will be different depending on medication type. Thus, the timing of medication is a critical clinical issue.

For DCS, timing of dose may explain mixed findings in the literature. In a general review of DCS augmentation across diagnoses, Hofmann (2014) highlighted that studies finding a positive effect for this augmentation strategy administer smaller doses of DCS (50–250 mg) earlier before (1–2 hours) less frequent exposure sessions (three to five). Moreover, this review suggested that positive effects for DCS may only occur when the exposure therapy is successful and that for nonsuccessful exposures, DCS may lead to negative effects (e.g., Litz et al., 2012). In a more recent review and meta-analysis of DCS across anxiety disorders, the optimal dosing was found to be 50 mg, administered at least 60 minutes prior to nine sessions of exposure therapy (Rosenfield et al., 2019). For PTSD, mixed results may be related to dosing, timing, and therapy factors. Or, it may be the case that DCS is not a beneficial augmentation strategy. Without stronger evidence supporting the augmentation benefits of DCS, clinical recommendations for its use cannot be developed.

For MDMA, the long duration and nature of the drug's effect impact the type of psychotherapy that can be administered. The only studies of MDMA for the treatment of PTSD tested a novel treatment designed specifically for MDMA-assisted therapy. This intervention involves two or three drug-assisted psychotherapy sessions of 6–8 hour duration, which are relatively unstructured. The participant is invited to focus their attention inward, use eye shades and music, and a 50% supplemental dose is offered after 2 hours to prolong the peak experience. Given the novel psychotherapy design, it is not possible to determine the efficacy of MDMA as an adjunct to evidence-based treatment for PTSD. More research is needed to determine whether MDMA-assisted psychotherapy is an effective, stand-alone treatment or if MDMA can augment evidence-based psychotherapy.

Future Developments

The literature for combination treatments for PTSD is underdeveloped. Studies replicating previous findings and identifying mechanisms of change are needed to provide strong clinical recommendations for or against combination approaches. Novel research methods will be needed to iden-tify whether any subpopulations may benefit from a certain combination approach to develop more precise and specialized clinical care for PTSD. Studies of daily-dosed medications should broaden their scope to examine other SSRIs and evidence-based psychotherapies and examine timing of the start-of-medication dose in a more systematic way. For example, a trial comparing different starting points for adding SSRIs to treatment within the same sample may be better able to identify not only the optimal timing for intervening with a combination approach, but also more precise indicators of who is less likely to respond and more amenable to a combination approach.

Alternatively, acute-acting augmentation agents to enhance specific components of psychotherapy demonstrate either consistently mixed findings in the literature (e.g., DCS) or are currently lacking in systematic study (e.g., yohimbine or propranolol). Because each augmentation agent is theorized to interact with different potential mechanisms of psychotherapy response (e.g., emotional engagement, cognitive rigidity, cortisol regulation), specific experimental designs are needed to understand these effects. For example, the theory that propranolol impacts memory consolidation has led researchers to study augmentation with a memory consolidation paradigm, which has specific implications for trauma-memory-focused interventions, like PE. Compared to other augmentation agents, DCS has the largest literature base examining its use in the treatment of PTSD. The mixed findings suggest that timing and dosage are important to efficacy for this approach. However, while future research may clarify these moderating factors, it may also be the case that DCS is not as strong a therapeutic enhancer as originally theorized, especially in heterogeneous PTSD patients. Given the large number of novel theorized augmentation agents, it is inevitable that agents will be found to not have an effect or possibly have a negative effect on psychotherapy. It is critical for future research to interpret and report these null findings to identify reliable and clinically meaningful augmentation strategies.

MDMA-assisted psychotherapy has demonstrated efficacy as a treatment for PTSD in three small clinical trials. Due to the unique psychotherapy delivered in these studies, it is difficult to determine the efficacy of MDMA as an augmentation strategy for evidence-based treatment for PTSD. Like other augmentation agents, MDMA has been studied in animal models that suggest specific mechanisms of change related to extinction learning (Young et al., 2017). Future studies are needed to determine whether MDMA is a feasible and effective augmentation agent for evidence-based psychotherapies. As psychedelics like MDMA and psilocybin gain prominence in the clinical literature as potential therapy-assisted interventions (see Mithoefer, Grob, & Brewerton, 2016), research will be needed to specify the type of therapy that should be provided with these medications as well as their safety and efficacy for treating PTSD.

Finally, future research should determine which medication and psychotherapy combinations are most effective, why they are effective, and for whom. Mechanisms of change in combination approaches have yet to be identified. Patient factors are likely to play a role, including preference for medication versus psychotherapy. A recently published study doubly randomized individuals to choose or be randomized to receive either sertraline or PE as monotherapies (Zoellner, Roy-Byrne, Mavissakalian, & Feeny,

2018). Findings indicated that being able to choose one's preferred treatment resulted in larger gains, regardless of the treatment received. Future research should test whether preference impacts combination treatment outcome.

Summary

Combination approaches for the treatment of PTSD have the potential to enhance treatment efficacy and improve response rates. The literature for augmenting exposure therapy with SSRIs is still underdeveloped, and combination strategies were not considered by the ISTSS *Posttraumatic Stress Disorder Prevention and Treatment Guidelines* and are not recommended by other recent PTSD treatment guidelines (American Psychological Association, 2017; U.S. Department of Veterans Affairs & Department of Defense, 2017). Combination approaches with medications like SSRIs are commonly practiced in clinical settings and warrant further study to determine best practices. Several novel augmentation agents designed to enhance psychotherapy for PTSD, such as DCS, methylene blue, dexamethasone, hydrocortisone, yohimbine, propranolol, MDMA, and rTMS, are being examined in clinical populations with the potential to impact future clinical recommendations and improve treatment for PTSD. Future research should focus on testing these and other potential augmentation strategies in novel experimental designs that can identify not only whether these agents convey additive benefits, but also who is most likely to benefit from them and what is the most optimal administration strategy.

REFERENCES

American Psychological Association. (2017). Clinical practice guideline for the treatment of posttraumatic stress disorder (PTSD) in adults. Retrieved from *www.apa.org/about/offices/directorates/guidelines/ptsd.pdf.*

Bouso, J. C., Doblin, R., Farre, M., Alcazar, M. A., & Gomez-Jarabo, G. (2008). MDMA-assisted psychotherapy using low doses in a small sample of women with chronic posttraumatic stress disorder. *Journal of Psychoactive Drugs, 40*(3), 225–236.

Brunet, A., Saumier, D., Liu, A., Streiner, D. L., Tremblay, J., & Pitman, R. K. (2018). Reduction of PTSD symptoms with pre-reactivation propranolol therapy: A randomized controlled trial. *American Journal of Psychiatry, 175*(5), 427–433.

Buhmann, C. B. O., Nordentoft, M., Ekstroem, M., Carlsson, J., & Mortensen, E. L. (2016). The effect of flexible cognitive–behavioural therapy and medical treatment, including antidepressants on post-traumatic stress disorder and depression in traumatised refugees: Pragmatic randomised controlled clinical trial. *British Journal of Psychiatry, 208*(3), 252–259.

Cusack, K., Jonas, D. E., Forneris, C. A., Wines, C., Sonis, J., Middleton, J. C., et al.

(2016). Psychological treatments for adults with posttraumatic stress disorder: A systematic review and meta-analysis. *Clinical Psychology Review, 43*, 128–141.

Davidson, J., Pearlstein, T., Londborg, P., Brady, K. T., Rothbaum, B., Bell, J., et al. (2001). Efficacy of sertraline in preventing relapse of posttraumatic stress disorder: Results of a 28-week double-blind, placebo-controlled study. *American Journal of Psychiatry, 158*(12), 1974–1981.

Davis, M., Ressler, K., Rothbaum, B. O., & Richardson, R. (2006). Effects of D-cycloserine on extinction: Translation from preclinical to clinical work. *Biological Psychiatry, 60*(4), 369–375.

de Kleine, R. A., Hendriks, G., Kusters, W. J. C., Broekman, T. G., & van Minnen, A. (2012). A randomized placebo-controlled trial of D-cycloserine to enhance exposure therapy for posttraumatic stress disorder. *Biological Psychiatry, 71*(11), 962–968.

Difede, J., Cukor, J., Wyka, K., Olden, M., Hoffman, H., Lee, F. S., et al. (2014). D-Cycloserine augmentation of exposure therapy for post-traumatic stress disorder: A pilot randomized clinical trial. *Neuropsychopharmacology, 39*(5), 1052–1058.

Difede, J., Rothbaum, B., Rizzo, A., Roy, M., & Reist, C. (2019). *Enhancing exposure therapy for PTSD: Virtual reality and imaginal exposure with a cognitive enhancer.* Manuscript in preparation.

Feeny, N. C., Mavissakalian, M., Roy-Byrne, P. P., Bedard-Gilligan, M., & Zoellner, L. A. (2020). *Optimizing posttraumatic stress disorder treatment: Prolonged exposure (PE) versus PE plus sertraline.* Manuscript in preparation.

Hien, D. A., Levin, F. R., Ruglass, L. M., López-Castro, T., Papini, S., Hu, M., et al. (2015). Combining seeking safety with sertraline for PTSD and alcohol use disorders: A randomized controlled trial. *Journal of Consulting and Clinical Psychology, 83*(2), 359–369.

Hofmann, S. G. (2014). D-Cycloserine for treating anxiety disorders: Making good exposures better and bad exposures worse. *Depression and Anxiety, 31*(3), 175–177.

Hoskins, M., Pearce, J., Bethell, A., Dankova, L., Barbui, C., Tol, W. A., et al. (2015). Pharmacotherapy for post-traumatic stress disorder: Systematic review and meta-analysis. *British Journal of Psychiatry, 206*(2), 93–100.

Hoskins, M., Sinnerton, R., Bridges, J., Slater, A., Underwood, J., & Bisson, J. (2020). *Drug-assisted therapies for PTSD: A systematic review and meta-analysis.* Manuscript submitted for publication.

Kline, A. C., Cooper, A. A., Rytwinski, N. K., & Feeny, N. C. (2018). Long-term efficacy of psychotherapy for posttraumatic stress disorder: A meta-analysis of randomized controlled trials. *Clinical Psychology Review, 59*, 30–40.

Kozel, F. A., Motes, M. A., Didehbani, N., DeLaRosa, B., Bass, C., Schraufnagel, C. D., et al. (2018). Repetitive TMS to augment cognitive processing therapy in combat veterans of recent conflicts with PTSD: A randomized clinical trial. *Journal of Affective Disorders, 229*, 506–514.

Lee, D. J., Schnitzlein, C. W., Wolf, J. P., Vythilingam, M., Rasmusson, A. M., & Hoge, C. W. (2016). Psychotherapy versus pharmacotherapy for posttraumatic stress disorder: Systemic review and meta-analyses to determine first-line treatments. *Depression and Anxiety, 33*(9), 792–806.

Litz, B. T., Salters-Pedneault, K., Steenkamp, M. M., Hermos, J. A., Bryant, R. A., Otto, M. W., et al. (2012). A randomized placebo-controlled trial of D-cycloserine and exposure therapy for posttraumatic stress disorder. *Journal of Psychiatric Research, 46*(9), 1184–1190.

Maples-Keller, J., Jovanovic, T., Dunlop, B. W., Rauch, S., Yasinski, C., Michopoulos, V., et al. (2019). When translational neuroscience fails in the clinic: Dexamethasone prior to virtual reality exposure therapy increases drop-out rates. *Journal of Anxiety Disorders, 61,* 89–97.

Mataix-Cols, D., Fernández de, L. C., Monzani, B., Rosenfield, D., Andersson, E., Pérez-Vigil, A., et al. (2017). D-Cycloserine augmentation of exposure-based cognitive behavior therapy for anxiety, obsessive-compulsive, and posttraumatic stress disorders: A systematic review and meta-analysis of individual participant data. *JAMA Psychiatry, 74*(5), 501–510.

Mithoefer, M. C., Grob, C. S., & Brewerton, T. D. (2016). Novel psychopharmacological therapies for psychiatric disorders: Psilocybin and MDMA. *Lancet Psychiatry, 3*(5), 481–488.

Mithoefer, M. C., Mithoefer, A. T., Feduccia, A. A., Jerome, L., Wagner, M., Wymer, J., et al. (2018). 3,4-Methylenedioxymethamphetamine (MDMA)–assisted psychotherapy for post-traumatic stress disorder in military veterans, firefighters, and police officers: A randomised, double-blind, dose-response, phase 2 clinical trial. *Lancet Psychiatry, 5*(6), 486–497.

Mithoefer, M. C., Wagner, M. T., Mithoefer, A. T., Jerome, L., & Doblin, R. (2011). The safety and efficacy of ±3,4-methylenedioxymethamphetamine-assisted psychotherapy in subjects with chronic, treatment-resistant posttraumatic stress disorder: The first randomized controlled pilot study. *Journal of Psychopharmacology, 25*(4), 439–452.

Mithoefer, M. C., Wagner, M. T., Mithoefer, A. T., Jerome, L., Martin, S. F., Yazar-Klosinski, B., et al. (2013). Durability of improvement in post-traumatic stress disorder symptoms and absence of harmful effects or drug dependency after 3,4-methylenedioxymethamphetamine-assisted psychotherapy: A prospective long-term follow-up study. *Journal of Psychopharmacology, 27*(1), 28–39.

Najavits, L. M. (2002). *Seeking safety: A treatment manual for PTSD and substance abuse.* New York: Guilford Press.

Oehen, P., Traber, R., Widmer, V., & Schnyder, U. (2013). A randomized, controlled pilot study of MDMA (±3,4-methylenedioxymethamphetamine)–assisted psychotherapy for treatment of resistant, chronic post-traumatic stress disorder (PTSD). *Journal of Psychopharmacology, 27*(1), 40–52.

Popiel, A., Zawadzki, B., Praglowska, E., & Teichman, Y. (2015). Prolonged exposure, paroxetine and the combination in the treatment of PTSD following a motor vehicle accident: A randomized clinical trial–The "TRAKT" study. *Journal of Behavior Therapy and Experimental Psychiatry, 48,* 17–26.

Rauch, S. A. M., Kim, H. M., Powell, C., Tuerk, P. W., Simon, N. M., Acierno, R., et al. (2019). Efficacy of prolonged exposure therapy, sertraline hydrochloride, and their combination among combat veterans with posttraumatic stress disorder: A randomized clinical trial. *JAMA Psychiatry, 76*(2), 117–125.

Rosenfield, D., Smits, J., Hofmann, S., Mataix-Cols, D., Fernández de la Cruz, L., Andersson, E., et al. (2019). Changes in dosing and dosing timing of D-cycloserine explain its apparent declining efficacy for augmenting exposure therapy for anxiety-related disorders: An individual participant-data meta-analysis. *Journal of Anxiety Disorders, 68.* [Epub ahead of print]

Rothbaum, B. O., Cahill, S. P., Foa, E. B., Davidson, J. R. T., Compton, J., Connor,

K. M., et al. (2006). Augmentation of sertraline with prolonged exposure in the treatment of posttraumatic stress disorder. *Journal of Traumatic Stress, 19*(5), 625–638.

Rothbaum, B. O., Price, M., Jovanovic, T., Norrholm, S. D., Gerardi, M., Dunlop, B., et al. (2014). A randomized, double-blind evaluation of D-cycloserine or alprazolam combined with virtual reality exposure therapy for posttraumatic stress disorder in Iraq and Afghanistan war veterans. *American Journal of Psychiatry, 171*(6), 640–648.

Schneier, F. R., Neria, Y., Pavlicova, M., Hembree, E., Sun, E. J., Amsel, L., et al. (2012). Combined prolonged exposure therapy and paroxetine for PTSD related to the World Trade Center attack: A randomized controlled trial. *American Journal of Psychiatry, 169*(1), 80–88.

Simon, N. M., Connor, K. M., Lang, A. J., Rauch, S., Krulewicz, S., LeBeau, R. T., et al. (2008). Paroxetine CR augmentation for posttraumatic stress disorder refractory to prolonged exposure therapy. *Journal of Clinical Psychiatry, 69*(3), 400–405.

Singewald, N., Schmuckermair, C., Whittle, N., Holmes, A., & Ressler, K. (2015). Pharmacology of cognitive enhancers for exposure-based therapy of fear, anxiety and trauma-related disorders. *Pharmacology and Therapeutics, 149,* 150–190.

Sonne, C., Carlsson, J., Bech, P., Elklit, A., & Mortensen, E. L. (2016). Treatment of trauma-affected refugees with venlafaxine versus sertraline combined with psychotherapy—A randomised study. *BMC Psychiatry, 16,* 383–396.

Tuerk, P. W., Wangelin, B. C., Powers, M. B., Smits, J. A. J., Acierno, R., Myers, U. S., et al. (2018). Augmenting treatment efficiency in exposure therapy for PTSD: A randomized double-blind placebo-controlled trial of yohimbine HCl. *Cognitive Behaviour Therapy, 47*(5), 351–371.

U.S. Department of Veterans Affairs & Department of Defense. (2017). VA/DoD clinical practice guideline for the management of posttraumatic stress disorder and acute stress disorder. Retrieved from *www.healthquality.va.gov/guidelines/MH/ptsd/VADoDPTSDCPGFinal082917.pdf.*

Watts, B. V., Schnurr, P. P., Mayo, L., Young-Xu, Y., Weeks, W. B., & Friedman, M. J. (2013). Meta-analysis of the efficacy of treatments for posttraumatic stress disorder. *Journal of Clinical Psychiatry, 74*(6), e551–e557.

Yehuda, R., Bierer, L. M., Pratchett, L. C., Lehrner, A., Koch, E. C., Van Manen, J. A., et al. (2015). Cortisol augmentation of a psychological treatment for warfighters with posttraumatic stress disorder: Randomized trial showing improved treatment retention and outcome. *Psychoneuroendocrinology, 51,* 589–597.

Young, M. B., Norrholm, S. D., Khoury, L. M., Jovanovic, T., Rauch, S. A. M., Reiff, C. M., et al. (2017). Inhibition of serotonin transporters disrupts the enhancement of fear memory extinction by 3,4-methylenedioxymethamphetamine (MDMA). *Psychopharmacology, 234*(19), 2883–2895.

Zoellner, L. A., Roy-Byrne, P. P., Mavissakalian, M., & Feeny, N. C. (2018). Doubly randomized preference trial of prolonged exposure versus sertraline for treatment of PTSD. *American Journal of Psychiatry, 176*(4), 287–296.

Zoellner, L. A., Telch, M., Foa, E. B., Farach, F. J., McLean, C. P., Gallop, R., et al. (2017). Enhancing extinction learning in posttraumatic stress disorder with brief daily imaginal exposure and methylene blue: A randomized controlled trial. *Journal of Clinical Psychiatry, 78*(7), e782–e789.

CHAPTER 18

E-Mental Health

Catrin Lewis and Miranda Olff

Despite robust evidence to indicate the best strategies for the assessment and treatment of posttraumatic stress disorder (PTSD) as reflected across the chapters of this volume, many factors limit the availability and uptake of these interventions. These logistical issues include the cost of interventions (National Institute for Health and Care Excellence, 2018); the perceived stigma associated with accessing support (Cuijpers, van Straten, & Andersson, 2008); and geographical variations in service provision (Griffiths & Christensen, 2007). In response, there has been a growing interest in electronic mental health (e-mental health) as an option for increasing access to appropriate care (Olff, 2015).

What Is E-Mental Health?

E-mental health has been defined as "mental health services and information delivered or enhanced through the Internet and related technologies" (Christensen, Griffiths, & Evans, 2002). It is a generic term that encompasses the use of digital technologies for screening and diagnosis, health promotion, prevention, monitoring, early intervention, treatment, or relapse prevention, as well as for improvement of health care delivery and professional development (Riper et al., 2010). It is a broader concept than tele-health or tele-medicine, which use technology to connect health care professionals with consumers for real-time delivery of standard care (Ashwick, Turgoose, & Murphy, 2019; Sood et al., 2007).

E-mental health may also be termed "computerized," "Internet-based," "Web-based," or "online" mental health. Various e-mental health applications have been developed, including information pages and portals; online support forums and social networks; blogs and podcasts; training modules for providers; and tools for assessment or diagnosis. Exciting developments also include virtual reality, which integrates real-time computer graphics with other sensory input devices to immerse a participant in a virtual environment and facilitate the processing of memories associated with the traumatic event (Rizzo, Reger, Gahm, Difede, & Rothbaum, 2009; Rothbaum, Hodges, Ready, Graap, & Alarcon, 2001). However, for the purpose of this chapter, we focus on the role of structured Internet-based therapeutic interventions that have been developed for the prevention and treatment of PTSD in adults, while acknowledging that e-mental health serves a broader function in the mental health sector and that rapid progress is being made in the field of online assessments (Price et al., 2018; van der Meer, Bakker, Schrieken, Hoofwijk, & Olff, 2017).

E-Mental Health Interventions for the Prevention of PTSD

There is little evidence to support the provision of preventative interventions to mitigate the psychological impact of trauma exposure (see O'Donnell, Pacella, Bryant, Olff, & Forbes, Chapter 8, this volume). It follows that relatively few attempts have been made to develop and evaluate Internet-based interventions for the prevention of PTSD (Ennis, Sijercic, & Monson, 2018). Here, we will summarize the preventative e-mental health interventions that have been developed to date.

Trauma TIPS

Developed in the Netherlands, Trauma TIPS is a self-guided intervention aimed at the prevention of PTSD in injury patients (Mouthaan, Sijbrandi, de Vries, et al., 2013; Mouthaan, Sijbrandij, Reitsma, Gersons, & Olff, 2011; Mouthaan, Sijbrandij, Reitsma, Luitse, et al., 2011). Based on cognitive-behavioral principles, Trauma TIPS incorporates psychoeducation, stress management, and *in vivo* exposure. It consists of six steps, including an introduction; video clips of a clinician and three patient stories; text describing common physical and psychological reactions after trauma; audio clips with instructions for stress management techniques; contact information for assistance/additional support for enduring symptoms; and a Web forum for peer support. The total duration of the program is approximately 30 minutes.

Afterdeployment.org

Afterdeployment.org and its accompanying app, LifeArmor, provide Internet-based self-assessment, self-management strategies, videos, and materials that address a number of topics in addition to PTSD, such as injury, alcohol and drug use, sleep, anger, military sexual abuse, and resilience after trauma exposure (Bush, Bosmajian, Fairall, McCann, & Ciulla, 2011). It is primarily intended as an adjunct to face-to-face therapy (Ruzek et al., 2011). It was designed to be used by health care professionals, military personnel, and their families. It includes psychoeducation as well as self-assessment tools and interactive content.

My Disaster Recovery

Although not specifically targeting PTSD, another Internet-based intervention designed for use in the aftermath of trauma, My Disaster Recovery, provides advice on seeking professional help, relaxation, social support, unhelpful ways of coping, self-talk, and trauma triggers and memories (Benight, Ruzek, & Waldrep, 2008). It consists of six interactive modules, which include self-tests and video vignettes.

Cancer Coping Online

Cancer Coping Online is another self-guided Internet-based program grounded in cognitive-behavioral principles (Beatty, Koczwara, & Wade, 2011). The six-session program focuses on teaching coping strategies for reducing cancer-specific traumatic-stress symptoms, depression, and anxiety.

RealConsent

Another approach is to develop interventions aimed at the prevention of trauma. RealConsent is an Internet-based bystander approach to the prevention of sexual violence (Salazar, Vivolo-Kantor, Hardin, & Berkowitz, 2014). It is based on social cognitive theory, social norms theory, and the bystander educational model, with the aims of increasing prosocial intervening behaviors and preventing sexually violent behavior toward women. The intervention consists of six 30-minute modules including interactivity, didactic activities, and episodes of a serial drama illustrating positive and negative behavior.

E-Mental Health Interventions for the Treatment of PTSD

E-mental health is said to be one of the most promising opportunities for more timely and effective treatment of common mental health problems (Christensen & Hickie, 2010). Internet-based psychological therapies have been developed and implemented for a range of disorders, with the aim of reducing health care expenditures and broadening access to psychological therapies. Since the emergence of the first e-mental health interventions for the treatment of mental disorders, a number of systematic reviews have supported their efficacy for depression (Spek et al., 2007), anxiety disorders (Lewis, Pearce, & Bisson, 2012; Olthuis, Watt, Bailey, Hayden, & Stewart, 2015), and eating disorders (Schlegl, Bürger, Schmidt, Herbst, & Voderholzer, 2015).

Internet-based interventions for the treatment of a mental disorder are highly structured online programs that aim to improve users' mental health by enhancing their knowledge and skills (Barak, Klein, & Proudfoot, 2009). These programs are commonly based on cognitive-behavioral therapy (CBT), but sometimes include components of other established psychological treatments, such as acceptance and commitment therapy (ACT) and mindfulness. The content of existing therapies is not usually altered, deviating from traditional psychological treatment only in terms of the method of delivery (Cuijpers, Donker, van Straten, Li, & Andersson, 2010).

Internet-based interventions vary in terms of the level of therapist assistance provided. They can be delivered with regular assistance from a highly engaged specialist therapist who provides input and feedback on homework, encourages engagement with the program, and provides technical assistance with the platform. They can also be delivered by a nonspecialist mental health professional who briefly introduces the program and intervenes to check on progress or provides input on demand, often by telephone or by e-mail. Finally, they can adopt a stand-alone approach, in which no therapist assistance is provided. There is evidence to support the superiority of interventions that include input from a therapist (Lewis et al., 2012; Lewis, Roberts, Bethell, Robertson, & Bisson, 2018; Spek et al., 2007).

The development and evaluation of e-mental health interventions for PTSD have lagged behind other disorders. The first RCT of a self-help-based intervention for PTSD preceded e-mental health (Ehlers et al., 2003). This intervention was found to be no more efficacious than repeated assessments; however, the self-help materials may not have been optimal and no therapist support or follow-up appointments were provided. This finding, however, may have discouraged the development of further interventions for a time. It is also likely that the potential for symptom worsening and adverse events has discouraged the development and implementation of interventions historically.

We know that psychological therapies are effective interventions for PTSD, and there is a substantial body of evidence in support of CBT-based treatment (see, in this volume, Chard, Kaysen, Galovski, Nixon, & Monson, Chapter 13; Ehlers, Chapter 15; Riggs, Tate, Chrestman, & Foa, Chapter 12). CBT protocols are structured, thereby lending themselves well to Internet-based delivery. Due to a combination of these factors, the majority of Internet-based interventions for the treatment of PTSD have been CBT-based.

Most Internet-based interventions for PTSD initiate treatment with psychoeducation and the rationale for CBT-based treatment (Improving Access to Psychological Therapies, 2010). These programs incorporate cognitive techniques, with the aim of identifying and modifying unhelpful patterns of cognition (Newman, Erickson, Przeworski, & Dzus, 2003). Usually, behavioral components are included; they generally encompass imaginal and *in vivo* exposure (Lewis et al., 2017). Trauma-focused programs involve activating the trauma memory, usually by writing about the traumatic event. Most conclude with a section on relapse prevention that focuses on staying well, recognizing signs of relapse, and offering advice on what to do if problems recur (Gega, Marks, & Mataix-Cols, 2004). There is a distinction between Internet-CBT and online psychoeducation. Although the two overlap in content, psychoeducation aims to increase knowledge, whereas Internet-CBT aims to teach skills and techniques that can be used to overcome specific PTSD symptoms. Internet-CBT programs are often based on existing face-to-face psychotherapy protocols and share many common features (Andersson & Cuijpers, 2009).

A number of e-mental health interventions have been developed for the treatment of PTSD. They are outlined here, followed by the findings with regard to efficacy in the next section (see Figure 18.1).

Interapy

The first formally evaluated e-mental health intervention to treat PTSD was developed in the Netherlands. Known as Interapy, it involves 10, 45-minute writing assignments completed over a period of 5 weeks. The intervention consists of three treatment phases: (1) self-confrontation, (2) cognitive reappraisal, and (3) social sharing. Initially, psychoeducation is presented in relation to the mechanisms of exposure. At the beginning of each writing phase, individuals plan when they are going to write. Halfway through and at the end of each treatment phase, the person with PTSD receives feedback and further writing instructions from his or her therapist via e-mail, which is based on a treatment manual that tailors feedback to specific needs. The e-mail feedback includes recognition and reinforcement of the person's work and motivation. In the first writing phase, the therapist helps the person with PTSD to write about the traumatic event, with a focus on his or

- Interapy
- PTSD Coach
- Spring
- Survivor to Thriver
- DElivery of Self-TRaining and Education for Stressful Situations (DESTRESS)

FIGURE 18.1. E-mental health interventions for the treatment of PTSD.

her most painful images and thoughts, in the first person and in the present tense, including sensory details. If necessary, the therapist supports the individual to address any avoided aspects of the trauma. During the second phase, psychoeducation in relation to the principles of cognitive change is presented. The aim is to form a new perspective on the traumatic event and to regain a sense of control. This involves writing a supportive letter to an imaginary friend who has been through the same experience, reflecting on the friend's feelings of guilt and shame and unrealistic thoughts. During the third phase, individuals receive psychoeducation about the positive effects of social sharing. In a final letter, the person with PTSD summarizes what happened, reflects on the therapeutic process, and describes how he or she plans to cope now and in the future. Warriors Internet Recovery and Education (WIRED) is a version of Interapy that has been adapted for use with veterans (Krupnick et al., 2017).

PTSD Coach

One of the most well-known e-mental health interventions for PTSD is PTSD Coach, developed jointly by the U.S. Department of Veterans Affairs (VA) and Department of Defense (DoD; Kuhn et al., 2014). PTSD Coach is a psychoeducational and self-management tool for acute distress related to PTSD (Kuhn et al., 2018). It targets military veterans as well as the broader civilian population. It consists of four core sections. The "Learn" section provides PTSD psychoeducation, information about professional support, and material related to PTSD and the family. The "Track Symptoms" feature allows users to complete the PTSD Checklist for the fifth edition of the *Diagnostic and Statistical Manual of Mental Disorders* (DSM-5; Blevins, Weathers, Davis, Witte, & Domino, 2015) and to receive feedback on their severity scores, with recommendations for treatment if indicated. This section also offers tracking of symptoms over time with the option of reminders and the ability to view a graph of changes in symptoms over time. The "Manage Symptoms" section offers the user the opportunity to learn coping tools that target different types of PTSD symptoms. The "Get Support" section contains crisis support resources, including supportive contacts added by the user. PTSD Coach is available free of charge from the iTunes and Google Play app stores for use with Apple and Android devices (Kuhn et al., 2014). The app has been translated and adapted into several languages, for example, Swedish (Cernvall, Sveen, Bergh Johannesson, & Arnberg, 2018). The slightly more generic Dutch version, called Support Coach, is now also available in app stores (van der Meer, Bakker, van Zuiden, Lok, & Olff, 2020).

Spring

Spring is a CBT-based program developed in the United Kingdom (Lewis, Roberts, Vick, & Bisson, 2013). It was systematically developed following

Medical Research Council (MRC; 2000) guidance for the development of a complex intervention. The work followed an iterative process incorporating qualitative work to model the intervention, followed by two pilot studies to refine it on the basis of quantitative and qualitative outcomes (Lewis et al., 2013). Collaboration with a software development company produced an interactive online version of the program. It includes eight online steps designed for delivery over 8 weeks. The eight steps are designed to be completed sequentially, with later steps relying on mastery of techniques taught in earlier steps. The program draws on active ingredients from trauma-focused CBT. Each of the eight steps activates a new tool or technique derived from CBT, which aims to reduce traumatic stress symptoms. The program is initiated with an hour-long appointment with a therapist, followed by fortnightly 30-minute sessions with a therapist. The aim of the guidance is to offer continued support, monitoring, motivation, and assistance with problem solving.

Survivor to Thriver

Survivor to Thriver was developed in the United States (Littleton, Grills, Kline, Schoemann, & Dodd, 2016). The intervention consists of nine modules. The first modules focus on psychoeducation, relaxation, grounding, and adaptive coping. The next modules introduce cognitive interventions. The final modules focus on using cognitive techniques to address specific concerns relevant to rape victims (e.g., self-blame, safety concerns). Modules are completed one at a time, and access to each subsequent module is granted by the therapist. Each module contains a video clip discussing the topic covered in the module, a written description of the skills or techniques being introduced, and written examples of women modeling the skills. The program also includes interactive exercises designed to help women think about the extent to which the particular issue raised in the module is a concern for them or to practice a described skill or technique and receive feedback on their practice. The interactive exercises provide information to enable the clinician to determine how long a client should spend on a particular module.

DElivery of Self-TRaining and Education for Stressful Situations (DESTRESS)

Also developed in the United States, DESTRESS-PC is a non-trauma-focused variant of CBT and stress inoculation training (Litz et al., 2007) designed for symptoms resulting from military trauma. The website allows access to psychoeducation about PTSD, stress, and trauma, as well as common comorbid problems and symptoms such as depression and survivor guilt. It also provides strategies for the management of stress, anger, and sleep disturbance. In addition, it teaches cognitive change techniques and strategies to alter self-talk. Individuals are asked to generate a hierarchy of avoided situations that trigger deployment memories. Each interaction with the website is intended to take 15–30 minutes, with related homework assignments taking another half hour. Clinicians are able to access a section of the DESTRESS website to monitor compliance and symptoms, and provide guidance as needed.

Advantages of E-Mental Health

Over the past decades, the Internet has altered most aspects of our day-to-day lives dramatically. It has become a basic tool for the dissemination of information, entertainment, communication, education, and knowledge transfer. Digital technologies have multifaceted attributes that lend themselves intrinsically to the delivery of mental health care. These attributes give rise to the numerous advantages of e-mental health, which are considered here (see Figure 18.2).

Timely Intervention

There is an inevitable delay between the onset of a mental disorder and the start of evidence-based psychotherapy (EBP) (Wang et al., 2007). Although some individuals are motivated and able to access timely intervention, the interval between symptoms arising and receipt of appropriate treatment varies substantially, and disorders including PTSD often go untreated for many years (Wang et al., 2005). If left untreated, PTSD is associated with functional and emotional impairment (Amaya-Jackson et al., 1999; Cloitre, Miranda, Stovall-McClough, & Han, 2005), reduced quality of life (Olatunji, Cisler, & Tolin, 2007; Zatzick et al., 2014), a predisposition for the development of other psychiatric and physical illnesses (Brady, Killeen, Brewerton, & Lucerini, 2000; Pacella, Hruska, & Delahanty, 2013), increased suicidal ideation (Krysinska & Lester, 2010), higher health care utilization (Domin Chan, Cheadle, Reiber, Unützer, & Chaney, 2009), and higher rates of alcohol abuse and dependence (Breslau, Davis, & Schultz, 2003; Jacobsen,

- Timely intervention
- Improved accessibility
- Anonymity
- Flexibility
- Standardization
- Empowerment
- Acceptability
- Potential for cost-effectiveness

FIGURE 18.2. Advantages of e-mental health.

Southwick, & Kosten, 2001). E-mental health may remove some of the barriers to EBP and allow earlier intervention, potentially preventing further sequelae of untreated PTSD.

Improved Accessibility

A distinct advantage of e-mental health is that it allows individuals living in geographically remote areas to access mental health care resources they might not otherwise be able to access (Griffiths & Christensen, 2007). There is evidence that individuals living in rural areas have a similar prevalence of mental health problems to those living in urban areas (Caldwell, Jorm, & Dear, 2004); however, fewer people in rural areas access services (Roberts, Battaglia, & Epstein, 1999). E-mental health interventions have the scope to reach users spread over a broader geographical area than traditional mental health services (Christensen & Hickie, 2010), breaking down barriers and supporting greater equity of care. E-mental health also offers a potentially crucial method of delivering mental health interventions to those exposed to war, ethnic conflict, and natural disasters on the basis that entire communities are often traumatized and may be difficult to access (Ruzek, Kuhn, Jaworski, Owen, & Ramsey, 2016).

Anonymity

E-mental health enables anonymous or discreet access to support and treatment for those who might not otherwise seek help (Williams, 2001). It enables access to mental health resources without visiting a health care professional. Because stigma creates a culture of secrecy and denial around mental health that impedes engagement with mental health services (Corrigan, Druss, & Perlick, 2014), this is a distinct advantage of the approach.

Flexibility

E-mental health resources are accessible 24 hours a day, allowing individuals to work through materials in their own time and at their own pace. For those accessing treatment online, it enables them to fit this in around other commitments (Williams & Whitfield, 2001). This may be especially advantageous to individuals who are employed, have family demands, or lead otherwise busy lives. It also negates or reduces the need to arrange child care to attend therapy sessions. E-mental health interventions enable access to treatment from home, which has several potential benefits (Carlbring, Westling, Ljungstrand, Ekselius, & Andersson, 2001). This flexibility may be appealing to individuals who experience difficulties concentrating or focusing on tasks. Furthermore, individuals may feel more comfortable and able to address their feelings at home, on their own, than in the presence of a therapist (Suler, 2004). Engaging in treatment at home is also useful to those who suffer mobility problems or difficulties leaving the house for psychological reasons (Lina, Isaac, & David, 2004). The opposite is also true, and at-home treatment may support an avoidance of leaving the house, or a tendency for individuals to avoid engaging with e-mental health materials.

Standardization

E-mental health services can be delivered with a high degree of fidelity (Christensen et al., 2002). The content of e-mental health programs is usually delivered to all users in broadly the same way. There is less reliance on therapist skill and less scope for clinicians to deviate from the treatment protocol if the intervention is guided. This may also act as a disadvantage. For more prescriptive and delineated intervention manuals, there may be less opportunity for tailoring interventions to the individual and his or her specific needs.

Empowerment

E-mental health supports a cultural shift in mental health services, giving consumers greater choice and the opportunity for input into care for their condition. E-mental health enables individuals to take more of an active role in addressing their illness and to claim responsibility for their recovery. Guided interventions create a therapeutic relationship based on collaboration consistent with policy focusing on increased involvement of consumers in all aspects of service delivery (Christensen & Petrie, 2013). E-mental health has been associated with empowerment, self-determination, self-control, confidence, and the development of personal coping strategies in effective recovery (Jacobson & Greenley, 2001). It introduces an approach whereby individuals work with their clinician to solve problems, drawing on their own expertise and experience. Although the approach allows an individual to attribute improvement to his or her own personal efforts, it is worth noting that the opposite is also true. There may be a tendency for lack of progress to be viewed as a personal failing (Fairburn, 1997).

Acceptability

There is public enthusiasm for psychological therapy, with it often favored over medication by individuals seeking treatment for a mental disorder. E-mental health offers a way to fulfill the demand for such therapies through an approach that has been found to be acceptable to users (Botella et al., 2009). There is also capacity for the development of bespoke resources to suit the needs of particular subgroups (e.g., military veterans, rape survivors), which may further enhance the acceptability of e-mental health.

Potential for Cost-Effectiveness

Scarcity of financial resources is a powerful rationale for the exploration of innovative alternatives for mental health care (Donker et al., 2015). Embracing the opportunities offered by e-mental health has the potential to alleviate some of the resource challenges faced by the mental health sector. From an economic perspective, e-mental health requires fewer personnel and less infrastructure, offering a potentially lower-cost alternative to standard mental health services (Hedman et al., 2014). E-mental health interventions aimed at the treatment of PTSD place less demand on therapist time, a costly and limited resource. Using the Internet to deliver EBP has the capacity to reduce the cost of effectively delivering EBP (Hedman et al., 2011; Hedman, Ljotsson, & Lindefors, 2012). However, the economic evaluation of e-mental health has not received sufficient attention (Donker et al., 2015), and further work is required before e-mental health interventions can be recommended not simply based on an assumption of cost-effectiveness.

Limitations of E-Mental Health

Ongoing work seeks to understand the role that e-mental health potentially has to play in the mental health sector. It is worth acknowledging the limitations of the delivery method and discussing the challenges that surround implementation of the approach (see Figure 18.3).

Ethical and Legal Responsibility

There is some resistance to e-mental health for fear of unethical practice or legal liability. Concern exists that information may be misinterpreted or used incorrectly (Christensen et al., 2002). The quality of information on websites is highly variable. It can be difficult for consumers to ascertain if a source is legitimate, or if information is reliable. Data security considerations are of importance and often overlooked or underestimated (Bennett, Bennett, & Griffiths, 2010).

> - Ethical and legal responsibility
> - Oversimplification
> - Difficulties using materials
> - Lack of evidence supporting acceptability to diverse groups

FIGURE 18.3. Limitations of e-mental health.

Oversimplification

Critics of the approach have suggested that e-mental health oversimplifies mental disorders and offers unsophisticated short-term solutions to difficult and complex issues. Others have commented that treatment delivered via e-mental health creates unrealistic expectations and the potential for individuals to feel as though they have failed when desired results are not attained. There is also the possibility for e-mental health to cause harm through improper use or misunderstanding. Others suggest the danger of self-help interventions being relied upon at times of crisis, in place of the individual seeking more appropriate support (Taylor & Luce, 2003). These issues might be avoided through thoughtful planning of e-mental health interventions, coupled with guidance for its responsible use.

Difficulties Using Materials

Gaining benefit from e-mental health resources may be challenging to those lacking motivation or the ability to concentrate. An inability to engage with the material may lead to perceived failure with an impact on self-esteem. The addition of guidance from a trained facilitator may alleviate this shortcoming to some extent. Materials written to motivate and reassure may also serve the same purpose when guidance is absent or limited.

Lack of Evidence Supporting Acceptability to Diverse Groups

When it comes to acceptability, we know little regarding the views of minority and culturally diverse groups (Richards, 2004). There is particular concern for those whose first language is not the language of the intervention. Ideally, culturally specific materials should be developed and evaluated in a range of languages. Cultural differences may exist in terms of optimal design, wording, and presentation of materials. Reliance on written text can also serve to exclude individuals who have difficulty reading. Presenting materials exclusively on the Internet may also raise questions of accessibility and potential exclusion, especially with regard to older generations.

Efficacy of E-Mental Health Interventions for the Prevention of PTSD

It is not possible to pool the available RCT data on preventative e-mental health approaches due to the small number of studies, which often adopted different primary outcome measures. The efficacy of existing interventions will be summarized narratively.

- *Trauma TIPS.* The results of the only RCT of Trauma TIPS, which randomized 300 injury patients to Trauma TIPS or usual care, did not support its efficacy (Mouthaan et al., 2013). Uptake of the intervention was low, with only one-fifth of participants logging in. The only significant decrease in PTSD symptoms occurred among a subgroup of patients with initially severe traumatic stress symptoms.

- *My Disaster Recovery.* An RCT of My Disaster Recovery found that worry was significantly reduced in comparison to an information-only control group. A similar, although not significant trend, emerged for depression (Steinmetz, Benight, Bishop, & James, 2012).

- *Cancer Coping Online.* Sixty individuals with cancer diagnosed in the previous 6 months and receiving treatment with curative intent were randomized to Cancer Coping Online or to Internet-based attention control. The findings did not support its efficacy in terms of reduction in cancer-related PTSD symptoms (Beatty, Koczwara, & Wade, 2016).

- *RealConsent.* An RCT randomized 743 male undergraduate students in the United States, ages 18–24, to RealConsent, or a general health promotion program. At 6-month follow-up, RealConsent participants intervened more often and engaged in less sexual violence than participants randomized to a general health promotion program. However, there was considerable attrition and the trial was forced to end prematurely, indicating the need for caution when interpreting the results.

Summary

Although the Internet provides a useful platform to widely disseminate preventative approaches, there is insufficient evidence to support the indiscriminate delivery of preventative e-mental health interventions to trauma-exposed populations. There may, however, be an argument for further exploration of targeted intervention, aimed only at those who are symptomatic on screening in the aftermath of a trauma. There is also scope for the use of e-mental health for widespread, low-cost screening of trauma survivors, which may serve a useful function in identifying those most likely to benefit. This, though, remains to be evaluated.

Efficacy of E-Mental Health in the Treatment of PTSD

A recent Cochrane review of Internet-based CBT (i-CBT) for PTSD found 10 RCTs that met eligibility criteria for the review (Lewis et al., 2018). Eight of the studies compared i-CBT delivered with therapist guidance to a wait-list control group. Two studies compared guided i-CBT with a non-CBT-based psychological therapy delivered on the Internet (see Table 18.1).

TABLE 18.1. Characteristics of Included Studies (Lewis et al., 2018)

	Country	N	Method of recruitment	Method of diagnosis	Trauma type	Duration of treatment	Experimental intervention	Therapist time	Control intervention	Relevant outcome measures
Engel et al. (2015)	U.S.	80	Ads	Clinician-rated	Military	6–8 wk	DElivery of SelfTRaining and Education for Stressful Situations (DESTRESS)	Nurse guidance; monitoring via website; guidance as necessary	Optimized usual care (i.e., usual primary care PTSD treatment with training of the clinic providers in management of PTSD)	PCL; PHQ-8; PHQ-15
Ivarsson et al. (2014)	Sweden	62	Ads	Clinician-rated	Various	8 wk	(unnamed)	Clinical psychology students; guidance once a week and occasional reminders via website	Attention control (i.e., answering weekly questions on well-being, stress, and sleep)	PDS; BDI-II; BAI; QOLI
Knaevelsrud, Brand, Lange, Ruwaard, & Wagner (2015)	Iraq	159	Ads	Self-reported	War related	5 wk	Interapy	Psychotherapists; weekly reminder e-mails and phone contact if no response	Wait list	PDS; HSCL-25; EUROHIS-QOL

(continued)

TABLE 18.1. (continued)

	Country	N	Method of recruitment	Method of diagnosis	Trauma type	Duration of treatment	Experimental intervention	Therapist time	Control intervention	Relevant outcome measures
Krupnick et al. (2017)	U.S.	34	Clinician referral	Self-reported	Military	10 wk	Warriors Internet Recovery and Education (WIRED); adapted from Interapy	Psychologists; short response after each writing exercise and as required	Treatment as usual	PCL-M; PHQ-9
Kuhn et al. (2017)	U.S.	120	Ads	Self-reported	Various	3 mo	PTSD Coach	None	Wait list	PCL-C; PHQ-8
Lewis et al. (2017)	UK	42	Clinician referral and ads	Clinician-rated	Various	8 wk	Spring	Trauma therapists; hour-long introductory session followed by fortnightly appointments face-to-face or by phone	Wait list	CAPS-5; BDI; BAI
Littleton et al. (2016)	U.S.	87	Ads	Clinician-rated	Rape	14 wk	From Survivor to Thriver	Brief check-ins by clinical psychology students	Website including psychoeducation, relaxation,	PSS-I; CES-D; FDAS

Study										Measures
							(approximately 5 min, approximately once every 2 wk)	grounding, and coping strategies		
Litz et al. (2007)	U.S.	45	Ads	Clinician-rated	Military	8 wk	DElivery of SelfTRaining and Education for Stressful Situations (DESTRESS)	2-hr-long introductory sessions (including basis assessment); phone and e-mail guidance as required	Non-CBT-based Internet intervention (monitoring non-trauma-related concerns, psycho-education, stress management); therapist contact as required, focused on non-trauma-related concerns	PSS-I; BDI; BAI
Miner et al. (2016)	U.S.	49	Ads	Self-reported	Various	4 wk	PTSD Coach	None	Wait list	PCL-C
Spence et al. (2011)	Australia	42	Ads	Clinician-rated	Various	8 wk	(unnamed)	Clinical psychologist via telephone, e-mail, and forum	Wait list	PCL-C; PHQ-9; GAD-7

Eligible studies were randomized controlled trials (RCTs); randomized cross-over trials; and cluster-randomized trials of i-CBT for the treatment of PTSD. Participants were required to be adults aged 16 years or older. At least 70% of study participants were required to meet full diagnostic criteria for PTSD according to DSM or ICD criteria, assessed by clinical interview or a validated self-report questionnaire. Studies were included regardless of the type of trauma experienced by the person with PTSD; the severity or duration of symptoms; or the length of time since trauma. No restrictions were applied on the basis of comorbidity as long as PTSD was the primary diagnosis and reduction in traumatic stress symptoms was the main aim of the intervention. I-CBTs with or without therapist guidance were eligible, including therapies delivered online and through mobile applications (apps). Programs that provided up to a maximum of 5 hours of therapist guidance were included, as well as programs that provided guidance delivered face-to-face or remotely. There were no restrictions related to the number of interactions with a therapist or length of the online program. Eligible comparator interventions were face-to-face psychological therapy; wait list/minimal attention/repeated assessment/treatment as usual (TAU); and non-CBT Internet-delivered psychological therapy. Sample size and publication status were not used to determine inclusion. Only English-language studies were eligible.

Outcomes

i-CBT versus Wait List/Treatment as Usual/Minimal Attention

There was evidence that i-CBT was more effective than wait list/treatment as usual/minimal attention in the reduction of PTSD symptoms postintervention (kappa = 8; n = 560; SMD = –0.60; CI = –0.97 to –0.24). However, these effects were not maintained at follow-up of 3–6 months (kappa = 3; n = 146; SMD = –0.0; CI = –0.64 to 0.04). The postintervention effect size was greater for studies in a subgroup analysis of only trauma-focused i-CBT (trauma focused [kappa = 4; n = 177; SMD = –1.04; CI = –1.57 to –0.51] vs. non-trauma-focused). There was also evidence for greater effect in a subgroup analysis of only guided i-CBT (kappa = 6; n = 391; SMD = –0.86; CI = –1.25 to –0.47). There was evidence of greater dropout from i-CBT than wait list/treatment as usual/minimal attention (kappa = 8; n = 585; RR = 1.39; CI = 1.03 to 1.88). There was evidence that i-CBT was more effective than wait list/treatment as usual/minimal attention in the reduction of symptoms of depression and anxiety postintervention and at follow-up of less than 6 months. There was also evidence that i-CBT was more effective than wait list/treatment as usual/minimal attention postintervention in terms of improvement in quality of life.

i-CBT versus i-Non-CBT

I-CBT showed no benefit when compared to i-non-CBT in the reduction of PTSD symptoms postintervention (kappa = 2; n = 82; *SMD* = –0.08; *CI* = –0.52 to 0.35), at follow-up of less than 6 months (kappa = 2; n = 65; *SMD* = 0.08; *CI* = –0.41 to 0.57), and at follow-up of 6–12 months (kappa = 1; n = 18; *SMD* = –8.83; *CI* = –17.32 to –0.34). There was also no evidence of greater dropout from i-CBT than i-non-CBT (kappa = 2; n = 132; *RR* = 2.14; *CI* = 0.97 to 4.73). There was insufficient data to conduct any subgroup analyses. There was no evidence of a difference between i-CBT and i-non-CBT on measures of depression or anxiety at postintervention or follow-up at less than 6 months. There was evidence from one study of a greater reduction in depression and anxiety at follow-up of over 6 months for the i-CBT group.

Summary

I-CBT may have been more effective than a wait list in reducing PTSD symptoms, depression, and anxiety posttreatment. However, there was no significant difference between the two groups on measures of quality of life. The magnitude of effect was smaller than that found in comparisons of therapist-administered trauma-focused CBT with wait list or usual care. There was no significant difference between i-CBT and i-non-CBT on any measure posttreatment. Only two small studies made this comparison; they showed that i-CBT was no more effective in reducing severity of PTSD symptoms, anxiety, and depression at 12-month follow-up. Although the review found some beneficial effects of i-CBT for PTSD, the quality of the evidence was very low due to the small number of included trials. It was concluded that further work is required to determine noninferiority to current EBPs.

Clinical Recommendations

Understanding and overcoming traditional barriers to treatment and providing alternatives that serve to maximize the number of individuals with PTSD who are able to quickly access and engage in EBP is an important public health concern. Demanding approximately 80% less therapist time than the EBPs delivered by a therapist, e-mental health interventions for PTSD have the potential to maximize the use of health care resources and widen access to effective treatment. They also have the potential to increase therapeutic capacity and reduce waiting lists, thereby enabling timely intervention and resolution of traumatic stress symptoms, which has numerous likely benefits including reduced distress and minimized interference with normal role functioning. E-mental health for PTSD also provides the scope to overcome many traditional barriers to treatment, including difficulties committing to weekly appointments due to work, family demands, child care commitments, or transport issues. There are many factors that need to be taken into account when considering the clinical use of e-mental health. While studies to date have found some beneficial effects of i-CBT for PTSD, the quality of the evidence is low. The approach shows promise. However, further work is required to establish noninferiority to current first-line interventions before they are used in routine clinical care.

Suitability

E-mental health interventions are not intended to replace face-to-face interventions. Since the effect of e-mental health interventions for the treatment of PTSD does not currently appear to be as strong as that found in reviews of face-to-face therapy, it is likely that careful selection of individuals is the best strategy for routine clinical use. E-mental health is particularly appropriate as an initial intervention in a stepped or stratified pathway of care. According to these models, additional treatment becomes available if and when the individual fails to benefit sufficiently from a less intense form of intervention, such as e-mental health (Bower & Gilbody, 2005). At least a proportion of individuals are likely to respond to e-mental health and require no further intervention, which fits well with the principles of prudent health care.

Maximizing Engagement

Despite initial easy access, many users do not fully engage with intervention content and may fail to receive an "adequate dose" of the intervention. Cost-effective means of encouraging full use of e-mental health interventions remain to be developed, whether these are human-administered or technological and automated. Further work is needed to explore rates of uptake and retention in trials of Internet-based interventions and to develop treatment protocols that maximize engagement.

Therapist Training

Internet-based interventions are delivered as stand-alone self-help therapies or with input from a trained professional or paraprofessional, with the greatest support for guided interventions (Lewis et al., 2012; Spek et al., 2007). There is a need for therapists to be appropriately trained in the delivery of e-mental health interventions (Ybarra & Eaton, 2005). Although the majority of interventions are based on cognitive-behavioral principles, methods of delivery diverge considerably from standard face-to-face therapy. For example, conveying information, encouragement, and instructions in a text-based format is very different to doing so verbally. There are many ways in which interventions may be facilitated. Some interventions require facilitators to monitor participants and only intervene when necessary or requested by the consumer. Other interventions incorporate more intensive face-to-face input from a facilitator that is more akin to delivering a brief form of therapy. Training needs to thereby vary according to the requirements of the specific intervention. We currently know very little in relation to therapist factors that affect the uptake and outcome of e-mental health (Lewis et al., 2018). It represents a different way of working, which is likely to suit some thera-peutic styles more than others. Studies have also found that therapists are less positive about e-mental health than individuals with PTSD (Waller & Gilbody, 2009). Work is required to engage clinicians and determine ways of optimally embedding e-mental health. Future work should ascertain the optimal balance between minimizing therapist input and maximizing out-come. It would also be useful to explore ways of augmenting programs with built-in self-reinforcement strategies (e.g., collection of rewards for comple-tion of assignments within a program) to reduce or eliminate the need for therapist assistance.

Intervention Development and Evolution

E-mental health interventions should be as visually appealing and techno-logically advanced as other websites (Ybarra & Eaton, 2005). Consumers are known to rate the credibility of information based partly on the look and functionality of websites. Technology evolves rapidly. Productive collabora-tions with Web developers are therefore necessary to ensure that interven-tions meet the needs of consumers from a technological point of view. Data security is also an important consideration. It is vital that researchers and providers have up-to-date knowledge of the security measures that will be necessary to protect the integrity of e-mental health interventions (Bennett et al., 2010). There is a need for the inclusion of a list of the risks and ben-efits in the consent forms for e-mental health interventions (Ybarra & Eaton, 2005).

Implementation

Implementation of effective e-mental health into routine care is an impor-tant consideration. There is discontinuity between academic-based innova-tions and their commercial application. This is partly due to problems with the ownership of intellectual property by universities and the need for com-panies to commercially develop and maintain the technology. A similar issue arises when technologies are developed with the intention of noncommer-cial access, due to problems of funding routine delivery when that is not the accepted role of individual investigators, research institutions, or funding organizations.

Research Recommendations

Here, we offer a number of recommendations in terms of the future research that will be required to advance the field.

Maximizing the Efficacy of i-CBT for PTSD

The findings of a smaller effect size than reviews of therapist-delivered CBT indicate that the interventions developed to date may not be optimal. A possible explanation is that the i-CBT programs evaluated to date have failed to deliver a sufficient "dose" of trauma processing. Previous research has indicated that PTSD sufferers were able to tolerate a larger dose of exposure than included in the original prototype, and later iterations of the program had a greater trauma focus with improved results and no reported adverse effects (Lewis et al., 2013). Further research is also needed to determine ways of merging the wide-ranging capabilities of e-mental health technologies (e.g., interactivity and automation) to maximize their influence (Ruzek et al., 2016). Further work is also needed to maximize the maintenance of treatment gains and improve longer-term outcomes.

Determining Factors Associated with Treatment Response and Dropout

There is a continued need to explore predictors of outcome and dropout, such as participant age, trauma type, levels of computer literacy, and symptom severity. This will provide a greater understanding of the individual characteristics that are likely to be associated with positive responses to e-mental health (Hamburg & Collins, 2010).

Exploring Mechanisms of Change

Little is known regarding the mechanisms of change associated with e-mental health interventions for PTSD (Andersson, Carlbring, Berger, Almlöv, & Cuijpers, 2009). Further work is needed to determine the moderators and mediators of treatment effects (Andersson, 2009). This is especially pertinent because the field has so far failed to find an advantage of CBT-based interventions in direct comparison with non-CBT-based approaches (Litz et al., 2007; Spence et al., 2014). This contradicts findings from the wider PTSD literature (Bisson, Roberts, Andrew, Cooper, & Lewis, 2013; Jonas et al., 2013) and warrants further scrutiny.

Establishing Effectiveness

Large multicenter effectiveness trials with nested process evaluation (aiming to explain how complex interventions work) are needed to improve the evidence base and for us to become able to more confidently recommend e-mental health for PTSD. More research is also needed to establish the efficacy and feasibility of e-mental health for those exposed to war or disaster (Ruzek et al., 2016).

Economic Evaluation

There have been no economic evaluations of e-mental health interventions for PTSD, and RCTs to date have not reported on costs incurred through delivery of the interventions (Lewis et al., 2018). Since cost is a major driving force behind the development and implementation of Web-based interventions, rigorous economic evaluations are needed to ascertain the cost-effectiveness of e-mental health. The initial investment required to create, implement, and evaluate e-mental health interventions is significant, and should not be underestimated (Donker et al., 2015). There are also costs associated with maintaining and updating websites and mobile phone apps (Christensen et al., 2002). Economic evaluations comparing the cost-effectiveness of different methods of delivering mental health services would serve a useful purpose. Only after thorough examination of the cost-effectiveness of e-mental health can we be certain that the approach makes good use of limited resources. There is also some concern that increased awareness of mental health due to e-mental health initiatives may have the short-term effect of overburdening already stretched services (Christensen et al., 2002).

Acceptability

We know little regarding the acceptability of e-mental health. Work is needed to determine the acceptability of this approach to both users and clinicians. There is also a need to measure and report adverse events arising from e-mental health. As outlined earlier, we know little regarding the acceptability of e-mental health to minority and culturally diverse groups (Richards, 2004). The use of e-mental health may raise questions of accessibility and potential exclusion, especially with regard to older generations, that also warrant attention.

Summary and Conclusions

Although a substantial body of literature supports trauma-focused psychological therapies as effective treatments for PTSD, numerous barriers, such as the cost of delivering therapies, the availability of suitably qualified therapists, and the availability of therapy in geographically remote areas, preclude timely intervention. In response, there has been a growing interest in using the Internet as a platform for the delivery of psychological therapy. This has the capacity to reduce the cost of effectively delivering evidence-based therapy and has the potential to overcome many other barriers that currently limit the availability and uptake of treatment. The collective evidence to date supports the promise of i-CBT as a treatment option for PTSD. However, further work is required to maximize the efficacy of programs, establish noninferiority to current first-line interventions, explore mechanisms of change, establish optimal levels of guidance, explore cost-effectiveness, measure adverse events, and determine predictors of efficacy and dropout.

REFERENCES

Amaya-Jackson, L., Davidson, J. R., Hughes, D. C., Swartz, M., Reynolds, V., George, L. K., et al. (1999). Functional impairment and utilization of services associated with posttraumatic stress in the community. *Journal of Traumatic Stress, 12*(4), 709–724.

Andersson, G. (2009). Using the Internet to provide cognitive behaviour therapy. *Behaviour Research and Therapy, 47*(3), 175–180.

Andersson, G., Carlbring, P., Berger, T., Almlöv, J., & Cuijpers, P. (2009). What makes Internet therapy work? *Cognitive Behaviour Therapy, 38*(S1), 55–60.

Andersson, G., & Cuijpers, P. (2009). Internet-based and other computerized psychological treatments for adult depression: A meta-analysis. *Cognitive Behaviour Therapy, 38*(4), 196–205.

Ashwick, R., Turgoose, D., & Murphy, D. (2019). Exploring the acceptabilavity of delivering cognitive processing therapy (CPT) to UK veterans with PTSD over Skype: A qualitative study. *European Journal of Psychotraumatology, 10*(1), 1573128.

Barak, A., Klein, B., & Proudfoot, J. G. (2009). Defining Internet-supported therapeutic interventions. *Annals of Behavioral Medicine, 38*(1), 4–17.

Beatty, L., Koczwara, B., & Wade, T. (2011). "Cancer Coping Online": A pilot trial of a self-guided CBT Internet intervention for cancer-related distress. *Sensoria: A Journal of Mind, Brain and Culture, 7*(2), 17–25.

Beatty, L., Koczwara, B., & Wade, T. (2016). Evaluating the efficacy of a self-guided Web-based CBT intervention for reducing cancer-distress: A randomised controlled trial. *Supportive Care in Cancer, 24*(3), 1043–1051.

Benight, C. C., Ruzek, J. I., & Waldrep, E. (2008). Internet interventions for traumatic stress: A review and theoretically based example. *Journal of Traumatic Stress: Official Publication of the International Society for Traumatic Stress Studies, 21*(6), 513–520.

Bennett, K., Bennett, A. J., & Griffiths, K. M. (2010). Security considerations for e-mental health interventions. *Journal of Medical Internet Research, 12*(5).

Bisson, J., Roberts, N., Andrew, M., Cooper, R., & Lewis, C. (2013). Psychological therapies for chronic post-traumatic stress disorder (PTSD) in adults. *Cochrane Database of Systematic Reviews,* Issue 12, Article No. CD003388.

Blevins, C. A., Weathers, F. W., Davis, M. T., Witte, T. K., & Domino, J. L. (2015). The posttraumatic stress disorder checklist for DSM-5 (PCL-5): Development and initial psychometric evaluation. *Journal of Traumatic Stress, 28*(6), 489–498.

Botella, C., Gallego, M. J., Garcia-Palacios, A., Banos, R. M., Quero, S., & Alcaniz,

M. (2009). The acceptability of an Internet-based self-help treatment for fear of public speaking. *British Journal of Guidance and Counselling, 37*(3), 297–311.

Bower, P., & Gilbody, S. (2005). Stepped care in psychological therapies: Access, effectiveness and efficiency: Narrative literature review. *British Journal of Psychiatry, 186*(1), 11–17.

Brady, K. T., Killeen, T. K., Brewerton, T., & Lucerini, S. (2000). Comorbidity of psychiatric disorders and posttraumatic stress disorder. *Journal of Clinical Psychiatry, 61*(Suppl. 7), 22–32.

Breslau, N., Davis, G. C., & Schultz, L. R. (2003). Posttraumatic stress disorder and the incidence of nicotine, alcohol, and other drug disorders in persons who have experienced trauma. *Archives of General Psychiatry, 60*(3), 289–294.

Bush, N. E., Bosmajian, C. P., Fairall, J. M., McCann, R. A., & Ciulla, R. P. (2011). afterdeployment.org: A web-based multimedia wellness resource for the post-deployment military community. *Professional Psychology: Research and Practice, 42*(6), 455.

Caldwell, T. M., Jorm, A. F., & Dear, K. B. (2004). Suicide and mental health in rural, remote and metropolitan areas in Australia. *Medical Journal of Australia, 181*(7), S10.

Carlbring, P., Westling, B. E., Ljungstrand, P., Ekselius, L., & Andersson, G. (2001). Treatment of panic disorder via the Internet: A randomized trial of a self-help program. *Behavior Therapy, 32*(4), 751–764.

Cernvall, M., Sveen, J., Bergh Johannesson, K., & Arnberg, F. (2018). A pilot study of user satisfaction and perceived helpfulness of the Swedish version of the mobile app PTSD Coach. *European Journal of Psychotraumatology, 9*(Suppl. 1), 1472990.

Christensen, H., Griffiths, K., & Evans, K. (2002). *e-Mental health in Australia: Implications of the Internet and related technologies for policy.* Canberra, Australia: Commonwealth Department of Health and Ageing.

Christensen, H., & Hickie, I. B. (2010). E-mental health: A new era in delivery of mental health services. *Medical Journal of Australia, 192*(11), S2.

Christensen, H., & Petrie, K. (2013). Information technology as the key to accelerating advances in mental health care. *Australian and New Zealand Journal of Psychiatry, 47*(2), 114–116.

Cloitre, M., Miranda, R., Stovall-McClough, K. C., & Han, H. (2005). Beyond PTSD: Emotion regulation and interpersonal problems as predictors of functional impairment in survivors of childhood abuse. *Behavior Therapy, 36*(2), 119–124.

Corrigan, P. W., Druss, B. G., & Perlick, D. A. (2014). The impact of mental illness stigma on seeking and participating in mental health care. *Psychological Science in the Public Interest, 15*(2), 37–70.

Cuijpers, P., Donker, T., van Straten, A., Li, J., & Andersson, G. (2010). Is guided self-help as effective as face-to-face psychotherapy for depression and anxiety disorders?: A systematic review and meta-analysis of comparative outcome studies. *Psychological Medicine, 40*(12), 1943–1957.

Cuijpers, P., van Straten, A., & Andersson, G. (2008). Internet-administered cognitive behavior therapy for health problems: A systematic review. *Journal of Behavioral Medicine, 31*(2), 169–177.

Domin Chan, P., Cheadle, A. D., Reiber, G., Unützer, J., & Chaney, E. F. (2009). Health care utilization and its costs for depressed veterans with and without comorbid PTSD symptoms. *Psychiatric Services, 60*(12), 1612–1617.

Donker, T., Blankers, M., Hedman, E., Ljotsson, B., Petrie, K., & Christensen, H.

(2015). Economic evaluations of Internet interventions for mental health: A systematic review. *Psychological Medicine, 45*(16), 3357–3376.

Ehlers, A., Clark, D. M., Hackmann, A., McManus, F., Fennell, M., Herbert, C., et al. (2003). A randomized controlled trial of cognitive therapy, a self-help booklet, and repeated assessments as early interventions for posttraumatic stress disorder. *Archives of General Psychiatry, 60*(10), 1024–1032.

Engel, C. C., Litz, B., Magruder, K. M., Harper, E., Gore, K., Stein, N., et al. (2015). Delivery of self training and education for stressful situations (DESTRESS-PC): A randomized trial of nurse assisted online self-management for PTSD in primary care. *General Hospital Psychiatry, 37*(4), 323–328.

Ennis, N., Sijercic, I., & Monson, C. M. (2018). Internet-delivered early interventions for individuals exposed to traumatic events: Systematic review. *Journal of Medical Internet Research, 20*(11), e280.

Fairburn, C. G. (1997). Self-help and guided self-help for binge eating problems. In D. M. Garner & P. E. Garfinkel (Eds.), *Handbook of treatment for eating disorders*. New York: Guilford Press.

Gega, L., Marks, I., & Mataix-Cols, D. (2004). Computer-aided CBT self-help for anxiety and depressive disorders: Experience of a London clinic and future directions. *Journal of Clinical Psychology, 60*(2), 147–157.

Griffiths, K. M., & Christensen, H. (2007). Internet-based mental health programs: A powerful tool in the rural medical kit. *Australian Journal of Rural Health, 15*(2), 81–87.

Hamburg, M. A., & Collins, F. S. (2010). The path to personalized medicine. *New England Journal of Medicine, 363*(4), 301–304.

Hedman, E., Andersson, E., Ljotsson, B., Andersson, G., Rück, C., & Lindefors, N. (2011). Cost-effectiveness of Internet-based cognitive behavior therapy vs. cognitive behavioral group therapy for social anxiety disorder: Results from a randomized controlled trial. *Behaviour Research and Therapy, 49*(11), 729–736.

Hedman, E., El Alaoui, S., Lindefors, N., Andersson, E., Rück, C., Ghaderi, A., et al. (2014). Clinical effectiveness and cost-effectiveness of Internet- vs. group-based cognitive behavior therapy for social anxiety disorder: 4-year follow-up of a randomized trial. *Behaviour Research and Therapy, 59*, 20–29.

Hedman, E., Ljotsson, B., & Lindefors, N. (2012). Cognitive behavior therapy via the Internet: A systematic review of applications, clinical efficacy and cost-effectiveness. *Expert Review of Pharmacoeconomics and Outcomes Research, 12*(6), 745–764.

Improving Access to Psychological Therapies. (2010). Good practice guidance on the use of self-help materials within IAPT services. Retrieved from *www.iapt. nhs.uk/silo/files/good-practice-guidance-on-the-use-of-selfhelp-materials-within-iapt-services.pdf/44fc608d-05b6-47a5-a68f-7599b2f312e0.*

Ivarsson, D., Blom, M., Hesser, H., Carlbring, P., Enderby, P., Nordberg, R., et al. (2014). Guided Internet-delivered cognitive behavior therapy for post-traumatic stress disorder: A randomized controlled trial. *Internet Interventions, 1*(1), 33–40.

Jacobsen, L. K., Southwick, S. M., & Kosten, T. R. (2001). Substance use disorders in patients with posttraumatic stress disorder: A review of the literature. *American Journal of Psychiatry, 158*(8), 1184–1190.

Jacobson, N., & Greenley, D. (2001). What is recovery?: A conceptual model and explication. *Psychiatric Services, 52*(4), 482–485.

Jonas, D., Cusack, K., Forneris, C., Wilkins, T., Sonis, J., Middleton, J., et al. (2013). *Psychological and pharmacological treatments for adults with posttraumatic stress disorder (PTSD)*. Rockville, MD: Agency for Healthcare Research and Activity. Retrieved from *www.ncbi.nlm.nih.gov/books/NBK137702/pdf/Bookshelf_NBK137702.pdf*.

Knaevelsrud, C., Brand, J., Lange, A., Ruwaard, J., & Wagner, B. (2015). Web-based psychotherapy for posttraumatic stress disorder in war-traumatized Arab patients: Randomized controlled trial. *Journal of Medical Internet Research, 17*(3).

Krupnick, J. L., Green, B. L., Amdur, R., Alaoui, A., Belouali, A., Roberge, E., et al. (2017). An Internet-based writing intervention for PTSD in veterans: A feasibility and pilot effectiveness trial. *Psychological Trauma: Theory, Research, Practice, and Policy, 9*(4), 461.

Krysinska, K., & Lester, D. (2010). Post-traumatic stress disorder and suicide risk: A systematic review. *Archives of Suicide Research, 14*(1), 1–23.

Kuhn, E., Greene, C., Hoffman, J., Nguyen, T., Wald, L., Schmidt, J., et al. (2014). Preliminary evaluation of PTSD Coach, a smartphone app for post-traumatic stress symptoms. *Military Medicine, 179*(1), 12–18.

Kuhn, E., Kanuri, N., Hoffman, J. E., Garvert, D. W., Ruzek, J. I., & Taylor, C. B. (2017). A randomized controlled trial of a smartphone app for posttraumatic stress disorder symptoms. *Journal of Consulting and Clinical Psychology, 85*(3), 267.

Kuhn, E., van der Meer, C., Owen, J. E., Hoffman, J. E., Cash, R., Carrese, P., et al. (2018). PTSD Coach around the world. *Mhealth, 4*(5).

Lewis, C., Farewell, D., Groves, V., Kitchiner, N. J., Roberts, N. P., Vick, T., et al. (2017). Internet-based guided self-help for posttraumatic stress disorder (PTSD): Randomized controlled trial. *Depression and Anxiety, 34*(6), 555–565.

Lewis, C., Pearce, J., & Bisson, J. (2012). Efficacy, cost-effectiveness and acceptability of self-help interventions for anxiety disorders: Systematic review. *British Journal of Psychiatry, 200*(1), 15–21.

Lewis, C., Roberts, N., Bethell, A., Robertson, L., & Bisson, J. (2018). Internet-based cognitive and behavioural therapies for post-traumatic stress disorder (PTSD) in adults. *Cochrane Database of Systematic Reviews,* Issue 12, Article No. CD011710.

Lewis, C., Roberts, N., Vick, T., & Bisson, J. I. (2013). Development of a guided self help (GSH) programme for the treatment of mild to moderate post traumatic stress disorder (PTSD). *Depression and Anxiety, 30*(11), 1121–1128.

Lina, G., Isaac, M., & David, M.-C. (2004). Computer-aided CBT self-help for anxiety and depressive disorders: Experience of a London clinic and future directions. *Journal of Clinical Psychology, 60*(2), 147–157.

Littleton, H., Grills, A. E., Kline, K. D., Schoemann, A. M., & Dodd, J. C. (2016). The From Survivor to Thriver program: RCT of an online therapist-facilitated program for rape-related PTSD. *Journal of Anxiety Disorders, 43*, 41–51.

Litz, B. T., Engel, C. C., Bryant, R. A., Papa, A., Litz, B. T., Engel, C. C., et al. (2007). A randomized, controlled proof-of-concept trial of an Internet-based, therapist-assisted self-management treatment for posttraumatic stress disorder. *American Journal of Psychiatry, 164*(11), 1676–1683.

Medical Research Council. (2000). *A framework for the development and evaluation of randomised controlled trials for complex interventions to improve health*. London: Author. Retrieved from *https://mrc.ukri.org/documents/pdf/rcts-for-complex-interventions-to-improve-health*.

Miner, A., Kuhn, E., Hoffman, J. E., Owen, J. E., Ruzek, J. I., & Taylor, C. B. (2016). Feasibility, acceptability, and potential efficacy of the PTSD Coach app: A pilot randomized controlled trial with community trauma survivors. *Psychological Trauma: Theory, Research, Practice, and Policy, 8*(3), 384.

Mouthaan, J., Sijbrandij, M., de Vries, G.-J., Reitsma, J. B., van de Schoot, R., Goslings, J. C., et al. (2013). Internet-based early intervention to prevent posttraumatic stress disorder in injury patients: Randomized controlled trial. *Journal of Medical Internet Research, 15*(8).

Mouthaan, J., Sijbrandij, M., Reitsma, J., Gersons, B. R., & Olff, M. (2011). Internet-based prevention of posttraumatic stress symptoms in injured trauma patients: Design of a randomized controlled trial. *European Journal of Psychotraumatology, 2*(1), 8294.

Mouthaan, J., Sijbrandij, M., Reitsma, J. B., Luitse, J. S., Goslings, J. C., & Olff, M. (2011). Trauma TIPS: An Internet-based intervention to prevent posttraumatic stress disorder in injured trauma patients. *Journal of Cybertherapy and Rehabilitation, 4*(3), 331–340.

National Institute for Health and Care Excellence. (2018). Post-traumatic stress disorder: NICE Guideline No. NG116. Retrieved from *www.nice.org.uk/guidance/ng116*.

Newman, M. G., Erickson, T., Przeworski, A., & Dzus, E. (2003). Self-help and minimal-contact therapies for anxiety disorders: Is human contact necessary for therapeutic efficacy? *Journal of Clinical Psychology, 59*(3), 251–274.

Olatunji, B. O., Cisler, J. M., & Tolin, D. F. (2007). Quality of life in the anxiety disorders: A meta-analytic review. *Clinical Psychology Review, 27*(5), 572–581.

Olff, M. (2015). Mobile mental health: A challenging research agenda. *European Journal of Psychotraumatology, 6*(1), 27882.

Olthuis, J. V., Watt, M. C., Bailey, K., Hayden, J. A., & Stewart, S. H. (2015). Therapist-supported Internet cognitive-behavioural therapy for anxiety disorders in adults. *BJPsych Advances, 21*(5), 290.

Pacella, M. L., Hruska, B., & Delahanty, D. L. (2013). The physical health consequences of PTSD and PTSD symptoms: A meta-analytic review. *Journal of Anxiety Disorders, 27*(1), 33–46.

Price, M., van Stolk-Cooke, K., Legrand, A. C., Brier, Z. M., Ward, H. L., Connor, J. P., et al. (2018). Implementing assessments via mobile during the acute post-trauma period: Feasibility, acceptability and strategies to improve response rates. *European Journal of Psychotraumatology, 9*(Suppl.1).

Richards, D. (2004). Self-help: Empowering service users or aiding cash strapped mental health services? *Journal of Mental Health, 13*, 117–123.

Riper, H., Andersson, G., Christensen, H., Cuijpers, P., Lange, A., & Eysenbach, G. (2010). Theme issue on e-mental health: A growing field in Internet research. *Journal of Medical Internet Research, 12*(5).

Rizzo, A., Reger, G., Gahm, G., Difede, J., & Rothbaum, B. O. (2009). Virtual reality exposure therapy for combat-related PTSD. In P. Shiromani, T. Keane, & J. E. LeDoux (Eds.), *Post-traumatic stress disorder* (pp. 375–399). New York: Springer.

Roberts, L. W., Battaglia, J., & Epstein, R. S. (1999). Frontier ethics: Mental health care needs and ethical dilemmas in rural communities. *Psychiatric Services, 50*(4), 497–503.

Rothbaum, B. O., Hodges, L. F., Ready, D., Graap, K., & Alarcon, R. D. (2001). Virtual reality exposure therapy for Vietnam veterans with posttraumatic stress disorder. *Journal of Clinical Psychiatry, 62*(8), 617–622.

Ruzek, J., Hoffman, J., Ciulla, R., Prins, A., Kuhn, E., & Gahm, G. (2011). Bringing Internet-based education and intervention into mental health practice: After-deployment.org. *European Journal of Psychotraumatology, 2*(1), 7278.

Ruzek, J. I., Kuhn, E., Jaworski, B. K., Owen, J. E., & Ramsey, K. M. (2016). Mobile mental health interventions following war and disaster. *Mhealth, 2.*

Salazar, L. F., Vivolo-Kantor, A., Hardin, J., & Berkowitz, A. (2014). A web-based sexual violence bystander intervention for male college students: Randomized controlled trial. *Journal of Medical Internet Research, 16*(9).

Schlegl, S., Bürger, C., Schmidt, L., Herbst, N., & Voderholzer, U. (2015). The potential of technology-based psychological interventions for anorexia and bulimia nervosa: A systematic review and recommendations for future research. *Journal of Medical Internet Research, 17*(3).

Sood, S., Mbarika, V., Jugoo, S., Dookhy, R., Doarn, C. R., Prakash, N., et al. (2007). What is telemedicine?: A collection of 104 peer-reviewed perspectives and theoretical underpinnings. *Telemedicine and e-Health, 13*(5), 573–590.

Spek, V., Cuijpers, P., Nyklícek, I., Riper, H., Keyzer, J., & Pop, V. (2007). Internet-based cognitive behaviour therapy for symptoms of depression and anxiety: A meta-analysis. *Psychological Medicine, 37*(3), 319–328.

Spence, J., Titov, N., Dear, B. F., Johnston, L., Solley, K., Lorian, C., et al. (2011). Randomized controlled trial of Internet-delivered cognitive behavioral therapy for posttraumatic stress disorder. *Depression and Anxiety, 28*(7), 541–550.

Spence, J., Titov, N., Johnston, L., Jones, M. P., Dear, B. F., & Solley, K. (2014). Internet-based trauma-focused cognitive behavioural therapy for PTSD with and without exposure components: A randomised controlled trial. *Journal of Affective Disorders, 162*, 73–80.

Steinmetz, S. E., Benight, C. C., Bishop, S. L., & James, L. E. (2012). My disaster recovery: A pilot randomized controlled trial of an Internet intervention. *Anxiety, Stress and Coping, 25*(5), 593–600.

Suler, J. (2004). The online disinhibition effect. *Cyberpsychology and Behavior, 7*(3), 321–326.

Taylor, C. B., & Luce, K. H. (2003). Computer and Internet based psychotherapy interventions. *Current Directions in Psychological Science, 12*(3), 18–22.

van der Meer, C. A., Bakker, A., Schrieken, B. A., Hoofwijk, M. C., & Olff, M. (2017). Screening for trauma-related symptoms via a smartphone app: The validity of smart assessment on your mobile in referred police officers. *International Journal of Methods in Psychiatric Research, 26*(3), e1579.

van der Meer, C. A. I., Bakker, A., van Zuiden, M., Lok, A., & Olff, M. (2020). Help in hand after traumatic events: The efficacy of the smartphone app "SUPPORT Coach" to reduce trauma-related symptoms in health care professionals. *European Journal of Psychotraumatology.*

Waller, R., & Gilbody, S. (2009). Barriers to the uptake of computerized cognitive behavioural therapy: A systematic review of the quantitative and qualitative evidence. *Psychological Medicine, 39*(5), 705–712.

Wang, P. S., Angermeyer, M., Borges, G., Bruffaerts, R., Chiu, W. T., De Girolamo, G., et al. (2007). Delay and failure in treatment seeking after first onset of mental disorders in the World Health Organization's World Mental Health Survey Initiative. *World Psychiatry, 6*(3), 177.

Wang, P. S., Berglund, P., Olfson, M., Pincus, H. A., Wells, K. B., & Kessler, R. C. (2005). Failure and delay in initial treatment contact after first onset of mental disorders in the National Comorbidity Survey Replication. *Archives of General Psychiatry, 62*(6), 603–613.

Williams, C. (2001). Use of written cognitive-behavioural therapy self-help materials to treat depression. *Advances in Psychiatric Treatment, 7,* 233–240.

Williams, C., & Whitfield, G. (2001). Written and computer-based self-help treatments for depression. *British Medical Bulletin, 57,* 133–144.

Ybarra, M. L., & Eaton, W. W. (2005). Internet-based mental health interventions. *Mental Health Services Research, 7*(2), 75–87.

Zatzick, D. F., Marmar, C. R., Weiss, D. S., Browner, W. S., Metzler, T. J., Golding, J. M., et al. (2014). Posttraumatic stress disorder and functioning and quality of life outcomes in a nationally representative sample of male Vietnam veterans. *American Journal of Psychiatry, 154*(12), 1690–1695.

CHAPTER 19

Complementary, Alternative, and Integrative Interventions

Ariel J. Lang and Barbara Niles

Treatments that are not part of standard Western medicine are typically classified as "complementary" (i.e., used in combination with established techniques) or "alternative" (i.e., used in place of typical practice) (National Center for Complementary and Integrative Health [NCCIH], 2018a). Internationally, estimates of all health-related use of complementary and alternative practices generally fall in the range of 20–30% (Kemppainen, Kemppainen, Reippainen, Salmenniemi, & Vuolanto, 2018; Peltzer, Pengpid, Puckpinyo, Yi, & Anh le, 2016; Rossler et al., 2007), with substantial differences noted based on regional and sociodemographic factors (Gureje et al., 2015; Thirthalli et al., 2016). Mental health care in low- and middle-income countries, for example, is heavily composed of alternative approaches, in part because of the lack of availability of pharmacotherapy or evidence-based psychotherapy (Gureje et al., 2015). Within the United States, the National Health Interview Survey 2017 documented generally stable rates of use over the past decade, with the exception of continued increases in yoga and meditation (NCCIH, 2018b). Both the U.S. military health care system (Herman, Sorbero, & Sims-Columbia, 2017) and U.S. Department of Veterans Affairs (VA; Taylor, Hoggatt, & Kligler, 2019) report providing complementary and alternative care to a substantial number of clients, with mental health and pain being the most common reasons for seeking such care. As use of these techniques becomes more common and they gain empirical support, however, approaches that are considered conventional medicine will change.

"Integrative" care has been defined by the National Center for Complementary and Integrative Health (2018a) as "a holistic, patient-focused approach to health care and wellness—often including mental, emotional,

343

functional, spiritual, social, and community aspects—and treating the whole person rather than, for example, one organ system." Although such programs exist and integrative care is an important aspiration, the empirical literature is particularly lacking in this area. To our knowledge, there has been no systematic evaluation of integrative care approaches, and assessment tools are much better developed for tracking symptom change than wellness.

The purpose of this chapter is to review the current evidence for mind–body interventions, which is the most commonly used class of complementary and alternative treatments for posttraumatic stress disorder (PTSD). In contrast to the Cartesian dualistic view of the mind and body as distinct and separable, mind–body therapies focus on treating the whole person with the intention to promote overall health and well-being. The NCCIH (2017b) further specifies that mind–body techniques are "administered or taught to others by a trained practitioner or teacher" such as a yoga instructor or acupuncturist. Dietary and herbal supplements, the other major class of complementary or integrative treatments defined by the NCCIH, are largely unstudied in PTSD; the single trial meeting criteria for this review is included here as well.

The rationale for the use of complementary, alternative, and integrative (CAI) approaches for PTSD is twofold. Pragmatically, these are interventions that individuals with PTSD are seeking out. The reasons for this may involve seeking alternatives to standard practices (e.g., to avoid pharmacotherapy or trauma-focused therapy) or the desire for a more holistic approach (Kroesen, Baldwin, Brooks, & Bell, 2002). As mental health professionals, we have a responsibility to understand the utility of these treatments so that we can responsibly guide clients in selecting an effective care plan. For some, an alternative intervention may provide sufficient symptom relief. For others, these techniques may be used in a complementary manner to facilitate entry into other types of care, for example, by enhancing one's perceived coping ability or trust in mental health professionals. Given that residual symptoms or continued functional impairment are common after even the most efficacious treatments (Schnurr & Lunney, 2015; Steenkamp, Litz, Hoge, & Marmar, 2015), there also may be a place for complementary interventions to target specific symptom types (e.g., reducing residual hyperarousal or enhancing positive affect) or functional areas (e.g., social connectedness) or to support coping with persistent symptoms. Theoretically, integrative approaches may be valuable for their ability to systematically target different mechanisms that maintain or are disrupted by the disorder. PTSD is increasingly understood as a systemic illness (McFarlane, 2017) associated with accelerated cellular aging and cardiometabolic morbidity (Wolf & Schnurr, 2016). Given the complex interplay of emotional, cognitive, and physical symptoms associated with PTSD, a whole-body treatment approach becomes necessary, an area in which CAI interventions show increasing promise.

The techniques reviewed in this chapter have been compiled into four groupings: meditation, acupuncture, yoga, and "other," which includes a variety of interventions for which only one study met the criteria for inclusion.

1. *Meditation* can be described as a process that cultivates greater awareness of or a different relationship to the mind. The broad term, however, encompasses a large variety of techniques that vary considerably in terms of the mechanisms by which PTSD may be affected (refer to Lang et al., 2012, for additional discussion).
2. *Acupuncture* involves stimulating specific points on the body, typically by applying thin needles that are manipulated by hand or using electrical current (NCCIH, 2017a).
3. *Yoga* describes a practice that typically combines physical postures, regulation of the breath, and techniques to cultivate attention (Gard et al., 2014), with the emphasis on each of these factors varying greatly among types of practice.
4. *Other*
   - Physical activity refers to various types of exercise, including aerobic and resistance-based activities, delivered for therapeutic benefit.
   - Music therapy may include creating or playing music, singing, moving to, or listening to music.
   - Nature–adventure includes a variety of adventure-based activities in natural outdoor settings.
   - Saikokeishikankyoto (SKK) is a traditional Japanese herbal formula.

Table 19.1 provides a summary of the interventions for which studies met criteria for inclusion within the *Posttraumatic Stress Disorder Prevention and Treatment Guidelines* advanced by the International Society for Traumatic Stress Studies (ISTSS) and the level of evidence for each approach.

Summary and Appraisal of the Evidence

Meditation

The mantram repetition program (MRP) is a practice that involves silent repetition of a spiritual word or phrase (called a *mantram*), slowing thoughts, and cultivation of "one-pointed attention" (Bormann, Thorp, Wetherell, & Golshan, 2008). Mantram repetition showed no benefit when compared with wait list or usual care. The initial feasibility study (Bormann et al., 2008) involved 31 veterans, who were assigned to MRP or a delayed treatment control. This pilot study was intended to assess feasibility, acceptability,

TABLE 19.1. Summary of ISTSS Guidelines for CAI Interventions

Meditation

Insufficient Evidence to Recommend–Mantram repetition, mindfulness-based stress reduction

Acupuncture

Intervention with Emerging Evidence–Acupuncture

Insufficient Evidence to Recommend–Electroacupuncture

Yoga

Intervention with Emerging Evidence–Sudarshan Kriya (SKY)/Kripalu/trauma informed

Other

Intervention with Emerging Evidence–Saikokeishikankyoto (SKK), somatic experiencing

Insufficient Evidence to Recommend–Group music therapy, nature adventure therapy, physical exercise

and initial clinical signal, and should be understood in this context. The second study (Bormannm Thorp, Wetherell, Golshan, & Lang, 2013) was also conducted with a veteran sample ($n = 146$), comparing MRP plus usual care to MRP alone. Strengths of the trial include its size and use of a gold standard outcome measure, the Clinician-Administered PTSD Scale (CAPS). A limitation, however, is the lack of control for the nonspecific effects of the group meetings.

MRP nevertheless showed a positive effect when compared with individual present-centered therapy (Bormann et al., 2018); it should be noted that this trial is not reflected in the evidence rating, which was based on performance as compared to wait list or treatment as usual. This most recent trial took place in two VA facilities ($n = 173$) and was designed to address some of the limitations of the previous studies (e.g., active comparison group, more than one site). The intervention was delivered on an individual basis in eight weekly 60-minute sessions by trained therapists. A primary limitation of the studies of MRP is generalizability. Because all three randomized trials have been conducted with veterans, it is unclear how the intervention would perform in different populations. Based on the findings from the two older studies that used wait-list or treatment-as-usual comparitors, there is *Insufficient Evidence to Recommend* MRP at this time. Because of the positive findings in the most methodologically rigorous study using an active treatment comparitor, however, additional studies of MRP are warranted.

Mindfulness-based stress reduction (MBSR) is a program that uses a variety of techniques to cultivate the state of mindfulness (i.e., nonjudgmental present-moment awareness; Kabat-Zinn, 1994). It is typically delivered in a series of weekly 2.5-hour group meetings along with a day-long retreat.

MBSR showed no benefit when compared with wait list or usual care in a veteran sample (Kearney, McDermott, Malte, Martinez, & Simpson, 2013).

Mindfulness training delivered via tele-health (two sessions in person and six by telephone) showed a positive effect for veterans when compared with psychoeducation also delivered via tele-health (Niles et al., 2012). This brief treatment was based on the tenets of MBSR but was delivered in individual sessions and did not include the full program. It is also notable that the improvements were not sustained over a 6-week follow-up.

There was no evidence of a difference between MBSR and present-centered therapy delivered in group sessions over three randomized controlled studies. A pilot study by Bremner and colleagues (2017) included 26 veterans, who were assessed using CAPS. The much larger trial by Polusny and colleagues (2015) involved 116 veterans. A limitation of this study is that treatment length was not matched, so those in the MBSR condition participated in 20 hours of group plus a daylong retreat, whereas those in present-centered groups received 13.5 hours of intervention. Finally, Davis and colleagues (2018) assigned 214 veterans from three VA clinics in the southeastern United States to eight 90-minute group sessions of MBSR or present-centered therapy. Only 55% of the consenting group in this trial completed the posttreatment assessment. Thus, the conclusion based on the trials of MBSR and related techniques is that there is *Insufficient Evidence to Recommend*. Given that two trials are large and methodologically rigorous, it is questionable whether additional study of MBSR in the veteran population would lead to a different conclusion. It is possible, however, that results would be different if the treatment were delivered to a different population of individuals with PTSD.

Three additional studies that were not published at the time of the meta-analysis warrant mention. Nidich and colleagues (2018) conducted a large ($n = 203$) randomized controlled trial (RCT) of transcendental meditation (TM), prolonged exposure (PE), and a health education control in a VA medical center. TM is a specific type of silent meditation developed by Maharishi Mahesh Yogi that involves repetition of a sound, that is, a mantra, to facilitate meditation (Travis & Shear, 2010). TM and the education control were delivered in groups, and PE was administered individually; all interventions took place over 12 weeks. The primary outcome was PTSD severity as measured by CAPS. The results suggest that TM was not inferior to PE, and both conditions were superior to health education. In addition, Bellehsen and colleagues recently completed a pilot study of TM compared to usual care in a sample of 40 veterans with PTSD. Those in the TM group showed significantly greater change in symptoms as measured by CAPS at posttreatment (Bellehsen, Stoycheva, Cohen, & Nidich, 2017).

Lang and colleagues (2019) conducted a small randomized trial of compassion meditation as compared to a relaxation control in a sample of 28 veterans. Compassion meditation is a contemplative meditation based on Buddhist philosophy, but operationalized in a secular way. It involves developing the heartfelt wish that others and oneself may be at peace and satisfied with their lives; such compassion is cultivated through recognition of common humanity. Both interventions were delivered in 10, 90-minute group sessions, and outcomes were assessed via CAPS. Compassion meditation led to significantly greater change in PTSD symptoms than the relaxation control condition.

In summary, meditation has received considerable empirical scrutiny in U.S. veteran populations, but it should be noted that randomized studies in civilian samples are absent. There is variability in outcomes based on the type of meditative practice that was implemented, so it is important to underscore that meditation is not a single intervention but rather a class of interventions. The consistent findings from large and methodologically sound trials of MBSR for PTSD suggest that it is unlikely to become a stand-alone PTSD intervention. That said, decades of research indicate that MBSR reduces depression and anxiety, improves quality of life and physical functioning, and is not associated with any notable adverse reactions (Grossman, Niemann, Schmidt, & Walach, 2004; Khoury, Sharma, Rush, & Fournier, 2015), so it may be a useful complement to PTSD care for certain comorbidities. Compassion meditation shows some preliminary clinical promise, suggesting that the contemplative framework supporting change in social connectedness may augment the effect of mindfulness-based meditation.

It is notable that some of the strongest results are associated with the mantra-based practices, MRP and TM. Although these practices share the repetition of a mantra, there are differences in the practices. In TM, the mantra is chosen by the course instructor and kept private, whereas the individual selects a personally meaningful spiritual word in MRP and may share the word as desired. In addition, TM is a sitting meditation (often operationalized as sitting quietly for 20 minutes twice per day), whereas mantram repetition can be accomplished in any position or location and for any amount of time. It is unclear the extent to which the mechanisms of change in PTSD symptoms are affected by these differences. The most recent evidence about MRP is very promising, and two papers now suggest that it is particularly effective at reducing hyperarousal (Bormann et al., 2013; Crawford, Talkovsky, Bormann, & Lang, 2019), which is the most common residual symptom type following current empirically supported treatments (Schnurr & Lunney, 2015). The effect of MRP has also been tied to spirituality (Bormann, Liu, Thorp, & Lang, 2011), which may be appealing for some treatment-seeking individuals. The recently published trials of TM are also quite promising. It has been conjectured that TM may be effective at reducing physiological arousal (Lang et al., 2012), although this was not examined in the recent trial. Ultimately, it will be important to standardize protocols so that they may be reliably evaluated and replicated, and to understand the mechanisms that differentiate the types of meditation to best apply meditation-based interventions to clinical problems.

Acupuncture

Acupuncture showed a positive effect when compared with wait list in a sample of community-dwelling adults based on a self-report measure of PTSD. In the same study, there was no evidence of a difference between acupuncture and cognitive-behavioral therapy with a trauma focus (CBT-T). The primary limitations of this study are that the sample was relatively small, intervention type is confounded with provider, and the highly educated, treatment-seeking sample may not represent the typical population of individuals with PTSD. A second study with an active comparator found no evidence of a difference between electroacupuncture and paroxetine. This study involved PTSD related to earthquake exposure in China. Thus, acupuncture is considered an *Intervention with Emerging Evidence*.

Of note, one additional study is relevant to the clinical use of acupuncture. Engel and colleagues (2014) randomized 55 U.S. military service members with PTSD to usual care or usual care plus acupuncture. Outcomes were evaluated using both CAPS and a self-report measure of symptomatology. The group that received acupuncture showed significantly greater clinical improvement, although the design does not disentangle the effect of additional intervention from that of acupuncture in particular. Nonetheless, the trial suggests generalizability of the aforementioned studies and supports the need for additional study of the practice.

Yoga

Yoga showed a positive effect when compared with wait list, assessment-only control, or attention control, leading to its designation as an *Intervention with Emerging Evidence*. The studies providing evidence for yoga, however, are largely pilot studies. Carter and colleagues (2013) implemented Sudarshan Kriya (SKY) yoga, a breath-based practice, as compared to wait list with 31 Australian Vietnam veterans. Seppala and colleagues (2014) similarly examined SKY versus wait list in 21 U.S. veterans. Both Mitchell and colleagues (2014) and Reinhardt and colleagues (2018) compared Kripalu yoga to an assessment-only control. Mitchell and colleagues' work involved 20 women and noted that change in hyperarousal may have been a key mechanism of change in the yoga condition. Reinhardt and colleagues enrolled a group of 51 U.S. veterans but had considerable attrition, resulting in a final analyzed group of 17. Both of these studies found no signficant differences in PTSD outcomes between the yoga and control groups. All studies have used standard interview-based or self-report tools. The largest trial was conducted by van der Kolk and colleagues (2014). They compared trauma-informed yoga to supportive health education with 64 women, using CAPS to evaluate outcomes, and found significantly greater symptom reductions for those in the yoga condition.

Although yoga is characterized as an emerging intervention, the heterogeneous nature of the practice limits the conclusions that can be drawn. There have been efforts to quantify key aspects of yoga (Groessl et al., 2015), and it will be important to utilize such tools to understand active ingredients and develop standardization to allow for replication and dissemination of efficacious protocols. The data on the use of yoga come from veterans and women, so future studies should consider issues of generalizability. Also of note is that only one trial utilized an active control condition. It will be important to examine whether or not yoga's effect is based on more than nonspecific therapeutic factors (e.g., expectancies, group support). Whether yoga's impact differs from that of other types of physical activity or relaxation may also help to understand mechanisms of action (for additional discussion of mechanisms of change, refer to Wells, Lang, Schmalzl, Groessl, & Strauss, 2016). Finally, yoga is an experiential practice, so the optimal frequency and duration of practice may vary considerably.

Other Techniques

Saikokeishikankyoto

Saikokeishikankyoto (SKK), a Japanese herbal formula, was compared to a no-treatment control with 47 Japanese outpatients diagnosed with PTSD (Numata et al., 2014). Participants in the SKK group received the herbal formula 3 times per day for 2 weeks. After treatment, the SKK group was significantly more improved than the control group on the Impact of Events Scale—Revised with no serious adverse events. The study was limited by use of a no-treatment rather than placebo control, and it did not include a follow-up assessment to determine whether the effects were lasting. On the basis of the aforementioned study, this herbal remedy is currently considered an *Intervention with Emerging Evidence* in the treatment of PTSD, although additional research is needed to confirm these findings and to examine the intervention's generalizability outside of Japan.

Somatic Experiencing

This therapeutic process focuses on awareness and regulation of internal sensations of physiological arousal within the context of psychotherapy (Levine, 2010; Payne, Levine & Crane-Godreau, 2015). The goal of the approach is to reduce physiological activation through increased ability to tolerate body sensations and related emotions. Clients acquire skills, such as body awareness, and focus on positive memories, which they are then directed to use to self-regulate their arousal and emotions. This therapy differs from psychotherapies with a trauma focus (such as PE; see Riggs, Tate, Chrestman, & Foa, Chapter 12, this volume) in that written or oral retelling of specific traumatic events is not required. However, this intervention contains elements that may be considered trauma exposure. Similar to interventions with a trauma focus, clients are instructed to engage with traumatic memories to elicit high arousal. Clients then practice using the skills to reduce the arousal, eventually leading to increased tolerance and reductions in distress related to posttraumatic arousal.

Brom and colleagues (2017) compared somatic experiencing to wait list in a sample of Israeli individuals with PTSD. The approach showed a positive effect when compared with wait list. This positive result and the good size of the trial ($n = 60$) led to it being classified as an *Intervention with Emerging Evidence*, although several limitations should be noted. Because of the lack of an active comparator, it is possible that nonspecific factors influenced the result. The single site of the trial also raises the possibility that results may not generalize. Somatic experiencing sits at the intersection between interventions with a trauma focus and CAI, incorporating elements of both in an integrative fashion. Future research can be designed to empirically evaluate the benefit of integrated programs and determine whether components combine in additive or synergystic ways to improve outcomes.

Group Music Therapy

Carr and colleagues (2012) compared group music therapy to wait list in a sample of 17 individuals in the United Kingdom who remained symptomatic after cognitive-behavioral therapy (CBT). Group music therapy showed a positive effect when compared with wait list, but there is *Insufficient Evidence to Recommend* the approach due to the small sample size.

Nature–Adventure Therapy

Although a number of programs purport to support recovery from PTSD through engagement with a variety of adventure-based activities in natural settings, only one study has employed a randomized design to evaluate the approach. Gelkopf, Hasson-Ohayon, Bikman, and Kravetz (2013) enrolled 22 Israeli veterans with combat-related PTSD in a year-long (delivered in weekly 3-hour meetings) program of sailing and other ocean-based activities and compared outcomes with those of 20 veterans who were on a wait list. Nature–adventure therapy showed no benefit when compared with wait list, leading to *Insufficient Evidence to Recommend*.

Physical Exercise

Physical activity interventions for PTSD showed no benefit when compared with wait list or usual care, leading to an *Insufficient Evidence* recommendation. Although the evidence to recommend physical activity is currently insufficient for the treatment of PTSD symptoms, physical activity should nonetheless be recommended universally as a part of health maintenance. PTSD is associated with increased morbidity and mortality (Boscarino, 2006), including cardiovascular disease (Ahmadi et al., 2011); poor physical fitness has been associated with increased symptomatology (Vancampfort et al., 2017); and evidence suggests that exercise supports physical health among those with mental health problems (Stubbs et al., 2018).

The current designation for exercise is based on two studies. Goldstein and colleagues (2018) conducted a pilot trial ($n = 47$) of a 12-week integrated (aerobic and resistance exercise with some mindfulness-based practices delivered in three weekly 1-hour classes) group exercise program as compared to wait list. The integrated exercise program showed greater reductions in PTSD symptoms. Rosenbaum, Sherrington, and Tiedemann (2015) examined the effect of the addition of an exercise program (six 30-minute sessions over 2 weeks involving resistance training and walking) to usual care in a sample of 81 individuals who were in an inpatient program for PTSD. Although they did not observe a benefit with regard to PTSD symptoms, their data suggest the possibility of additional benefits such as reduced waist circumference and improved sleep quality.

It is critically important to consider broader health impacts in future studies of exercise for PTSD; future recommendations about the inclusion of exercise in a recovery plan should be considered based on both physical and mental health outcomes, particularly given the increased morbidity and mortality associated with PTSD. In addition, a good deal remains to be understood about the impact of physical activity of individuals with PTSD. Both of the exercise studies included aerobic and resistance-based exercise, and it is unknown whether different types of exercise have a different impact on symptomatology. A recent review suggested several possible mechanisms by which aerobic exercise might reduce PTSD symptoms (Hegberg, Hayes, & Hayes, 2019): exposure and desensitization to interoceptive arousal, enhanced cognitive function, exercise-induced neuroplasticity, normalization of endocrine function, and reductions in inflammation. Future studies can elucidate which of these mechanisms are at play to guide how to successfully integrate exercise with traditional psychotherapies for PTSD. For example, Fetzner and Asmundson (2015) examined ways in which exercise may be best delivered to enhance exposure and desensitization. They compared the impact of aerobic exercise (six sessions in 2 weeks) across three conditions: attention to somatic arousal, distraction from somatic arousal, or no distractions/prompts. Although all groups showed reductions in symptoms, this was attenuated in the interoceptively focused group. We caution against concluding that distraction is useful, however, as longer-term outcomes may differ. In addition, systematic exposure to interoceptive cues, which may differ based on the type and intensity of exercise, has been suggested as a way to augment treatment response (Wald & Taylor, 2007), meaning that exercise could play an important complementary role when engaging in therapy with a trauma focus.

Practical Delivery of the Recommendations

Despite the paucity of empirical evidence presented in the ISTSS guidelines to support the use of CAI approaches in the treatment of PTSD, three treatments—acupuncture, yoga, and somatic experiencing—are cautiously recommended as interventions with emerging evidence. Although there remains insufficient evidence to recommend meditation, several approaches show clinical promise and recommendations may change as evidence accumulates. Given the nascent state of the literature on CAI therapies for PTSD, it is premature to recommend any as first-line treatments for PTSD, and additional research is needed to determine how and when these treatments might be most efficacious when used adjunctively. Yoga and acupuncture are mind–body treatments that could be delivered to complement standard psychotherapies, such as treatments with a trauma focus (i.e., prior to, during, or following standard therapies) or as stand-alone treatments (for individuals who choose not to pursue psychological therapies). In a different approach, somatic experiencing therapy integrates mind–body components with more traditional "talk therapy" components within the treatment. With a focus on the body sensations and emotions that arise with trauma memories, individuals learn to tolerate negative feelings and to regulate their physiological reactions.

As the evidence base of methodologically rigorous trials of CAI treatments continues to grow, it is likely that additional CAI treatments soon will accrue sufficient evidence to recommend them. For example, as noted previously, since the review of evidence for these guidelines was completed, a methodologically rigorous study of transcendental meditation was published (Nidich et al., 2018) that indicates it may be a promising treatment for PTSD. Similarly, the strongest evidence to date for mantram repetition involves a study with a nonspecific psychotherapy control (Bormann et al., 2018), which falls outside the a priori procedures for recommendation in these treatment guidelines.

It is important to acknowledge, however, that many CAI therapies do not target reductions in specific symptoms. Because change in PTSD symptoms is a critical metric for evaluating PTSD treatments, it is possible that their contributions are underestimated. Mindfulness, which is a component of many of these approaches, encourages present-moment awareness and aims to reduce the struggle against distressing sensations. A major focus of these therapies is on changing one's *relation to* one's physical and mental states, rather than changing symptoms themselves. For example, the number of intrusive trauma memories one has over a week may not change substantially, but the distress associated with the memories may recede and the ability to engage in other life activities may improve. Thus, a shift in the methods used to evaluate outcomes for CAI therapies may be required to capture changes such as distress tolerance, sense of well-being, or enhancement of valued life goals. The need for such standards for the evaluation of CAI may, in turn, prompt broader understanding of the impact of other types of interventions to the benefit of individuals looking to recover from traumatic experiences.

An important caveat to the use of CAI interventions is that they may foster avoidance and/or cultivate dependence if applied inappropriately. A well-meaning instructor, for example, may communicate that stimuli triggering strong emotions (e.g., certain asanas or vigorous exercise) should be avoided, inadvertently reinforcing the fear that internal experiences are harmful. Similarly, a technique may be misapplied in an attempt to avoid internal experience, rather than as a way to cope while expanding functionality. Thus, it is critical that CAI practitioners be provided with a basic understanding of processes that contribute to the development and maintenance of PTSD. Alternatively, an individual might misattribute change to a particularly skilled instructor rather than the individual's efforts and become reliant on seeing that instructor several times per week. In such cases, clients should be encouraged to accept responsibility for their own recovery, such as developing their own practice outside of session or using the skills developed (e.g., mindful awareness) to face other life challenges. Therapists should be alert to the possibility that, in some cases, client engagement in CAI interventions can distract from, rather than augment, the work of evidence-based psychological treatments for PTSD, such as therapies with a trauma focus.

Despite the potential drawbacks of using CAI therapies in the treatment of PTSD, there are important reasons to consider this category of interventions as part of a treatment plan for PTSD. First, the current patient-centered care focus in health care obliges providers to respond to client preferences, and CAI interventions are well utilized and gaining popularity (NCCIH, 2018b). Surveys indicate that 20% of those diagnosed with PTSD (Bystritsky et al., 2012) and approximately half of U.S. veterans and military personnel use CAI modalities to address symptoms such as stress and chronic pain and to promote relaxation and well-being (Libby, Pilver, & Desai, 2013; Taylor et al., 2019). Second, CAI interventions are freely available in many settings. They are frequently offered and promoted in health care systems, community organizations, or workplace wellness programs as part of larger preventive health promotion efforts, often at little to no cost to the individual. For example, the Veterans Health Administration (VHA), the largest integrated health care system in the United States, offers CAI health services "such as acupuncture, mind-body techniques, yoga, and massage" at many of its 1,250 health care facilities as part of a strategic goal to "empower veterans to improve their well-being" (U.S. Department of Veterans Affairs, 2016). Third, there are few drawbacks to many of the treatments that fall under the category of CAI: side effects are frequently absent or positive (i.e., improved strength and fitness, enhanced sense of well-being), and client satisfaction ratings are generally high. Therefore, in many clinical settings it is reasonable to encourage these adjunctive treatments as part of the treatment plan for individuals with PTSD who seek them.

Treatment planning can be challenging when clients with PTSD request CAI treatments in place of psychotherapies with more robust empirical evidence to support them. It is recommended that clinicians always begin treatment planning discussions by communicating the evidence available to support various treatment options. Based on that shared understanding, providers can then collaboratively move toward treatment planning, considering client preferences and previous experiences. Establishing measurable goals is equally important when considering CAI interventions as with traditional interventions; providers should not persist with treatments that show little measurable benefit and should use shared goals as a way to encourage exploration of approaches that were not initially preferred. In this way, CAI treatments may be a "foot in the door" to facilitate future engagement in evidence-based psychotherapies or other treatment if the CAI does not provide the desired effects. By developing a positive alliance with a provider or health care system and fostering discussion of holistic goals, engaging in CAI interventions may increase openness to considering other treatment modalities.

For both individual clinicians and health-care systems, determining the quality and legitimacy of available treatments is one of the biggest challenges. We know to be wary of nostrums; expensive, heavily advertised interventions that claim to cure all ills in a short amount of time are likely to disappoint. There is emerging evidence provided by this review to support several approaches, but definitive guidance is lacking. If the treatments cited here are unavailable, it can be difficult to determine how to guide clients in choosing. Clinicians can look to other mental health research to evaluate the legitimacy of interventions that may be offered to their clients. Some CAI interventions have solid empirical bases for disorders that are frequently comorbid with PTSD, such as depression, chronic pain, or management of physical disorders. If the research has been conducted by a variety of objective researchers who do not have strong interests in the success of a particular intervention, this offers additional confidence that claims of the intervention's success are not exaggerated. In such cases, we reiterate the importance of maintaining an evidence-based stance: establish mutually agreed-upon, measurable goals to be reevaluated according to a set schedule. If goals are met, continue course and speed. If not, engage in collaborative discussion of which untested approaches would be a next reasonable step.

Characteristics of CAI Interventions to Consider

Group versus Individual

Some PTSD clients seek treatment groups with people who have had similar traumatic experiences, while socially avoidant clients may steadfastly refuse any group program. Group interventions can be very helpful in ameliorating isolation and depression that commonly accompany PTSD, and therapists should encourage clients to consider the added benefits of participating in

CAI therapies with others. At this time, the literature on CAI cannot support one modality over another.

Treatment Targets and Individual Preferences

One strategy that clinicians may adopt could be to match strategies to individual symptom profiles; meditative therapies may be preferable for those with high hyperarousal symptoms, whereas group exercise may provide interaction for those who are isolative or activation for those with concurrent low mood/low energy. Individuals who have participated in sports in their youth and veterans who engaged in physical training in the military also may find a group exercise intervention immediately appealing. Although the CAI interventions included in these guidelines are largely secular, some CAI treatments have spiritual components that may either augment or conflict with religious practices. Clients with a background in martial arts may be drawn to tai chi, a form of martial arts composed of slow, gentle movements, or those who have played an instrument may be drawn to music therapy. Anecdotal reports of success experiences with CAI therapies, from public figures in the media or friends and relatives, may inspire individuals to try certain treatments. Such factors reasonably may be incorporated in treatment planning given the importance of client preference in outcomes and the lack of data to guide individual treatment matching.

Instructor Match

Information about the expertise, personality, and "match" of a specific instructor also may be utilized in choosing an intervention. A compelling, dynamic instructor can draw in and motivate hesitant individuals. Many CAI programs have certification and training criteria for teachers, so certified instructors should be sought to support client safety. For example, yoga teachers have 200-, 300-, or 500-hour yoga therapist certifications, so clinicians should familiarize themselves with the training and experience of providers in their area. Instructors should be cognizant of the need for some modifications in their procedures to accommodate individuals with PTSD, such as suggesting to individuals with high levels of vigilance that they may prefer to keep their eyes half open during a meditation, or using verbal cues rather than manual adjustments to guide proper body positions in yoga or tai chi. As an example, Emerson, Sharma, Chaudhry, and Turner (2009) have described a set of trauma-sensitive modifications for yoga practice. As noted before, however, providers should use caution that modifications do not foster avoidance.

Practical and Logistical Considerations

Aspects of accessibility are predictive of follow-through with exercise programs (e.g., Morgan et al., 2016). Thus, practical concerns for individuals, such as financial costs, distance to travel, access to public transportation, or availability of parking, and whether the environment is welcoming should be weighted in decision making. Practical considerations are relevant for health care systems also, as interventions such as yoga that require large, empty spaces may not be feasible in some settings and specialized equipment such as treadmills or acupuncture tables may not be available or affordable. On the other hand, many CAI interventions are delivered in groups and do not require special equipment or large spaces, making them less financially burdensome to facilities. There are also online or app-based delivery options for some of these techniques; clinicians should consider compiling a resource list if there is sufficient demand within their practice. In weighing the costs and benefits for a health care system, the costs are often low. Even if the benefit of a particular approach is not yet established, it may be useful to consider other potential benefits for health care systems, such as responding to patient preferences, promoting a positive image to the community, and promoting wellness broadly. Ultimately, satisfaction with a health care system should be driven not only by a reduction in target symptoms but also by improved functioning and quality of life.

Resources for Maintenance

At the end of a 10-week yoga program or a 12-session meditation course, clients may have difficulty continuing to practice on their own. It is important to incorporate relapse prevention strategies from the outset and to encourage clients to access resources that will assist them with home practice both during and following the intervention. Online videos and/or smartphone applications can augment between-session practice during the intervention and increase the likelihood that individuals will continue to utilize these resources after the intervention ends. Local resources, such as yoga classes at a neighborhood gym or drop-in meditation groups, have the potential to provide a supportive community to encourage a new practice to develop into a lifestyle routine; again, it can be helpful to clinicians to maintain lists of good options.

Active versus Passive

Given the heterogeneity of the therapies considered to be CAI, one useful classification in CAI treatments is the extent to which they are "active" versus "passive." In active therapies, instructors teach skills in session that clients are encouraged to practice and hone on their own outside of sessions. These treatments require agency from clients as they are expected to initiate home practice, to use the skills taught as they live their lives outside of session, and to maintain these skills beyond the termination of the formal sessions. Examples include yoga, meditation, and physical exercise, which typically can be delivered in group settings with minimal need for equipment. They often have resources available (i.e., written materials, audio or video recordings, links to smartphone applications) to facilitate practice outside of sessions. Benefits of active approaches therefore may include a sense of agency for the client and low-cost barriers for the provider or health care system.

By contrast, in therapies such as acupuncture or massage, clients passively receive the treatment as they are delivered one-on-one from a therapist. In addition, specialized equipment (e.g., acupuncture needles, massage table) may be required. Thus, passive techniques can create some risk of dependence on the provider or external attribution of change. Passive treatments also may not be financially feasible as ongoing, long-term practices for clients. To avoid such pitfalls, these therapies may best be applied in the short term to "jump start" additional lifestyle changes and cognitive shifts to sustain positive effects. Passive treatments also may allow reluctant participants to experience benefits without a great deal of initial effort, thereby generating hope for clients that their symptoms can improve or there is sufficient symptom relief to allow engagement in other approaches.

Figure 19.1 provides tips for the application of CAI therapies in the treatment of PTSD.

Future Developments

The current evidence for CAIs is limited; none of the approaches have more than emerging evidence to support them. Interest is high in this area, however, leading to the hope that future guidelines will be able to provide more definitive recommendations. Along with potentially leading to important advancements in recovery from PTSD, CAIs also bring new scientific challenges. The outcomes of CAI interventions are often expected to be broader

---

1. Employ evidence-based practices, including objective assessment of outcomes.

2. Help clients to make informed choices, set objective markers of success, and plan to revisit progress.

3. Identify and use high-quality strategies that have been used before (e.g., existing classes, apps) and that are inexpensive or in the public domain, rather than inventing or recommending untested yet expensive products.

4. Coordinate with other providers to consider the total burden for the client and to consider any unintended effects (e.g., fostering avoidance).

5. Only deliver interventions directly with proper training and supervision.

6. Encourage open-minded exploration: a client may try a variety of techniques to determine the best match in terms of sustainability and response.

7. Plan for posttreatment maintenance of new practices.

FIGURE 19.1. Tips for application of CAI therapies in the treatment of PTSD.

than a reduction in PTSD symptoms, so investigators should determine the best ways to assess recovery in a more holistic way. Broader outcome assessment will benefit consumers of PTSD treatment more broadly because all interventions share the goal of restoring optimal functioning.

With a seemingly endless number of approaches and numerous variants within each approach, we risk stalling advances in care for the sake of evaluating every approach. We encourage reductionist strategies: identify and apply key change agents (e.g., nonreactivity to internal experience, focused attention, reduced arousal) that are shared by multiple approaches. In this way, we may develop thoughtfully integrated care, although we will be left with the challenge of developing methodologies to evaluate personalized approaches and outcomes. Ultimately, this process may lead to the development of empirically based integrated programs, an elusive entity at this juncture.

To the extent that protocols are developed, this should be done with adequate specificity to allow for replication (e.g., meditation protocols, prescribed acupuncture points) and clear criteria for training and certifying instructors/providers. Within a given approach, studies will be necessary to determine optimal dose and timing. Although this process may seem antithetical to CAI providers who are accustomed to individually tailoring treatments, it is critical to building an evidence base to guide care. In some instances, an approach may not lend itself to manualization. Examples include exercise and yoga, which are taught in thousands of venues and are available online. In such cases, it may be more useful to develop guidelines (e.g., types of exercise or supporting instructions) to guide consumers to apply the practice to their recovery.

In spite of the nontraditional nature of some of the interventions, methodologically rigorous studies should be strongly encouraged, which is a call for the research community to support such endeavors. Studies should be appropriate to the level of evidence about the approach (NCCIH, 2017c). RCTs should include equally appealing, active control conditions. Researchers should use common data elements so that results can be compared across studies. Longer-term outcome assessment will be necessary to assess durability of change and whether maintenance of practice is critical to durability of improvements. We may need to borrow from colleagues who are experts in studying lifestyle change for health outcomes to apply the techniques to supporting long-term mental wellness.

Summary

Complementary, alternative, and integrative practices describe a set of intervention techniques that are not currently part of traditional Western practice. Although highly utilized worldwide for amelioration of physical and mental health problems, evidence of their efficacy for the treatment of

PTSD is just emerging. This chapter describes four approaches with emerging evidence—yoga, acupuncture, SKK, and somatic experiencing—as well as others that may be promising, such as certain types of meditation, for which there is not yet sufficient support to make a recommendation. Although not recommended as first-line PTSD interventions, their high degree of safety and demonstrated benefits in other areas (e.g., stress reduction, pain, physical wellness) lead us to encourage their thoughtful use to complement standard care within an evidence-based framework. We strongly encourage additional empirical evaluation of CAI interventions.

REFERENCES

Ahmadi, N., Hajsadeghi, F., Mirshkarlo, H. B., Budoff, M., Yehuda, R., & Ebrahimi, R. (2011). Post-traumatic stress disorder, coronary atherosclerosis, and mortality. *American Journal of Cardiology, 108*(1), 29–33.

Bellehsen, M., Stoycheva, V., Cohen, B., & Nidich, S. (2017, November). *Effect of transcendental meditation as a treatment for PTSD in veterans: A randomized controlled study.* Paper presented at the annual conference of the International Society for Traumatic Stress Studies, Chicago.

Bormann, J. E., Liu, L., Thorp, S., & Lang, A. J. (2011). Spiritual wellbeing mediates PTSD change in veterans with military-related PTSD. *International Journal of Behavioral Medicine, 19,* 496–502.

Bormann, J. E., Thorp, S. R., Smith, E., Glickman, M., Beck, D., Plumb, D., et al. (2018). Individual treatment of posttraumatic stress disorder using mantram repetition: A randomized clinical trial. *American Journal of Psychiatry, 175*(10), 979–988.

Bormann, J. E., Thorp, S., Wetherell, J. L., & Golshan, S. (2008). A spiritually based group intervention for combat veterans with posttraumatic stress disorder: Feasibility study. *Journal of Holistic Nursing, 26,* 109–116.

Bormann, J. E., Thorp, S. R., Wetherell, J. L., Golshan, S., & Lang, A. J. (2013). Meditation-based mantram intervention for veterans with posttraumatic stress disorder: A randomized trial. *Psychological Trauma: Theory, Research, Practice, and Policy, 5*(3), 259–267.

Boscarino, J. A. (2006). Posttraumatic stress disorder and mortality among US Army veterans 30 years after military service. *Annals of Epidemiology, 16*(4), 248–256.

Bremner, J. D., Mishra, S., Campanella, C., Shah, M., Kasher, N., Evans, S., et al. (2017). A pilot study of the effects of mindfulness-based stress reduction on post-traumatic stress disorder symptoms and brain response to traumatic reminders of combat in Operation Enduring Freedom/Operation Iraqi Freedom combat veterans with post-traumatic stress disorder. *Frontiers in Psychiatry, 8,* 157.

Brom, D., Stokar, Y., Lawi, C., Nuriel-Porat, V., Ziv, Y., Lerner, K., et al. (2017). Somatic experiencing for posttraumatic stress disorder: A randomized controlled outcome study. *Journal of Traumatic Stress, 30*(3), 304–312.

Bystritsky, A., Hovav, S., Sherbourne, C., Stein, M. B., Rose, R. D., Campbell-Sills, L., et al. (2012). Use of complementary and alternative medicine in a large sample of anxiety patients. *Psychosomatics, 53*(3), 266–272.

Carr, C., d'Ardenne, P., Sloboda, A., Scott, C., Wang, D., & Priebe, S. (2012). Group music therapy for patients with persistent post-traumatic stress disorder–an exploratory randomized controlled trial with mixed methods evaluation. *Psychology and Psychotherapy: Theory, Research and Practice, 85*(2), 179–202.

Carter, J. J., Gerbarg, P. L., Brown, R. P., Ware, R. S., D'Ambrosio, C., Anand, L., et al. (2013). Multi-component yoga breath program for Vietnam veteran post-traumatic stress disorder: Randomized controlled trial. *Journal of Traumatic Stress Disorders and Treatment, 2*, 1–10.

Crawford, J. N., Talkovsky, A. M., Bormann, J. E., & Lang, A. J. (2019). Targeting hyperarousal: Mantram repetition program for PTSD in US veterans. *European Journal of Psychotraumatology, 10*(1), 1665768.

Davis, L. L., Whetsell, C., Hamner, M. B., Carmody, J., Rothbaum, B. O., Allen, R. S., et al. (2018). A multisite randomized controlled trial of mindfulness-based stress reduction in the treatment of posttraumatic stress disorder. *Psychiatric Research and Clinical Practice.*

Emerson, D., Sharma, R., Chaudhry, S., & Turner, J. (2009). Trauma-sensitive yoga: Principles, practice, and research. *International Journal of Yoga Therapy, 19*(1), 123–128.

Engel, C. C., Cordova, E. H., Benedek, D. M., Liu, X., Gore, K. L., Goertz, C., et al. (2014). Randomized effectiveness trial of a brief course of acupuncture for posttraumatic stress disorder. *Medical Care, 52*(12, Suppl. 5), S57–S64.

Fetzner, M. G., & Asmundson, G. J. (2015). Aerobic exercise reduces symptoms of posttraumatic stress disorder: A randomized controlled trial. *Cognitive Behaviour Therapy, 44*(4), 301–313.

Gard, T., Taquet, M., Dixit, R., Holzel, B. K., de Montjoye, Y. A., Brach, N., et al. (2014). Fluid intelligence and brain functional organization in aging yoga and meditation practitioners. *Frontiers in Aging Neuroscience, 6*, 76.

Gelkopf, M., Hasson-Ohayon, I., Bikman, M., & Kravetz, S. (2013). Nature adventure rehabilitation for combat-related posttraumatic chronic stress disorder: A randomized control trial. *Psychiatry Research, 209*(3), 485–493.

Goldstein, L. A., Mehling, W. E., Metzler, T. J., Cohen, B. E., Barnes, D. E., Choucroun, G. J., et al. (2018). Veterans group exercise: A randomized pilot trial of an integrative exercise program for veterans with posttraumatic stress. *Journal of Affective Disorders, 227*, 345–352.

Groessl, E. J., Maiya, M., Elwy, A. R., Riley, K. E., Sarkin, A. J., Eisen, S. V., et al. (2015). The essential properties of yoga questionnaire: Development and methods. *International Journal of Yoga Therapy, 25*(1), 51–59.

Grossman, P., Niemann, L., Schmidt, S., & Walach, H. (2004). Mindfulness-based stress reduction and health benefits: A meta-analysis. *Journal of Psychosomatic Research, 57*(1), 35–43.

Gureje, O., Nortje, G., Makanjuola, V., Oladeji, B. D., Seedat, S., & Jenkins, R. (2015). The role of global traditional and complementary systems of medicine in the treatment of mental health disorders. *Lancet Psychiatry, 2*(2), 168–177.

Hegberg, N. J., Hayes, J. P., & Hayes, S. M. (2019). Exercise intervention in PTSD: A narrative review and rationale for implementation. *Frontiers in Psychology, 10*, 133.

Herman, P. M., Sorbero, M. E., & Sims-Columbia, A. C. (2017). Complementary and alternative medicine services in the military health system. *Journal of Alternative and Complementary Medicine, 23*(11), 837–843.

Kabat-Zinn, J. (1994). *Wherever you go, there you are: Mindfulness meditation in everyday life*. New York: Hyperion.

Kearney, D. J., McDermott, K., Malte, C., Martinez, M., & Simpson, T. L. (2013). Effects of participation in a mindfulness program for veterans with posttraumatic stress disorder: A randomized controlled pilot study. *Journal of Clinical Psychology, 69*(1), 14–27.

Kemppainen, L. M., Kemppainen, T. T., Reippainen, J. A., Salmenniemi, S. T., & Vuolanto, P. H. (2018). Use of complementary and alternative medicine in Europe: Health-related and sociodemographic determinants. *Scandinavian Journal of Public Health, 46*(4), 448–455.

Khoury, B., Sharma, M., Rush, S. E., & Fournier, C. (2015). Mindfulness-based stress reduction for healthy individuals: A meta-analysis. *Journal of Psychosomatic Research, 78*(6), 519–525.

Kroesen, K., Baldwin, C. M., Brooks, A. J., & Bell, J. R. (2002). US military veterans' perceptions of the conventional medical care system and their use of complementary and alternative medicine. *Family Practice, 19*, 57–64.

Lang, A. J., Malaktaris, A. L., Casmar, P., Baca, S. A., Golshan, S., Harrison, T., et al. (2019). Compassion meditation for posttraumatic stress disorder in veterans: A randomized proof of concept study. *Journal of Traumatic Stress, 32*(2), 299–309.

Lang, A. J., Strauss, J. L., Bomyea, J., Bormann, J. E., Hickman, S. D., Good, R. C., et al. (2012). The theoretical and empirical basis for meditation as an intervention for PTSD. *Behavior Modification, 36*(6), 759–786.

Levine, P. A. (2010). *In an unspoken voice: How the body releases trauma and restores goodness*. Berkeley, CA: North Atlantic Books.

Libby, D. J., Pilver, C. E., & Desai, R. (2013). Complementary and alternative medicine use among individuals with posttraumatic stress disorder. *Psychological Trauma: Theory, Research, Practice, and Policy, 5*(3), 277–285.

McFarlane, A. C. (2017). Post-traumatic stress disorder is a systemic illness, not a mental disorder: Is Cartesian dualism dead? *Medical Journal of Australia, 206*(6), 248–249.

Mitchell, K. S., Dick, A. M., DiMartino, D. M., Smith, B. N., Niles, B., Koenen, K. C., et al. (2014). A pilot study of a randomized controlled trial of yoga as an intervention for PTSD symptoms in women. *Journal of Traumatic Stress, 27*(2), 121–128.

Morgan, F., Battersby, B., Weightman, A. L., Searchfield, L., Turley, R., Morgan, H., et al. (2016). Adherence to exercise referral schemes by participants—what do providers and commissioners need to know?: A systematic review of barriers and facilitators. *BMC Public Health, 16*(1), 227–211.

National Center for Complementary and Integrative Health. (2017a, September 24). Acupuncture. Retrieved April 12, 2019, from *https://nccih.nih.gov/health/acupuncture*.

National Center for Complementary and Integrative Health. (2017b, September 24). Mind and body practices. Retrieved April 12, 2019, from *https://nccih.nih.gov/health/mindbody*.

National Center for Complementary and Integrative Health. (2017c, September 24). The range of research questions. Retrieved April 12, 2019, from *https://nccih.nih.gov/about/research/range-research-questions*.

National Center for Complementary and Integrative Health. (2018a, July).

Complementary, alternative, or integrative health: What's in a name? Retrieved April 12, 2019, from *https://nccih.nih.gov/health/integrative-health.*

National Center for Complementary and Integrative Health. (2018b, November 14). National Health Interview Survey 2017. Retrieved April 12, 2019, from *https:// nccih.nih.gov/research/statistics/NHIS/2017.*

Nidich, S., Mills, P. J., Rainforth, M., Heppner, P., Schneider, R. H., Rosenthal, N. E., et al. (2018). Non-trauma-focused meditation versus exposure therapy in veterans with post-traumatic stress disorder: A randomised controlled trial. *Lancet Psychiatry, 5*(12), P975–P986.

Niles, B. L., Klunk-Gillis, J., Ryngala, D. J., Silberbogen, A. K., Paysnick, A., & Wolf, E. J. (2012). Comparing mindfulness and psychoeducation treatments for combat-related PTSD using a telehealth approach. *Psychological Trauma: Theory, Research, Practice, and Policy, 4,* 538–547.

Numata, T., Gunfan, S., Takayama, S., Takahashi, S., Monma, Y., Kaneko, S., et al. (2014). Treatment of posttraumatic stress disorder using the traditional Japanese herbal medicine saikokeishikankyoto: A randomized, observer-blinded, controlled trial in survivors of the great East Japan earthquake and tsunami. *Evidence-Based Complementary and Alternative Medicine,* 683293.

Payne, P., Levine, P. A., & Crane-Godreau, M. A. (2015). Somatic experiencing: Using interoception and proprioception as core elements of trauma therapy. *Frontiers in Psychology, 6,* 93.

Peltzer, K., Pengpid, S., Puckpinyo, A., Yi, S., & Anh le V. (2016). The utilization of traditional, complementary and alternative medicine for non-communicable diseases and mental disorders in health care patients in Cambodia, Thailand and Vietnam. *BMC Complementary Alternative Medicine, 16,* 92.

Polusny, M. A., Erbes, C. R., Thuras, P., Moran, A., Lamberty, G. J., Collins, R. C., et al. (2015). Mindfulness-based stress reduction for posttraumatic stress disorder among veterans: A randomized clinical trial. *Journal of the American Medical Association, 314*(5), 456–465.

Reinhardt, K. M., Noggle Taylor, J. J., Johnston, J., Zameer, A., Cheema, S., & Khalsa, S. B. S. (2018). Kripalu yoga for military veterans with PTSD: A randomized trial. *Journal of Clinical Psychology, 74*(1), 93–108.

Rosenbaum, S., Sherrington, C., & Tiedemann, A. (2015). Exercise augmentation compared with usual care for post-traumatic stress disorder: A randomized controlled trial. *Acta Psychiatrica Scandinavica, 131*(5), 350–359.

Rossler, W., Lauber, C., Angst, J., Haker, H., Gamma, A., Eich, D., et al. (2007). The use of complementary and alternative medicine in the general population: Results from a longitudinal community study. *Psychological Medicine, 37*(1), 73–84.

Schnurr, P. P., & Lunney, C. A. (2015). Differential effects of prolonged exposure on posttraumatic stress disorder symptoms in female veterans. *Journal of Consulting and Clinical Psychology, 83*(6), 1154–1160.

Seppala, E. M., Nitschke, J. B., Tudorascu, D. L., Hayes, A., Goldstein, M. R., Nguyen, D. T., et al. (2014). Breathing-based meditation decreases posttraumatic stress disorder symptoms in US military veterans: A randomized controlled longitudinal study. *Journal of Traumatic Stress, 27*(4), 397–405.

Steenkamp, M. M., Litz, B. T., Hoge, C. W., & Marmar, C. R. (2015). Psychotherapy for military-related PTSD: A review of randomized clinical trials. *Journal of the American Medical Association, 314*(5), 489–500.

Stubbs, B., Vancampfort, D., Hallgren, M., Firth, J., Veronese, N., Solmi, M., et al. (2018). EPA guidance on physical activity as a treatment for severe mental illness: A meta-review of the evidence and position statement from the European Psychiatric Association (EPA), supported by the International Organization of Physical Therapists in Mental Health (IOPTMH). *European Psychiatry, 54,* 124–144.

Taylor, S. L., Hoggatt, K., & Kligler, B. (2019). Complementary and integrated health approaches: What do veterans use and want. *Journal of General Internal Medicine, 34*(7), 1192–1199.

Thirthalli, J., Zhou, L., Kumar, K., Gao, J., Vaid, H., Liu, H., et al. (2016). Traditional, complementary, and alternative medicine approaches to mental health care and psychological wellbeing in India and China. *Lancet Psychiatry, 3*(7), 660–672.

Travis, F., & Shear, J. (2010). Focused attention, open monitoring and automatic self-transcending: Categories to organize meditations from Vedic, Buddhist and Chinese traditions. *Consciousness and Cognition, 19*(4), 1110–1118.

U.S. Department of Veterans Affairs. (2016). Advancing complementary and integrative health in VHA [Under Secretary for Health memorandum]. Retrieved from *http://projects.hsl.wisc.edu/SERVICE/courses/whole-health-for-pain-and-suffering/M1-Advancing-Complementary-and-Integrative-Health-in-VHA.pdf.*

van der Kolk, B. A., Stone, L., West, J., Rhodes, A., Emerson, D., Suvak, M., et al. (2014). Yoga as an adjunctive treatment for posttraumatic stress disorder: A randomized controlled trial. *Journal of Clinical Psychiatry, 75*(6), e559–e565.

Vancampfort, D., Stubbs, B., Richards, J., Ward, P. B., Firth, J., Schuch, F. B., et al. (2017). Physical fitness in people with posttraumatic stress disorder: A systematic review. *Disability Rehabilitation, 39*(24), 2461–2467.

Wald, J., & Taylor, S. (2007). Efficacy of interoceptive exposure therapy combined with trauma-related exposure therapy for posttraumatic stress disorder: A pilot study. *Journal of Anxiety Disorders, 21*(8), 1050–1060.

Wells, S. Y., Lang, A. J., Schmalzl, L., Groessl, E. J., & Strauss, J. (2016). Yoga as an intervention for PTSD: A theoretical rationale and review of the literature. *Current Treatment Options in Psychiatry, 3,* 60–72.

Wolf, E. J., & Schnurr, P. P. (2016). Posttraumatic stress disorder-related cardiovascular disease and accelerated cellular aging. *Psychiatric Annals, 46*(9), 527–532.

CHAPTER 20

Treatment of Complex PTSD

Marylene Cloitre, Thanos Karatzias, and Julian D. Ford

Complex posttraumatic stress disorder (CPTSD) was formally recognized as a mental disorder with the release of the 11th revision of the *International Classification of Diseases* (ICD-11; World Health Organization, 2018). CPTSD is listed under the parent category "disorders specifically associated with stress" (code 6B41), and diagnosis requires traumatic exposure and at least one symptom from each of six clusters. The first three, shared with posttraumatic stress disorder (PTSD), are reexperiencing in the here and now, avoidance of traumatic reminders, and a sense of current threat. The second three clusters, reflecting "disturbances in self-organization" (DSO), are affective dysregulation, negative self-concept, and difficulties in forming and maintaining interpersonal relationships. CPTSD also requires that the PTSD and DSO symptoms cause significant impairment in functioning.

CPTSD represents the spectrum of problems that follow from traumatic exposures that are typically of a chronic and repeated nature, particularly, but not exclusively, interpersonal trauma during the developmental years of childhood and adolescence. Unlike previous formulations of the concept of complex PTSD, however, type of trauma is a risk factor not a requirement, for consideration of the CPTSD diagnosis. This recognizes the presence of personal (e.g., genetic or dispositional) and environmental (e.g., social support or lack thereof) factors that can create increased risk for or protection against the disorder. For example, a person who has experienced sustained childhood sexual abuse might develop PTSD rather than CPTSD, or might not develop any trauma-related disorder, depending on dispositional strengths and the presence of protective resources, such as caregivers who have effectively safeguarded development. Alternatively, an individual who experiences a single traumatic event in adulthood (e.g., witnessing the murder of his or her child) might develop CPTSD given dispositional vulnerabilities, poor social support, a nonresponsive or negative social environment, or a history of adverse childhood events.

As CPTSD is a new disorder, no studies have as yet been reported that directly test the effectiveness of psychological therapies or pharmacotherapies for ICD-11 CPTSD. In the absence of published treatment studies, the Guidelines Committee of the International Society for Traumatic Stress Studies (ISTSS) identified a range of CPTSD treatment options for investigation, including current evidence-based PTSD therapies, interventions derived from cognitive, behavioral, mindfulness, emotion regulation, psychodynamic, interpersonal, pharmacological, or technology-based formulations and combination or sequential therapies incorporating these interventions (ISTSS Guidelines Committee, 2018). This chapter presents broadly framed treatment recommendations consistent with the guidelines and supported by published studies that have included the assessment and treatment of individuals with histories of chronic exposure to multiple types of interpersonal trauma. This chapter provides basic principles for therapeutic work with adults with CPTSD and empirically informed best practices in the assessment and treatment of ICD-11 CPTSD. The CPTSD diagnosis is applicable to children and adolescents as well, and the treatment of CPTSD in these samples is addressed by Berliner, Meiser-Stedman, and Danese (Chapter 5, this volume).

Therapeutic Frame

Treatment of CPTSD begins with the establishment of a therapeutic frame by obtaining a fully informed consent for participation from the patient following a collaborative discussion of his or her rights, the procedures that will be involved, the potential outcomes and limitations of treatment, and the responsibilities of the therapist. Although this introduction is a requirement in all forms of psychological and medical treatment, it has special significance with persons with complex trauma histories that may have involved sustained victimization, deception, exploitation, or betrayal by trusted others (Courtois & Ford, 2013).

A fundamental principle guiding both the assessment and treatment of individuals with CPTSD is the assumption that many of the symptoms resulting from sustained and multiple forms of interpersonal trauma begin as adaptive efforts under conditions of extreme adversity. Dissociation and emotional numbing are protective reactions to overwhelming experiences. Avoidance of relationships and intimacy can be strategies for staying physically and emotionally safe. Mistrust and aggressive behaviors such as those that occur in combat or in environments of chronic violence (e.g., multigenerational civil war) are necessary for survival. These reactions transition from adaptive to nonadaptive when the traumatic threats no longer are present but the affective, cognitive, and behavioral adaptations continue, creating a mismatch between an environment and responses to it. Alternatively, some traumatic exposures continue for extended periods of time (e.g., warfare, domestic violence, community violence) and overtax the individual such that repertoires for managing trauma and stress convert into less flexible and less adaptive responses (chronic dissociation, learned helplessness).

Psychoeducation is an important component of the theoretical frame for treatment. This includes explaining how CPTSD symptoms develop as adaptive responses to a traumatic event, with the goal of normalizing the patient's experience of his or her symptoms and reducing stigma. During the assessment and throughout all phases of the treatment process, the therapist instills hope by describing how the treatment will address the specific problems that the patient is presenting, by identifying the specific personal and relational resources the patient is bringing to the treatment, and by describing the collaborative nature of decision making in the therapy. The therapist listens carefully and without assumptions about which problems bother the patient most and respects that individual's interests and preferences. Emphasis on the collaborative nature of the work, responsiveness to the patient's concerns, and flexibility in implementing the treatment all support the therapeutic alliance, which has been consistently demonstrated as a significant contributor to engaging, retaining, and achieving positive outcomes with adults with a wide range of psychosocial problems.

Tasks of Treatment

Three important tasks of treatment are identified in this section and include assessment, treatment planning and implementation, and follow-up care or supportive reintegration of the patient into his or her community and life activities (see Courtois & Ford, 2013).

1. *Assessment.* Creating an appropriate treatment plan includes assessing the life circumstances of the patient with regard to safety and stability and conducting a good differential diagnosis, particularly between CPTSD and borderline personality disorder (BPD). Individuals with CPTSD who are living in chaotic and disruptive conditions (e.g., ongoing domestic violence, homelessness) should be provided services that address their needs for safety and stability as a first step, and such services must be maintained as needed throughout the course of treatment. For patients who are not currently exposed but are at risk for exposure to violence or victimization, the development and maintenance of a safety plan will be integral to the treatment.

2. *Treatment planning and implementation.* Consistent with the definition of CPTSD, treatment focuses on resolution of both PTSD and DSO symptoms. The goal of treatment includes reducing intrusive reexperiencing and

avoidance of trauma memories and the associated sense of fear and inescapable threat that represent the PTSD symptoms, while also increasing the core self-competencies of affect regulation, interpersonal skills and security, and positive self-concept.

3. *Follow-up care and reintegration.* Due to the chronicity and severity of their traumas as well as their symptoms, individuals with CPTSD may have become disconnected from or never participated in family or community life, have limited social support and few relationships, and have limited education or employment prospects. Common underlying factors driving these circumstances are a sense of being somehow "damaged" or "different" from members of the surrounding community, fear of being stigmatized, or having actually been stigmatized due to their trauma and significant limitations or a deterioration in their functional capacities related to relationships, social engagement, and work.

Follow-up care can include continued contact with patients via "booster" sessions and the opportunity to return to treatment during times of stress. Additional resources can be recommended, such as support groups with other survivors to address stigma and increase their sense of community, and where they can share resources to support education, employment, housing, health care, parenting, and addiction recovery. These resources encourage and help maintain a sense of normality, efficacy, and social connectedness that patients might have never experienced in the past, and offer an opportunity to develop a sense of purpose in life and to commit to life goals and objectives.

Assessment

Assessment of CPTSD includes the evaluation of CPTSD symptoms as well as associated biopsychosocial symptoms (e.g., suicidality, self-harm, addictions, guilt, shame, sexuality, sleep), adverse life circumstances and stressors, and personal and relational resources and strengths. Comorbidity and co-occurring stressors or adversities are common in CPTSD; hence, these are important to identify using empirically validated measures.

In adult patient populations, special attention is given to the differential diagnosis of CPTSD as compared to BPD. At least four studies have demonstrated that CPTSD and BPD are distinct disorders, with distinct symptom profiles and patient populations (see Hyland, Karatzias, Shevlin, & Cloitre, 2019). BPD and CPTSD have conceptual overlap in the type of problems that are included in each diagnosis, namely, difficulties in affect regulation, self-concept, and interpersonal relationships. However, there are important phenomenological differences in *how* these symptoms manifest across the disorders.

CPTSD and BPD are most similar in the domains of affect disturbances of emotional reactivity and numbing. However, in addition and central to the BPD diagnosis is the presence of suicide attempts and self-injurious behavior, which are priority targets in treatment. Individuals with CPTSD may have a history of suicide attempts and self-injurious behaviors, but this is not central to their presentation and indeed is not part of the diagnosis. In BPD, self-concept difficulties reflect an unstable sense of self, whereas in CPTSD, it reflects a persistent, negative view of the self. Relational difficulties in BPD are characterized by volatile patterns of interactions, whereas in CPTSD, they reflect a persistent tendency to avoid relationships. There are other relevant features that differentiate BPD and CPTSD, most notably the fact that CPTSD requires the presence of trauma-specific PTSD symptoms and BPD does not require traumatic exposure for diagnosis. A diagnosis of BPD can be made via several validated measures currently available. At this time, there are two reliable and validated measures to assess CPTSD. One is a brief self-report measure, the International Trauma Questionnaire (ITQ; Cloitre et al., 2018), and the other an interview, the International Trauma Interview (ITI; Roberts, Cloitre, Bisson, & Brewin, 2018).

Treatment Approach

Commitment to Best Practices

CPTSD is a new diagnosis, and there is to date no direct evidence about how to treat it. ISTSS guidelines, consistent with those of several other professional societies (e.g., American Psychological Association, 2017), recommend that the decision for how to treat a particular individual with a particular disorder follow from the available empirical evidence as well as several other considerations, including the patient's values and preferences, individual differences (cultural values, previous successes and failures in treatment), and the clinician's expertise. All four factors—empirical evidence, patient preferences, individual differences, and clinician expertise—are applied to develop a treatment plan that has the highest likelihood of achieving the identified goals of therapy. This three-factor approach, particularly attention to patient needs and preferences, is especially important when empirical evidence is limited.

Evidence from Meta-Analyses

Karatzias and colleagues (2019) and Coventry (2018) conducted meta-analyses to identify whether current evidence-based therapies for PTSD were equally appropriate for patient populations that were representative of those who might meet criteria for the newly established CPTSD diagnosis. In both meta-analyses, the authors identified randomized controlled trials (RCTs) for PTSD that included (1) samples that had experienced sustained exposure to interpersonal trauma (e.g., childhood abuse, domestic violence, combat, genocide campaigns) and (2) measures corresponding to the CPTSD symptom clusters related to the PTSD factor (reexperiencing, avoidance, and heightened sense of threat) and to the DSO factor (emotion dysregulation, negative self-concept, and interpersonal difficulties).

Karatzias and colleagues (2019) found that trauma-focused therapies were effective in reducing symptoms in all six CPTSD domains. However, moderator analyses determined that the trauma-focused therapies were consistently less positive for persons with histories of childhood trauma compared to those who had experienced trauma only in adulthood, and this was true for each of the six CPTSD symptom clusters. The Coventry (2018) meta-analysis found that both trauma-focused and non-trauma-focused therapies provided substantial benefits for PTSD symptoms but noted that the positive effects for the DSO symptom clusters were modest. There was some suggestion that multicomponent therapies provided a better outcome, particularly among childhood sexual abuse survivors. In sum, the results of these meta-analyses suggest that current therapies for PTSD are not likely to be optimal for CPTSD patient populations and that one strategy for improving outcomes is a multimodular approach.

A multimodular approach that is made up of empirically supported interventions is consistent with, and supports use of, the treatment guidelines. Multimodular approaches provide flexibility with regard to the selection and implementation of interventions so that they can be organized to be responsive to the presenting problems, needs, and preferences of patients. This approach takes advantage of the availability of validated trauma memory processing (TMP) therapies to treat symptoms of the PTSD cluster (such as reexperiencing, nightmares, and avoidance) but also allows consideration of interventions that focus on emotion regulation (ER), identity issues, or relationship problems. There are a variety of ways multiinterventions or multimodal interventions can be implemented, including sequenced (phase-based), combination, or integrative strategies. Examples of therapies that implement each of these strategies are provided later in the chapter.

Important Symptoms of CPTSD to Target

CPTSD is by definition a relatively complex disorder, and it is not necessarily the case that all symptoms or symptom clusters are of equal importance. Identification of the symptoms that are central to the disorder and have the most influence in exacerbating or maintaining other symptoms provides guidance on how to conceptualize the goals of treatment.

A recent network analysis of CPTSD symptoms in four nationally representative samples (Knefel et al., 2019) found that negative self-concept was the most central aspect of the CPTSD formulation, followed by affect dysregulation. Negative self-concept has been defined in terms of persistent beliefs about one's self as diminished, defeated, or worthless, accompanied by deep and pervasive feelings of shame, guilt, or failure. The network analyses indicated that interpersonal problems were related to emotion regulation (ER) difficulties (particularly numbing) and negative self-concept (Knefel et al., 2019), suggesting these as the most complex and potentially challenging problems to resolve. The PTSD symptoms were less central to the disorder and significantly influenced by the DSO symptoms. To address the limited information about, and past attention to, how best to treat DSO symptoms, several empirically supported interventions that directly target each of the three DSO clusters are presented next.

Negative Self-Concept

"Third-wave" cognitive-behavioral therapies focus on exercising mindfulness or developing a more compassionate attitude toward one's self for the purposes of ameliorating psychological distress by changing the client's relationship to his or her problems. Mindfulness approaches may be effective for the treatment of CPTSD per se as there is some evidence that mindfulness can reduce avoidance and enable ER, symptoms of the PTSD and DSO cluster, respectively (see Banks, Newman, & Saleem, 2015; Follette, Palm, & Pearson, 2006).

However, of most relevance to the problem of negative self-concept are interventions that focus on the development of self-compassion. Self-compassion has been described as involving three distinct elements, including (1) being kind and understanding toward oneself in times of difficulty, (2) being mindfully aware of painful thoughts and feelings to prevent over-identification, and (3) seeing one's struggles as part of a broader human experience rather than as a unique and isolating experience (Neff, 2011). Thus, self-compassion can be particularly helpful with symptoms of negative self-concept and disrupted relations by reducing self-judgment, rumination, and feelings of isolation (Gilbert & Irons, 2004). For example, Karatzias and colleagues (2018) found direct relationships between dimensions of self-compassion and CPTSD symptoms; specifically, self-judgment and isolation significantly predicted negative self-concept, while self-judgment and common humanity significantly predicted hypoactive affect dysregulation. These data suggest that adding compassion-based interventions to the treatment of CPTSD might be particularly useful for symptoms of disrupted sense of self.

Emotion Regulation Difficulties

In light of the salient role of affect dysregulation in CPTSD, systematic interventions to enhance ER are a logical component of treatment. Two therapies are provided as example interventions. They are relatively brief and have been tested with complex trauma populations and shown to reduce ER problems and interpersonal difficulties.

Trauma Affect Regulation: Guide for Education and Therapy (TARGET) is a 4- to 20-session treatment that has been implemented with diverse trauma populations in several studies (Ford, 2020b). As relevant to adults with CPTSD, a 10-session version of the treatment was found to be effective in reducing ER and interpersonal problems as well as PTSD symptoms when evaluated among low-income mothers with extensive histories of multiple forms of victimization beginning in childhood and chronic PTSD, as compared to a present-centered interpersonal therapy (IPT) or treatment as usual (TAU; Ford, Steinberg, & Zhang, 2011). The treatment teaches a seven-step sequence of self-regulation skills summarized by the acronym FREEDOM. The first two skills, Focusing and Recognizing triggers, provide a foundation for shifting from stress reactions driven by hypervigilance to proactive ER. The following four skills provide a dual-processing approach to differentiating stress-related and core value-grounded Emotions, Evaluative thoughts, client-Defined goals, and behavioral Options. The final skill is designed to promote application of the skills set in everyday life as well as enhance self-esteem and self-efficacy by purposeful allocation of attention to recognizing how being emotionally regulated when experiencing stressors (including reminders of past traumatic events and intrusive memories) is a way to Make an important positive contribution in relationships, at school/work, and in the pursuit of personal goals. The results suggest that although the treatment focused heavily on ER difficulties, it provided positive significant benefits to the remainder of the DSO and PTSD symptoms.

Skills Training in Affect and Interpersonal Regulation (STAIR) is a brief (5- to 12-session) treatment that can be used in individual or group format and has been applied to different types of trauma populations. As relevant to adults, the efficacy of 5-session STAIR as a stand-alone treatment has been evaluated in an RCT of veterans with diverse traumas and, as compared to wait list, was found to improve ER, interpersonal, and social engagement strategies and to reduce PTSD symptoms (Jain et al., in press). More relevant to "complex trauma," an open trial of a 10-session version of the treatment delivered via tele-mental health to women veterans with military sexual trauma and high rates of childhood abuse was found to improve the same symptom sets. The treatment provides psychoeducation on the impact of trauma on ER and relationships, followed by successive sessions on ER (emotional awareness, ER, distress tolerance, and positive activities) and concluding with interpersonal skills training. The interpersonal work includes recognizing and modifying maladaptive expectations in relationships as well as improving communication skills to enhance assertiveness, interpersonal flexibility, and closeness with others.

Interpersonal Difficulties

STAIR directly addresses interpersonal difficulties, and both STAIR and TARGET have demonstrated effectiveness in reducing interpersonal difficulties and improving social functioning. However, IPT is entirely dedicated to interpersonal difficulties. IPT is a 14- to 16-week treatment that focuses on four areas of interpersonal difficulties: interpersonal disputes, role transitions, grief/loss or interpersonal sensitivity, and social deficits. Although IPT has not been tested with a complex trauma population in individual format, it has been tested in group format among women with PTSD who had experienced multiple interpersonal traumas (Krupnick et al., 2008). An RCT found that compared to wait list, the group treatment provided superior reductions in interpersonal problems as well as PTSD symptoms. Additionally, a 14-session version of IPT delivered as individual therapy was compared to prolonged exposure (PE) and relaxation therapy (RT) among those with PTSD related to various types of trauma. IPT was found to yield comparably positive results overall for adults diagnosed with PTSD and lower dropouts for the entire sample; for the subgroup who had histories of chronic sexual assault, however, IPT was superior to both PE and RT (Markowitz, Neria, Lovell, Van Meter, & Petkova, 2017). While not directly assessing CPTSD, this study further suggests that IPT may be beneficial for adults with complex trauma histories and symptoms.

Summary

This review has highlighted the relative centrality of the DSO symptoms in the CPTSD diagnosis and described several interventions that successfully address them. A further important question is how to organize selected interventions into a program of treatment.

Treatment Delivery: Ordering Interventions

Flexible Problem-Focused Multimodular Approach

The flexible problem-focused treatment model sequences treatment by addressing symptoms based on priorities collaboratively identified by the patient and therapist. The use of flexible, problem-driven multimodular interventions has been shown to be highly effective and superior to single module treatments in mental health services for children and adolescents (Weisz et al., 2012). This approach is particularly useful for patients who have moderate to high heterogeneity in symptom presentation, as is true with CPTSD.

Sequential Multimodular Treatment

Sequential treatments are protocols that deliver treatment modules ordered in a set fashion. Patients and therapists may select particular interventions within each treatment component, but the components themselves are fixed. Sequential treatments for CPTSD have traditionally used three sequential components: first, interventions to ensure safety and enhance personal, social, and environmental resources and self-regulation capacities; second, interventions for TMP; and third, interventions for generalizing therapeutic gains to daily life (Courtois & Ford, 2013). Four RCT studies of sequential treatments have been reported. All four studies enrolled women who had experienced significant interpersonal trauma and had either a diagnosis of PTSD related to childhood abuse or BPD and PTSD. The studies varied in outcomes of interest, but all studies indicated that this approach provided benefit to patients.

An RCT of a two-module treatment, STAIR followed by narrative therapy (derived from PE), was conducted among women with PTSD related to childhood abuse and found that compared to wait list, the treatment provided significant and superior improvements in ER, social support, interpersonal functioning, and PTSD symptoms (Cloitre, Koenen, Cohen, & Han, 2002). Moreover, improvements in ER and the quality of the therapeutic alliance established during STAIR facilitated effective use of the narrative work as measured by PTSD symptom reduction, providing a rationale for this treatment order. A second RCT compared the sequential treatment to two comparator conditions, each of which tested one active component by replacing the partner component with supportive counseling. Results indicated that the STAIR/narrative therapy combination provided superior outcomes as compared to the other two conditions (Cloitre et al., 2010). This finding suggests the particular benefits of specific interventions tailored to ER and interpersonal disturbances.

The two other RCTs enrolled women with BPD plus PTSD, and the treatments involved the sequencing of dialectical behavioral therapy preceding trauma-focused work. A pilot RCT by Harned and colleagues (Harned, Korslund, & Linehan, 2014) reported that women assigned to DBT plus PE compared to DBT alone showed better outcomes in PTSD symptoms as well as reduced suicide attempts and self-injury, the latter two being key targets of BPD treatment. The introduction of the exposure work was flexible and initiated, on average, 24 weeks into the treatment, contingent on the patient's ability to achieve high-priority treatment targets (emotional self-control, no suicide or self-injurious behaviors for 2 months). In a recently completed RCT, Bohus (2018) compared DBT plus CPT as compared to CPT alone. In the CPT-alone treatment, trauma-focused work was initiated at about the 15th week of treatment, while the DBT plus CPT treatment started TMP at approximately 24 weeks. Both treatments were of equal duration (approximately 1 year). Findings indicated superior outcomes on measures of PTSD as well as important outcomes of ER, beliefs about self, and interpersonal/social engagement in the sequenced treatment as compared to CPT alone.

There has been some concern that sequencing treatments where the trauma-focused work comes after other treatment modules may result in adverse effects, specifically in reinforcing avoidance of TMP or undermining the patient's confidence in mastery over traumatic material (De Jongh et al., 2016). However, no evidence supports this concern. Indeed, the data thus far indicate that treatment dropout and symptom exacerbation are reduced when treatments are sequenced with skills-training interventions preceding TMP (Cloitre et al., 2010).

Sequential treatments have the benefit of limiting the amount of new learning and behavioral practice that occurs at any one time, in contrast to combination treatments where the presence of multiple interventions presented simultaneously may create a burden in the assimilation of new information and practice of new behaviors. Nevertheless, requiring a particular sequencing structure may be inconsistent with the principle of "patient-centered" care. For example, reversing the order described previously—that is, TMP first—may be clinically appropriate and of greater therapeutic value for some patients. Examples include situations where patients wish to immediately address their trauma memories, patients whose most salient symptoms are nightmares or reexperiencing (including flashbacks), or whose avoidance of trauma-related stimuli significantly impairs daily functioning (e.g., cannot drive a car or travel to their work location).

Investigations evaluating which sequences work best and for whom are an important next step in research. Similarly, it would be of interest to conduct comparative effectiveness trials assessing the benefits of patient-driven compared to protocol- or algorithm-determined approaches in sequencing interventions.

Combination Treatments

Combination treatments refer to those where multiple intervention components are delivered relatively simultaneously over a period of time. This approach is often used and relatively easily implemented in residential or inpatient settings. An open trial of a DBT-PTSD program was tested in a residential treatment setting for women who had PTSD related to childhood sexual abuse (Steil, Dyer, Priebe, Kleindienst, & Bohus, 2011). The treatment comprised several groups (skills training, self-esteem, mindfulness, and PTSD psychoeducation) as well as two weekly 35-minute individual therapy sessions, about a quarter of which were dedicated to exposure techniques. The duration of the treatment across the participants was approximately 3 months; treatment outcomes indicated significant reductions in PTSD as well as depression and anxiety. The treatment did not assess changes in ER, negative self-concept, or interpersonal functioning.

Another example of a combination approach is Concurrent Treatment of PTSD and Substance Use Disorders Using Prolonged Exposure (COPE). The treatment has been evaluated in an RCT where it was compared to relapse prevention therapy (RPT) and an active monitoring control group (AMCG) in a sample of adults with PTSD and a co-occurring substance use disorder (SUD) (Ruglass et al., 2017). Results indicated that COPE and RPT were superior to AMCG for PTSD and SUD symptom reduction, and COPE was superior to RPT in PTSD symptom reduction for persons with a full PTSD diagnosis. The organization of the treatment was innovative: different components were layered one on top of the other across time. The 13-session treatment began with 4 sessions devoted to enhancing motivation and CBT for SUD; *in vivo* exposure was incorporated in Sessions 5–12, imaginal exposure in Sessions 6–12, and CBT for PTSD in Sessions 8–12, with a review and aftercare program in the 13th session. The treatment did not evaluate psychiatric or psychosocial symptoms other than PTSD and did not identify patients who might have had CPTSD. However, the treatment model presents an interesting "layering" strategy for introducing interventions that may be useful for CPTSD where treatment components have some overlapping goals (e.g., improvement in ER, then using ER skills to facilitate TMP and to improve interpersonal and social skills).

Group Therapy

Group therapies are a practical way to provide interventions to large numbers of patients and can have a number of benefits for CPTSD sufferers. Group therapies might be particularly useful for treating the relationship/interpersonal problems of CPTSD by enabling participants to exercise existing skills or acquire new interpersonal skills by participating in a group that promotes safety, respect, honesty, and privacy (Karatzias, Ferguson, Gullone, & Cosgrove, 2016). By being in a group of individuals who share similar experiences but are at different stages of recovery, group therapy can instill hope that recovery is possible. Group therapies can also provide opportunities for interpersonal learning (e.g., effective communication, the difference between safe and supportive vs. victimizing or exploitive relationships) that patients who have lived in chronically traumatizing environments may not have had the opportunity to experience. Therapeutic group interactions also can provide opportunities to observe how others are able to modulate and recover from negative emotional states, and to safely experience positive emotions that may have been prohibited or punished in past traumatic experiences.

There are several group therapy models that may be applicable to CPTSD. These include cognitive-behavioral therapy (CBT)—with or without TMP—ER, IPT, as well as psychodynamic, feminist, and relational/supportive therapeutic approaches. TMP in group therapy may be implemented using a CBT approach, as an intensive first-person or narrative retelling of a specific trauma memory with or without cognitive restructuring, or in a relational and testimonial manner in which a group member describes the past and current impact that such traumatic events had, and continue to have, on his or her life, including emotions, self-concept, relationships, achievements, self-defined failures or disappointments, and view of the future (Ford, 2020a).

A recent meta-analysis identified 36 RCT studies of group therapy: 10 studies with TMP group therapies and 26 with trauma-focused group therapies that did not involve TMP (Mahoney, Karatzias, & Hutton, 2019). Participants were predominantly women with histories of childhood abuse or violence at the hands of an intimate partner. Trauma-focused group therapies achieved greater improvements in PTSD symptoms than wait-list controls or TAU but were not superior to active non-trauma-focused group therapies. The trauma-focused group therapies had comparable benefits in improving PTSD and dissociation symptoms regardless of whether TMP was included. However, trauma-focused group therapy yielded the best outcomes for depression and psychological distress if TMP was *not* included. Thus, psychoeducation and skills for affect and interpersonal regulation may be of particular value in group therapy for adults with CPTSD.

The effectiveness of phased interventions offered in a group format for adults with CPTSD-like trauma histories and symptoms also was examined in meta-analysis (Mahoney et al., 2019). Phase 1 (delivered first) psychoeducational interventions were associated with reductions in symptoms of general distress (e.g., anxiety and depression), whereas Phase 2 (delivered second) memory processing group interventions were associated with reductions in PTSD symptoms. Thus, interventions representing both phases in the sequential treatment paradigm can be useful for the treatment of CPTSD. Research evaluating the relative efficacy of differently ordered treatment components and whether specific sequences may be of particular benefit to certain types of patients is important for optimizing outcomes.

Treatment Challenges

Development of a Treatment Plan

Treatment planning for CPTSD involves identification of the specific forms of dysregulation of emotion, relationships, and sense of self that are causing impairment and are of primary concern to the individual patient. Therefore, a collaborative attitude toward the patient as a partner in identifying the key treatment problems and selection of evidence-based intervention, as well as a measurement-based approach assessing change over time in the primary goals of the patient's therapy, is essential to guiding treatment. Regular assessment will help determine how well target problems in each domain of CPTSD are resolving and importantly whether new problems are emerging, in order to update the treatment plan as therapy proceeds. Given the complexity of CPTSD, and the variable presentation with different patients, the formulation and updating of a correspondingly complex and individualized treatment plan that accounts for all significant CPTSD symptoms and impairments is essential in order to fully address the needs in each unique case.

Length of Treatment

Length of treatment is likely to be highly variable depending on the severity, number, and diversity of clients' symptoms, the strengths and skills they bring to the therapy, the specific goals of treatment, and the emergence of crises that disrupt treatment. Many clients achieve substantial symptom reduction and other gains within a few months. However, more extended involvement of a year or beyond followed by periodic check-ins (particularly if stressors lead to symptom exacerbation or recurrence) is likely to be beneficial, enabling the client to make fundamental and enduring changes in core beliefs, relational choices and working models, coping and goal-attainment styles, and ER and crisis prevention/management skills.

Tempo of Treatment

Establishing a steady tempo of sustained therapeutic work is often difficult. Clients with CPTSD are likely to live with high levels of fear, anxiety, shame, and dysphoria that interfere with self-reflection and learning and with applying new skills and knowledge. It is important to choose a tempo that matches the client's capacity for learning and to engage in a deliberate pace that neither pushes for overly rapid results nor slows to a standstill due to fear, dysphoria, or other emotional or interpersonal problems. Helping the client to make steady progress even when crises or "stuck points" occur provides a corrective learning experience that represents an important contrast with previous life experiences (e.g., failure or relapse into old behaviors). Engaging in what may seem to be small talk or listening with interest while the client talks about current or past events provides essential basic human contact that often has been missing in his or her experiences and can open the door to spontaneous disclosures by the client, thus offering opportunities for empathic reflection and teaching by the therapist.

Maintaining Focus While Adjusting the Tasks of Treatment

It is important to maintain a coherent treatment focus based on the treatment plan, while also flexibly moving between the two primary tasks of CPTSD treatment: processing memories of past traumas and dealing with current stressors or life activities. Past-focused (processing of trauma) and present-focused (dealing with daily life stressors) interventions are complementary rather than competing tasks that together help clients become aware of and able to actively process (rather than avoid) trauma reminders and trauma-related emotions, thoughts, and behavior patterns. Both of these therapeutic tasks typically may need to be repeated over time, potentially causing the therapy to occasionally appear to be "going backward," to enable clients to consolidate and sustain their gains going forward in treatment and in life.

Severe Dissociation

Severe dissociation can lead to great discomfort for the therapist as well as the client. A proactive approach to working with dissociation is to help the client recognize triggers for dissociation and proactively use ER skills and a growing trust in relationships (initially the therapeutic relationship and gradually other relationships) to either interrupt or transition out of dissociative states. A key therapeutic task therefore is to assist the client in developing reflective self-awareness and confidence in recognizing and managing the distress that leads to dissociation. Interventions helpful in the management of dissociation include body self-awareness and grounding as well as enhancement of the client's understanding of why dissociation occurs and how to process rather than avoid distressing emotions, thoughts, and impulses. If a diagnosis of dissociative identity disorder (DID) is present, the therapist should focus on validating the client's experience of distinct self-states while maintaining the perspective that the client is a single self with multiple aspects. Consultation with or referral to a clinician with specialized training in treating DID and other severe and sustained forms of dissociation is recommended in such cases.

Concurrent Problems and Team Work

Clients with CPTSD may present with co-occurring health problems, including physical injuries from traumatic exposures (e.g., combat, sexual assault) and chronic health disorders (e.g., chronic pain, gynecological disturbances, heart or gastrointestinal disorders). These types of problems are best treated through collaboration with trauma-informed health care specialists in other disciplines, where an integrated treatment plan is developed and tracked over time, potentially including the use and management of medications for both mental and physical health problems. Individuals with CPTSD may have several providers for different diagnoses, and there is thus a risk of treatment becoming "siloed" and the client experiencing what seem to be contradictory or conflicting treatment plans. The presence of providers from primary care or other disciplines should be explicitly highlighted as part of all treatment plans, both in discussions with clients and in the final reports of treatment outcomes. In addition, there may be a potential role or need for the mental health clinician to provide respectful and sensitive education to other providers involved in the client's care, including primary health providers, concerning the client's possible cues and triggers, attitudes and concerns (e.g., distrust of authority figures), and symptoms (e.g., dissociation, reduced attentional capacities) that will facilitate collaborative and effective management of the client's multiple health problems.

Crises and Chaotic Lives

Individuals with CPTSD may experience a substantial number of crises and ongoing exposure to major life stressors, including traumatic events such as domestic violence, accidents, new illnesses and diagnoses, and family members in crisis, injured, or dying. Although crises cannot always be anticipated, the therapist can help the client to identify stressor events and resultant reactions that are likely and may be anticipated or coped with using skills learned in treatment and support from healthy relationships. Applying treatment concepts and skills to proactively anticipate and constructively debrief crisis or symptom escalation episodes can help clients increase their confidence and sense of competence or mastery. In addition, the clinician can help the client develop a network of services that are readily accessible.

Role of the Therapeutic Alliance

Clinician awareness of the beneficial role of the therapeutic alliance can facilitate progress and consolidate gains, while lack of attention to the therapeutic alliance can hinder or undermine progress. The therapeutic alliance is an important foundation for coregulation between therapist and client, and for helping the client to move from coregulation to self-regulation and mutuality rather than dependence or avoidance in relationships (Courtois & Ford, 2013). It also can enable clients to safely process reexperiencing or reenactments of the trauma-related dynamics of past victimization, betrayal, or other interpersonal traumas, providing the client with role modeling and guidance in the exploration of painful emotions and memories with confidence and self-compassion. Lastly, clients can learn from the therapist via role modeling of various skills, such as authentic self-regulation, acknowledgment of mistakes and misunderstandings, and maintaining professional limits within a therapeutically boundaried relationship.

Conclusion

The development and clinical and scientific evaluation of best practices and replicable therapeutic interventions for adults with CPTSD are nascent. However, innovative treatment models, and approaches to the sequencing and delivery of treatment, for this challenging clinical population are emerging and show promise in empirical studies. The codification of a CPTSD diagnosis in ICD-11 provides a much-needed foundation for systematic treatment development and randomized clinical trial studies that will guide therapists and patients as they collaboratively develop and implement treatment designed to promote recovery from the combination of PTSD and disturbances of self-organization that constitute CPTSD.

REFERENCES

American Psychological Association. (2017). *Clinical practice guidelines for the treatment of PTSD*. Washington, DC: Author.

Banks, K., Newman, E., & Saleem, J. (2015). An overview of the research on mindfulness-based interventions for treating symptoms of posttraumatic stress disorder: A systematic review. *Journal of Clinical Psychology, 71*(10), 935–963.

Bohus, M. (2018, November). Evaluation of DBT for complex PTSD—A multicomponent program to treat the sequelae of interpersonal violence during childhood and adolescence. In M. Cloitre (Chair), *Innovations in complex trauma treatment: Trauma-focused or not?* Symposium presented at the annual conference of the International Society for Traumatic Stress Studies, Washington, DC.

Cloitre, M., Koenen, K. C., Cohen, L. R., & Han, H. (2002). Skills training in affective and interpersonal regulation followed by exposure: A phase-based treatment for PTSD related to childhood abuse. *Journal of Consulting and Clinical Psychology, 70*(5), 1067–1074.

Cloitre, M., Shevlin, M., Brewin, C. R., Bisson, J. I., Roberts, N. P., Maercker, A., et al. (2018). The International Trauma Questionnaire (ITQ): Development of a self-report measure of ICD-11 PTSD and complex PTSD. *Acta Psychiatrica Scandinavica, 138*, 536–546.

Cloitre, M., Stovall-McClough, K. C., Nooner, K., Zorbas, P., Cherry, S., Jackson, C. L., et al. (2010). Treatment for PTSD related to childhood abuse: A randomized controlled trial. *American Journal of Psychiatry, 167*(8), 915–924.

Courtois, C. A., & Ford, J. D. (2013). *Treating complex trauma: A sequenced relationship-based approach.* New York: Guilford Press.

Coventry, P. (2018, November). INterventions for Complex Traumatic Events (INCiTE): A systematic review and research prioritisation exercise. In M. Cloitre (Chair), *Innovations in complex trauma treatment: Trauma-focused or not?* Symposium presented at the annual conference of the International Society for Traumatic Stress Studies, Washington, DC.

De Jongh, A., Resick, P. A., Zoellner, L. A., van Minnen, A., Lee, C. W., Monson, C. M., et al. (2016). Critical analysis of the current treatment guidelines for complex PTSD in adults. *Depression and Anxiety, 33*(5), 359–369.

Follette, V., Palm, K. M., & Pearson, A. N. (2006). Mindfulness and trauma: Implications for treatment. *Journal of Rational-Emotive and Cognitive-Behavior Therapy, 24*(1), 45–61.

Ford, J. D. (2020a). Group therapy. In J. D. Ford & C. A. Courtois (Eds.), *Treating complex traumatic stress disorders: An evidence-based guide* (2nd ed., pp. 415–439). New York: Guilford Press.

Ford, J. D. (2020b). Trauma affect regulation: Guide for education and therapy. In J. D. Ford & C. A. Courtois (Eds.), *Treating complex traumatic stress disorders: An evidence-based guide* (2nd ed., pp. 390–412). New York: Guilford Press.

Ford, J. D., Steinberg, K. L., & Zhang, W. (2011). A randomized clinical trial comparing affect regulation and social problem-solving psychotherapies for mothers with victimization-related PTSD. *Behavior Therapy, 42*(4), 560–578.

Gilbert, P., & Irons, C. (2004). A pilot exploration of the use of compassionate images in a group of self-critical people. *Memory, 12*, 507–516.

Harned, M. S., Korslund, K. E., & Linehan, M. M. (2014). A pilot randomized controlled trial of dialectical behavior therapy with and without the dialectical behavior therapy prolonged exposure protocol for suicidal and self-injuring women with borderline personality disorder and PTSD. *Behaviour Research and Therapy, 55*, 7–17.

Hyland, P., Karatzias, T., Shevlin, M., & Cloitre, M. (2019). Examining the discriminant validity of complex posttraumatic stress disorder and borderline personality disorder symptoms: Results from a United Kingdom population sample. *Journal of Traumatic Stress, 32*, 855–863.

ISTSS Guidelines Committee. (2018). ISTSS guidelines position paper on complex PTSD in adults. Retrieved April 14, 2019, from *www.istss.org/getattachment/ Treating-Trauma/New-ISTSS-Prevention-and-Treatment-Guidelines/ISTSS_CPTSD-Position-Paper-(Adults)_FNL.pdf.aspx.*

Jain, S., Ortigo, K., Gimeno, J., Baldour, D. A., Weiss, B. J., & Cloitre, M. (in press). A randomized controlled trial of brief Skills Training in Affective and Interpersonal Regulation (STAIR) for veterans in primary care. *Journal of Traumatic Stress.*

Karatzias, T., Ferguson, S., Gullone, A., & Cosgrove, K. (2016). Group psychotherapy for adult survivors of interpersonal psychological trauma: A preliminary study in Scotland. *Journal of Mental Health, 25*(6), 512–519.

Karatzias, T., Hyland, P., Bradley, A., Fyvie, C., Logan, K., Easton, P., et al. (2018). Is self-compassion a worthwhile therapeutic target for ICD-11 complex PTSD (CPTSD)? *Behavioural and Cognitive Psychotherapy, 47*(30), 1–13.

Karatzias, T., Murphy, P., Cloitre, M., Bisson, J., Roberts, N., Shevlin, M., et al. (2019). Psychological interventions for ICD-11 complex PTSD symptoms: Systematic review and meta-analysis. *Psychological Medicine, 49*(11), 1761–1775.

Knefel, M., Karatzias, T., Ben-Ezra, M., Cloitre, M., Lueger-Schuster, B., & Maercker, A. (2019). The replicability of ICD-11 complex post-traumatic stress disorder system networks in adults. *British Journal of Psychiatry, 214*(6), 361–368.

Krupnick, J. L., Green, B. L., Stockton, P., Miranda, J., Krause, E., & Mete, M. (2008). Group interpersonal psychotherapy for low-income women with posttraumatic stress disorder. *Psychotherapy Research, 18*(5), 497–507.

Mahoney, A., Karatzias, T., & Hutton, P. (2019). A systematic review and meta-analysis of group treatments for adults with symptoms associated with complex post-traumatic stress disorder. *Journal of Affective Disorders, 15*(243), 305–321.

Markowitz, J. C., Neria, Y., Lovell, K., Van Meter, P. E., & Petkova, E. (2017). History of sexual trauma moderates psychotherapy outcome for posttraumatic stress disorder. *Depression and Anxiety, 34*(8), 692–700.

Neff, K. D. (2011). Self-compassion, self-esteem, and well-being. *Social and Personality Psychology Compass, 5*(1), 1–12.

Roberts, N., Cloitre, M., Bisson, J. I., & Brewin, C. (2018). PTSD and complex PTSD diagnostic interview schedule for ICD-11. Unpublished interview.

Ruglass, L. M., Lopez-Castro, T., Papini, S., Killeen, T., Back, S. E., & Hien, D. A. (2017). Concurrent treatment with prolonged exposure for co-occurring full or subthreshold posttraumatic stress disorder and substance use disorders: A randomized clinical trial. *Psychotherapy and Psychosomatics, 86*(3), 150–161.

Steil, R., Dyer, A., Priebe, K., Kleindienst, N., & Bohus, M. (2011). Dialectical behaviour therapy for posttraumatic stress disorder related to childhood sexual abuse: A pilot study of an intensive residential treatment program. *Journal of Traumatic Stress, 24*(1), 102–106.

Weisz, J. R., Chorpita, B. F., Palinkas, L. A., Schoenwald, S. K., Miranda, J., Bearman, S. K., et al. (2012). Testing standard and modular designs for psychotherapy treating depression, anxiety, and conduct problems in youth: A randomized effectiveness trial. *Archives of General Psychiatry, 69*, 274–282.

World Health Organization. (2018). The ICD-11 for mortality and morbidity statistics. Retrieved from *https://icd.who.int/browse11/l-m/en.*

PART V

TREATMENTS FOR CHILDREN AND ADOLESCENTS

CHAPTER 21

Treatment of PTSD and Complex PTSD

Tine Jensen, Judith Cohen, Lisa Jaycox, and Rita Rosner

This chapter covers recommendations for the treatment of posttraumatic stress disorder (PTSD) in children and adolescents including pharmacological interventions. We review the summary of evidence and provide a theoretical basis for understanding change processes in child trauma treatment. A review of common elements across treatments and developmental considerations are highlighted, as well as treatments for different settings such as school and war-torn countries. Lastly, clinical guidelines for working with complex PTSD (CPTSD), newly identified as a disorder in the 11th revision of the *International Classification of Diseases* (ICD-11), are discussed along with recommendations for future research.

Summary of the Evidence

As reviewed in Forbes, Bisson, Monson, and Berliner (Chapter 1, this volume), the scoping questions for children were slightly modified from scoping questions for adults due to fewer studies and to acknowledge differences between children and adults affected by trauma. The scoping question was the following: For children and adolescents with clinically relevant posttraumatic stress symptoms, do psychological treatments when compared to treatment as usual, waiting list, no treatment, or other psychological treatments result in a clinically important reduction of symptoms, improved functioning/quality of life, presence of disorder, or adverse effects? For pharmacological interventions, the scoping question was this: For children and adolescents with clinically relevant posttraumatic stress symptoms, do pharmacological treatments when compared to placebo, other pharmacological, or psychosocial interventions result in a clinically important reduction of symptoms, improved functioning/quality of life, presence of disorder, or adverse effects?

The recommendations are thus based on studies that explicitly target PTSD and significant posttraumatic stress symptoms as the primary outcome(s). It is nonetheless recognized that other outcomes may be just as important for children and adolescents, such as depression, anxiety, disruptive and externalizing behaviors, substance abuse, and school functioning. Within this framework, a *Strong* recommendation has been given to cognitive-behavioral therapy with a trauma focus (CBT-T), provided either alone with the child or with the child and caregiver. There was *Insufficient Evidence to Recommend* CBT-T only with the caregiver. Eye movement desensitization and reprocessing (EMDR) therapy also received a *Strong* recommendation. The work group decided to include an *Intervention with Emerging Evidence* category to recognize novel treatment approaches. These recommendations were usually based on one or two randomized controlled trials (RCTs) with lower-quality ratings. Although such interventions are not recommended as frontline approaches for the treatment of PTSD, there may be other considerations that warrant their use. For example, although group CBT-T with children is classified as an *Intervention with Emerging Evidence*, it may be a very helpful treatment to make available to reach children who may not otherwise receive services, especially in low- and middle-income countries. It is also noteworthy that of all the treatment interventions reviewed for children and adolescents, none received an *Insufficient Evidence to Recommend* rating. This means that there are many different interventions that may prove helpful and many promising new ones.

This chapter focuses on recommended treatments and their common elements.

Cognitive-Behavioral Models of PTSD

Most of the recommended interventions in the guidelines issued by the International Society for Traumatic Stress Studies (ISTSS) are based on cognitive-behavioral theory (CBT), which has provided a primary theoretical foundation for understanding trauma impact and serves as the basis for trauma-focused interventions (TF-CBT; Brewin, Dalgleish, & Joseph, 1996; Ehlers & Clark, 2000). CBT is based on the idea that thoughts, feelings, and behaviors are interconnected and mutually influence each other, and that targeting thoughts, feelings, and/or behavior in therapy can bring about positive change. Although initially developed for adults, several scholars have argued that the same theoretical approach can be used to explain and understand the development of posttraumatic responses in children and youth (Ehlers, Mayou, & Bryant, 2003; Hayes et al., 2017; Meiser-Stedman, 2002; Meiser-Stedman, Dalgleish, Smith, Yule, & Glucksman, 2007; Salmond et al., 2011).

In particular, the cognitive theory proposed by Ehlers and Clark (2000) has been applied in the child trauma field (Meiser-Stedman, 2002; Smith, Perrin, Yule, & Clark, 2010). According to this model, two processes are central in the development and maintenance of PTSD: (1) disturbances in the memory processing of the traumatic event(s) and (2) negative appraisals and interpretations of the trauma and/or its sequelae that often become global and overgeneralized. According to this theory, PTSD becomes persistent if the traumatic memories are poorly elaborated and contextualized and are not well integrated with other autobiographical memories. Due to impaired processing and storing of the traumatic memories, the memories remain in a sensory format. Consequently, trauma reminders (e.g., trauma-related cues or stimuli reminding the child of the trauma) can easily trigger these memories. Trauma reminders may evoke intense psychological and physiological reactivity and arousal, leading to distress and unpleasant emotions (Cohen, Mannarino, Deblinger, & Berliner, 2009). Disturbance in the memory processing of the trauma can thus explain the intrusive and involuntary characteristics of trauma memories, resulting in increased activation, avoidance, intrusive symptoms, and reexperiencing (Brewin et al., 1996; Ehlers & Clark, 2000; Foa & Rothbaum, 2001).

The other central aspect of Ehlers and Clark's model is related to how negative appraisals of the trauma and/or thoughts and reactions in the aftermath of trauma affect an individual's beliefs about his or her self and the world. When experiencing one or more terrifying and overwhelming events, children search for an explanation or reason for why such an event happened to them. This is often an attempt to gain and restore some sense of control or predictability in life. However, if no rational explanation can be found, they may develop inaccurate and dysfunctional beliefs and cognitions to make the world predictable and understandable once again. Thus, traumatic experiences may profoundly change the way children see themselves and the world, and trauma-related cognitions often become global and overgeneralized. Such negative and maladaptive cognitions are commonly observed among traumatized children and youth (Meiser-Stedman et al., 2009; Nixon et al., 2010). Negative posttraumatic cognitions can threaten an individual's view of the self (e.g., "I must be a bad person since these things keep happening to me") and the world (e.g., "Something bad can happen at any time"; "No one can be trusted"), causing a subjective sense of persistent and current threat, and encourage the use of maladaptive coping strategies (Meiser-Stedman et al., 2009). Inaccurate and dysfunctional cognitions and beliefs about causation and responsibility might also result in feelings of shame and guilt, helplessness and hopelessness. A child who struggles with these emotions will likely have thoughts of being worthless and damaged, leading to depression and increasing the risk for withdrawal, isolation, and interpersonal and behavioral problems (Cohen, Mannarino, & Deblinger, 2017). Thus, posttraumatic cognitions can contribute to the development and maintenance of posttraumatic stress symptoms, but also lead to depression and anxiety (Beck, 2005).

Behavioral aspects of the development of PTSD focus on the way that avoidance of trauma memories and trauma reminders produces an immediate reduction in distress, and therefore is reinforced over time (via negative reinforcement). Such avoidance can reinforce the negative appraisals as well as create limitations in daily functioning.

Thus, global and overgeneralized trauma-related appraisals and behaviors may explain many of the characteristics of persistent PTSD, such as perception of current threat, avoidance, symptoms of arousal, negative emotions, and lack of trust in others. These experiences often lead to a range of coping strategies that may be maladaptive and contribute to the maintenance of PTSD (Bryant, Salmon, Sinclair, & Davidson, 2007; Ehlers et al., 2003; Meiser-Stedman et al., 2007; Mitchell, Brennan, Curran, Hanna, & Dyer, 2017; Stallard & Smith, 2007).

Possible Change Processes in Child Trauma Treatment

There is emerging evidence that cognitive processes are important in not only the development and maintenance of posttraumatic stress reactions in youth, but also for treatment outcomes. Several youth studies have now demonstrated that changing cognitions is an important mechanism for reducing posttraumatic stress symptoms in treatment (Jensen, Holt, Mørup Ormhaug, Fjermestad, & Wentzel-Larsen, 2018; Meiser-Stedman et al., 2017; Pfeiffer, Sachser, de Haan, Tutus, & Goldbeck, 2017; Smith et al., 2007). For instance, Meiser-Stedman and colleagues (2017) found in one RCT comparing CBT-T to wait list that changes in posttraumatic cognitions mediated the beneficial effects of CBT-T on posttraumatic stress symptoms among children and adolescents exposed to a single-event trauma. This is in line with two other treatment studies that found evidence for the same cognitive mediation effect on posttraumatic stress symptoms in TF-CBT for multitraumatized youth (Jensen et al., 2018; Pfeiffer et al., 2017). It is, however, still unclear whether reductions in posttraumatic stress early in treatment contribute to more adaptive and helpful cognitions, or if cognitive changes precede the reduction in posttraumatic stress. To date, only two published studies have examined the longitudinal directional relationship between changes in posttraumatic cognitions and posttraumatic stress symptoms in a clinical sample of traumatized youth, with both showing that changes in cognitions precede changes in posttraumatic stress (Knutsen, Czajkowski, & Ormhaug, 2018; McLean, Yeh, Rosenfield, & Foa, 2015). Taken together, these studies indicate that changing maladaptive cognitions in traumatized youth should be a primary target of treatment. What the mechanisms of change are is still unclear, and it may be that several components or techniques contribute to altering cognitions. For instance, providing psychoeducation and using Socratic methods can alter negative or unhelpful thoughts. Teaching coping skills when facing trauma reminders and trauma exposure work may reduce a sense of ongoing threat, and the belief that the world is a dangerous place. Having new positive personal experiences may alter feelings of mistrust in adults.

In a series of studies, Hayes and colleagues sought to understand more about the change processes in TF-CBT by examining the role of overgeneralizations, rumination, and avoidance in the processing of traumatic experiences in youth. They found that more overgeneralization during the narrative phase predicted less improvement in internalizing symptoms at posttreatment and a worsening of externalizing symptoms at follow-up (Ready et al., 2015). Overgeneralization was associated with more rumination, less decentering, and more negative emotion (Hayes et al., 2017). Interestingly, they did not find that changes in these cognitive processes were related to a decrease in posttraumatic stress symptoms for these youth. Thus, more studies are needed to fully understand such complicated change processes.

A central element in all treatment is engaging the youth in the therapy process. The therapeutic alliance predicts treatment outcomes in child and adolescent therapy (Murphy & Hutton, 2018), but is less explored in child trauma treatment studies. Some studies have, however, determined that a strong therapeutic alliance is related to trauma treatment outcomes (Ormhaug, Jensen, Wentzel-Larsen, & Shirk, 2014; Zorzella, Muller, & Cribbie, 2015). One study examining the therapeutic alliance in TF-CBT and therapy as usual (TAU) found that the alliance predicted outcome in TF-CBT but not TAU. Since treatment outcomes were significantly higher in TF-CBT, this indicates that both a good alliance and trauma focus are necessary for good outcomes (Ormhaug et al., 2014). Also, rapport-building behaviors in early sessions of TF-CBT are associated with a stronger alliance, and having a focus on trauma experiences does not appear to undermine alliance formation, but rather facilitates the alliance with youth who are passively disengaged (Ovenstad, Ormhaug, Shirk, & Jensen, 2020).

Developmental Considerations in Treatment

Developmental considerations should always play a role in the treatment of children and adolescents. However, what may be a common, appropriate, and "normal" behavior in early childhood might be regarded as abnormal in adolescence. Boundaries are usually not sharply defined for developmental stages and determining what is abnormal needs to factor in age, gender, developmental stage, and societal and cultural norms at a minimum. Younger children may show less specific symptoms. Development may come to a rest in specific areas so that children may be judged as younger or not adequately developed for their age.

Age-specific reactions to traumatic events are known, including separation anxiety, temper tantrums, and enuresis for toddlers and preschool children, while school-age children may display oppositional behavior or stress-reactive somatic complaints. Recent research shows that type and timing of traumatic events in childhood and adolescence may affect the severity of not only PTSD but also of other (comorbid) syndromes, such as major depression, substance abuse, and anxiety disorders (for a review, see Teicher & Samson, 2016). This points to possible underlying neurodevelopmental processes and epigenetic modifications. Psychosocial development and all its components such as emotion regulation, personality development, attachment, morality, and many more may be affected negatively by early trauma.

Diagnostic considerations are discussed in other chapters of this book (see Berliner, Meiser-Stedman, & Danese, Chapter 5, and Cloitre, Cohen, & Schnyder, Chapter 23). In addition to diagnostics, developmental considerations are vital in treatment planning. The most relevant aspects are (1) whether and how much parents and caregivers should be included, (2) dosage, and (3) the adaptation of interventions in a developmentally appropriate way.

For children under 3 years, interventions might be almost exclusively directed at caregivers (i.e., parent–child relationship enhancement); in preschool and school-age children, an equal distribution of time for parents and children is advisable, that is, TF-CBT (Cohen, Deblinger, & Mannarino, 2016) and preschool PTSD treatment (PPT; Scheeringa, 2015). Interventions for adolescents and young adults include parents and caregivers significantly less or not at all (Foa, McLean, Capaldi, & Rosenfield, 2013; Rosner et al., 2019). This reflects the adolescents' need to become more independent and autonomous, while at the same time parents and caretakers are still legally responsible.

In terms of dosage, younger children may need shorter sessions, whereas the session length for adolescents is often the same as for adults. Thus, the amount of time spent with the caregiver may be adapted to the child's developmental age. Also, interventions for preschoolers should include more childlike modes of interventions such as playing, storytelling, and drawing, whereas interventions for teenagers can be more language-driven. In addition, treatment for adolescents should consider specific developmental tasks in this age group, for example, autonomy, romantic relationships, or career choices.

Finally, and in terms of the evidence base, although most of the child- and adolescent-specific manuals are adapted to developmental age, empirical comparisons of developmentally adapted manuals with not adapted manuals do not exist, thus leaving these developmental considerations on the level of clinical recommendations.

Yet, there is some empirical support stemming from previous meta-analyses (Gutermann et al., 2016; Morina, Koerssen, & Pollet, 2016) that do report age effects. Depending on the analysis subset (e.g., when looking at RCTs only), Gutermann and colleagues (2016) determined that older children benefit more than younger children in terms of posttraumatic symptom severity reduction. Similarly, Morina and colleagues (2016) found a correlation between age and treatment efficacy (only for comparisons with wait lists). But the median age in both meta-analyses was around 12 years, and only a handful of studies on preschoolers as well as adolescents (above 14 years of age) were included. Thus, these age groups are underrepresented in the two meta-analyses and the age-related findings are only valid for a very restricted age range.

Common Elements across Recommended Treatments

The majority of trauma treatments with empirical support for improving posttraumatic stress and PTSD are CBT-based models. In part, this may be the case because CBT-based approaches generally use and are guided by standardized assessments, are easy to systematically describe in a treatment manual, and are easy to replicate across treatment settings with clearly established standards of fidelity. Thus, CBT-based models readily meet requirements for use in RCTs for many childhood disorders.

Treatments based on CBT typically include certain common elements: *psychoeducation*, various types of *coping skills*, *cognitive restructuring* for unhelpful thoughts, and *behavioral components* (e.g., exposure for anxiety; behavioral activation or problem solving for depression; contingency management for disruptive behavior). Different CBT models may sequence the delivery of the common elements in different ways and emphasize some elements more than others.

Some core underlying CBT principles as related to trauma-focused treatment include the following:

1. Thoughts, feelings, and behaviors are interconnected: untrue/unhelpful trauma-related beliefs (self-blame, dangerous world, untrustworthy others) lead to negative emotional states and/or unhelpful behaviors. The unhelpful behaviors may have a legitimate function (e.g., relief, reduction of distress, avoidance of perceived danger), but can interfere with recovery and functioning.

2. Trauma avoidance is a hallmark of posttraumatic stress and PTSD and interferes with recovery and functioning. Common CBT components address and reduce avoidance (e.g., psychoeducation, coping skills, exposure, and cognitive processing).

3. Behavior has a purpose and typically functions to get a desired result or avoid a negative outcome. Behavior is influenced by antecedents and consequences (A $\rightarrow$ B $\rightarrow$ C); positive or negative reinforcement will serve to perpetuate the behavior even when the behavior is unhelpful or

not functional. Behaviors such as avoidance, withdrawal, reactivity, or acting out may arise in children affected by trauma because they bring relief, reduce risk for rejection, or lead to needed attention even if negative. Antecedents to traumatized children's traumatic behavioral problems are often trauma reminders (e.g., a loud voice, perceived rejection, parental scolding for misbehavior). The consequences may inadvertently reinforce the unhelpful behaviors. For example, parents may allow children to not go to school or make exceptions about behavioral expectations as a form of being supportive for trauma impact. But this may lead to functional problems and parent–child conflict. Effective CBT strategies, especially positive parenting techniques, can modify these child traumatic behavioral problems.

The common elements found in most of the recommended models and their application to trauma impact are listed next.

Psychoeducation

The goal of psychoeducation is to empower children and their families to understand more about posttraumatic reactions (i.e., make sense of their symptoms), and to become a collaborative partner in treatment. Psychoeducation provides information about posttraumatic stress and PTSD and the prevalence of trauma, and stresses that recovery is possible. Through psychoeducation, youth learn to connect their symptoms to their trauma experiences rather than to think there is something inherently wrong with them (e.g. "I'm bad"; "I'm crazy"). All trauma-focused child trauma treatments include some form of psychoeducation to explain, validate, and normalize.

Coping Skills

Many models typically include teaching a variety of coping skills (relaxation, controlled breathing, emotion identification and monitoring, cognitive coping, distraction, mindfulness, and positive parenting) to address the youth's physical, emotional, cognitive, and behavioral dysregulation. Trauma-specific child models often encourage youth to not only use these skills for everyday stressors, but also to apply them in response to trauma-specific cues (trauma reminders), and in therapy to prepare for the exposure and restructuring activities that may evoke distress as well as *in vivo*. The goal of coping skills in trauma-specific therapy is to forestall avoidance and teach mastery. Children learn to regulate negative trauma-related emotions and behaviors by recognizing feelings and changing maladaptive beliefs. Different trauma models emphasize teaching coping skills to a greater or lesser degree. The evidence does not show that extensive coping skills practice is always necessary before directly addressing the trauma and, in some cases, it can prolong avoidance of the imaginal exposure and restructuring components. Teaching coping skills in itself without further trauma-related work does not seem to be efficient for reducing posttraumatic stress in adults, but the child literature has not yet examined this issue.

One big challenge for teaching coping skills is that they are typically taught in the low-stress, supportive environment of a clinic office. Many clients can demonstrate proficiency of a skill in that context, especially with modeling and role-play practice. However, the key is to focus on the successful use of coping skills in real-life stressful contexts whether they are trauma-related or not. The focus on between-session practice is often essential for the acquisition of coping skills that may be used effectively in real life.

Exposure and Cognitive Restructuring

The goals of exposure and cognitive restructuring for traumatized youth are to master trauma avoidance, fear, and other negative trauma-related symptoms by directly confronting feared trauma memories and nondangerous trauma reminders, and to identify and correct trauma-related maladaptive cognitions. Techniques include trauma narration in different forms. As with adult approaches, many models for children differentially emphasize imaginal/*in vivo* exposure and cognitive processing. For example, prolonged exposure (PE) adapted for adolescent sexual assault victims primarily uses exposure (Foa et al., 2013). In EMDR therapy, imaginal exposure is used by asking the youth to internally remember his or her worst traumatic experience without describing or recording it aloud. Other models incorporate both exposure and processing through creating a written narrative of the youth's trauma "story" (e.g., TF-CBT, Cognitive-Behavioral Intervention for Trauma in Schools [CBITS]) or use a life narrative or timeline utilizing stones to represent traumas and flowers to represent positive experiences (e.g., KidNET). In each of these models, therapists work with youth to identify and correct trauma-related maladaptive cognitions.

Parenting Support and Skills

Most child interventions incorporate parents in the treatment. There are several potential goals and benefits of incorporating an active parenting component into treatment for traumatized youth. Parental involvement can enhance their understanding of the youth's trauma experiences and increase emotional support for the youth. Engaging parents may facilitate treatment through reinforcement and support in practicing the skills in real life that are taught during therapy. Inclusion of effective parent management training may be especially important for youth exhibiting traumatic behavior problems, which can lead to negative parent–child interactions, reduced emotional support for the child, and functional impairment (e.g., school or community problems).

Not all of the recommended treatments fully integrate parents into treatment. Recommendations are listed in Table 21.1.

TABLE 21.1. Recommendations for Psychological Treatment

Strong Recommendation—CBT-T *(caregiver and child)*, CBT-T *(child)*, and EMDR *therapy* are recommended for the treatment of children and adolescents with clinically relevant posttraumatic stress symptoms.

Intervention with Emerging Evidence—Group *CBT-T (child)*, *group psychoeducation*, and *parent–child relationship enhancement* have emerging evidence of efficacy for the treatment of children and adolescents with clinically relevant posttraumatic stress symptoms.

Insufficient Evidence to Recommend—There is insufficient evidence to recommend *CBT-T (caregiver)*, *family therapy*, *group CBT-T (caregiver and child)*, *KidNET*, *nondirective counseling*, or *stepped-care CBT-T (caregiver and child)* for the treatment of children and adolescents with clinically relevant posttraumatic stress symptoms.

Strongly Recommended Treatments

Trauma-Focused Cognitive-Behavioral Therapy

TF-CBT (Cohen et al., 2017) has the most RCT studies for effectively treating child and adolescent posttraumatic stress and PTSD as well as related trauma symptoms. To date, 20 RCTs of TF-CBT have been published (reviewed in Cohen et al., 2017, pp. 74–80). These studies have focused on different index traumas—for example, sexual abuse, domestic violence, commercial sexual exploitation, war, disaster, and diverse traumas—although as is typical, most children in TF-CBT treatment studies have experienced multiple traumas (e.g., Cohen, Deblinger, Mannarino, & Steer, 2004; Cohen, Mannarino, & Iyengar, 2011; Goldbeck, Muche, Sachser, Tutus, & Rosner, 2016; Jensen et al., 2014; O'Callaghan, McMullen, Shannon, Rafferty, & Black, 2013). TF-CBT studies have been conducted for youth across development, in diverse settings and across different countries and cultures (e.g., in the United States, Europe, Australia, Africa), and have been provided in individual and group formats. These studies have consistently documented the efficacy of TF-CBT in improving children's posttraumatic stress and PTSD, with multiple studies also showing the superiority of TF-CBT to comparison or control conditions for improving children's anxiety, depression, externalizing behavior problems, and/or trauma-related maladaptive cognitions. Additionally, TF-CBT has been shown to be superior to comparison conditions for improving participating parents' support of the child, parental emotional distress, parental PTSD symptoms, and effective parenting practices.

TF-CBT is CBT-based; the core principles include (1) a structured, components- and phase-based approach with defined pacing of components; (2) collaborative empiricism and an assessment-driven approach in which the therapist, youth, and parent monitor the youth's trauma and other relevant symptoms throughout treatment and adjust the implementation of TF-CBT components accordingly; (3) gradual exposure incorporated into all components to enhance the youth's and parent's mastery of trauma reminders;

and (4) parent or caregiver inclusion throughout treatment to support the youth's practice and mastery of skills, enhance positive parenting and parental support, address trauma-related behavior problems, improve the parent's understanding of trauma impact, and minimize parental emotional distress related to the youth's trauma experiences (Cohen et al., 2017). TF-CBT consists of individual sessions provided in parallel to youth and parent, with half of each treatment session provided to the youth and parent, respectively, with several joint child–parent sessions also included in the model. Treatment duration is 12–16 sessions (this may be extended to 16–24 sessions for more complex trauma situations).

The core components of TF-CBT are summarized by the acronym PRACTICE and include the following: psychoeducation, parenting skills, relaxation skills, affective regulation skills, cognitive processing skills, trauma narration and processing, in vivo mastery (the only TF-CBT optional component, reserved for youth who have overgeneralized fear and avoidance of safe situations), conjoint child–parent sessions, and enhancing safety and future developmental trajectory. TF-CBT also includes traumatic grief components, described in detail at *www.musc.edu/ctg*.

Preschool PTSD Treatment

PPT (Scheeringa, 2015) is a CBT-based model that includes all of the PRACTICE components described above. It differs from TF-CBT for preschoolers in that (1) this model is more highly structured following a session-by-session format; (2) the parent views the child's sessions behind a one-way mirror to better understand and support the child's trauma responses; (3) treatment addresses one identified primary trauma experience, rather than the full range of experienced traumas; and (4) there is relatively more focus on fear desensitization than on cognitive processing. One RCT (Scheeringa, Weems, Cohen, Amaya-Jackson, & Guthrie, 2011) documented significant efficacy of the model in improving preschool children's PTSD symptoms relative to a comparison condition.

Cognitive Therapy for PTSD

Cognitive therapy for PTSD (CT-PTSD; Smith et al., 2010) shares many of the same features as TF-CBT and is based on Ehlers and Clark's (2000) cognitive model of PTSD and their treatment program for adults (Ehlers, Clark, Hackmann, McManus, & Fennell, 2005). Two studies have shown the model to have good effects on children who have experienced single-event traumas (Meiser-Stedman et al., 2017; Smith et al., 2007). CT-PTSD emphasizes an integration of cognitive restructuring with reliving. The protocol differs from TF-CBT in that it typically does not include relaxation training or other arousal reduction techniques for decreasing stress. The use of *in vivo* exposure is more common, and changing unhelpful cognitions is highly emphasized as the hallmark of this model. Sessions are typically conducted with the child alone. Parents are often included to review interventions from the child sessions and to plan homework tasks. The treatment targets are (1) elaborating and developing the trauma memory into a coherent account, (2) identifying problematic appraisals of the trauma and its consequences, (3) helping the child to not use unhelpful cognitive and behavioral strategies. The treatment components include the following:

1. *Psychoeducation.* The child and usually the parents are provided with information about PTSD and the cognitive model. The child's symptoms are reviewed, and the child is helped to identify unhelpful strategies he or she has been using.

2. *Reclaiming your life.* The child and parents are asked to identify activities that give the child a sense of fun, social connectedness, and meaning that he or she may have dropped after the trauma. The child is encouraged, with support from the parents, to identify and return to normal activities.

3. *Imaginal reliving.* The child is guided through an imaginal reliving to help access the moments in the trauma memory that are linked to the problematic meanings of the trauma without using any form of relaxation or anxiety management strategies. If the child becomes upset, the therapist provides empathy and encourages the child to talk about his or her feelings and normalizes these. The child is asked to talk about the trauma from its beginning until the point when the child felt safe again. The primary focus is to identify areas of confusion and/or emotional "hot spots." These are then specifically targeted.

4. *Cognitive restructuring.* The therapist helps the child identify idiosyncratic appraisals about the trauma and/or the child's reactions.

5. *Updating the trauma memory.* Hotspots in the narrative are often accompanied by appraisals about feared outcomes. The therapist discusses hotspots with the child and helps the child to identify alternative and more functional appraisals that are then incorporated into the reliving. The child is asked to include the new information in the trauma narrative by speaking it out loud during imaginal reliving of the hotspot or writing it into the relevant spot in the narrative script.

6. *Working with triggers (stimulus discrimination).* The therapist and child work together to identify stimuli that trigger unwanted intrusions. The child is then encouraged to confront these triggers and make a conscious effort to focus on everything about the present that is different from the memory while remaining aware of the present. This is done initially in-session and then practiced as homework.

7. *Site visit.* A visit to where the trauma happened is used to help the child understand that the trauma is over. The child is asked to remind

him- or herself of the trauma while at the site and then to notice everything that has changed since the trauma. The first time the site visit is carried out, the therapist is present and usually the parents are too.

8. *Parent work.* Parents of younger children are involved in treatment, dependent on the clinical need. Older adolescents may come to treatment without their parents. However, all parents are provided with psychoeducation and a description of the treatment. During therapy, the parents are frequently invited to discuss their child's progress, and parents can also request sessions alone to alleviate their own stress related to their child's trauma.

The treatment components are administered in a flexible and developmentally sensitive manner and do not follow a prescribed session-by-session approach but are administered throughout treatment as necessary to address the model-derived targets. (For further details, see Perrin et al., 2017; Smith et al., 2010.)

Prolonged Exposure for Adolescents

Prolonged exposure for adolescents (PE-A) is an adaption of PE (see Riggs, Tate, Chrestman, & Foa, Chapter 12, this volume). PE is based on the theory that successful emotional processing of traumatic memories is the mechanism of change and leads to a reduction in PTSD symptoms. Emotional processing is primarily achieved through repeated imaginal exposure both in the clinical office and between sessions. The adolescent adaptions specifically include increased family involvement in the treatment program by providing caregivers with psychoeducational information and tips to support their children. There is additional focus on the social and developmental considerations associated with adolescence. The model also has adjusted the therapeutic exercises to be more developmentally congruent.

The treatment model is phase-based and consists of the following components:

- *Phase 1: Pretreatment preparation.* A motivational interview is used to enhance attendance and engagement if needed and address concrete barriers to participation with case management.
- *Phase 2: Psychoeducation and treatment preparation.* Clients are provided with information about trauma, trauma impact, and the therapeutic rationale. Breathing retraining is introduced for coping with anxiety.
- *Phase 3: Exposures.* These modules are the majority of the treatment focus (5–8 sessions). They include *in vivo* exposure to trauma reminders, repeated imaginal exposure to the memory, and a worst moment's module. Imaginal exposure is tape-recorded and youth are instructed to listen to the tapes daily at home.
- *Phase 4: Relapse prevention.* In this phase the focus is on generalizing the skills learned and preventing relapse.

Two studies with adolescents who have experienced single-event traumas have shown PE-A to be more effective in reducing posttraumatic stress than time-limited dynamic therapy (mostly related to motor-vehicle accidents; Gilboa-Schechtman et al., 2010) and supportive counseling (related to rape; Foa et al., 2013).

EMDR Therapy

EMDR therapy is an eight-phase approach that has some similar components to CBT-T treatments but is unique in including rapid eye movement as an important aspect of the intervention. During processing, the child is asked to concentrate on the worst moment of the memory along with the concomitant negative belief and physical sensation, while visually following the therapist's moving fingers. This is repeated with different aspects of the memory until the child reports no further distress. Moving their eyes rapidly while focusing on the traumatic memory may be difficult for younger children, so tactile stimulation such as hand-tapping or drumming is recommended. The first two phases of EMDR therapy consist of assessing the child's trauma history, understanding the current trauma symptoms, and helping the child cope. For example, relaxation exercises include visualizing a "safe place" or other positive affect-generating image. Assessment includes visualizing aspects of the trauma, identifying negative body sensations and negative thoughts associated with the traumatic event, and identifying a desired positive thought. Processing addresses all these elements related to the trauma and current triggers. The treatment ends with addressing coping needs for the future. Developmental modifications are recommended for young children, such as the use of pictures and involving caregivers in treatment.

EMDR therapy is based on the adaptive information processing (AIP) model, which posits that memories of disturbing events may be physiologically stored in unprocessed form, leading to problems in day-to-day functioning. Information-processing systems facilitate the interpretation of current experiences by linking them with previously established memory networks of similar events. When confronted with a disturbing life experience, the processing system does not always function optimally. The result is a failure to process the event and it becomes "frozen in time," incorporating the negative affects, sensations, and beliefs experienced at the time of the event. The underlying basis for this dysfunction may be a failure of episodic memory to be integrated into the semantic memory system so that inadequately processed events are easily activated by both internal and external stimuli. In contrast to behavioral models, the AIP model does not view negative self-characterizations as causes of emotional dysfunction but rather as symptoms. In contrast to CBT where therapeutic change occurs via behavioral, narrative, and cognitive tasks, with EMDR therapy, change is conceptualized as a consequence of memory processing through the internal associations that are elicited during sets of bilateral stimulation (eye movements, taps, or tones). For a more detailed description, see the work of Shapiro and colleagues (Shapiro, Russell, Lee, & Schubert, Chapter 14, this volume; Shapiro, Wesselmann, & Mevissen, 2017).

Although there has been more research conducted on the effectiveness of EMDR therapy for adults (see Lee & Cuijpers, 2013, for an overview) than for children and adolescents, evidence now exists that EMDR therapy is also effective for youth (Rodenburg, Benjamin, de Roos, Meijer, & Stams, 2009). One study compared EMDR therapy and cognitive-behavioral writing therapy (CBWT) for youth seeking treatment tied to a single trauma. At posttreatment, 92.5% of those receiving EMDR therapy and 90.2% of those receiving CBWT no longer met the diagnostic criteria for PTSD, and all gains were maintained at follow-up (de Roos et al., 2017). In one study, 48 Dutch children who had experienced single- or multiple-event traumas were randomized to receive eight sessions of TF-CBT or EMDR therapy. Both treatments were equally effective in reducing posttraumatic stress symptoms. On comorbid problems, parents of children in the TF-CBT condition reported more positive treatment effects than parents of children in the EMDR therapy condition, possibly due to the inclusion of parents in TF-CBT (Diehle, Opmeer, Boer, Mannarino, & Lindauer, 2015).

Recommended Treatments in School and Group Settings

Applications of CBT-based trauma-focused treatment elements for schools and school-like group settings (summer camps, after-school programs) have been under development for the past few decades. Socioeconomically disadvantaged children have the greatest difficulty accessing mental health services (U.S. Public Health Service, 2000), and traumatized individuals are also less likely to seek health services than their nontraumatized counterparts (Guterman, Hahm, & Cameron, 2002). Thus, the most vulnerable youth are those least likely to ever receive traditional clinic-based mental health care. An example from trauma-focused treatment comes from a study conducted following a disaster (Jaycox et al., 2010). Children were randomized to receive the school-based group intervention (CBITS) or TF-CBT delivered at a community clinic. All children benefited from the interventions. However, far more children accessed the school-based treatment than the clinic-based treatment despite extensive efforts to support TF-CBT participation during the study. Schools can serve an important role in addressing unmet mental health needs following trauma, especially when the trade-off might be no treatment.

The school-/group-based interventions tend to take two forms: (1) interventions designed for "at-risk" students or (2) school-based treatment for children with trauma-related symptoms (traumatic stress).

Most school programs developed to date are intended for at-risk students and include a screening or identification process to determine which students might benefit from the intervention. School intervention programs for traumatic stress (including PTSD and related symptoms) are trauma-focused, developmentally oriented, and incorporate the core components common to many trauma-focused interventions as described earlier. Moreover, they are designed to fit into the school culture and meet logistical constraints. To date, there have been few rigorous evaluations of such programs. Of over 30 programs reviewed, only five have evidence of impact from randomized or quasi-experimental controlled trials. Five programs have been developed specifically for use in schools and focus on a broad array of traumas:

1. The *Cognitive-Behavioral Intervention for Trauma in Schools* (CBITS; Jaycox et al., 2010; Kataoka et al., 2003; Stein et al., 2003) was evaluated first in a quasi-experimental study with students who were recent immigrants to Los Angeles (Kataoka et al., 2003) and then in a randomized trial (Stein et al., 2003). Results demonstrated a significant decrease in PTSD and depressive symptoms in the group of students who received CBITS as compared to those on a waiting list, as well as improved grades among those who received CBITS earlier in the year compared to those who received it later in the year (Kataoka et al., 2011). A field trial in New Orleans following Hurricane Katrina showed comparable results in terms of reductions in PTSD and depression scores among those randomized to CBITS as well as those who received trauma-focused CBT (Jaycox et al., 2010). The addition of a family component showed that parent functioning can be improved alongside child improvements (Santiago, Lennon, Fuller, Brewer, & Kataoka, 2014).

2. An adaptation of CBITS for younger elementary students (grades K–5) called *Bounce Back* has demonstrated improved child outcomes (in terms of PTSD and anxiety symptoms) in an RCT as compared to a wait-list group (Langley, Gonzalez, Sugar, Solis, & Jaycox, 2015).

3. An adaptation of CBITS for delivery by nonclinical school personnel called *Support for Students Exposed to Trauma* has demonstrated improved outcomes (reductions in PTSD symptoms and depression), but no changes in parent- or teacher-reported behavior problems, in one randomized pilot study (Jaycox et al., 2009).

4. *Trauma-Focused Coping in Schools* (previously known as Multimodality Trauma Treatment) was evaluated with a staggered start date control design and showed decreases in PTSD, depressive, and anxiety symptoms among 14 treated students (March, Amaya-Jackson, Murray, & Schulte, 1998). These effects were replicated in subsequent studies (Amaya-Jackson et al., 2003).

5. The *UCLA Trauma and Grief Component Therapy for Adolescents Program* showed reductions in PTSD and grief symptoms and improvements in GPA among 26 participants in an open trial, but did not exhibit changes in depressive symptoms (Layne, Pynoos, & Cardenas, 2001; Saltzman, Pynoos,

Layne, Steinberg, & Aisenberg, 2001). A brief version of the program demonstrated reductions in PTSD symptoms in two field trials following an earthquake in Armenia (Goenjian, Karayan, & Pynoos, 1997; Goenjian et al., 2005). In addition, the program was implemented in postwar Bosnia (Layne, Pynoos, & Saltzman, 2001), showing greater reductions in PTSD, depression, and maladaptive grief within the full program as compared to an active comparison condition, with both groups improving significantly (Layne et al., 2008). All five draw on evidence-based practices for trauma, largely cognitive-behavioral techniques, and all have empirical support for the reduction of trauma-related symptoms.

There also have been some notable international efforts of school-based interventions in regions affected by disaster or ongoing terrorist threat. These are typically CBT-based trauma treatments containing the common CBT elements. An eight-session program for grades 2–6 called *Overshadowing the Threat of Terrorism* (OTT) has been used and evaluated in Israel (Berger, Pat-Horenczyk, & Gelkopf, 2007), showing reduced PTSD, somatic, and anxiety symptoms 2 months after the intervention among children who took part. A related program, more curricular in nature, is *Enhancing Resilience among Students Experiencing Stress* (ERASE-S), designed to mitigate the effects of ongoing terrorism. ERASE-S uses teachers to deliver the material and has demonstrated improved outcomes in terms of PTSD and anxiety, as well as reduced stereotypes and discriminatory behaviors (Berger, Gelkopf, & Heineberg, 2012; Berger, Gelkopf, Heineberg, & Zimbardo, 2016; Gelkopf & Berger, 2009). Another study of children exposed to continuing violence in Palestine examined teaching recovery techniques and found a positive impact on PTSD symptoms (Barron, Abdallah, & Smith, 2013).

On the other hand, some studies have not shown positive effects on posttraumatic stress symptoms but have other positive outcomes. A cluster-randomized school study of intervention for war-exposed migrants in Australia did not show improvement in PTSD symptoms, but on depressive symptoms (Ooi et al., 2016), and several studies of war-exposed children show mixed or null findings on PTSD symptoms (Tol et al., 2008, 2014).

In addition to interventions developed specifically for use in schools, it is also possible to bring clinical services onto school campuses or into school-like settings, and to adapt them somewhat to fit the institution's context and culture. Implementing these types of interventions comes with its challenges, including more intensive training and supervision for clinicians, fitting the sessions into the school day, and handling logistical issues such as space and privacy. Despite these challenges, such interventions can be good options for students with demonstrated clinical needs. Interventions currently and commonly implemented in schools and school-like settings include an adaptation of a TF-CBT (Cohen et al., 2004) described earlier. Another example of efforts to bring clinical treatments into schools or other nonclinic settings is *Community Outreach Program–Esperanza* (COPE;

de Arellano et al., 2005), which integrates the core components of a TF-CBT package with enhanced support for parents, active outreach and case management for children ages 4–18. *Life Skills, Life Stories* (Cloitre, Koenen, Cohen, & Han, 2002) is a clinical program for women that was adapted for female high school students with a history of sexual victimization and child abuse. A version for adolescents, called *STAIR-A*, was tested within schools in a quasi-experimental study and found to reduce depressive symptoms and improve some aspects of functioning (Gudiño, Leonard, & Cloitre, 2016).

In juvenile justice settings and schools, *Trauma Adaptive Recovery Group Education and Therapy for Adolescents* (TARGET-A; Ford, Mahoney, & Russo, 2001) focuses on body self-regulation, memory, interpersonal problem solving, and stress management for youths ages 10–18 affected by physical or sexual abuse, domestic or community violence, or traumatic loss.

Finally, there is work adapting interventions for residential treatment settings and schools. For instance, *Structured Psychotherapy for Adolescents Responding to Chronic Stress* (SPARCS; DeRosa & Pelcovitz, 2009) for teens exposed to chronic interpersonal traumas combines CBT and dialectical behavior therapy approaches (including mindfulness) to improve coping, affect regulation, relationships, and functioning in the present.

Complex PTSD

During the last two decades, there have been a number of attempts to define a broader category of trauma-related psychopathological sequelae, most of them referring to adults. Of the few definitions attempted for children and adolescents, some focused on specific traumatic events, for example, recurring sexual child abuse, and others comprised a broader range of symptoms beyond specific PTSD symptoms. Developmental trauma disorder was proposed for inclusion in DSM-5, but it was finally not included on the basis of insufficient empirical support (Schmid, Petermann, & Fegert, 2013). ICD-11 includes a new category of complex PTSD, which is meant to be applicable to children and adolescents as well. Beyond the three unique PTSD symptom clusters (reexperiencing, avoidance, startle/hypervigilance), at least one symptom is needed to be present in each of the three CPTSD-specific symptom clusters referred to as disturbances in self-organization: affect dysregulation, negative self-concept, and interpersonal problems (World Health Organization, 2018). Yet, given the developmental considerations discussed previously, some of the described symptoms are not to be regarded as psychopathological at a certain age. For example, temper tantrums (dysregulation) may be considered normal or pathological depending on the child's age. As we do not have strictly defined diagnostic boundaries (e.g., exactly when temper tantrums become psychopathological), some of the CPTSD criteria will remain difficult to disentangle from the developmental stage. Furthermore, the symptoms contained in the disturbances of self-organization are not necessarily specific to trauma impact but may be better and more parsi-moniously explained by other disorders or comorbidities, or be premorbid risk factors for more severe and pervasive trauma impact (see ISTSS, 2018).

At present, there are neither specific instruments available for assess-ing CPTSD, nor do we have treatment studies for children and adolescents based on the respective diagnostic criteria. Thus, currently most research focuses on *post hoc* analyses.

Publications concerning diagnosing CPTSD use items extracted from a number of instruments, interviews, and self-report measures, and are there-fore best regarded as approximations. First results support the notion that PTSD and CPTSD can be differentiated, based on data from an RCT com-paring TF-CBT with a wait-list control (Goldbeck et al., 2016) in children and adolescents with PTSD associated with mixed traumatic events. Latent class analysis resulted in two distinct classes, PTSD and CPTSD (Sachser, Keller, & Goldbeck, 2017). Considering the small data pool and that the measures were not specifically adapted to cover CPTSD, these are promising first results that CPTSD may be a relevant diagnostic category.

Yet, the final and more important test of this construct is whether we need specific interventions for CPTSD as compared to PTSD in children and adolescents. As young people with CPTSD were included in treatment studies on pediatric PTSD, secondary analysis should reveal if there is a differential outcome. Sachser and colleagues (2017) did not find a differential treatment response in the above-mentioned trial by Goldbeck and colleagues (2016). Overall, participants benefited from TF-CBT, with participants with CPTSD beginning and finishing treatment with a higher symptom load. This would be consistent with other childhood disorders where children with more severe clinical presentations tend to benefit by the standard evidence-based treatments but have higher symptoms at the end of treatment trials. From a clinician's view, the question arises whether CPTSD patients need a higher treatment dose or a different treatment model.

Treatment models applying a phase-based approach that begins with emotion regulation skills and then is followed by the trauma-focused CBT have thus far mostly been tested in adults. They assume that fostering emo-tion regulation techniques before starting a trauma-focused intervention is beneficial in the treatment of CPTSD. Yet, many phase-based interventions were developed before the CPTSD definition became available (for instance, TF-CBT) and therefore targeted other definitions of complex trauma-related disorders. One of these phase-based interventions is Skills Training in Affect and Interpersonal Regulation (STAIR; Cloitre, Cohen, & Koenen, 2006), which was developed for adults with PTSD related to sexual abuse in child-hood. STAIR was then adapted to adolescents (STAIR narrative therapy for adolescents [SNT-A]). SNT-A is a cognitive-behavioral intervention begin-ning with a skills training module (about 8–12 sessions), followed by four to eight sessions of a narrative therapy module (Gudiño, Leonard, Stiles, Havens, & Cloitre, 2017). Although some studies support STAIR, there is ongoing discussion on how to appraise these findings (De Jongh et al., 2016). Concerning the adaptation of STAIR to adolescents, only two studies have been published to date (Gudiño et al., 2014, 2016), one of them with a controlled design, where no significant improvement in PTSD symptoms was found (Guidiño et al., 2016).

Another stepped treatment approach is a developmentally adapted version of cognitive processing therapy (CPT), where CPT was not only adapted to the respective age group but preceded by a commitment phase to enhance treatment motivation and therapeutic alliance and by an emotion regulation training phase. The approach was tested in an uncontrolled pilot study (Matulis, Resick, Rosner, & Steil, 2014), showing large effect sizes, and in an RCT (Rosner et al., 2019). In the RCT, young people with PTSD related to sexual and/or physical abuse were compared with a usual care condition. The developmentally adapted CPT was highly effective in reducing posttraumatic symptom severity as well as comorbid symptoms compared to usual care. An analysis of treatment course revealed that changes in posttraumatic symptom severity occurred during the core CPT phase. Further studies are needed to clarify whether such preceding modules (e.g., emotion regulation or skills training) are necessary before starting trauma-focused interventions in young patients with CPTSD.

Summarizing the currently available empirical literature, no recommendation concerning the treatment of CPTSD can be given at the moment, other than that the first-line interventions for PTSD described in this chapter may be helpful.

Pharmacological Interventions for PTSD

The list of recommendations for pharmacological interventions in children and adolescents can be seen in Table 21.2. Several neurotransmitter systems are implicated in the development and maintenance of pediatric PTSD, and

---

TABLE 21.2. Recommendation for Psychopharmacological Treatment

Prevention/early intervention

Insufficient Evidence to Recommend—There is insufficient evidence to recommend *propranolol*, within the first 3 months of a traumatic event, as an early pharmacological intervention to prevent clinically relevant posttraumatic stress symptoms in children and adolescents.

Treatment

Insufficient Evidence to Recommend—There is insufficient evidence to recommend *sertraline* for the treatment of children and adolescents with clinically relevant posttraumatic stress symptoms.

---

pharmacological treatment for pediatric PTSD is widespread. However, there have been only a few RCTs examining the efficacy of pharmacological agents to treat pediatric PTSD, and to date none of these has documented the efficacy of medication for this population. Due to developmental differences, adult pharmacological studies cannot be extrapolated to children and adolescents. In PTSD, this has been shown with the SSRI antidepressant sertraline that, although efficacious for adult PTSD, was not superior to placebo in improving PTSD in children and adolescents in a multisite RCT (Robb, Cueva, Sporn, Yang, & Vanderburg, 2010). This finding was reinforced in a small RCT that examined TF-CBT + sertraline versus TF-CBT + placebo, which did not find significant differences between conditions in improving PTSD (Cohen, Mannarino, Perel, & Staron, 2007). Two additional RCTs in youth evaluated the beta-adrenergic blocking agent propranolol versus placebo and determined no significant differences (Nugent et al., 2010; Sharp, Thomas, Rosenberg, Rosenberg, & Meyer, 2010), although the former study found a significant interaction between gender and treatment group among medication-adherent youth, with males responding better to propranolol treatment. Another study similarly found no differences between the NMDA partial agonist D-cycloserine + CBT versus placebo + CBT (Scheeringa & Weems, 2014), although there was a trend toward the active medication group speeding recovery during the exposure sessions. More studies with larger pediatric samples are needed to clarify what medications may be helpful for which subsamples of youth with PTSD. At the current time, evidence-based trauma-focused psychotherapy is the first line of treatment for pediatric PTSD. Psychopharmacology should only be used to treat co-occurring conditions with evidence-based pharmacological treatments, or to target specific symptoms that are carefully and systematically tracked.

Future Developments

In summary, the ISTSS *Posttraumatic Stress Disorder Prevention and Treatment Guidelines'* scientific review of treatments of PTSD and clinically significant posttraumatic stress in children strongly recommend different models of CBT with a trauma focus and EMDR therapy. This means we can confidently recommend these treatments to children and families with an expectation of good results.

It seems likely that other versions of trauma-focused treatments that may not have quite the same level of empirical support but contain some or all of the common elements as the recommended CBT interventions could be potentially beneficial when the strongly recommended approaches are not available. The main differences among the recommended treatments are (1) the relative emphasis on exposure and cognitive processing and how they are implemented, (2) the timing and amount of focus on teaching coping skills of various kinds, (3) the degree to which (if at all) parents are included in treatment. Due to the similarities in outcomes across CBT models, it is unlikely that research resources will be allocated for large head-to-head comparisons of different models, although more head-to-head studies of trauma-focused CBT models and EMDR therapy may be warranted.

School and group interventions do not reach the same level of effect sizes as treatments delivered individually. They may, however, be beneficial in situations where many are affected or where services are limited. CBT for parents alone does not have a *Strong* recommendation, and studies show that improving parent stress does not improve child posttrauma symptoms (Holt, Jensen, & Wentzel-Larsen, 2014).

We need to know more about the relative importance, temporal ordering, and dosage of the different components for the different presentations of children affected by trauma. Some children will not need the full course of the recommended treatments, so stepped care may be the better option, and current studies are examining stepped-care models of TF-CBT to evaluate "who needs what" components (Salloum et al., 2016). Gender effects and the sequencing of interventions targeting comorbid syndromes such as substance abuse or prolonged grief need to be examined, too. We also need to better understand what the mechanisms of change may be in different interventions. Dismantling studies and therapy process analysis could help us understand what components are necessary and help target interventions for the individual child and family. In the future, it is possible that such efforts will enable clinicians to optimally tailor treatment to best fit the needs of individual traumatized children and families. Some children do not benefit sufficiently from the standard recommended approaches. It will be especially important to confirm if CPTSD exists as a separate clinical phenomenon versus representing a more severe version of PTSD, if entirely new treatments or treatment components are needed, or if increasing the dosage of certain components or extending standard treatments will be effective. And finally, we need more studies on the implementation of interventions. Having several effective treatments is not helpful if they cannot be delivered in real-world settings.

REFERENCES

Amaya-Jackson, L., Reynolds, V., Murray, M. C., McCarthy, G., Nelson, A., Cherney, M. S., et al. (2003). Cognitive-behavioral treatment for pediatric posttraumatic stress disorder: Protocol and application in school and community settings. *Cognitive and Behavioral Practice, 10*(3), 204–213.

Barron, I. G., Abdallah, G., & Smith, P. (2013). Randomized control trial of a CBT trauma recovery program in Palestinian schools. *Journal of Loss and Trauma, 18*(4), 306–321.

Beck, A. T. (2005). The current state of cognitive therapy: A 40-year retrospective. *Archives of General Psychiatry, 62*(9), 953–959.

Berger, R., Gelkopf, M., & Heineberg, Y. (2012). A teacher-delivered intervention for adolescents exposed to ongoing and intense traumatic war-related stress: A quasi-randomized controlled study. *Journal of Adolescent Health, 51*(5), 453–461.

Berger, R., Gelkopf, M., Heineberg, Y., & Zimbardo, P. (2016). A school-based intervention for reducing posttraumatic symptomatology and intolerance during political violence. *Journal of Educational Psychology, 108*(6), 761–771.

Berger, R., Pat-Horenczyk, R., & Gelkopf, M. (2007). School-based intervention for prevention and treatment of elementary-students' terror-related distress in Israel: A quasi-randomized controlled trial. *Journal of Traumatic Stress, 20*(4), 541–551.

Brewin, C. R., Dalgleish, T., & Joseph, S. (1996). A dual representation theory of posttraumatic stress disorder. *Psychological Review, 103*(4), 670–686.

Bryant, R. A., Salmon, K., Sinclair, E., & Davidson, P. (2007). A prospective study of appraisals in childhood postraumatic stress disorder. *Behaviour Research and Therapy, 45*(11), 2502–2507.

Cloitre, M., Cohen, L. R., & Koenen, K. C. (2006). *Treating survivors of childhood abuse: Psychotherapy for the interrupted life.* New York: Guilford Press.

Cloitre, M., Koenen, K., Cohen, L. R., & Han, H. (2002). Skills training in affective and interpersonal regulation followed by exposure: A phase-based treatment for PTSD related to childhood abuse. *Journal of Consulting and Clinical Psychology, 70,* 1067–1074.

Cohen, J. A., Deblinger, E., & Mannarino, A. P. (2016). Trauma-focused cognitive behavioral therapy for children and families. *Psychotherapy Research, 28*(1), 47–57.

Cohen, J. A., Deblinger, E., Mannarino, A. P., & Steer, R. A. (2004). A multisite, randomized controlled trial for children with sexual abuse-related PTSD symptoms. *Journal of the American Academy of Child and Adolescent Psychiatry, 43*(4), 393–402.

Cohen, J. A., Mannarino, A. P., & Deblinger, E. (2017). *Treating trauma and traumatic grief in children and adolescents.* New York: Guilford Press.

Cohen, J. A., Mannarino, A. P., Deblinger, E., & Berliner, L. (2009). Cognitive-behavioral therapy for children and adolescents. In E. B. Foa, T. M. Keane, M. J. Friedman, & J. A. Cohen (Eds.), *Effective treatments for PTSD: Practice guidelines from the International Society for Traumatic Stress Studies* (pp. 223–244). New York: Guilford Press.

Cohen, J. A., Mannarino, A. P., & Iyengar, S. (2011). Community treatment of posttraumatic stress disorder for children exposed to intimate partner violence: A randomized controlled trial. *Archives of Pediatrics Adolescent Medicine, 165*(1), 16–21.

Cohen, J. A., Mannarino, A. P., Perel, J. M., & Staron, V. (2007). A pilot randomized controlled trial of combined trauma-focused CBT and sertraline for childhood PTSD symptoms. *Journal of the American Academy of Child and Adolescent Psychiatry, 46*(7), 811–819.

de Arellano, M. A., Waldrop, A. E., Deblinger, E., Cohen, J. A., Danielson, C. K., & Mannarino, A. P. (2005). Community outreach program for child victims of traumatic events: A community-based project for underserved populations (Special issue). *Behavior Modification: Beyond Exposure for Posttraumatic Stress Disorder Symptoms: Broad Spectrum PTSD Treatment Strategies, 29*(1), 130–155.

De Jongh, A., Resick, P. A., Zoellner, L. A., Minnen, A., Lee, C. W., Monson, C. M., et al. (2016). Critical analysis of the current treatment guidelines for complex PTSD in adults. *Depression and Anxiety, 33*(5), 359–369.

de Roos, C., Oord, S., Zijlstra, B., Lucassen, S., Perrin, S., Emmelkamp, P., et al. (2017). Comparison of eye movement desensitization and reprocessing therapy, cognitive behavioral writing therapy, and wait-list in pediatric posttraumatic stress disorder following single-incident trauma: A multicenter randomized clinical trial. *Journal of Child Psychology and Psychiatry, and Allied Disciplines, 58*(11), 1219–1228.

DeRosa, R., & Pelcovitz, D. (2009). Group treatment methods for traumatized children: Igniting SPARCS of change. In J. Ford, R. Pat-Horenczyk, & D. Brom (Eds.), *Treating traumatized children: Risk, resilience, and recovery* (pp. 225–239). New York: Routledge.

Diehle, J., Opmeer, B. C., Boer, F., Mannarino, A. P., & Lindauer, R. J. L. (2015). Trauma-focused cognitive behavioral therapy or eye movement desensitization and reprocessing: What works in children with posttraumatic stress symptoms?: A randomized controlled trial. *European Child and Adolescent Psychiatry, 24*(2), 227–236.

Ehlers, A., & Clark, D. M. (2000). A cognitive model of posttraumatic stress disorder. *Behaviour Research and Therapy, 38*(4), 319–345.

Ehlers, A., Clark, D. M., Hackmann, A., McManus, F., & Fennell, M. (2005). Cognitive therapy for post-traumatic stress disorder: Development and evaluation. *Behaviour Research and Therapy, 43*(4), 413–431.

Ehlers, A., Mayou, R., & Bryant, B. (2003). Cognitive predictors of posttraumatic stress disorder in children: Results of a prospective longitudinal study. *Behaviour Research and Therapy, 41*(1), 1–10.

Foa, E. B., McLean, C. P., Capaldi, S., & Rosenfield, D. (2013). Prolonged exposure vs supportive counseling for sexual abuse–related PTSD in adolescent girls: A randomized clinical trial. *Journal of the American Medical Association, 310*(24), 2650–2657.

Foa, E. B., & Rothbaum, B. O. (2001). *Treating the trauma of rape: Cognitive-behavioral therapy for PTSD.* New York: Guilford Press.

Ford, J., Mahoney, K., & Russo, E. (2001). *TARGET and FREEDOM (for children).* Farmington: University of Connecticut Health Center.

Gelkopf, M., & Berger, R. (2009). A school-based, teacher-mediated prevention program (ERASE-Stress) for reducing terror-related traumatic reactions in Israeli youth: A quasi-randomized controlled trial. *Journal of Child Psychology and Psychiatry, and Allied Disciplines, 50*(8), 962–971.

Gilboa-Schechtman, E., Foa, E. B., Shafran, N., Aderka, I. M., Powers, M. B., Rachamim, L., et al. (2010). Prolonged exposure versus dynamic therapy for adolescent PTSD: A pilot randomized controlled trial. *Journal of the American Academy of Child and Adolescent Psychiatry, 49*(10), 1034–1042.

Goenjian, A. K., Karayan, I., & Pynoos, R. S. (1997). Outcome of psychotherapy among early adolescents after trauma. *American Journal of Psychiatry, 154,* 536–542.

Goenjian, A. K., Walling, D., Steinberg, A. M., Karayan, I., Najarian, L. M., & Pynoos, R. S. (2005). A prospective study of posttraumatic stress and depressive reactions among treated and untreated adolescents 5 years after a catastrophic disaster. *American Journal of Psychiatry, 162,* 2302–2308.

Goldbeck, L., Muche, R., Sachser, C., Tutus, D., & Rosner, R. (2016). Effectiveness of trauma-focused cognitive behavioral therapy for children and adolescents: A randomized controlled trial in eight German mental health clinics. *Psychotherapy and Psychosomatics, 85*(3), 159–170.

Gudiño, O., Leonard, S., & Cloitre, M. (2016). STAIR-A for girls: A pilot study of a skills-based group for traumatized youth in an urban school setting. *Journal of Child and Adolescent Trauma, 9*(1), 67–79.

Gudiño, O. G., Leonard, S., Stiles, A. A., Havens, J. F., & Cloitre, M. (2017). STAIR narrative therapy for adolescents. In M. A. Landolt, M. Cloitre, & U. Schnyder (Eds.), *Evidence-based treatments for trauma related disorders in children and adolescents* (pp. 251–271). New York: Springer.

Gudiño, O. G., Weis, J. R., Havens, J. F., Biggs, E. A., Diamond, U. N., Marr, M., et al. (2014). Group trauma-informed treatment for adolescent psychiatric inpatients: A preliminary uncontrolled trial. *Journal of Traumatic Stress, 27*(4), 496–500.

Guterman, N. B., Hahm, H. C., & Cameron, M. (2002). Adolescent victimization and subsequent use of mental health counseling services. *Journal of Adolescent Health, 30*(5), 336–345.

Gutermann, J., Schreiber, F., Matulis, S., Schwartzkopff, L., Deppe, J., Steil, R. J. C. C., et al. (2016). Psychological treatments for symptoms of posttraumatic stress disorder in children, adolescents, and young adults: A meta-analysis. *Clinical Child and Family Psychology Review, 19*(2), 77–93.

Hayes, A. M., Yasinski, C., Grasso, D., Ready, C. B., Alpert, E., McCauley, T., et al. (2017). Constructive and unproductive processing of traumatic experiences in trauma-focused cognitive-behavioral therapy for youth. *Behavior Therapy, 48*(2), 166–181.

Holt, T., Jensen, T. K., & Wentzel-Larsen, T. (2014). The change and the mediating role of parental emotional reactions and depression in the treatment of traumatized youth: Results from a randomized controlled study. *Child and Adolescent Psychiatry and Mental Health, 8,* 11.

International Society for Traumatic Stress Studies. (2018). New ISTSS prevention and treatment guidelines. Retrieved from *www.istss.org/treating-trauma/new-istss-prevention-and-treatment-guidelines.aspx*.

Jaycox, L. H., Cohen, J. A., Mannarino, A. P., Walker, D. W., Langley, A. K., Gegenheimer, K. L., et al. (2010). Children's mental health care following Hurricane Katrina: A field trial of trauma-focused psychotherapies. *Journal of Traumatic Stress, 23*(2), 223–231.

Jaycox, L. H., Langley, A. K., Stein, B. D., Wong, M., Sharma, P., Scott, M., et al. (2009). Support for students exposed to trauma: A pilot study. *School Mental Health, 1*(2), 49–60.

Jensen, T. K., Holt, T., Mørup Ormhaug, S., Fjermestad, K. W., & Wentzel-Larsen, T. (2018). Change in post-traumatic cognitions mediates treatment effects for traumatized youth—A randomized controlled trial. *Journal of Counseling Psychology, 65*(2), 166.

Jensen, T. K., Holt, T., Ormhaug, S. M., Egeland, K., Granly, L., Hoaas, L. C., et al. (2014). A randomized effectiveness study comparing trauma-focused cognitive behavioral therapy with therapy as usual for youth. *Journal of Clinical Child and Adolescent Psychology, 43*(3), 356–369.

Kataoka, S., Jaycox, L. H., Wong, M., Nadeem, E., Langley, A., Tang, L., et al. (2011).

Effects on school outcomes in low-income minority youth: Preliminary findings from a community-partnered study of a school-based trauma intervention. *Ethnicity and Disease, 21*(3), S1–S7.

Kataoka, S. H., Stein, B. D., Jaycox, L. H., Wong, M., Escudero, P. I. A., Tu, W., et al. (2003). A school-based mental health program for traumatized Latino immigrant children. *Journal of the American Academy of Child and Adolescent Psychiatry, 42*(3), 311–318.

Knutsen, M. L., Czajkowski, N. O., & Ormhaug, S. M. (2018). Changes in posttraumatic stress symptoms, cognitions, and depression during treatment of traumatized youth. *Behaviour Research and Therapy, 111,* 119–126.

Langley, A. K., Gonzalez, A., Sugar, C. A., Solis, D., & Jaycox, L. (2015). Bounce back: Effectiveness of an elementary school-based intervention for multicultural children exposed to traumatic events. *Journal of Consulting and Clinical Psychology, 83*(5), 853–865.

Layne, C. M., Pynoos, R. S., & Cardenas, J. (2001). Wounded adolescence: School-based group psychotherapy for adolescents who sustained or witnessed violent injury. In M. Shafii & S. Shafii (Eds.), *School violence: Contributing factors, management, and prevention* (pp. 163–180). Washington, DC: American Psychiatric Press.

Layne, C. M., Pynoos, R. S., & Saltzman, W. R. (2001). Trauma/grief focused group psychotherapy: School based post-war intervention with traumatized Bosnian adolescents *Group Dynamics, 5,* 277–290.

Layne, C. M., Saltzman, W. R., Poppleton, L., Burlingame, G. M., Pašalić, A., Duraković, E., et al. (2008). Effectiveness of a school-based group psychotherapy program for war-exposed adolescents: A randomized controlled trial. *Journal of the American Academy of Child and Adolescent Psychiatry, 47*(9), 1048–1062.

Lee, C. W., & Cuijpers, P. (2013). A meta-analysis of the contribution of eye movements in processing emotional memories. *Journal of Behavior Therapy and Experimental Psychiatry, 44*(2), 231–239.

March, J. S., Amaya-Jackson, L., Murray, M. C., & Schulte, A. (1998). Cognitive-behavioral psychotherapy for children and adolescents with posttraumatic stress disorder after a single-incident stressor. *Journal of American Academy of Child and Adolescent Psychiatry, 37*(6), 585–593.

Matulis, S., Resick, P. A., Rosner, R., & Steil, R. (2014). Developmentally adapted cognitive processing therapy for adolescents suffering from posttraumatic stress disorder after childhood sexual or physical abuse: A pilot study. *Clinical Child and Family Psychology Review, 17*(2), 173–190.

McLean, C. P., Yeh, R., Rosenfield, D., & Foa, E. B. (2015). Changes in negative cognitions mediate PTSD symptom reductions during client-centered therapy and prolonged exposure for adolescents. *Behaviour Research and Therapy, 68,* 64–69.

Meiser-Stedman, R. (2002). Towards a cognitive–behavioral model of PTSD in children and adolescents. *Clinical Child and Family Psychology Review, 5*(4), 217–232.

Meiser-Stedman, R., Dalgleish, T., Smith, P., Yule, W., & Glucksman, E. (2007). Diagnostic, demographic, memory quality, and cognitive variables associated with acute stress disorder in children and adolescents. *Journal of Abnormal Psychology, 116*(1), 65–79.

Meiser-Stedman, R., Smith, P., Bryant, R., Salmon, K., Yule, W., Dalgleish, T., et al. (2009). Devlopment and validation of the Child Post-Traumatic Cognitions Inventory (CPTCI). *Journal of Child Psychology and Psychiatry, 50*(4), 432–440.

Meiser-Stedman, R., Smith, P., McKinnon, A., Dixon, C., Trickey, D., Ehlers, A., et al. (2017). Cognitive therapy as an early treatment for post-traumatic stress disorder in children and adolescents: A randomized controlled trial addressing preliminary efficacy and mechanisms of action. *Journal of Child Psychology and Psychiatry, 58*(5), 623–633.

Mitchell, R., Brennan, K., Curran, D., Hanna, D., & Dyer, K. F. (2017). A meta-analysis of the association between appraisals of trauma and posttraumatic stress in children and adolescents. *Journal of Traumatic Stress, 30*, 88–93.

Morina, N., Koerssen, R., & Pollet, T. V. (2016). Interventions for children and adolescents with posttraumatic stress disorder: A meta-analysis of comparative outcome studies. *Clinical Psychology Review, 47*, 41–54.

Murphy, R., & Hutton, P. (2018). Practitioner review: Therapist variability, patient-reported therapeutic alliance, and clinical outcomes in adolescents undergoing mental health treatment—a systematic review and meta-analysis. *Journal of Child Psychology and Psychiatry, 59*(1), 5–19.

Nixon, R. D. V., Nehmy, T. J., Ellis, A. A., Ball, S.-A., Menne, A., & McKinnon, A. C. (2010). Predictors of posttraumatic stress in children following injury: The influence of appraisals, heart rate, and morphine use. *Behaviour Research and Therapy, 48*(8), 810–815.

Nugent, N. R., Christopher, N. C., Crow, J. P., Browne, L., Ostrowski, S., & Delahanty, D. L. (2010). The efficacy of early propranolol administration at reducing PTSD symptoms in pediatric injury patients: A pilot study. *Journal of Traumatic Stress, 23*(2), 282–287.

O'Callaghan, P., McMullen, J., Shannon, C., Rafferty, H., & Black, A. (2013). A randomized controlled trial of trauma-focused cognitive behavioral therapy for sexually exploited, war-affected Congolese girls. *Journal of the American Academy of Child and Adolescent Psychiatry, 52*(4), 359–369.

Ooi, C. S., Rooney, R. M., Roberts, C., Kane, R. T., Wright, B., & Chatzisarantis, N. (2016). The efficacy of a group cognitive behavioral therapy for war-affected young migrants living in Australia: A cluster randomized controlled trial. *Frontiers in Psychology, 7*, 1641.

Ormhaug, S. M., Jensen, T. K., Wentzel-Larsen, T., & Shirk, S. R. (2014). The therapeutic alliance in treatment of traumatized youths: Relation to outcome in a randomized clinical trial. *Journal of Consulting and Clinical Psychology, 82*(1), 52–64.

Ovenstad, K. S., Ormhaug, S. M., Shirk, S. R., & Jensen, T. K. (2020). Therapists' behaviors and youths' therapeutic alliance during trauma-focused cognitive behavioral therapy. *Journal of Consulting and Clinical Psychology*. [Epub ahead of print]

Perrin, S., Leigh, E., Smith, P., Yule, W., Ehlers, A., & Clark, D. M. (2017). Cognitive therapy for PTSD in children and adolescents. In M. A. Landolt, M. Cloitre, & U. Schnyder (Eds.), *Evidence-based treatments for trauma related disorders in children and adolescents* (pp. 187–207). New York: Springer.

Pfeiffer, E., Sachser, C., de Haan, A., Tutus, D., & Goldbeck, L. (2017). Dysfunctional posttraumatic cognitions as a mediator of symptom reduction in trauma-focused cognitive behavioral therapy with children and adolescents: Results of a randomized controlled trial. *Behaviour Research and Therapy, 97*, 178–182.

Ready, C. B., Hayes, A. M., Yasinski, C. W., Webb, C., Gallop, R., Deblinger, E., et al. (2015). Overgeneralized beliefs, accommodation, and treatment outcome in youth receiving trauma-focused cognitive behavioral therapy for childhood trauma. *Behavior Therapy, 46*(5), 671–688.

Robb, A. S., Cueva, J. E., Sporn, J., Yang, R., & Vanderburg, D. G. (2010). Sertraline treatment of children and adolescents with posttraumatic stress disorder: A double-blind, placebo-controlled trial. *Journal of Child and Adolescent Psychopharmacology, 20*(6), 463–471.

Rodenburg, R., Benjamin, A., de Roos, C., Meijer, A. M., & Stams, G. J. (2009). Efficacy of EMDR in children: A meta-analysis. *Clinical Psychology Review, 29*(7), 599–606.

Rosner, R., Rimane, E., Frick, U., Guterman, J., Hagl, M., Renneberg, B., et al. (2019). Developmentally adapted cognitive processing therapy for youth with PTSD symptoms after sexual and physical abuse: A randomized clinical trial. *JAMA Psychiatry, 76*(5), 484–491.

Sachser, C., Keller, F., & Goldbeck, L. (2017). Complex PTSD as proposed for ICD-11: Validation of a new disorder in children and adolescents and their response to trauma-focused cognitive behavioral therapy. *Journal of Child Psychology and Psychiatry, 58*(2), 160–168.

Salloum, A., Wang, W., Robst, J., Murphy, T. K., Scheeringa, M. S., Cohen, J. A., et al. (2016). Stepped care versus standard trauma-focused cognitive behavioral therapy for young children. *Journal of Child Psychology and Psychiatry, 57*(5), 614–622.

Salmond, C. H., Meiser-Stedman, R., Glucksman, E., Thompson, P., Dalgleish, T., & Smith, P. (2011). The nature of trauma memories in acute stress disorder in children and adolescents. *Journal of Child Psychology and Psychiatry, 52*(5), 560–570.

Saltzman, W. R., Pynoos, R. S., Layne, C. M., Steinberg, A. M., & Aisenberg, E. (2001). Trauma- and grief-focused intervention for adolescents exposed to community violence: Results of a school-based screening and group treatment protocol. *Group Dynamics: Theory, Research and Practice, 5,* 291–303.

Santiago, C. D., Lennon, J. M., Fuller, A. K., Brewer, S. K., & Kataoka, S. H. (2014). Examining the impact of a family treatment component for CBITS: When and for whom is it helpful? *Journal of Family Psychology, 28*(4), 560–570.

Scheeringa, M. S. (2015). *Treating PTSD in preschoolers: A clinical guide.* New York: Guilford Press.

Scheeringa, M. S., & Weems, C. F. (2014). Randomized placebo-controlled D-cycloserine with cognitive behavior therapy for pediatric posttraumatic stress. *Journal of Child and Adolescent Psychopharmacology, 24*(2), 69–77.

Scheeringa, M. S., Weems, C. F., Cohen, J. A., Amaya-Jackson, L., & Guthrie, D. (2011). Trauma-focused cognitive-behavioral therapy for posttraumatic stress disorder in three through six year-old children: A randomized clinical trial. *Journal of Child Psychology and Psychiatry, 52*(8), 853–860.

Schmid, M., Petermann, F., & Fegert, J. (2013). Developmental trauma disorder: Pros and cons of including formal criteria in the psychiatric diagnostic systems. *BMC Psychiatry, 13*(1), 1–12.

Shapiro, F., Wesselmann, D., & Mevissen, L. (2017). Eye movement desensitization and reprocessing therapy (EMDR). In M. A. Landolt, M. Cloitre, & U. Schnyder (Eds.), *Evidence-based treatments for trauma related disorders in children and adolescents* (pp. 273–297). New York: Springer.

Sharp, S., Thomas, C., Rosenberg, L., Rosenberg, M., & Meyer, W. (2010). Propranolol does not reduce risk for acute stress disorder in pediatric burn trauma. *Journal of Trauma: Injury, Infection, and Critical Care, 68*(1), 193–197.

Smith, P., Perrin, S., Yule, W., & Clark, D. M. (Eds.). (2010). *Post traumatic stress disorder: Cognitive therapy with children and young people*. London: Routledge.

Smith, P., Yule, W., Perrin, S., Tranah, T., Dalgleish, T., & Clark, D. (2007). Cognitive behavior therapy for PTSD in children and adolescents: A preliminary randomized controlled trial. *Journal of American Academy of Child and Adolescent Psychiatry, 46*(8), 1051–1061.

Stallard, P., & Smith, E. (2007). Appraisals and cognitive coping styles associated with cronic post-traumatic symptoms in child road traffic accident survivors. *Journal of Child Psychology and Psychiatry, 48*(2), 194–201.

Stein, B. D., Jaycox, L. H., Kataoka, S. H., Wong, M., Tu, W., Elliott, M. N., et al. (2003). A mental health intervention for schoolchildren exposed to violence: A randomized controlled trial. *Journal of the American Medical Assocation, 290*(5), 603–611.

Teicher, M. H., & Samson, J. A. (2016). Annual research review: Enduring neurobiological effects of childhood abuse and neglect. *Journal of Child Psychology and Psychiatry, and Allied Disciplines, 57*(3), 241–266.

Tol, W. A., Komproe, I. H., Jordans, M. J. D., Ndayisaba, A., Ntamutumba, P., Sipsma, H., et al. (2014). School-based mental health intervention for children in war-affected Burundi: A cluster randomized trial. *BMC Medicine, 12*(1).

Tol, W. A., Komproe, I. H., Susanty, D., Jordans, M. D., Macy, R. D., & De Jong, J. M. (2008). School-based mental health intervention for children affected by political violence in indonesia: A cluster randomized trial. *Journal of the American Medical Association, 300*(6), 655–662.

U.S. Public Health Service. (2000). Report of the Surgeon General's Conference on Children's Mental Health: A national action agenda. Retrieved from *www.surgeongeneral.gov/CMH/default.htm*.

World Health Organization. (2018). ICD-11 for mortality and morbidity statistics. Retrieved from *https://icd.who.int/browse11/l-m/en*.

Zorzella, K. P. M., Muller, R. T., & Cribbie, R. A. (2015). The relationships between therapeutic alliance and internalizing and externalizing symptoms in trauma-focused cognitive behavioral therapy. *Child Abuse and Neglect, 50*, 171–181.

PART VI

APPLICATION, IMPLEMENTATION, AND FUTURE DIRECTIONS

CHAPTER 22

Treatment Considerations
for PTSD Comorbidities

Neil P. Roberts, Sudie E. Back, Kim T. Mueser,
and Laura K. Murray

Comorbidity is the norm for posttraumatic stress disorder (PTSD). It is estimated that, in the general population, over 80% of individuals with PTSD will experience at least one additional lifetime mental health disorder, and around 50% will experience three or more comorbidities (Kessler, Sonnega, Bromet, Hughes, & Nelson, 1995). Among clinical populations, the rates of comorbidity can exceed 90% (Brown, Campbell, Lehman, Grisham, & Mancil, 2001; Richardson et al., 2017).

Conceptual, clinical, and causal relationships between PTSD and other conditions are complex and multifaceted (Lockwood & Forbes, 2014). A range of factors have been implicated as conferring vulnerability or playing a causal role in PTSD comorbidity, including gender, socioeconomic status, genetics, childhood trauma, and certain personality traits (e.g., Lockwood & Forbes, 2014; Müller et al., 2014). PTSD is often perceived as mediating the relationship between trauma experience and the onset of a comorbidity (van Minnen, Zoellner, Harned, & Mills, 2015), but evidence from a number of studies suggests that the relationship between PTSD and other disorders is often bidirectional and includes a range of shared common features and underlying vulnerabilities (Lockwood & Forbes, 2014). Mental and physical health comorbidities have been shown to have a major impact on PTSD symptom trajectories and are associated with poor health-related quality of life (Li, Zweig, Brackbill, Farfel, & Cone, 2018). Network approaches suggest that there may be "many roads to comorbidity," such that for a given person, the causal chain of symptom interactions is likely to be highly individualized and shaped by specific personal factors and events (Borsboom, Cramer, Schmittmann, Epskamp, & Waldrop, 2011).

There is increasingly robust evidence for a range of psychological and pharmacological interventions for PTSD. These psychological treatments, designed for one specific/primary disorder, PTSD, are often referred to as "disorder-specific treatments." Historically, disorder-specific treatments have been evaluated in more tightly controlled efficacy trials and have significantly advanced the field by generating a body of research leading to the availability of evidence-based treatments (EBTs). However, many trials exclude individuals with more clinically challenging comorbidities, such as substance use disorders, psychosis, personality disorders, persistent self-harming, and suicidality, because these individuals tend to have more severe clinical profiles (Roberts, Roberts, Jones, & Bisson, 2015; van Minnen et al., 2015). Individuals with multiple comorbidities tend to have poorer functioning and well-being, and inferior treatment outcomes (Müller et al., 2014; Roberts et al., 2015; Schäfer & Najavits, 2007). Clinicians are often reluctant to use some EBTs because they fear that PTSD or comorbid symptoms will become exacerbated (van Minnen, Harned, Zoellner, & Mills, 2012; van Minnen et al., 2015). Comorbidity therefore can provide a particular challenge for clinicians in terms of prioritizing treatment goals, how to manage risk, and how to deliver an optimal intervention.

There has been growing research on a single comorbid condition with PTSD, or PTSD plus one other disorder (recognizing that individuals with the comorbidity for inclusion may have other comorbidities as well). Some emerging options for treatment of PTSD plus comorbid conditions include (1) utilizing a PTSD-focused EBT and examining the effects of the comorbid *conditions* (e.g., how much a PTSD treatment affects depression), (2) using EBTs for the two conditions sequentially, (3) integration of two EBTs to address both conditions simultaneously (e.g., PTSD and panic), and (4) transdiagnostic models that address multiple problem areas (e.g., Mansell, Harvey, Watkins, & Shafran, 2009; Marchette & Weisz, 2017).

Specific scoping questions related to comorbidity issues were not included in the current revised *Posttraumatic Stress Disorder Prevention and Treatment Guidelines* released by the International Society for Traumatic Stress Studies (ISTSS) (see Bisson, Lewis, & Roberts, Chapter 6 and Bisson et al., Chapter 7, this volume), so the guidelines may have limitations when it comes to generalizing recommendations for some comorbid disorders (Lugtenberg, Burgers, Clancy, Westert, & Schneider, 2011). In this chapter, we consider some of the challenges and debates related to PTSD comorbidities, the relationship between PTSD and other disorders, comorbid treatment approaches and their evidence, and recommendations for future research. We focus on six types of PTSD and a comorbidity among adult populations: depression, panic, substance use disorders, psychosis, borderline personality disorder, and chronic pain, as these are among the most common and challenging comorbidities faced by clinicians treating individuals with PTSD. We briefly review child comorbidity, focusing on internalizing and externalizing symptoms overlapping with PTSD, rather than paired comorbidities.

For each comorbidity, we review EBTs that are commonly used, which have historically been disorder-specific treatments, and, where available, review the use of sequential or integrated approaches. Finally, we briefly review emerging research on transdiagnostic interventions for PTSD and its comorbidities.

Adult Comorbidity

Depression

Depression is the most common PTSD comorbidity, with around 50% of PTSD sufferers meeting the diagnosis for major depressive disorder (MDD; Rytwinski, Scur, Feeny, & Youngstrom, 2013). PTSD sufferers also demonstrate elevated suicide risk (e.g., Panagioti, Gooding, & Tarrier, 2012). Individuals with depression are not usually excluded from PTSD trials, except when there is a significant suicide risk, but the comorbidity is associated with increased symptom severity and poorer functioning as compared to either disorder alone (van Minnen et al., 2012). Clinicians are sometimes concerned that it will be more difficult to engage patients with co-occurring depression in trauma processing work and to address rigid negative beliefs reflecting feelings of hopelessness and guilt (van Minnen et al., 2012).

A range of explanations has been proposed to explain the association between PTSD and depression. Prominent among these is that the relationship is a result of symptom overlap, particularly through symptoms of dysphoria (e.g., poor sleep, concentration difficulties, anger, loss of interest, negative appraisals about the self and world; see Flory & Yehuda, 2015; Lockwood & Forbes, 2014). PTSD and depression also share common components, such as negative cognitions, negative affect, restricted affect, and avoidant behaviors (Horesh et al., 2017). Other explanations include PTSD as the antecedent disorder (e.g., Ginzburg, Ein-Dor, & Solomon, 2010); a depressogenic model, where depression leads to subsequent PTSD (e.g., King, King, McArdle, Shalev, & Doron-LaMarca, 2009); and the argument that each disorder is an independent consequence of trauma (Horesh et al., 2017; Lockwood & Forbes, 2014). It has also been proposed that PTSD and depression may be subclusters of a larger syndrome (Flory & Yehuda, 2015). Evidence from prospective studies suggests that there is a complex temporal relationship between the two disorders involving bidirectional causality and a range of common risk factors (e.g., Ginzburg et al., 2010; Horesh et al., 2017; Stander, Thomsen, & Highfill-McRoy, 2014).

There is little literature on specific models of treatment for this comorbidity (Stander et al., 2014). Antidepressants can play a role in improving symptoms of PTSD alongside depression, but their effects tend to be small (see Bisson, Hoskins, & Stein, Chapter 16, this volume). The available evidence also suggests that individuals with PTSD make only limited gains from psychological interventions primarily aimed at treating depression (see

Bisson et al., Chapter 7, this volume). However, depressive symptoms typically show medium to large pre- to posttreatment effect size improvements alongside symptoms of PTSD with evidence-based PTSD interventions, such as prolonged exposure (PE; see Riggs, Tate, Chrestman, & Foa, Chapter 12, this volume), cognitive processing therapy (CPT; see Chard, Kaysen, Galovski, Nixon, & Monson, Chapter 13, this volume), and eye movement desensitization and reprocessing (EMDR) therapy (see Shapiro, Russell, Lee, & Schubert, Chapter 14, this volume), in comparison to control conditions (Bisson, Roberts, Andrew, Cooper, & Lewis, 2013; van Minnen et al., 2015). There is some indication that improvement in depressive symptoms tends to follow PTSD symptom improvement (van Minnen et al., 2015). However, there is also some evidence from two studies in veteran populations investigating heterogeneity of treatment responses through latent class analysis showing that higher depression scores predict poorer treatment outcomes (Murphy & Smith, 2018; Phelps et al., 2018). This work points to the importance of careful assessment of depressive symptoms and of the development of individualized treatment planning, which may sometimes indicate the need for treatment of more severe depressive symptoms with medication or an EBT for depression prior to engagement in EBT for PTSD when depressive symptoms are severe and likely to inhibit engagement in PTSD treatment. At such times, clinicians may want to give particular consideration to treatment approaches that target both PTSD and depression symptoms, such as CPT and cognitive therapy, particularly when problems like chronic guilt are indicated (Phelps et al., 2018).

Panic Disorder

Data from the National Comorbidity Survey (Kessler et al., 1995) estimate a lifetime prevalence of comorbid panic disorder and PTSD of around 11%, with a higher prevalence for women than men. Other studies have found far higher rates of panic symptoms in PTSD and traumatized populations, with rates as high as 35% (e.g., Cougle, Feldner, Keough, Hawkins, & Fitch, 2010; Hinton, Pollack, Pich, Fama, & Barlow, 2005). Rates of comorbid PTSD of around 30% have also been reported in panic disorder–diagnosed populations (e.g., Craske et al., 2006). Individuals with PTSD–panic disorder comorbidity have been shown to be increasingly vulnerable to other comorbidities, such as substance abuse, suicidal behavior, chronic pain, and medically unexplained symptoms, as well as interpersonal and occupational impairments (see Cougle et al., 2010; Teng et al., 2013). The comorbidity is also a unique predictor of more severe psychiatric disability compared to those without panic attacks (Cougle et al., 2010).

PTSD and panic disorder share several overlapping features in hypervigilance, autonomic reactivity, heightened perception of danger, and avoidance of internal and external reminders (Teng et al., 2013). Panic attacks in PTSD sufferers are often triggered by trauma-related reminders (Teng et al., 2013), and there is some indication that panic and agoraphobia tend to develop following the onset of PTSD, rather than vice versa (Brown et al., 2001). Surprisingly, there is a paucity of research aimed at understanding the relationship between PTSD and panic disrder (Cougle et al., 2010; Liness, 2009; Teng et al., 2013). One explanation for this relationship that has some empirical support is "anxiety sensitivity" (Vujanovic, Zvolensky, & Bernstein, 2008). Anxiety sensitivity is conceptualized as a fear of anxiety and anxiety-related physiological arousal, alongside fearful cognitions related to somatic, psychological, and social concerns (Vujanovic et al., 2008). It is argued that individuals who are prone to anxiety sensitivity have a predisposition to become "emotionally alarmed" when they experience anxiety, leading to an escalation in their symptoms (Vujanovic et al., 2008). Anxiety sensitivity is therefore thought to be a contributory factor in the development and maintenance of both disorders (Teng et al., 2013). From a classical conditioning perspective, it has been argued that, in addition to external cues, internal cues such as thoughts, feelings, and physiological responses experienced at the time of a trauma may trigger activation of the trauma memory network, resulting in panic responses (Falsetti, Resnick, Dansky, Lydiard, & Kilpatrick, 1995; Hinton, Hofmann, Pitman, Pollock, & Barlow, 2008). When an individual is unable to attribute a panic attack to a triggering event, he or she may therefore believe that it has "come out of the blue." As a result of chronic hyperarousal from PTSD, small increases in arousal may be sufficient to trigger a panic response (Falsetti et al., 1995). The association between conditioned cues and responses is thought to be further reinforced by avoidance behaviors that inhibit the opportunity for new learning.

Individuals with PTSD–panic disorder are sometimes reluctant to engage in trauma processing because of fears that their panic will escalate and become uncontrollable (Liness, 2009). These fears can result in avoidance of treatment sessions and dropout. Empirical evidence about the potential benefits of adapting existing PTSD therapies or developing alternative treatment models remains limited (Teng et al., 2013). Anxiety symptoms tend to improve in line with other symptoms in most clinical trials of psychological interventions for PTSD (see Bisson et al., 2013; van Minnen et al., 2015). However, few trials have reported on panic disorder as a diagnostic outcome (Teng et al., 2013). In the small number of trials where panic disorder diagnostic status has been examined, a significant minority of participants did not experience improvement in panic symptoms (Teng et al., 2013). Treatments for the two disorders share some common features (e.g., psychoeducation, cognitive restructuring, exposure to feared situations; Teng et al., 2013), and in some models, such as cognitive therapy, it may be possible to incorporate intervention for panic into a PTSD-related treatment formulation (Liness, 2009). Drawing on common treatment processes, Falsetti and colleagues (e.g., Falsetti, Resnick, & Davis, 2008) developed multiple channel exposure therapy (M-CET) to specifically treat PTSD–panic disorder. M-CET is a combined treatment, adapted from CPT and CBT for panic, that addresses both disorders concurrently over 12 sessions (Falsetti et al., 2008). Early sessions help patients reduce their fear of the physical features of panic through interoceptive exposure to physiological reactions to panic symptoms (i.e., inducing panic symptoms to facilitate habituation to feared internal physical symptoms), which, it is argued, leads to a subsequent decrease in physiological arousal associated with these symptoms as well as trauma-related fear. This then allows therapy to address distorted PTSD- and panic-related appraisals simultaneously in subsequent sessions (Falsetti et al., 2008). A culturally adapted version of M-CET has also been developed for use with Southeast Asian refugees (Hinton, Pollack, et al., 2005). Preliminary findings from several small randomized controlled trials (RCTs; e.g., Falsetti et al., 2008; Hinton, Chhean, et al., 2005) are encouraging, although it is not clear if this combined treatment improves panic and PTSD outcomes beyond those of established PTSD therapies.

Substance Use Disorders

One of the most common co-occurring mental health disorders among individuals with PTSD is substance use disorders (SUDs). A strong association between PTSD and SUD is evidenced by data from large-scale epidemiological studies as well as clinical studies on treatment-seeking populations (e.g., Blanco et al., 2013; Gielen, Krumeich, Havermans, Smeets, & Jansen, 2014). Data from the National Epidemiological Survey on Alcohol and Related Conditions (N = 36,309) indicate that the lifetime prevalence of alcohol and drug use disorders is 29% and 10%, respectively, in the United States (Grant et al., 2016). Rates of SUD are significantly higher among individuals with PTSD (Mills, Teesson, Ross, & Peters, 2006; Pietrzak, Goldstein, Southwick, & Grant, 2012). In comparison to the general population, military veterans are at increased risk for developing both PTSD and SUD (e.g., Petrakis, Rosenheck, & Desai, 2011; Sabella, 2012). In a recent study of 26,754 newly enlisted U.S. soldiers (N = 30,583), rates of PTSD were found to increase in a dose-response fashion as severity of substance use increased. Among soldiers who binge-drink, rates of PTSD were approximately 15%, whereas among soldiers with probable alcohol use disorder, rates of PTSD increased to approximately 23% (Stein et al., 2017). Taken together, these data indicate a high prevalence of co-occurring PTSD and SUD across various populations.

Various hypotheses and theories have been proposed to help explain the common co-occurrence of PTSD and SUD. While no single theoretical model has received unequivocal empirical support, the self-medication hypothesis is among the most prominent. This hypothesis is that individuals with PTSD use alcohol and drugs in an attempt to alleviate distressing PTSD symptoms, such as trouble sleeping and intrusive memories (e.g., Back, 2010; Back, Foa, et al., 2014; Khantzian, 1997). Support for the self-medication theory comes from daily diary studies that show individuals consume more alcohol on days that they experience more PTSD symptoms (e.g., Dvorak, Pearson, & Day, 2014; Kaysen, Stappenbeck, Rhew, & Simpson, 2014). In addition, research on the temporal order of onset demonstrates that the onset of PTSD typically precedes the development of SUD (e.g., Back, Jackson, Sonne, & Brady, 2005; Mills et al., 2006). On average, adults with PTSD-SUD report exposure to their first traumatic event around age 8–10 (Mills et al., 2012; Persson et al., 2017). Furthermore, compelling data in support of the self-medication hypothesis are provided by studies showing that improvements in PTSD severity have a greater impact on improvements in SUD than vice versa (Back, Brady, Sonne, & Verduin, 2006; Hien et al., 2010).

Several other theories have been put forward to help shed light on the complex relationship between PTSD and SUD. One theory posits that individuals with SUD are at increased risk for experiencing potentially traumatic events, which may lead to PTSD, such as car accidents or sexual assault (Schäfer & Najavits, 2007; Testa & Livingston, 2009). This increased risk could be due to cognitive impairment as a result of chronic substance use and factors associated with a high-risk lifestyle. In addition, a growing body of literature identifies shared neurobiological factors associated with both conditions (Brady & Sinha, 2005; Gilpin & Weiner, 2017). For example, both PTSD and SUD are associated with dysregulation in corticolimbic structures, in particular, the amygdala (associated with emotional valance and fear extinction) and the prefrontal cortex (associated with executive functioning, decision making, and response inhibition). Dysregulation in these areas may reduce the ability to use "top-down control" to regulate intrusive memories, cravings, and thoughts about using substances. Alternations in the hypothalamic–pituitary–adrenal (HPA) axis and noradrenergic systems have also been identified as key components in the development and maintenance of PTSD and SUD (Brady & Sinha, 2005). While the contribution of neurobiological and genetic factors to the etiology of PTSD-SUD is not completely understood, there is evidence of shared underlying processes that may increase the risk of developing both conditions and serve as important prevention and treatment targets.

PTSD-SUD presents numerous clinical challenges, even to the most seasoned mental health professional. Patients with PTSD-SUD present with a more severe clinical profile, including a greater number of mental health comorbidities, more functional impairment (e.g., physical, cognitive), increased violence, higher rates of homelessness, and poorer treatment outcomes (Barrett, Teesson, & Mills, 2014; Blanco et al., 2013; Bowe & Rosenheck, 2015; Mills et al., 2006; Norman, Haller, Hamblen, Southwick, & Pietrzak, 2018; Roberts et al., 2015). In addition, patients with PTSD-SUD have high rates of suicidal ideation and attempts (Back et al., 2019; Norman et al., 2018; Mills et al., 2012). Given the severity of mental, physical, and functional impairment that is often characteristic of patients with PTSD-SUD, it is not surprising that clinicians perceive the dual diagnosis to be substantially more difficult to treat than either disorder alone (Back, Waldrop, & Brady, 2009; Gielen et al., 2014; Schäfer & Najavits, 2007). Common difficulties reported by clinicians in treating patients with PTSD-SUD include self-destructive behaviors and heavy case management needs (e.g., housing).

Clinicians also report the challenge of uncertainty regarding how to implement treatment. Questions on whether to refer PTSD-SUD patients to addiction treatment first and knowing when to initiate EBTs for PTSD are common (Adams et al., 2016; Back et al., 2009). This relates to a larger debate concerning which approaches, sequential or integrated focal treatments, are optimal. Historically, patients with PTSD-SUD have been referred to SUD-only treatment first and, following successful completion of SUD-only treatment, are then referred for PTSD treatment (van Dam, Vedel, Ehring, & Emmelkamp, 2012). Indeed, only a minority of treatment facilities have been found to provide integrated PTSD and SUD care (Substance Abuse and Mental Health Services Administration [SAMHSA], 2016). In a study investigating the reasons why clinicians do not implement integrated treatments, Gielen and colleagues (2014) found that many SUD clinicians underestimated the prevalence of comorbid PTSD-SUD, and expressed practical barriers such as lack of time, limited facility funds, and lack of expertise. In addition, clinicians expressed the belief that integrated treatment of PTSD and SUD would "cause more misery," increase craving, and impede addiction treatment. However, the majority of patients with PTSD-SUD perceive their symptoms to be related and prefer integrated treatment in which both their PTSD and SUD are addressed concurrently (Back, Killeen, et al., 2014). Importantly, empirical data from the past two decades support the safety and efficacy of integrated treatments in significantly reducing PTSD, SUD severity, and associated areas of impairment, such as depression (Back et al., 2019; Norman et al., 2019; Roberts et al., 2015; Simpson, Lehavot, & Petrakis, 2017; van Dam et al., 2012).

Retention is another salient challenge in treating PTSD-SUD. In a meta-analysis of 42 studies examining treatments for PTSD, Imel, Laska, Jakupcak, and Simpson (2013) found that the average dropout rate was 18%. Dropout rates for PTSD treatment may be higher among military veterans (Myers, Haller, Angkaw, Harik, & Norman, 2019). Data from the Substance Abuse and Mental Health Services Administration indicate that, across various types of addiction services (e.g., outpatient, residential, detoxification), approximately 45–65% complete treatment (SAMHSA, 2015; Stahler, Mennis, & DuCette, 2016). And, in a recent review of PTSD-SUD patients receiving three types of treatments (exposure based, coping based, and addiction focused), approximately 50% of patients overall completed treatment (Simpson et al., 2017). Interestingly, studies examining treatment dropout reveal that a substantial proportion (36–68%) of patients who drop out before completing treatment evidence clinically significant improvement or meet good end-state functioning with regard to PTSD and/or SUD symptoms prior to dropping out (Szafranski et al., 2017, 2018), suggesting that dropout is not always due to a worsening or lack of symptom improvement. Nonetheless, attrition is a common problem in treating PTSD-SUD, and more effective methods for retaining patients are needed.

To date, patients presenting with co-occurring PTSD-SUD have often received *sequential treatment* in which patients first complete SUD-only treatment and are then referred to PTSD-only treatment, generally provided by a different clinician. There is significant potential within the sequential treatment model, however, for patients to "fall through the cracks" and not complete either the SUD or PTSD treatment sequence. Proponents of the integrated treatment model assert that PTSD symptoms may, at least in part, contribute to alcohol and drug use problems, and that untreated PTSD symptoms increase the risk of relapse. In so far as co-occurring SUD represents a form of self-medication of PTSD symptoms, addressing the PTSD early in treatment may help optimize long-term outcomes (Hien et al., 2010; McCauley, Killeen, Gros, Brady, & Back, 2012). Furthermore, as noted, a substantial proportion of patients with PTSD and SUD prefer an integrated treatment.

Integrated treatment efforts are often categorized into one of two groups using various terminology: (1) exposure-based, trauma-focused, or past-focused treatments; and (2) coping-based, non-trauma-focused, or present-focused treatments. Treatments from the first category incorporate PE (Back, Foa, et al., 2014; Foa, Gillihan, & Bryant, 2013; Mills et al., 2012; Norman et al., 2019; Persson et al., 2017; Ruglass et al., 2017) or components of PE, such as imaginal, *in vivo*, or written exposure exercises (e.g., van Dam, Ehring, Vedel, & Emmelkamp, 2013). Other integrated interventions include psychoeducation and components of CPT to address both PTSD and SUD (McGovern, Lambert-Harris, Alterman, Xie, & Meier, 2011; Vujanovic, Smith, Green, Lane, & Schmitz, 2018). In contrast, treatments from the second category do not discuss or talk about the traumatic event, but rather focus on present-day coping skills, such as self-care, increasing compassion and honesty, and detaching from emotional pain (e.g., Boden, Bonn-Miller, Kashdan, Alvarez, & Gross, 2012; Frisman, Ford, Hsiu-Ju, Mallon, & Chang, 2008; Hien et al., 2009; Myers, Browne, & Norman, 2015). The most commonly researched coping-based treatment is Seeking Safety, a 25-session manualized intervention (Najavits, 2002).

In the most recent and comprehensive review of psychological interventions for PTSD-SUD, Simpson and colleagues (2017) examined 24 randomized clinical trials (N = 2,294). Among exposure-based treatments, the findings revealed significantly better PTSD outcomes with exposure-based treatment as compared to the control group in six out of seven studies. SUD outcomes were comparable, though not significantly better, in most studies of exposure-based integrated treatments. Among coping-based studies, no between-group differences in PTSD outcomes between the coping-based treatment and the control condition were revealed. Similar findings were reported in an earlier review of 14 studies (N = 1,506 participants), which found more favorable PTSD treatment outcomes and comparable SUD outcomes for individual-based, trauma-focused interventions delivered concurrently alongside a SUD intervention (Roberts et al., 2015). The findings from these reviews and other investigations (Back et al., 2019; Norman et al., 2019) provide evidence that exposure-based integrated treatments are effective for PTSD-SUD, and that the addition of trauma-focused interventions does not increase substance use or risk for relapse. Hence, patients presenting with co-occurring PTSD-SUD should be offered integrated treatment or EBT for PTSD without waiting for abstinence. Of note, one study found that only about half of PTSD-SUD patients endorse a goal of abstinence (Lozano et al., 2015), and outcomes from the integrated studies mentioned here indicate that, even for patients who do not achieve abstinence, a significant reduction in PTSD symptoms can be attained.

Although important advances have been made in the development of integrated treatments for comorbid PTSD-SUD, much work remains to optimize interventions and to identify the underlying mechanisms of action. Exploration of novel pharmacological interventions that may help further reduce SUD symptomatology, such as cravings and substance use, would be beneficial. More work on the shared neurobiology associated with PTSD and SUD is needed to help elucidate the biological underpinnings of this comorbidity and identify novel treatment targets. Finally, research on the development of novel ways to enhance retention is needed for patients with PTSD-SUD.

Severe Mental Illness

The term "psychotic disorders" is used most often to refer to schizophrenia-spectrum disorders (schizophrenia; schizoaffective disorder; schizophreniform disorder, hereafter referred to as schizophrenia) and other relatively uncommon disorders such as brief psychotic disorder or psychotic disorder not otherwise specified (American Psychiatric Association, 2013). However, this term is somewhat of a misnomer because it implies that psychotic symptoms (e.g., hallucinations, delusions, bizarre behavior) are the most important clinical feature distinguishing these disorders from others. In fact, grandiosity is included as a criterion for the diagnosis of a manic episode in bipolar disorder, and loss of insight is a common problem. Additionally, other psychotic symptoms (e.g., hallucinations, delusions) are often present during manic and depressive episodes of bipolar disorder or major depression, including depression with comorbid PTSD (Gottlieb, Mueser, Rosenberg, Xie, & Wolfe, 2011). Furthermore, episodes of depression or mania can occur in schizophrenia. What distinguishes the two groups of disorders is that there must be some evidence for the presence of psychotic symptoms when mood is normal for a diagnosis of schizophrenia, whereas psychotic symptoms must remit for a diagnosis of major mood disorder.

This section focuses primarily on PTSD comorbidity with schizophrenia and bipolar disorder. However, some attention will be given to the more broadly defined group of people with severe mental illness (SMI), typically defined as those having a major mental health disorder (schizophrenia, bipolar disorder, major depression) that has a profound and persistent impact on psychosocial functioning in areas such as ability to fulfill role functions (e.g., work, school, parenting), participation in social relationships, and independent living and self-care. The relevance of the broader SMI category to the topic of PTSD comorbidity is that, despite high rates of comorbidity, individuals with SMI have historically been excluded from PTSD treatment trials based on narrow study exclusion criteria (e.g., psychotic symptoms, cognitive impairments, suicidal ideation), and because most trials have not been conducted at community mental health centers where persons with SMI receive their treatment.

There is ample evidence that schizophrenia and bipolar disorder are both associated with increased rates of comorbid PTSD. Three meta-analyses indicate rates of PTSD in schizophrenia of 12.4–29% (Achim et al., 2011; Buckley, Miller, Lehrer, & Castle, 2009; Zammit et al., 2018), and one meta-analysis of bipolar disorder reported a 16% rate of comorbidity with PTSD (Otto et al., 2004). Even higher rates of PTSD comorbidity have been reported in inpatient and outpatient samples of persons with SMI, with most reports ranging between 25 and 50% (Grubaugh, Zinzow, Paul, Egede, & Frueh, 2011; Mueser et al., 1998), but with low levels of comorbidity documented in patients' charts. Thus, PTSD is a common but frequently undetected comorbid disorder in people with these disorders (Zammit et al., 2018).

A variety of reasons may account for the high comorbidity of PTSD with schizophrenia and bipolar disorder. First, in addition to increasing the risk of developing PTSD, exposure to traumatic events in childhood increases vulnerability to the development of psychotic symptoms and illness (Varese et al., 2012) and the broad range of mental health disorders in adulthood (Carr, Martins, Stingel, Lemgruber, & Juruena, 2013), including schizophrenia (Husted, Ahmed, Chow, Brzustowicz, & Bassett, 2012; Matheson, Shepherd, Pinchbeck, Laurens, & Carr, 2013) and bipolar disorder (Etain, Henry, Bellivier, Mathieu, & Leboyer, 2008). Thus, trauma may serve as a "third variable" increasing vulnerability to both PTSD and psychotic disorders. Second, the diagnosis of PTSD is predictive of subsequent hospitalization and treatment for schizophrenia and bipolar disorder (Okkels, Trabjerg, Arendt, & Pedersen, 2017), suggesting that the stress associated with PTSD may trigger the onset of psychotic symptoms for some. Third, individuals with schizophrenia are more likely to be traumatized and interpersonally victimized in the community after developing their mental illness (Desmarais et al., 2014; Maniglio, 2009), thereby increasing their risk of developing PTSD. Fourth, there is evidence for shared genetic vulnerability to the development of PTSD and schizophrenia and bipolar disorder (Duncan et al., 2018). Fifth, psychotic symptoms may occur secondary to PTSD (Seow et al., 2016; Shevlin, Armour, Murphy, Houston, & Adamson, 2011), leading to the possible misdiagnosis of PTSD as a psychotic disorder.

The treatment of PTSD in people with schizophrenia and bipolar disorder has lagged far behind treatment advances for the primary PTSD population, for two primary reasons. First, some clinicians believed that reports of patients with psychotic symptoms about their traumatic experiences and PTSD symptoms were unreliable, and likely to reflect distorted or delusional thinking. Contrary to this concern, research has shown that the assessment of trauma history and PTSD symptoms with standardized measures yields reliable and valid diagnoses of PTSD in patients with SMI (Meyer, Muenzenmaier, Cancienne, & Struening, 1996; Mueser et al., 2001). Second, some clinicians were concerned that the assessment of trauma history and PTSD could be upsetting to people with psychotic symptoms, and that the stress of trauma-based treatment of PTSD could precipitate relapse of symptoms. Early efforts to assess trauma and PTSD in persons with schizophrenia and bipolar disorder found no basis for these concerns, nor did early work on treatment.

Interest in treating PTSD in persons with schizophrenia and bipolar disorder emerged out of a growing awareness of the high prevalence of undiagnosed PTSD in this population (Cusack, Grubaugh, Knapp, & Frueh, 2006), coupled with research suggesting that PTSD contributes to a worse course of the illness (Mueser, Rosenberg, Goodman, & Trumbetta, 2002). The importance of this work was amplified in a review of 34 published RCTs of PTSD treatment for adults that found severe comorbid psychopathology was the single most common reason for excluding patients from studies, and called for research on treatments for PTSD that were flexible and could be adapted to characteristics of those patients most likely to have the disorder (Spinazzola, Blaustein, & van der Kolk, 2005). In the intervening years, growing evidence has supported the feasibility and beneficial effects of treating PTSD in people with schizophrenia and bipolar disorder.

Several research groups have evaluated the delivery of established treatment methods for PTSD in the general population to individuals with schizophrenia and/or bipolar disorder. Mueser, Rosenberg, and Rosenberg (2009) developed a 12- to 16-session individual program for vulnerable populations with PTSD, based primarily on cognitive restructuring, but also including psychoeducation about PTSD and breathing retraining. After demonstrating the safety, feasibility, and clinical promise of the intervention in an uncontrolled trial (Rosenberg, Mueser, Jankowski, Salyers, & Acker, 2004), the program was evaluated in two RCTs of persons with SMI and PTSD. The first trial compared the cognitive restructuring program with usual services in 108 patients with SMI (39% schizophrenia or bipolar), and found significantly greater improvements in PTSD and depression at the end of treatment, with gains maintained at 3- and 6-month follow-ups (Mueser et al., 2008). The second RCT compared the full cognitive restructuring program with just the psychoeducation and breathing retraining components delivered over three sessions in 201 patients with SMI (68% schizophrenia or bipolar) and PTSD (Mueser et al., 2015). Patients in the cognitive restructuring program improved more than those in the brief program in PTSD symptoms and psychosocial functioning (both groups improved similarly in depression), with gains maintained at 6- and 12-month follow-ups. In neither study was there a significant treatment group by diagnosis interaction, indicating that people with schizophrenia and bipolar disorder benefited as much from the cognitive restructuring program as those with major depression. A third small RCT compared the cognitive restructuring program with usual treatment in 61 patients with schizophrenia and PTSD. Both groups of patients showed significant improvements in PTSD symptoms, but there were no differences between the groups (Steel et al., 2017). An important difference between this third study and the previous two studies was that the patients had less severe PTSD symptoms, suggesting that the benefits of the cognitive restructuring program may be strongest for persons with schizophrenia or bipolar disorder with more severe PTSD.

Some research also supports the feasibility and beneficial effects of evidence-based exposure therapy and EMDR therapy in patients with schizophrenia. Frueh, Grubaugh, and colleagues developed a treatment model for patients with schizophrenia-PTSD that combines social skills training and exposure therapy (Frueh et al., 2009), and it has been shown to be feasible and associated with improvements in PTSD and related outcomes in two uncontrolled clinical trials (Frueh et al., 2009; Grubaugh et al., 2016). Van den Berg and colleagues (2015) conducted an RCT comparing a nine-session exposure therapy program with a nine-session EMDR therapy program, with usual services in 151 patients with schizophrenia-PTSD, and found greater reductions in PTSD symptoms within both active treatment groups, which were maintained at 6-month follow-up. Furthermore, patients who received either of the trauma-focused interventions were significantly less likely to experience symptom exacerbations, adverse events, or revictimization (van den Berg et al., 2016), suggesting that delaying trauma-focused treatment could actually expose patients to worse clinical and psychosocial outcomes. Together, these studies provide preliminary evidence that PTSD can be treated in people with comorbid schizophrenia or bipolar disorder, and that trauma-focused interventions with this population are both safe and effective.

Borderline Personality Disorder

Borderline personality disorder (BPD) has been conceptualized by some to have its origins in early life traumatic experiences and to overlap with PTSD (Gunderson & Sabo, 1993; McLean & Gallop, 2003). Several studies have found that BPD is particularly associated with childhood abuse and neglect (see Cattane, Rossi, Lanfredi, & Cattaneo, 2017), although childhood trauma is not universally reported and biological vulnerabilities and neurobiologi-cal processes have also been found to be important to the development of BPD. Research indicates high rates of PTSD comorbidity in patients with BPD, ranging from 25 to 56% (see Golier et al., 2003; Mueser et al., 1998; Pagura et al., 2010). However, despite the high comorbidity of these two disorders, only limited research has examined the treatment of PTSD in patients with BPD.

Historically, the high level of affective instability in patients with BPD, their low tolerance for negative emotions, and in particular the parasuicidal and self-injurious behavior patterns that characterize the disorder have dis-couraged clinicians from attempting to treat comorbid PTSD for fear of worsening these behaviors and increasing the risk of a completed suicide. The prevailing clinical approach to BPD, dialectical behavior therapy (DBT; Linehan, 1993), has been to focus initial treatment on teaching personal self-management and social skills to reduce parasuicidal and self-injurious behav-iors, regardless of whether comorbid PTSD is also present. More recently along these lines, a formal stage model was developed for treating people with BPD and PTSD over a 1-year period, in which DBT is implemented first in order for the patient to achieve a sufficient level of self-control, and then followed by PE (Harned, Korslund, Foa, & Linehan, 2012). A small ($N = 27$) pilot RCT in patients with BPD and PTSD comparing DBT with DBT plus PE reported that 59% of patients assigned to the staged treatment completed the treatment, and that patients in the staged group had better PTSD outcomes than those who received DBT alone (Harned, Korslund, & Linehan, 2014).

Two RCTs of trauma-focused PTSD treatments in general population samples have explored whether patients with PTSD and BPD benefit less from treatment than those with PTSD only. In an RCT of 72 rape survivors with PTSD randomized to PE, stress inoculation (SI), PE + SI, or wait-list control, the outcomes of 12 women who met criteria for BPD or partial BPD were explored (Feeny, Zoellner, & Foa, 2002). The general observation was that the patients with PTSD and BPD (or partial BPD) benefited from the treatments, but the sample size prevents definitive conclusions. A second RCT compared the effectiveness of PE and CPT in 131 rape victims with PTSD who were also administered a self-report measure of BPD at base-line (Clarke, Rizvi, & Resick, 2008). Patients with higher scores on the self-reported BPD measure had more severe PTSD symptoms than those with PTSD alone but did not differ in rates of dropout from treatment or in ben-efit from treatment. This study suggests that women with BPD-PTSD may benefit from trauma-focused treatment, although it is limited by self-report measurement of BPD.

Finally, the results from two RCTs of the cognitive restructuring pro-gram for PTSD in special populations (Mueser et al., 2009) have bearing on the effects of trauma-focused treatments on patients with BPD. The two RCTs described in the previous section included patients with SMI-PTSD and compared the cognitive restructuring program in the first study with treatment as usual (TAU; Mueser et al., 2008) and in the second study with a brief (three-session) intervention (Mueser et al., 2015). In addition to meeting criteria for SMI and PTSD, participants were also evaluated at baseline for BPD with the SCID-II, with 27/108 (25%) and 55/201 (27%) meeting criteria for BPD, respectively. Of note, at baseline, nearly 60% of patients in both samples endorsed recently having suicidal thoughts (Kredlow Acunzo et al., 2017). Separate analyses of the patients with BPD indicated that in both studies those who received cognitive restructuring had greater improvements in PTSD symptoms and diagnosis than the usual treatment group, who actually worsened over the treatment period in general psychiatric symptoms in Study 1 (Kredlow Acunzo et al., 2017). Across both studies, rates of PTSD symptom exacerbation for patients with BPD in the cognitive restructuring group were very low (Kredlow Acunzo et al., 2017), suggesting the trauma-focused intervention was tolerated well by this group.

Taken together, the findings provide some evidence that patients with PTSD-BPD can safely participate in trauma-focused treatment, and that receipt of such treatment is associated with improvements in PTSD and related outcomes.

Chronic Pain

Chronic pain is one of the most commonly reported problems for people with PTSD (Sharp & Harvey, 2001). Individuals with chronic pain resulting from a variety of pathologies frequently present with PTSD symptoms (Asmundson, Coons, Taylor, & Katz, 2002; Sharp & Harvey, 2001). High levels of chronic pain have been found especially among some populations with PTSD, such as veterans (Fishbain, Pulikal, Lewis, & Gao, 2017), torture survivors (Dibaj, Halvorsen, Kennair, & Stenmark, 2017), and refugees (Rometsch-Ogioun El Sount et al., 2019). Two systematic reviews (Brennenstuhl, Tarquinio, & Montel, 2015; Fishbain et al., 2017) found PTSD rates far higher than in the general population for most pain types. Other work has pointed to frequent reporting of childhood abuse in some chronic pain populations (Coppens et al., 2017).

There is evidence from several sources that the co-occurrence of chronic pain and PTSD has a major impact on the evolution of both disorders (Asmundson, 2014; Asmundson et al., 2002). The presence of pain is associated with poorer treatment outcomes in some populations, although the treatment literature for co-occurring PTSD and chronic pain is very limited (Asmundson, 2014). Clinical experience suggests that some patients will avoid trauma-focused therapy for fear of exacerbating their pain. The use of analgesics has been found to be particularly high in PTSD sufferers, compared to other mental health disorders (Schwartz et al., 2006).

Pain is recognized as a complex phenomenon involving biological, psychological, and social factors (Asmundson et al., 2002; Brennenstuhl et al., 2015). PTSD and chronic pain share some overlapping features (e.g., heightened anxiety, hypervigilance and attentional bias for potential threats, avoidance behaviors) and some vulnerabilities such as anxiety sensitivity (Asmundson, 2014; Asmundson et al., 2002; Bosco, Gallinati, & Clark, 2013). Pain and PTSD are also thought be involved in mutual maintenance (Asmundson et al., 2002; Bosco et al., 2013). Pain can represent a trauma cue, acting as a reminder of the traumatic experience. Pain is also emotionally distressing and may aggravate hyperarousal symptoms, which are, in turn, associated with muscular tension and spasms, contributing to increased pain and leading to a "self-perpetuating vicious cycle" (Asmundson, 2014). Pain can also feature as a sensory component of reexperiencing (Bosco et al., 2013). As a result, chronic pain sufferers are likely to avoid pain triggers, which inhibits natural processing of trauma memories. There is some research to suggest that PTSD influences the perception of pain, such that individuals with PTSD experience greater pain severity and report more pain complaints (see Fishbain et al., 2017).

In routine practice, clinicians from a mental health background often fail to screen for chronic pain (Asmundson, 2014). Clinicians treating individuals with PTSD should ensure that they investigate for co-occurring pain symptoms with the aim of understanding their relationship to PTSD symptoms (Asmundson et al., 2002; Asmundson & Hadjistavropolous, 2006; Fishbain et al., 2017). Key aspects of pain that clinicians should explore include pain intensity and location, patient beliefs and attitudes in relation to their pain, patterns of coping, pain-related emotional distress, and resulting physical limitations (Asmundson & Hadjistavropolous, 2006). Similarly, trauma history and PTSD symptoms should be screened for on a routine basis in chronic pain settings (Coppens et al., 2017). Cognitive-behavioral interventions for pain and PTSD share some common features. Reduction of cognitive and behavioral avoidance, via exposure, and aiming to increase activity levels are central to the treatment of both conditions (Sharp & Harvey, 2001). When the two disorders co-occur, it is important to help the patient understand how they are connected and to consider whether treatment needs to be adapted to enhance engagement and address maintaining cycles (Asmundson et al., 2002). The treatment literature for co-occurring PTSD and chronic pain is very limited. There is some indication that chronic pain can interfere with engagement in trauma-focused therapy but also some work suggesting that many individuals can improve with PTSD therapy (Asmundson, 2014). To date, there is no evidence that CBT for pain management has any significant impact on PTSD symptoms (Asmundson, 2014). Very little literature exists on distinctive models of treatment for PTSD-chronic pain comorbidity (Asmundon, 2014; Brennenstuhl et al., 2015). Some experts in the field (e.g., Asmundson, 2014; Otis, Keane, Kerns, Monson, & Scioli, 2009) have suggested that integrated PTSD and pain approaches might be helpful for many patients. Potential common components of integrated therapy may include psychoeducation, cognitive restructuring, emotion regulation strategies such as progressive muscle relaxation, *in vivo* and graded *in vivo* exposure, activity planning, and weight training (Asmundon, 2014; Bosco et al., 2013). Data evaluating such approaches are very limited. Some very preliminary work suggests the potential benefit of co-delivered exercise and physiotherapy, in conjunction with trauma-focused therapy (Dibaj et al., 2017; Manger & Motta, 2005). Otis and colleagues (2009) developed a pilot integrated model incorporating components of CPT for PTSD with CBT for pain management, but this is yet to be tested in a comparison study. Further research into interventions that might improve this comorbidity is clearly required.

Addressing Comorbidity in Children and Adolescents

Although clinicians are often less concerned with establishing specific diagnostic status for child and adolescent populations than for adults, comorbidity is also the rule. A clear sign of this is the common reference to either overall "internalizing" or "externalizing" symptoms in children and adolescent populations. Research reports high rates of comorbidity for childhood anxiety disorders, which could include PTSD, generalized anxiety disorder (GAD), specific and social phobia, panic disorder, and obsessive–compulsive disorder. Studies have shown overlap with depression (17–69%), externalizing disorders (8–69%), attention-deficit hyperactivity disorder (ADHD), oppositional defiant disorder (ODD), and conduct disorder (CD) (Angold, Costello, & Erkanli, 1999). Studies of children and adolescents show that exposure to traumatic events, especially violence and polyvictimization, and PTSD diagnoses are associated with behavior problems and SUDs (e.g., Carliner et al., 2016; Moffitt & Caspi, 2001). Maltreatment and interpersonal violence experiences in childhood are consistently associated with externalizing problems in children and adolescents (e.g., Dube et al., 2006; Widom, Schuck, & White, 2006) with estimated prevalence rates of ODD, CD, and SUD two to four times higher in trauma-exposed populations, relative to those with no exposure and higher rates following exposure to interpersonal violence (Carliner, Gary, McLaughlin, & Keyes, 2017; Lubman, Allen, Rogers, Cementon, & Bonomo, 2007). Comorbidity is often associated with increased symptom variation, severity and impairment, more frequent and severe negative correlates and sequelae, differential treatment response, and distinct courses (Ollendick, Jarrett, Grills-Taquechel, Hovey, & Wolff, 2008).

Trauma-focused cognitive-behavioral therapies and EMDR therapy have the strongest evidence base for children and adolescents with PTSD (see Kenardy, Kassam-Adams, & Dyb, Chapter 10, and Jensen, Cohen, Jaycox, & Rosner, Chapter 21, this volume). Given the frequent comorbidity found in trauma-exposed children and adolescents, many studies evaluating PTSD treatments measure both internalizing and externalizing symptoms. In a review by Silverman and colleagues (2008), two interventions were determined to be effective for symptoms of PTSD, depression, anxiety, and externalizing behavior problems: trauma-focused cognitive-behavioral therapy (TF-CBT; for further information, go to *www.musc.edu/tfcbt*) and Cognitive Behavioral Intervention for Trauma in Schools (CBITS). TF-CBT has the most extensive evidence of effectiveness for children and adolescents with trauma-related symptoms, with multiple RCTs, longer-term follow-up (12 months out), and a large number of quasi-experimental studies (see Dorsey, Briggs, & Woods, 2011, for a review). TF-CBT also has been evaluated in trials in low- and middle-income countries, showing strong effectiveness even when delivered by lay providers without formal mental health training (Murray et al., 2015). Evidence of reduced PTSD symptoms has also been reported for CBITS in one RCT and two uncontrolled studies (see Dorsey et al., 2011, for a review). Ollendick and colleagues (2008) examined comorbidity and its potential effects on treatment outcomes of focal EBTs. The authors concluded that, although many treatment studies with children and adolescents included comorbid samples, very few studies examined whether comorbidity was a moderator of treatment outcome.

Transdiagnostic Interventions

Addressing comorbidity, from the perspectives of public health, efficiency, and implementation science (e.g., Martin, Murray, Darnell, & Dorsey, 2018), has led to growing interest and research in transdiagnostic treatments for children, adolescents, and adults. Transdiagnostic approaches are those that aim to address multiple problem areas or diagnoses. In the early 2000s, researchers hypothesized the ability for one focal treatment to alleviate symptoms of a comorbid disorder—suggesting that some of the processes that maintain one disorder also maintain comorbid disorders (Mansell et al., 2009; Tsao, Mystkowski, Zucker, & Craske, 2005). Researchers have cited a number of potential advantages of transdiagnostic treatment approaches, such as more efficient training and dissemination, reduced training costs for organizations, improved fit for comorbid presentations, and better clinician and client satisfaction (e.g., Mansell et al., 2009; Marchette & Weisz, 2017). A number of transdiagnostic approaches have now been developed (see Boustani, Gellatly, Westman, & Chorpita, 2017) and evaluated compared to disorder-specific treatments. Transdiagnostic approaches are designed in a number of different ways. For example, some models utilize the same elements conceptualizing comorbidities as resulting from a shared mechanism (e.g., the Unified Protocol for the Treatment of Emotional Disorders [UP]; Barlow et al., 2017). A variation on these models is a modular treatment, which chooses and prioritizes different elements depending on the symptom/problem presentation (e.g., Modular Approach to Therapy for Children with Anxiety, Depression, Trauma, or Conduct Problems [MATCH-ADTC]; Chorpita & Weisz, 2009).

UP is a transdiagnostic treatment based on the shared mechanisms approach, targeting a range of anxiety and mood disorders in adults (Barlow et al., 2017). The shared underlying mechanism targeted by UP is the biologically based propensity to experience strong negative emotions. UP includes elements on increasing tolerance of negative emotions, decreasing avoidant coping that maintains negative emotional experiences, and teaching patients more adaptive ways to respond to negative emotions. UP has shown strong effectiveness across depression and anxiety disorders through multiple trials (Barlow et al., 2017; Farchione et al., 2012). In the large 2017 RCT (N = 223), UP had treatment equivalence with disorder-specific treatment protocols for four anxiety disorders on severity of principal diagnosis at the end of treatment and a 6-month follow-up (Barlow et al., 2017). UP has shown effectiveness for panic disorder along with other mood and emotional disorders, including PTSD (Barlow et al., 2017; Farchione et al., 2012).

Focused in low- and middle-income countries globally, the Common Elements Treatment Approach (CETA; Murray et al., 2014) has been evaluated in three published RCTs with populations who have experienced trauma, and two additional RCTs that have been completed (Bolton et al., 2014; Bonilla-Escobar et al., 2018; Weiss et al., 2015). CETA is a cognitive-behavioral, modular, flexible, multiproblem transdiagnostic treatment model that was developed based on advances in high-income settings and built for implementation in low- and middle-income countries with lay providers. Traumatic stress symptoms could be a key focus of treatment in CETA through cognitive and exposure-based elements. On the Thailand/Myanmar border, CETA's effect sizes (Cohen's d) were strong for improving depression (d = 1.16) and posttraumatic stress (d = 1.19). In Iraq, there were large effect sizes for improving depression (d = 1.78) and posttraumatic stress (d = 2.38; Weiss et al., 2015). In Iraq, CETA outperformed two disorder-specific treatments: behavioral activation for depression and CPT for trauma (Bolton et al., 2014).

For children and adolescents, Chorpita and colleagues introduced the idea of common practice elements *within* different focal treatments with the Distillation and Matching Model (DMM; Chorpita, Daleiden, & Weisz, 2005). They went on to develop the Modular Approach to Therapy for Children with Anxiety, Depression, Trauma, or Conduct Problems (MATCH-ADTC), which is the most evaluated transdiagnostic approach in the United States. MATCH-ADTC addresses high-prevalence clusters of problems among children and adolescents from 6 to 15 years of age, including PTSD, which include elements such as exposure (Chorpita & Weisz, 2009). The effectiveness of MATCH-ADTC over both usual care and disorder-specific treatments has been established through two large RCTs in community settings (Chorpita et al., 2017; Weisz et al., 2012), with effects maintained at 2-year follow-up (Chorpita et al., 2013). Compared to usual care, MATCH-ADTC was associated with shorter treatment duration, lower use of other mental health services, and lower rates of psychotropic medication use. Another transdiagnostic model for children and adolescents is principle-guided, which focuses on the principles of therapeutic change that underlie common procedures (Weisz & Bearman, 2020). This approach was only recently introduced and is in the early stages of testing (Weisz, Bearman, Santucci, & Jensen-Doss, 2017). UP was recently adapted for adolescents and children (Ehrenreich-May et al., 2017) and is also based on a core dysfunction or maintaining process that leads to multiple problems or disorders (Barlow et al., 2017). This approach shows promise for children and young people, with clinical several effectiveness trials under way. CETA (Murray et al., 2014) has been evaluated for children and adolescents living in refugee camps in East Africa in an open trial and showed significant reductions in externalizing and internalizing symptoms, and PTSD (Murray et al., 2018).

Additional studies are warranted on transdiagnostic models from different approaches (shared mechanism, common elements, and principle-guided), perhaps specifically to compare disorder-specific treatments' impact on comorbid problems with that of emerging transdiagnostic models.

Conclusions

Clinical Considerations

The presence of comorbidity presents a challenge to clinicians, researchers, and providers. This chapter presents evidence establishing that trauma-focused therapies can be effective for PTSD with a number of comorbidities, although manualized interventions may sometimes require adaptation. Increasingly, evidence favors combined/integrated approaches for SUD comorbidity, with some support for similar approaches with other comorbidities such as chronic pain and panic disorder. For children and adolescents, transdiagnostic approaches are being increasingly advocated. From a clinical standpoint, thorough screening and assessment of comorbidities are clearly key to good treatment planning. Clinicians should seek to elicit a detailed history of the unfolding of symptoms both pre- and post-event (Lockwood & Forbes, 2014) so that they can fully understand the relationship between events, symptom development, and maintaining factors to formulate a treatment plan appropriate to the patient's needs. In many cases, it should be possible to treat patients with many comorbidities successfully—sometimes with minor adaptations to existing treatment protocols. However, in cases of severe comorbidity, clinicians should consider integrated or concurrent treatment.

The realities of clinical practice are that many patients present for help with multiple comorbidities, often alongside related clinical problems, such as relationship problems, problematic anger, interpersonal violence perpetration, parenting issues, housing problems, and employment-related difficulties. In complex cases, it can be difficult to decide what problems should be prioritized, and sometimes addressing conditions such as PTSD may not be the immediate concern. For those with complex needs, a case management approach is often required to plan and coordinate a response to primary needs. For some individuals, a period of building a trusting relationship with a service or team may be an important foundation for engagement with EBTs (Holdsworth, Bowen, Brown, & Howat, 2014; Kehle-Forbes & Kimerling, 2017). Ambivalence about engaging in trauma-focused therapy is a significant issue in the field, even for those without significant comorbidities (Kehle-Forbes & Kimerling, 2017). Psychoeducation and motivational interventions are often an important part of the engagement process, although evidence of the benefits of interventions aimed at enhancing motivation to engage in EBTs is mixed (Kehle-Forbes & Kimerling, 2017). Figure 22.1 identifies some of the key principles of treatment planning when multiple comorbidities are indicated.

- PTSD sufferers should be screened for common comorbidities on a routine basis, with further detailed assessment as indicated.
- PTSD is a common comorbidity with many other disorders and should be screened for in all mental health settings.
- Clinicians should routinely develop a biopsychosocial case formulation (e.g., Lee, 2016) to support their understanding of the development and maintenance of PTSD and comorbid conditions. Particular attention should be given to precipitating factors, current stressors and triggers, and mutual maintaining factors and cycles of symptom interaction.
- Clinicians should not exclude patients with a diagnosis of psychotic disorders, substance use disorders, and borderline personality disorders from trauma-focused psychological therapy. Readiness to engage in evidence-based treatment should be evaluated on an individual basis.
- Intervention should be guided by current evidence.
- High-risk concerns should normally be the priority for intervention.
- Psychoeducation adapted to the individual's level of comprehension is often an important component of engagement. Promoting an understanding of the relationship between PTSD and other relevant comorbidities can also help the engagement process.
- During the assessment process, clinicians should consider whether comorbid disorders and symptoms are likely to obstruct engagement in trauma-focused therapy and consider offering concurrent interventions, such as COPE or M-CET, when indicated.
- When significant comorbidities are present, clinicians should consider evidence-based interventions that may address common cycles of symptom maintenance.
- When therapeutic blocks occur, clinicians should reformulate.

FIGURE 22.1. Principles for treating PTSD and comorbidities.

Future Research

From the current treatment literature, it is unclear to what extent comorbidities such as depression, panic disorder, and chronic pain impede the success of EBT for PTSD. To better understand the impacts of comorbidities, it would be helpful if future treatment trials could investigate comorbidity effects and report outcomes by comorbidity so that data can be aggregated across studies to establish clearer comorbidity effects. Outcomes for co-occurring conditions should be evaluated throughout the course of treatment (Teng et al., 2013). Future studies would need to be adequately powered and resourced to achieve this goal. Reporting of this kind would also help to give a clearer understanding of the need for integrated approaches (Asmundson, 2014; Stander et al., 2014). Although this chapter focused on mental health disorders as comorbidities, continued research is necessary to identify and target other co-occurring clinical problems such as anger, interpersonal violence perpetration, intimate relationship and parenting problems, and difficulties returning to work (Monson & Fredman, 2012; Stergiopoulos, Cimo, Cheng, Bonato, & Dewa, 2011; Taft, Creech, & Murphy, 2017).

In future work, it will be helpful to identify critical treatment mechanisms that may mediate outcomes across disorders (Stander et al., 2014). Future research must also seek to identify modifiable risks and vulnerabilities, which might be targets for prevention and treatment approaches (Stander et al., 2014). In this vein, anxiety sensitivity has been indicated as a vulnerability factor for both panic disorder and chronic pain (Asmundson, 2014; Teng et al., 2013), and interventions aimed at reducing anxiety sensitivity may merit further exploration as a possible early psychological intervention or in conjunction with established treatments. Finally, although there is evidence of the benefits of transdiagnostic approaches for young people, such approaches have not been given as much attention in the adult PTSD literature, despite some evidence of their benefit in trauma-exposed populations living in low- and middle-income countries (Bolton et al., 2014; Weiss et al., 2015). Transdiagnostic approaches may be beneficial in addressing underlying shared core vulnerabilities in PTSD and its comorbidities (Gutner, Galovski, Bovin, & Schnurr, 2016) and should therefore be investigated further.

REFERENCES

Achim, A. M., Maziade, M., Raymond, E., Olivier, D., Mérette, C., & Roy, M. A. (2011). How prevalent are anxiety disorders in schizophrenia?: A meta-analysis and critical review on a significant association. *Schizophrenia Bulletin, 37*(4), 811–821.

Adams, Z. W., McCauley, J. L., Back, S. E., Hellmuth, J. C., Hanson, R. F., Killeen, T. K., et al. (2016). Clinician perspectives on treating adolescents with co-occurring posttraumatic stress disorder, substance use, and other problems. *Journal of Child and Adolescent Substance Abuse, 25*, 575–583.

American Psychiatric Association. (2013). *Diagnostic and statistical manual of mental disorders* (5th ed.). Alexandria, VA: Author.

Angold, A., Costello, E. J., & Erkanli, A. (1999). Comorbidity. *Journal of Child Psychology and Psychiatry and Allied Disciplines, 40,* 57–87.

Asmundson, G. J. G. (2014). The emotional and physical pains of trauma: Contemporary and innovative approaches for treating co-occurring PTSD and chronic pain. *Depression and Anxiety, 31*(9), 717–720.

Asmundson, G. J. G., Coons, M. J., Taylor, S., & Katz, J. (2002). PTSD and the experience of pain: Research and clinical implications of shared vulnerability and mutual maintenance models. *Canadian Journal of Psychiatry, 47,* 930–937.

Asmundson, G. J. G., & Hadjistavropolous, H. D. (2006). Addressing shared vulnerability for comorbid PTSD and chronic pain: A cognitive-behavioral perspective. *Cognitive and Behaviour Practice, 13,* 8–16.

Back, S. E. (2010). Toward an improved model of treating co-occurring PTSD and substance use disorders. *American Journal of Psychiatry, 167*(1), 11–13.

Back, S. E., Brady, K. T., Sonne, S. C., & Verduin, M. L. (2006). Symptom improvement in co-occurring PTSD and alcohol dependence. *Journal of Nervous and Mental Disease, 194*(9), 690–696.

Back, S. E., Foa, E. B., Killeen, T. K., Mills, K. L., Teesson, M., Carroll, K. M., et al. (2014). *Concurrent treatment of PTSD and substance use disorders using prolonged exposure (COPE) therapist manual.* New York: Oxford University Press.

Back, S. E., Jackson, J. L., Sonne, S., & Brady, K. T. (2005). Alcohol dependence and posttraumatic stress disorder: Differences in clinical presentation and response to cognitive–behavioral therapy by order of onset. *Journal of Substance Abuse Treatment, 29*(1), 29–37.

Back, S. E., Killeen, T., Badour, C. L., Flanagan, J. C., Allan, N. P., Ana, E. S., et al. (2019). Concurrent treatment of substance use disorders and PTSD using prolonged exposure: A randomized clinical trial in military veterans. *Addictive Behaviors, 90,* 369–377.

Back, S. E., Killeen, T. K., Teer, A. P., Hartwell, E. E., Federline, A., Beylotte, F., et al. (2014). Substance use disorders and PTSD: An exploratory study of treatment preferences among military veterans. *Addictive Behaviors, 39,* 369–373.

Back, S. E., Waldrop, A. E., & Brady, K. T. (2009). Treatment challenges associated with comorbid substance use and posttraumatic stress disorder: Clinicians' perspectives. *American Journal on Addictions, 18*(1), 15–20.

Barlow, D. H., Farchione, T. J., Bullis, J. R., Gallagher, M. W., Murray-Latin, H., Sauer-Zavala, S., et al. (2017). The unified protocol for transdiagnostic treatment of emotional disorders compared with diagnosis-specific protocols for anxiety disorders. *JAMA Psychiatry, 74,* 875–884.

Barrett, E. L., Teesson, M., & Mills, K. L. (2014). Associations between substance use, post-traumatic stress disorder and the perpetration of violence: A longitudinal investigation. *Addictive Behaviors, 39*(6), 1075–1080.

Bisson, J. I., Roberts, N. P., Andrew, M., Cooper, R., & Lewis, C. (2013). Psychological therapies for chronic post-traumatic stress disorder (PTSD) in adults. *Cochrane Database of Systematic Reviews,* Issue 12, Article No. CD003388.

Blanco, C., Xu, Y., Brady, K., Pérez-Fuentes, G., Okuda, M., & Wang, S. (2013). Comorbidity of posttraumatic stress disorder with alcohol dependence among US adults: Results from National Epidemiological Survey on Alcohol and Related Conditions. *Drug and Alcohol Dependence, 132*(3), 630–638.

Boden, M. T., Bonn-Miller, M. O., Kashdan, T. B., Alvarez, J., & Gross, J. J. (2012). The interactive effects of emotional clarity and cognitive reappraisal in post-traumatic stress disorder. *Journal of Anxiety Disorders, 26*(1), 233–238.

Bolton, P., Lee, C., Haroz, E. E., Murray, L. K., Dorsey, S., Robinson, C., et al. (2014). Transdiagnostic community based mental health treatment for comorbid disorders: Development and outcomes of a randomized controlled trial among Burmese refugees in Thailand. *PLOS Medicine, 11*(11), e1001757.

Bonilla-Escobar, F. J., Fandino-Losada, A., Martinez-Buitrago, D. M., Santaella-Tenorio, J., Tobon-Garcia, D., Munoz-Morales, E. J., et al. (2018). A randomized controlled trial of a transdiagnostic cognitive-behavioral intervention for Afrodescendants' survivors of systemic violence in Colombia. *PLOS ONE, 13*(12), e0208483.

Borsboom, D., Cramer, A. O. J., Schmittmann, V. D., Epskamp, S., & Waldorp, L. J. (2011). The small world of psychopathology. *PLOS ONE, 6*(11), e27407.

Bosco, M. A., Gallinati, J. L., & Clark, M. E. (2013). Conceptualizing and treating comorbid chronic pain and PTSD. *Pain Research and Treatment*. [Epub ahead of print]

Boustani, M. M., Gellatly, R., Westman, J. G., & Chorpita, B. F. (2017). Advances in cognitive behavioral treatment design: Time for a glossary. *The Behavior Therapist, 40*(6), 199–208.

Bowe, A., & Rosenheck, R. (2015). PTSD and substance use disorder among veterans: Characteristics, service utilization and pharmacotherapy. *Journal of Dual Diagnosis, 11*(1), 22–32.

Brady, K. T., & Sinha, R. (2005). Co-occurring mental and substance use disorders: The neurobiological effects of chronic stress. *American Journal of Psychiatry, 162*(8), 1483–1493.

Brennenstuhl, M. J., Tarquinio, C., & Montel, S. (2015). Chronic pain and PTSD: Evolving views on their comorbidity. *Perspectives in Psychiatric Care, 51*(4), 295–304.

Brown, T. A., Campbell, L. A., Lehman, C. L., Grisham, J. R., & Mancill, R. B. (2001). Current and lifetime comorbidity of the DSM-IV anxiety and mood disorders in a large clinical sample. *Journal of Abnormal Psychology, 110*(4), 585–599.

Buckley, P. F., Miller, B. J., Lehrer, D. S., & Castle, D. J. (2009). Psychiatric comorbidities and schizophrenia. *Schizophrenia Bulletin, 35*(2), 383–402.

Carliner, H., Gary, D., McLaughlin, K. A., & Keyes, K. M. (2017). Trauma exposure and externalizing disorders in adolescents: Results from the National Comorbidity Survey Adolescent Supplement. *Journal of the American Academy of Child and Adolescent Psychiatry, 56*, 755–764.

Carliner, H., Keyes, K. M., McLaughlin, K. A., Meyers, J. L., Dunn, E. C., & Martins, S. S. (2016). Childhood trauma and illicit drug use in in adolescence: A population-based national comorbidity survey replication-adolescent supplement study. *Journal of the American Academy of Child and Adolescent Psychiatry, 55*, 701–708.

Carr, C. P., Martins, C. M., Stingel, A. M., Lemgruber, V. B., & Juruena, M. F. (2013). The role of early life stress in adult psychiatric disorders: A systematic review according to childhood trauma subtypes. *Journal of Nervous and Mental Disease, 201*, 1007–1020.

Cattane, N., Rossi, R., Lanfredi, M., & Cattaneo, A. (2017). Borderline personality disorder and childhood trauma: Exploring the affected biological systems and mechanisms. *BMC Psychiatry, 17*(1), 221.

Chorpita, B. F., Daleiden, E. L., Park, A. L., Ward, A. M., Levy, M. C., Cromley, T., et al. (2017). Child STEPs in California: A cluster randomized effectiveness trial comparing modular treatment with community implemented treatment for youth with anxiety, depression, conduct problems, or traumatic stress. *Journal of Consulting and Clinical Psychology, 85*(1), 13–25.

Chorpita, B. F., Daleiden, E. L., & Weisz, J. R. (2005). Identifying and selecting the common elements of evidence based interventions: A distillation and matching model. *Mental Health Services Research, 7*(1), 5–20.

Chorpita, B. F., & Weisz, J. R. (2009). *MATCH-ADTC: Modular approach to therapy for children with anxiety, depression, trauma, or conduct problems*. Satellite Beach, FL: PracticeWise.

Chorpita, B. F., Weisz, J. R., Daleiden, E. L., Schoenwald, S. K., Palinkas, L. A., Miranda, J., et al. (2013). Long-term outcomes for the Child STEPs randomized effectiveness trial: A comparison of modular and standard treatment designs with usual care. *Journal of Consulting and Clinical Psychology, 81*(6), 999–1009.

Clarke, S. B., Rizvi, S. L., & Resick, P. A. (2008). Borderline personality characteristics and treatment outcome in cognitive-behavioral treatments for PTSD in female rape victims. *Behavior Therapy, 39,* 72–78.

Coppens, E., van Wambeke, P., Morlion, B., Weltens, N., Giao Ly, H., Tack, J., et al. (2017). Prevalence and impact of childhood adversities and post-traumatic stress disorder in women with fibromyalgia and chronic widespread pain. *European Journal of Pain, 21,* 1582–1590.

Cougle, J. R., Feldner, M. T., Keough, M. E., Hawkins, K. A., & Fitch, K. E. (2010). Comorbid panic attacks among individuals with posttraumatic stress disorder: Associations with traumatic event exposure history, symptoms, and impairment. *Journal of Anxiety Disorders, 24,* 183–188.

Craske, M. G., Roy-Byrne, P., Stein, M. B., Sullivan, G., Hazlett-Stevens, H., & Bystritsky, A. (2006). CBT intensity and outcome for panic disorder in a primary care setting. *Behavior Therapy, 37,* 112–119.

Cusack, K. J., Grubaugh, A. L., Knapp, R. G., & Frueh, B. C. (2006). Unrecognized trauma and PTSD among public mental health consumers with chronic and severe mental illness. *Community Mental Health Journal, 42,* 478–500.

Desmarais, S. L., Van Dorn, R. A., Johnson, K. L., Grimm, K. J., Douglas, K. S., & Swartz, M. S. (2014). Community violence perpetration and victimization among adults with mental illnesses. *American Journal of Public Health, 104,* 2342–2349.

Dibaj, I., Halvorsen, J. Ø., Kennair, L. E. O., & Stenmark, H. I. (2017). An evaluation of combined narrative exposure therapy and physiotherapy for comorbid PTSD and chronic pain in torture survivors, *Torture, 27,* 13–27.

Dorsey, S., Briggs, E. C., & Woods, B. A. (2011). Cognitive-behavioral treatment for posttraumatic stress disorder in children and adolescents. *Child and Adolescent Psychiatric Clinics of North America, 20*(2), 255–269.

Dube, S. R., Miller, J. W., Brown, D. W., Giles, W. H., Felitti, V. J., Dong, M., et al. (2006). Adverse childhood experiences and the association with ever using alcohol and initiating alcohol use during adolescence. *Journal of Adolescent Health, 38,* 444.e1–444.e10.

Duncan, L. E., Ratanatharathorn, A., Aiello, A. E., Almli, L. M., Amstadter, A. B., Ashley-Koch, A. E., et al. (2018). Largest GWAS of PTSD (N = 20,070) yields genetic overlap with schizophrenia and sex differences in heritability. *Molecular Psychiatry, 23,* 666–673.

Dvorak, R. D., Pearson, M. R., & Day, A. M. (2014). Ecological momentary assessment of acute alcohol use disorder symptoms: Associations with mood, motives, and use on planned drinking days. *Experimental and Clinical Psychopharmacology, 22,* 285–297.

Ehrenreich-May, J., Rosenfield, D., Queen, A. H., Kennedy, S. M., Remmes, C. S., & Barlow, D. H. (2017). An initial waitlist-controlled trial of the Unified Protocol for the treatment of emotional disorders in adolescents. *Journal of Anxiety Disorders, 46,* 46–55.

Etain, B., Henry, C., Bellivier, F., Mathieu, F., & Leboyer, M. (2008). Beyond genetics: Childhood affective trauma in bipolar disorder. *Bipolar Disorders, 10,* 867–876.

Falsetti, S. A., Resnick, H. S., Dansky, B. S., Lydiard, R. B., & Kilpatrick, D. G. (1995). The relationship of stress to panic disorder: Cause or effect? In C. M. Mazure (Ed.), *Does stress cause psychiatric illness?* (pp. 111–147). Washington, DC: American Psychiatric Press.

Falsetti, S., Resnick, H., & Davis, J. (2008). Multiple channel exposure therapy for women with PTSD and comorbid panic attacks. *Cognitive Behaviour Therapy, 37,* 117–130.

Farchione, T. J., Fairholme, C. P., Ellard, K. K., Boisseau, C. L., Thompson-Hollands, J., Carl, J. R., et al. (2012). Unified Protocol for transdiagnostic treatment of emotional disorders: A randomized controlled trial. *Behavior Therapy, 43*(3), 666–678.

Feeny, N. C., Zoellner, L. A., & Foa, E. B. (2002). Treatment outcome for chronic PTSD among female assault victims with borderline personality characteristics: A preliminary examination. *Journal of Personality Disorders, 16,* 30–40.

Fishbain, A., Pulikal, J., Lewis, J., & Gao, J. (2017). Chronic pain types differ in their reported prevalence of post-traumatic stress disorder (PTSD) and there is consistent evidence that chronic pain is associated with PTSD: An evidence-based structured systematic review. *Pain Medicine, 18,* 711–735.

Flory, J. D., & Yehuda, R. (2015). Comorbidity between post-traumatic stress disorder and major depressive disorder: Alternative explanations and treatment considerations. *Dialogues in Clinical Neuroscience, 17*(2), 141–150.

Foa, E. B., Gillihan, S. J., & Bryant, R. A. (2013). Challenges and successes in dissemination of dvidence-based treatments for posttraumatic stress. *Psychological Science in the Public Interest, 14*(2), 65–111.

Frisman, L., Ford, J., Hsiu-Ju, L., Mallon, S., & Chang, R. (2008). Outcomes of trauma treatment using the TARGET model. *Journal of Groups in Addiction and Recovery, 3,* 285–303.

Frueh, B. C., Grubaugh, A. L., Cusack, K. J., Kimble, M. O., Elhai, J. D., & Knapp, R. G. (2009). Exposure-based cognitive-behavioral treatment of PTSD in adults with schizophrenia or schizoaffective disorder: A pilot study. *Journal of Anxiety Disorders, 23,* 665–675.

Gielen, N., Krumeich, A., Havermans, R. C., Smeets, F., & Jansen, A. (2014). Why clinicians do not implement integrated treatment for comorbid substance use disorder and posttraumatic stress disorder: A qualitative study. *European Journal of Psychotraumatology, 5*(1), 22821.

Gilpin, N. W., & Weiner, J. L. (2017). Neurobiology of comorbid post-traumatic stress disorder and alcohol-use disorder. *Genes, Brain and Behavior, 16*(1), 15–43.

Ginzburg, K., Ein-Dor, T., & Solomon, Z. (2010). Comorbidity of posttraumatic stress disorder, anxiety and depression: A 20-year longitudinal study of war veterans. *Journal of Affective Disorders, 123*(1–3), 249–257.

Golier, J. A., Yehuda, R., Bierer, L. M., Mitropoulou, V., New, A. S., Schmeidler, J., et al. (2003). The relationship of borderline personality disorder to posttraumatic stress disorder and traumatic events. *American Journal of Psychiatry, 160,* 2018–2024.

Gottlieb, J. D., Mueser, K. T., Rosenberg, S. D., Xie, H., & Wolfe, R. (2011). Psychotic depression, posttraumatic stress disorder, and engagement in cognitive-behavioral therapy within an outpatient sample of adults with serious mental illness. *Comprehensive Psychiatry, 52,* 41–49.

Grant, B. F., Saha, T. D., Ruan, W. J., Goldstein, R. B., Chou, S. P., Jung, J., et al. (2016). Epidemiology of *DSM-5* drug use disorder. *JAMA Psychiatry, 73*(1), 39.

Grubaugh, A. L., Clapp, J. D., Frueh, B. C., Tuerk, P. W., Knapp, R. G., & Egede, L. E. (2016). Open trial of exposure therapy for PTSD among patients with severe and persistent mental illness. *Behaviour Research and Therapy, 78,* 1–12.

Grubaugh, A. L., Zinzow, H. M., Paul, L., Egede, L. E., & Frueh, B. C. (2011). Trauma exposure and posttraumatic stress disorder in adults with severe mental illness: A critical review. *Clinical Psychology Review, 31,* 883–899.

Gunderson, J. G., & Sabo, A. N. (1993). The phenomenological and conceptual interface between borderline personality disorder and PTSD. *American Journal of Psychiatry, 150,* 19–27.

Gutner, C. A., Galovski, T., Bovin, M. J., & Schnurr, P. P. (2016). Emergence of transdiagnostic treatments for PTSD and posttraumatic distress. *Current Psychiatry Reports, 18,* 95.

Harned, M. S., Korslund, K. E., Foa, E. B., & Linehan, M. M. (2012). Treating PTSD in suicidal and self-injuring women with borderline personality disorder: Development and preliminary evaluation of a dialectical behavior therapy prolonged exposure protocol. *Behaviour Research and Therapy, 50,* 381–386.

Harned, M. S., Korslund, K. E., & Linehan, M. M. (2014). A pilot randomized controlled trial of dialectical behavior therapy with and without the dialectical behavior therapy prolonged exposure protocol for suicidal and self-injuring women with borderline personality disorder and PTSD. *Behaviour Research and Therapy, 55,* 7–17.

Hien, D. A., Jiang, H., Campbell, A. N. C., Hu, M.-C., Miele, G. M., Cohen, L. R., et al. (2010). Do treatment improvements in PTSD severity affect substance use outcomes?: A secondary analysis from a randomized clinical trial in NIDA's Clinical Trials Network. *American Journal of Psychiatry, 167*(1), 95–101.

Hien, D. A., Wells, E. A., Jiang, H., Suarez-Morales, L., Campbell, A. N. C., Cohen, L. R., et al. (2009). Multisite randomized trial of behavioral interventions for women with co-occurring PTSD and substance use disorders. *Journal of Consulting and Clinical Psychology, 77*(4), 607–619.

Hinton, D., Chhean, D., Pich, V., Safren, S., Hofmann, S., & Pollack, M. A. (2005). A randomized controlled trial of cognitive-behavior therapy for Cambodian refugees with treatment-resistant PTSD and panic attacks: A cross-over design. *Journal of Traumatic Stress, 18,* 617–629.

Hinton, D. E., Hofmann, S. G., Pitman, R. K., Pollack, M. H., & Barlow, D. H. (2008). The Panic Attack-Posttraumatic Stress Disorder Model: Applicability to orthostatic panic among Cambodian refugees. *Cognitive Behaviour Therapy, 37,* 101–116.

Hinton, D. E., Pollack, M. H., Pich, V., Fama, J. M., & Barlow, D. H. (2005). Orthostatically induced panic attacks among Cambodian refugees: Flashbacks, catastrophic cognitions, and associated psychopathology. *Cognitive and Behavioral Practice, 12,* 301–311.

Holdsworth, E., Bowen, E., Brown, S., & Howat, D. (2014). Client engagement in psychotherapeutic treatment and associations with client characteristics, therapist characteristics, and treatment factors. *Clinical Psychology Review, 34,* 428–450.

Horesh, D., Lowe, S. R., Galea, S., Aiello, A. E., Uddin, M., & Koenen, K. C. (2017). An in-depth look into PTSD-depression comorbidity: A longitudinal study of chronically-exposed Detroit residents. *Journal of Affective Disorders, 208,* 653–661.

Husted, J. A., Ahmed, R., Chow, E. W., Brzustowicz, L. M., & Bassett, A. S. (2012). Early environmental exposures influence schizophrenia expression even in the presence of strong genetic predisposition. *Schizophrenia Research, 137,* 166–168.

Imel, Z. E., Laska, K., Jakupcak, M., & Simpson, T. L. (2013). Meta-analysis of dropout in treatments for posttraumatic stress disorder. *Journal of Consulting and Clinical Psychology, 81*(3), 394–404.

Kaysen, D., Stappenbeck, C., Rhew, I., & Simpson, T. (2014). Proximal relationships between PTSD and drinking behavior. *European Journal of Psychotraumatology, 5*(1), 26518.

Kehle-Forbes, S., & Kimerling, R. (2017). Patient engagement in PTSD treatment. *PTSD Research Quarterly, 28*(3), 1–10.

Kessler, R. C., Sonnega, A., Bromet, E., Hughes, M., & Nelson, C. B. (1995). Posttraumatic stress disorder in the National Comorbidity Survey. *Archives of General Psychiatry, 52,* 1048–1060.

Khantzian, E. J. (1997). The self-medication hypothesis of substance use disorders: A reconsideration and recent applications. *Harvard Review of Psychiatry, 4,* 231–244.

King, D. W., King, L. A., McArdle, J. J., Shalev, A., & Doron-LaMarca, S. (2009). Sequential temporal dependencies in associations between symptoms of depression and posttraumatic stress disorder: An application of bivariate latent difference score structural equation modeling. *Multivariate Behavioral Research, 44,* 437–464.

Kredlow Acunzo, M. A., Szuhany, K. L., Lo, S., Xie, X., Gottlieb, J. D., Rosenberg, S. D., et al. (2017). Cognitive behavioral therapy for posttraumatic stress disorder in individuals with severe mental illness and borderline personality disorder. *Psychiatry Research, 249,* 86–93.

Lee, D. (2016). Case conceptualisation in complex PTSD: Integrating theory with practice. In N. Tarrier & J. Johnson (Eds.), *Case formulation in cognitive behaviour therapy: The treatment of challenging and complex cases* (pp. 142–166). New York: Routledge.

Li, J., Zweig, K. C., Brackbill, R. M., Farfel, M. R., & Cone, J. E. (2018). Comorbidity amplifies the effects of post-9/11 posttraumatic stress disorder trajectories on health-related quality of life. *Quality of Life Research, 27,* 651–660.

Linehan, M. M. (1993). *Cognitive-behavioral treatment of borderline personality disorder.* New York: Guilford Press.

Liness, S. (2009). Cognitive therapy for PTSD and panic attacks. In N. Grey (Ed.), *A casebook of cognitive therapy for traumatic stress reactions* (pp. 147–163). Abingdon, UK: Routledge.

Lockwood, E., & Forbes, D. (2014). Posttraumatic stress disorder and comorbidity: Untangling the Gordian knot. *Psychological Injury and Law, 7*(2), 108–121.

Lozano, B. E., Gros, D. F., Killeen, T., Jaconis, M., Beylotte, F. M., Boyd, S., et al. (2015). To reduce or abstain?: Substance use goals in the treatment of veterans with substance use disorders and comorbid PTSD. *American Journal on Addictions, 24*(7), 578–581.

Lubman, D. I., Allen, N. B., Rogers, N., Cementon, E., & Bonomo, Y. (2007). The impact of co-occurring mood and anxiety disorders among substance abusing youth. *Journal of Affective Disorders, 103,* 105–112.

Lugtenberg, M., Burgers, J. S., Clancy, C., Westert, G. P., & Schneider, E. C. (2011). Current guidelines have limited applicability to patients with comorbid conditions: A systematic analysis of evidence-based guidelines. *PLOS ONE, 6*(10), e25987.

Manger, T. A., & Motta, R. W. (2005). The impact of an exercise program on posttraumatic stress disorder, anxiety and depression. *International Journal of Emergency Mental Health, 7,* 49–57.

Maniglio, R. (2009). Severe mental illness and criminal victimization: A systematic review. *Acta Psychiatrica Scandinavia, 119,* 180–191.

Mansell, W., Harvey, A., Watkins, E., & Shafran, R. (2009). Conceptual foundations of the transdiagnostic approach to CBT. *Journal of Cognitive Psychotherapy: An International Quarterly, 23,* 6–19.

Marchette, L. K., & Weisz, J. R. (2017). Practitioner review: Empirical evolution of youth psychotherapy toward transdiagnostic approaches. *Journal of Child Psychology and Psychiatry, 58,* 970–984.

Martin, P., Murray, L. K., Darnell, D., & Dorsey, S. (2018). Transdiagnostic treatment approaches for greater public health impact: Implementing principles of evidence-based mental health interventions. *Clinical Psychology: Science and Practice, 25*(4), e12270.

Matheson, S. L., Shepherd, A. M., Pinchbeck, R. M., Laurens, K. R., & Carr, V. J. (2013). Childhood adversity in schizophrenia: A systematic meta-analysis. *Psychological Medicine, 43,* 225–238.

McCauley, J. L., Killeen, T., Gros, D. F., Brady, K. T., & Back, S. E. (2012). Posttraumatic stress disorder and co-occurring substance use disorders: Advances in assessment and treatment. *Clinical Psychology, 19*(3), 283–304.

McGovern, M. P., Lambert-Harris, C., Alterman, A. I., Xie, H., & Meier, A. (2011). A randomized controlled trial comparing integrated cognitive behavioral therapy versus individual addiction counseling for co-occurring substance use and posttraumatic stress disorders. *Journal of Dual Diagnosis, 7*(4), 207–227.

McLean, L. M., & Gallop, R. (2003). Implications of childhood sexual abuse for adult borderline personality disorder and complex posttraumatic stress disorder. *American Journal of Psychiatry, 160,* 369–371.

Meyer, I. H., Muenzenmaier, K., Cancienne, J., & Struening, E. L. (1996). Reliability and validity of a measure of sexual and physical abuse histories among women with serious mental illness. *Child Abuse and Neglect, 20,* 213–219.

Mills, K. L., Teesson, M., Back, S. E., Brady, K. T., Baker, A. L., Hopwood, S., et al. (2012). Integrated exposure-based therapy for co-occurring posttraumatic stress disorder and substance dependence: A randomized controlled trial. *Journal of the American Medical Association, 308*(7), 690–699.

Mills, K., Teesson, M., Ross, J., & Peters, L. (2006). Trauma, PTSD, and substance use disorders: Findings from the Australian National Survey of Mental Health and Well-Being. *American Journal of Psychiatry, 163*(4), 652.

Moffitt, T. E., & Caspi, A. (2001). Childhood predictors differentiate life-course persistent and adolescence-limited antisocial pathways among males and females. *Development and Psychopathology, 13,* 355–375.

Monson, C. M., & Fredman, S. J. (2012). *Cognitive-behavioural conjoint therapy for posttraumatic stress disorder: Harnessing the healing power of relationships.* New York: Guilford Press.

Mueser, K. T., Goodman, L. A., Trumbetta, S. L., Rosenberg, S. D., Osher, F. C., Vidaver, R., et al. (1998). Trauma and posttraumatic stress disorder in severe mental illness. *Journal of Consulting and Clinical Psychology, 66,* 493–499.

Mueser, K. T., Gottlieb, J. D., Xie, H., Lu, W., Yanos, P. T., Rosenberg, S. R., et al. (2015). Evaluation of cognitive restructuring for PTSD in people with severe mental illness. *British Journal of Psychiatry, 206,* 501–508.

Mueser, K. T., Rosenberg, S. D., Goodman, L. A., & Trumbetta, S. L. (2002). Trauma, PTSD, and the course of schizophrenia: An interactive model. *Schizophrenia Research, 53,* 123–143.

Mueser, K. T., Rosenberg, S. D., & Rosenberg, H. J. (2009). *Treatment of posttraumatic stress disorder in special populations: A cognitive restructuring program.* Alexandria, VA: American Psychological Association.

Mueser, K. T., Rosenberg, S. D., Xie, H., Jankowski, M. K., Bolton, E. E., Lu, W., et al. (2008). A randomized controlled trial of cognitive-behavioral treatment of posttraumatic stress disorder in severe mental illness. *Journal of Consulting and Clinical Psychology, 76,* 259–271.

Mueser, K. T., Salyers, M. P., Rosenberg, S. D., Ford, J. D., Fox, L., & Carty, P. (2001). A psychometric evaluation of trauma and PTSD assessments in persons with severe mental illness. *Psychological Assessment, 13,* 110–117.

Müller, M., Vandeleur, C., Rodgers, S., Rössler, W., Castelao, E., Preisig, M., et al. (2014). Factors associated with comorbidity patterns in full and partial PTSD: Findings from the PsyCoLaus study. *Comprehensive Psychiatry, 55*(4), 837–848.

Murphy, D., & Smith, K. V. (2018). Treatment efficacy for veterans with posttraumatic stress disorder: Latent class trajectories of treatment response and their predictors. *Journal of Traumatic Stress, 31,* 753–763.

Murray, L. K., Dorsey, S., Haroz, E., Lee, C., Alsiary, M. M., Haydary, A., et al. (2014). A common elements treatment approach for adult mental health problems in low- and middle-income countries. *Cognitive and Behavioral Practice, 21*(2), 111–123.

Murray, L. K., Hall, B. J., Dorsey, S., Ugueto, A. M., Puffer, E. S., Sim, A., et al. (2018). An evaluation of a common elements treatment approach for youth in Somali refugee camps. *Global Mental Health, 5,* e16.

Murray, L. K., Skavenski, S., Kane, J. C., Mayeya, J., Dorsey, S., Cohen, J. A., et al. (2015). Effectiveness of trauma-focused cognitive behavioral therapy among trauma-affected children in Lusaka, Zambia: A randomized clinical trial. *JAMA Pediatrics, 169*(8), 761–769.

Myers, U. S., Browne, K. C., & Norman, S. B. (2015). Treatment engagement: Female survivors of intimate partner violence in treatment for PTSD and alcohol use disorder. *Journal of Dual Diagnosis, 11*(3–4), 238–247.

Myers, U. S., Haller, M., Angkaw, A. C., Harik, J. M., & Norman, S. B. (2019). Evidence-based psychotherapy completion and symptom improvement among returning combat veterans with PTSD. *Psychological Trauma, 11*(2), 216–223.

Najavits, L. M. (2002). *Seeking Safety: A treatment manual for PTSD and substance abuse.* New York: Guilford Press.

Norman, S. B., Haller, M., Hamblen, J. L., Southwick, S. M., & Pietrzak, R. H. (2018). The burden of co-occurring alcohol use disorder and PTSD in U.S. military veterans: Comorbidities, functioning, and suicidality. *Psychology of Addictive Behaviors, 32*(2), 224–229.

Norman, S. B., Trim, R., Haller, M., Davis, B. C., Myers, U. S., Colvonen, P. J., et al. (2019). Efficacy of integrated exposure therapy vs integrated coping skills therapy for comorbid posttraumatic stress disorder and alcohol use disorder: A randomized clinical trial. *JAMA Psychiatry, 76*(8), 791–799.

Okkels, N., Trabjerg, B., Arendt, M., & Pedersen, C. B. (2017). Traumatic stress disorders and risk of subsequent schizophrenia spectrum disorder or bipolar disorder: A nationwide cohort study. *Schizophrenia Bulletin, 43,* 180–186.

Ollendick, T. H., Jarrett, M. A., Grills-Taquechel, A. E., Hovey, L. D., & Wolff, J. C. (2008). Comorbidity as a predictor and moderator of treatment outcome in youth with anxiety, affective, attention deficit/hyperactivity disorder, and oppositional/conduct disorders. *Clinical Psychology Review, 28,* 1447–1471.

Otis, J. D., Keane, T. M., Kerns, R. D., Monson, C., & Scioli, E. (2009). The development of an integrated treatment for veterans with comorbid chronic pain and posttraumatic stress disorder. *Pain Medicine, 10,* 1300–1311.

Otto, M. W., Perlman, C. A., Wernicke, R., Reese, H. E., Bauer, M. S., & Pollack, M. H. (2004). Posttraumatic stress disorder in patients with bipolar disorder: A review of prevalence, correlates, and treatment strategies. *Bipolar Disorder, 6,* 470–479.

Pagura, J., Stein, M. B., Bolton, J. M., Cox, B. J., Grant, B., & Sareen, J. (2010). Comorbidity of borderline personality disorder and posttraumatic stress disorder in the U.S. population. *Journal of Psychiatric Research, 44,* 1190–1198.

Panagioti, M., Gooding, P. A., & Tarrier, N. (2012). Hopelessness, defeat, and entrapment in posttraumatic stress disorder: Their association with suicidal behavior and severity of depression. *Journal of Nervous and Mental Disease, 200*(8), 676–683.

Persson, A., Back, S. E., Killeen, T. K., Brady, K. T., Schwandt, M. L., Heilig, M., et al. (2017). Concurrent Treatment of PTSD and Substance Use Disorders Using Prolonged Exposure (COPE): A pilot study in alcohol-dependent women. *Journal of Addiction Medicine, 11*(2), 119–125.

Petrakis, I. L., Rosenheck, R., & Desai, R. (2011). Substance use comorbidity among veterans with posttraumatic stress disorder and other psychiatric illness. *American Journal on Addictions, 20*(3), 185–189.

Phelps, A., Steel, Z., Metcalf, O., Alkemade, N., Kerr, K., O'Donnell, M., et al. (2018). Key patterns and predictors of response to treatment for military veterans with post-traumatic stress disorder: A growth mixture modelling approach. *Psychological Medicine, 48*(1), 95–103.

Pietrzak, R. H., Goldstein, R. B., Southwick, S. M., & Grant, B. F. (2012). Psychiatric comorbidity of full and partial posttraumatic stress disorder among older adults in the United States: Results from Wave 2 of the National Epidemiologic Survey on Alcohol and Related Conditions. *American Journal of Geriatric Psychiatry, 20,* 380–390.

Richardson, J. D., Ketcheson, F., King, L., Shnaider, P., Marlborough, M., Thompson

A., et al. (2017). Psychiatric comorbidity pattern in treatment-seeking veterans. *Psychiatry Research, 258,* 488–493.

Roberts, N. P., Roberts, P. A., Jones, N., & Bisson, J. I. (2015). Psychological interventions for post-traumatic stress disorder and comorbid substance use disorder: A systematic review and meta-analysis. *Clinical Psychology Review, 38,* 25–38.

Rometsch-Ogioun El Sount, C., Windthorst, P., Denkinger, J., Ziser, K., Nikendei, C., & Junne, F. (2019). Chronic pain in refugees with posttraumatic stress disorder (PTSD): A systematic review on patients' characteristics and specific interventions. *Journal of Psychosomatic Research, 118,* 83–97.

Rosenberg, S. D., Mueser, K. T., Jankowski, M. K., Salyers, M. P., & Acker, K. (2004). Cognitive-behavioral treatment of posttraumatic stress disorder in severe mental illness: Results of a pilot study. *American Journal of Psychiatric Rehabilitation, 7,* 171–186.

Ruglass, L. M., Lopez-Castro, T., Papini, S., Killeen, T., Back, S. E., & Hien, D. A. (2017). Concurrent treatment with prolonged exposure for co-occurring full or subthreshold posttraumatic stress disorder and substance use disorders: A randomized clinical trial. *Psychotherapy and Psychosomatics, 86*(3), 150–161.

Rytwinski, N. K., Scur, M. D., Feeny, N. C., & Youngstrom, E. A. (2013). The co-occurrence of major depressive disorder among individuals with posttraumatic stress disorder: A meta-analysis. *Journal of Traumatic Stress, 26*(3), 299–309.

Sabella, D. (2012). PTSD among our returning veterans. *American Journal of Nursing, 112*(11), 48–52.

Schäfer, I., & Najavits, L. M. (2007). Clinical challenges in the treatment of patients with posttraumatic stress disorder and substance abuse. *Current Opinion in Psychiatry, 20,* 614–618.

Schwartz, A. C., Bradley, R., Penza, K. M., Sexton, M., Jay, D., Haggard, P. J., et al. (2006). Pain medication use among patients with posttraumatic stress disorder. *Psychosomatics, 47*(2), 136–142.

Seow, L. S. E., Ong, C., Mahesh, M. V., Sagayadevan, V., Shafie, S., Chong, S. A., et al. (2016). A systematic review on comorbid post-traumatic stress disorder in schizophrenia. *Schizophrenia Research, 176,* 441–451.

Sharp, T. J., & Harvey, A. G. (2001). Chronic pain and posttraumatic stress disorder: Mutual maintenance? *Clinical Psychology Review, 21,* 857–877.

Shevlin, M., Armour, C., Murphy, J., Houston, J. E., & Adamson, G. (2011). Evidence for a psychotic posttraumatic stress disorder subtype based on the National Comorbidity Survey. *Social Psychiatry and Psychiatric Epidemiology, 46,* 1069–1078.

Silverman, W. K., Ortiz, C. D., Viswesvaran, C., Burns, B. J., Kolko, D. J., Putnam, F. W., et al. (2008). Evidence-based psychosocial treatments for children and adolescents exposed to traumatic events. *Journal of Clinical Child and Adolescent Psychology, 37*(1), 156–183.

Simpson, T. L., Lehavot, K., & Petrakis, I. L. (2017). No wrong doors: Findings from a critical review of behavioral randomized clinical trials for individuals with co-occurring alcohol/drug problems and posttraumatic stress disorder. *Alcoholism: Clinical and Experimental Research, 41*(4), 681–702.

Spinazzola, J., Blaustein, M., & van der Kolk, B. A. (2005). Posttraumatic stress disorder treatment outcome research: The study of unrepresentative samples? *Journal of Traumatic Stress, 18,* 425–436.

Stahler, G. J., Mennis, J., & DuCette, J. P. (2016). Residential and outpatient treatment completion for substance use disorders in the U.S.: Moderation analysis by demographics and drug of choice. *Addictive Behaviors, 58,* 129–135.

Stander, V. A., Thomsen, C. J., & Highfill-McRoy, R. M. (2014). Etiology of depression comorbidity in combat-related PTSD: A review of the literature. *Clinical Psychology Review, 34,* 87–98.

Steel, C., Hardy, A., Smith, B., Wykes, T., Rose, S., Enright, S., et al. (2017). Cognitive behaviour therapy for posttraumatic stress in schizophrenia: A randomised controlled trial. *Psychological Medicine, 47,* 43–51.

Stein, M. B., Campbell-Sills, L., Gelernter, J., He, F., Heeringa, S. G., Nock, M. K., et al. (2017). Alcohol misuse and co-occurring mental disorders among new soldiers in the U.S. Army. *Alcoholism: Clinical and Experimental Research, 41*(1), 139–148.

Stergiopoulos, E., Cimo, A., Cheng, C., Bonato, S., & Dewa, C. S. (2011). Interventions to improve work outcomes in work-related PTSD: A systematic review. *BMC Public Health, 11,* 838–847.

Substance Abuse and Mental Health Services Administration. (2015). *Treatment Episode Data Set (TEDS): Discharges from substance abuse treatment services* (BHSIS Series S-81, HHS Publication No. [SMA] 16-4976). Rockville, MD: Author.

Substance Abuse and Mental Health Services Administration. (2016). National Survey on Drug Use and Health. In *National Survey on Drug Use and Health: Quality assessment of the 2002 to 2013 NSDUH public use files.* Rockville, MD: Author.

Szafranski, D. D., Gros, D. F., Acierno, R., Brady, K. T., Killeen, T. K., & Back, S. E. (2018). Heterogeneity of treatment dropout: PTSD, depression, and alcohol use disorder reductions in PTSD and AUD/SUD treatment noncompleters. *Clinical Psychology and Psychotherapy, 26,* 218–226.

Szafranski, D. D., Snead, A., Allan, N. P., Gros, D. F., Killeen, T., Flanagan, J., et al. (2017). Integrated, exposure-based treatment for PTSD and comorbid substance use disorders: Predictors of treatment dropout. *Addictive Behaviors, 73,* 30–35.

Taft, C. T., Creech, S. K., & Murphy, C. M. (2017). Anger and aggression in PTSD. *Current Opinion in Psychology, 14,* 67–71.

Teng, E. J., Hiatt, E. L., McClair, V., Kunik, M. E., Frueh, B. C., & Stanley, M. A. (2013). Efficacy of posttraumatic stress disorder treatment for comorbid panic disorder: A critical review and future directions for treatment research. *Clinical Psychology Science and Practice, 20,* 268–284.

Testa, M., & Livingston, J. A. (2009). Alcohol consumption and women's vulnerability to sexual victimization: Can reducing women's drinking prevent rape? *Substance Use and Misuse, 44*(9–10), 1349–1376.

Tsao, J. C. I., Mystkowski, J. L., Zucker, B. G., & Craske, M. G. (2005). Impact of cognitive-behavioural therapy for panic disorder on comorbidity: A controlled investigation. *Behaviour Research and Therapy, 43,* 959–970.

van Dam, D., Ehring, T., Vedel, E., & Emmelkamp, P. M. (2013). Trauma-focused treatment for posttraumatic stress disorder combined with CBT for severe substance use disorder: A randomized controlled trial. *BMC Psychiatry, 13*(1), 172.

van Dam, D., Vedel, E., Ehring, T., & Emmelkamp, P. M. G. (2012). Psychological treatments for concurrent posttraumatic stress disorder and substance use disorder: A systematic review. *Clinical Psychology Review, 32*(3), 202–214.

van den Berg, D. P. G., de Bont, P. A. J. M., van der Vleugel, B. M., de Roos, C., de Jongh, A., van Minnen, A., et al. (2015). Prolonged exposure versus eye movement desensitization and reprocessing versus waiting list for posttraumatic stress disorder in patients with a psychotic disorder. *JAMA Psychiatry, 72,* 259–267.

van den Berg, D. P., de Bont, P. A., van der Vleugel, B. M., de Roos, C., de Jonge, A., van Minnen, A., et al. (2016). Trauma-focused treatment in PTSD patients with psychosis: Symptom exacerbation, adverse events, and revictimization. *Schizophrenia Bulletin, 42,* 693–702.

van Minnen, A., Harned, M. S., Zoellner, L., & Mills, K. (2012). Examining potential contraindications for prolonged exposure therapy for PTSD. *European Journal of Psychotraumatology, 3,* 18805.

van Minnen, A., Zoellner, L. A., Harned, M. S., & Mills, K. (2015). Changes in comorbid conditions after prolonged exposure for PTSD: A literature review. *Current Psychiatry Reports, 17*(3), 549.

Varese, F., Smeets, F., Drukker, M., Lieverse, R., Lataster, T., Viechtbauer, W., et al. (2012). Childhood adversities increase the risk of psychosis: A meta-analysis of patient-control, prospective- and cross-sectional cohort studies. *Schizophrenia Bulletin, 38,* 661–671.

Vujanovic, A. A., Smith, L. J., Green, C. E., Lane, S. D., & Schmitz, J. M. (2018). Development of a novel, integrated cognitive-behavioral therapy for co-occurring posttraumatic stress and substance use disorders: A pilot randomized clinical trial. *Contemporary Clinical Trials, 65,* 123–129.

Vujanovic, A. A., Zvolensky, M. J., & Bernstein, A. (2008). Incremental associations between facets of anxiety sensitivity and posttraumatic stress and panic symptoms among trauma-exposed adults. *Cognitive Behaviour Therapy, 37*(2), 76–89.

Weiss, W. M., Murray, L. K., Zangana, G. A., Mahmooth, Z., Kaysen, D., Dorsey, S., et al. (2015). Community-based mental health treatments for survivors of torture and militant attacks in Southern Iraq: A randomized control trial. *BMC Psychiatry, 15,* 249.

Weisz, J. R., & Bearman, S. K. (2020). *Principle-guided psychotherapy for children and adolescents: The FIRST Program for Behavioral and Emotional Problems.* New York: Guilford Press.

Weisz, J. R., Bearman, S. K., Santucci, L. C., & Jensen-Doss, A. (2017). Initial test of a principle-guided approach to transdiagnostic psychotherapy with children and adolescents. *Journal of Clinical Child and Adolescent Psychology, 46*(1), 44–58.

Weisz, J. R., Chorpita, B. F., Palinkas, L. A., Schoenwald, S. K., Miranda, J., Bearman, S. K., et al. (2012). Testing standard and modular designs for psychotherapy treating depression, anxiety, and conduct problems in youth: A randomized effectiveness trial. *Archives of General Psychiatry, 69*(3), 274–282.

Widom, C. S., Schuck, A. M., & White, H. R. (2006). An examination of pathways from childhood victimization to violence: The role of early aggression and problematic alcohol use. *Violence and Victims, 21,* 675–690.

Zammit, S., Lewis, C., Dawson, S., Colley, H., McCann, H., Piekarski, A., et al. (2018). Undetected post-traumatic stress disorder in secondary-care mental health services: Systematic review. *British Journal of Psychiatry, 212*(1), 11–18.

CHAPTER 23

Building a Science of Personalized Interventions for PTSD

Marylene Cloitre, Zachary Cohen, and Ulrich Schnyder

This chapter is dedicated to exploring "next steps" in improving treatment outcomes for people with posttraumatic stress disorder (PTSD). Over the past decade, there has been growing attention to the development of *personalized interventions* to improve treatment response rates. Personalized interventions consider at least three factors for the refinement and tailoring of treatment: the individual patient, his or her specific problem, and the particular set of circumstances under which the individual is treated. This idea was proposed by psychotherapy researchers over a half-century ago (e.g., Luborsky, Crits-Christoph, Mintz, & Auerbach, 1988; Paul, 1967), but the methodological and statistical means by which to reach this goal were lacking. More recently, there have been advances in the conceptualization of personalized interventions along with advances in research and analytic methods that are likely to allow this goal to be realized.

This chapter reviews several evolving strategies for personalizing mental health interventions that are relevant to the treatment of PTSD. These include adaptation of treatments for specific populations and environments, modular therapies, sequential multiple assignment randomized trials (SMART), and individualized metrics. We also report on the literature regarding personalized treatments in the context of neurobiological findings.

Therapies Adapted for Specific Populations and Environments

The most common example of adaptations of evidence-based therapies (EBTs) lies in their application to different cultures. Because most EBTs have been developed and tested mainly with Caucasian and Western samples, the concepts and examples used in the treatments may not be relevant to and are potentially discordant with other cultures. Adaptations may involve not only a translation to a different language but also reformulation of the treatment to attend to culturally relevant trauma-related experiences and concepts as well as reformulation of the interventions themselves so that the treatment is consistent with the patient's experience and perspective (Bernal, Jimenez-Chafey, & Domenech Rodriguez, 2009; Hinton, Field, Nickerson, Bryant, & Simon, 2013).

To date, most adaptations have been developed for culturally distinct subgroups of a population of interest. The process by which adaptations are made typically involves collaboration with providers, patients, and community stakeholders to assess the content validity of the treatment, to revise the treatment, and to engage in iterative modifications throughout the initial delivery of the protocol (Dixon, Ahles, & Marques, 2016; Hinton, Rivera, Hofmann, Barlow, & Otto, 2012).

The most conservative study design assesses whether the cultural adaptation of the protocol confers added benefit relative to the standard approach. Evaluations using this type of design with regard to adaptations of cognitive-behavioral therapy (CBT) for Latino populations in the United States have found mixed results, with benefit associated only with some adaptations depending on the specific treatment, type of problem, and strength of identification with the subculture (Ng & Weisz, 2016). The results thus far suggest that culturally sensitive perceptions of mental health disturbances as well as their solutions vary from subgroup to subgroup and from culture to culture, indicating the importance of utilizing qualitative data derived from multiple sources to formulate adaptations and of developing reliable means by which to make generalizations (see Riggs et al., Chapter 24, this volume, on implementation science).

Several recent studies of traumatized populations have described collaborative processes between researchers and stakeholders who represent minority populations or cultures different from the researchers to develop more appropriate and effective engagement strategies, assessment measures, and therapies (e.g., Kaysen et al., 2013; Tay & Silove, 2017; Valentine, Dixon, Borba, Shtasel, & Marques, 2016), providing good examples of implementation science principles. Clinical trials have evaluated the feasibility and efficacy of adapted cognitive-behavioral therapies relative to wait list or treatment as usual in several non-Western cultures. Probably the most well-studied intervention used in non-Western settings is narrative exposure therapy (NET). NET was initially developed by Western clinician-researchers mainly using "Western" cognitive-behavioral concepts to address PTSD in African refugees. A number of randomized controlled trials (RCTs) have successfully been conducted in a variety of cultural settings, demonstrating NET's effectiveness in both Western and non-Western countries (e.g., Hijazi et al., 2014; Neuner, Schauer, Klaschik, Karunakara, & Elbert, 2004; Neuner et al., 2008).

At least three adaptations of cognitive processing therapy (CPT) have been tested in RCT designs (Bass et al., 2013; Bolton et al., 2014; Weiss et al.,

2015). As an example of the adaptation of CPT for the Kurdish population in Iraq, initial review indicated that two traditional CPT themes considered related to trauma, impact on *self-esteem* and *intimacy*, did not have a direct translation in the Kurdish language, so alternative themes of *respect* and *caring* were identified and used in the treatment. The adapted version of CPT was found to show moderate to strong effect sizes relative to wait list on depression, posttraumatic stress symptoms, and dysfunction (Bolton et al., 2014). A similar process of adaptation has been applied to trauma-focused cognitive-behavioral therapy (TF-CBT) for delivery to Congolese female adolescent victims of sexual violence. Adaptations included the use of familiar games and songs to convey concepts and visits to the girls' guardians, with the goal of reducing the family's perception of stigma and fostering family acceptance of and reconnection with the victim. Results of an RCT comparing TF-CBT to wait list found that the treatment group reported significant reductions in trauma symptoms and increased prosocial behavior (O'Callaghan, McMullen, Shannon, Rafferty, & Black, 2013). Both of these studies indicate that an evidence-based treatment can successfully be adapted to very different cultures. There have been several other evidence-based interventions that demonstrated successful adaptation to other cultures, including an open trial of eye movement desensitization and reprocessing (EMDR) therapy in the Congo (Allon, 2015) and behavioral activation treatment for depression among Kurds in Northern Iraq (Bolton et al., 2014).

Several questions can be posed when considering the adaptation of evidence-based treatments across different environments. With regard to any treatment, one might ask how much a specific therapy can be adapted and still be considered the same treatment, or how many changes can be made to a protocol before it becomes unrecognizable and evolves into another treatment. These types of questions highlight the need for caution regarding assumptions that the benefits in an adapted version will be similar to those of the established protocol. If an established treatment is substantially changed, the empirical evidence that provided the rationale for the application of the treatment to the new population may no longer provide a credible basis for predictions of beneficial outcomes. An alternative approach may be to identify the key common elements of effective trauma treatments (see Schnyder et al., 2015) and to develop treatments based on general principles of recovery instantiated in the language, idioms, beliefs, and behaviors of the specific culture or population.

Modular Therapies

Modular therapies describe psychotherapies in which evidence-based modules known to address and resolve specific problems are selected and organized to create a treatment plan tailored to a particular patient's most significant symptoms and concerns. This approach reduces the risk of including interventions and concepts that are not particularly relevant to the individual patient, potentially leading to greater willingness to engage in treatment, better treatment attendance, increased use of interventions, and ultimately better outcomes. The approach is particularly attractive considering the potential heterogeneity of the symptom profiles of patients diagnosed with DSM-5 PTSD or alternatively diagnosed with either PTSD or complex PTSD (CPTSD) as delineated in the 11th revision of the *International Classification of Diseases and Related Health Problems* (ICD-11). Moreover, it could be helpful in creating a streamlined treatment plan that is inclusive of the common comorbid symptoms and disorders, such as depression, chronic pain, and substance use. Thus, a modular therapy is an approach that can be conceptualized as an efficient and effective way to address all and only the problems presented by a particular patient.

Current treatment protocols offer a standardized sequence of interventions, with treatment generally focusing on processing of the trauma memory (e.g., CPT, NET, prolonged exposure [PE], cognitive therapy for PTSD [CT-PTSD]). Other therapies present or include resource-building interventions, such as social support enhancements, relationship strengthening, and emotion regulation interventions (e.g., brief eclectic psychotherapy for PTSD [BEPP], EMDR therapy, interpersonal therapy [IPT], skills training in affective and interpersonal regulation [STAIR] narrative therapy), and still others that have been identified as relevant to commonly occurring comorbidities, such as behavioral activation for depression, biofeedback for chronic pain, and relapse prevention for substance use. In addition, the introduction or integration of other types of interventions like medication, mindfulness, or psychodynamic interventions can be considered. The specific interventions or series of interventions to be selected for investigating a modular therapy approach remain to be considered and may vary as different researchers use protocols with which they are experienced as the reference or standard treatment to which the modularized treatment will be compared.

The infrastructure supporting the implementation of flexible modular therapies typically includes assessment measures and decision-making flowcharts (Chorpita & Weisz, 2009). The therapist and patient collaborate to review the initial assessment results and to identify the primary problem; this information is used, in turn, to select a module or series of modules for the treatment plan. A critical aspect of the work is regular symptom assessment, identifying progress made on target symptoms. The results of these assessments guide next-step decision making about whether to repeat the module, go on to the next planned module, or revise plans for the next module if the secondary symptoms have resolved or new symptoms or problems have emerged.

Relevant to this discussion is consideration of the potential benefits of the flexible multimodular treatment approach broadly conceived and evidence for its success. In studies of child and adolescent mental health programming, the flexible sequencing of self-contained modules has been demonstrated to be more effective compared to the use of full protocols for a single disorder (Daleiden, Chorpita, Donkervoet, Arensdorf, & Brogan,

2006) or to the sequencing of full protocols for different disorders (Weisz et al., 2012). There are no published data regarding patient preferences or administrator preferences between protocol-driven versus modular selection in PTSD. However, treatment duration for modular as compared to standard protocols tends to be shorter, suggesting greater benefit for the patient with regard to time commitment and potentially for the health care system in terms of staff resources and clinician time (Weisz et al., 2012). Lastly, clinicians report more positive attitudes about adopting modular therapies compared to standard protocol therapies (Borntrager, Chorpita, Higa-McMillan, & Weisz, 2009; Chorpita et al., 2015), suggesting the potential for greater ease of adoption and dissemination and uptake of these evidence-based interventions. Demonstration of the feasibility, effectiveness, and satisfaction associated with the flexible modular approach suggests its potential for PTSD patients and value in future research.

Sequential Multiple Assignment Randomized Trial Designs

Research to date on modular therapies has been structured so that the formulation of the treatment to be implemented is generally made at the initial assessment following a flowchart, with the selection of the modules and their sequence having been predetermined. The assessment of interest occurs at the end of the trial (posttreatment and at follow-up) to determine if the modular treatment outcome is superior to a standard treatment. An alternative approach is a sequential multiple assignment randomized trial (SMART; Collins, Murphy, & Strecher, 2007; Lei, Nahum-Shani, Lynch, Oslin, & Murphy, 2012; Murphy, 2005). In SMART designs, assessments critical to the process and outcome of a study are conducted at several points across the treatment, there are repeated randomizations into alternative interventions based on the periodic assessment results, and the comparator treatment is not an established standard but another multiple randomization sequence. SMART designs are useful when no established standard treatment exists and empirical and/or theoretical guides are not available to create hypotheses about a preferred treatment approach. SMART designs are not tests of adapted treatments but are used to inform the development of adaptive treatments, which then can be compared to standard treatments.

To provide a relevant example from the PTSD literature, it is known that Web-based PTSD programs have better outcomes when there is some level of therapist involvement, but studies had varied widely regarding the number of sessions and amount of time that therapists have engaged with patients (Olthuis et al., 2016). To gather information about the relative benefits of differing amounts of therapist support, a SMART trial could be designed such that the amount of therapist involvement is adjusted systematically from lower to higher amounts contingent on the results of periodic assessments. This approach would provide answers to many more questions and much more quickly compared to RCTs, which are highly controlled and do not propose contingency-based changes for individual participants across the course of treatment. In SMART designs, there are typically at least two stages, each with its own randomization procedure, hypotheses, and outcome evaluation. In this investigation, for example, Stage 1 participants are randomized into either a no-therapist Web-based treatment condition (nWBT) or a biweekly therapist-supported (bWBT) condition. After 6 weeks, each participant is classified as a responder or nonresponder (e.g., someone who has experienced less than a 10-point drop in his or her PTSD score). Stage 2 is the initiation phase where responders continue in their assigned condition while the nonresponders in each condition are rerandomized. In the nWBT condition, nonresponders are randomly assigned to either biweekly or weekly Web-based treatment (bWBT or wWBT). In the original bWBT, nonreponders are assigned to weekly WBT or weekly WBT with an additional phone call as needed (wWBT or w + WBT). The trial is completed at the end of a second 6 weeks.

This design allows comparison of the two first-stage treatments, nWBT and bWBT, with regard to their nonresponse rates at the 6th week as well as the differential benefit observed among the responders at both the 6th and 12th weeks. It also tests four adaptive interventions in the second stage (or randomization) of the trial. Determination of the relative benefits of one adaptation over another can be assessed by comparing outcomes of the pair of adaptations to which nonresponders have been randomized (bWBT vs. wWBT, wWBT vs. w + WBT) and as relative to the initial responders.

This type of design can be applied to explore several other types of treatment questions. For example, the first phase of a SMART RCT might compare a trauma-focused (TF) versus non-trauma-focused (NTF) treatment. At the end of this phase, nonresponders in each condition would be randomized again, where, for example, nonresponders to TF receive either more TF or switch to an NTF, while nonresponders to NTF might either obtain more NTF or switch to TF. Similarly, two different medications might be tested in the first randomization phase, and in the second phase, nonresponders could be randomized to an increased dose of the same medication or a switch to another drug. In both of these examples, the relative efficacy of two treatments is being assessed in the first randomization, the relative proportion of nonresponders is being identified, and preliminary data regarding options for nonresponders are being obtained.

Treatment Selection

One of the most common approaches to personalized mental health is treatment selection, defined as using patient factors to identify the optimal intervention for an individual among a set of available treatments (see Cohen & DeRubeis, 2018, for an extensive review).

Historically, treatment selection in mental health and in medicine more broadly has been practiced through the use of diagnoses. Patients are given a diagnosis to identify an appropriate and effective treatment. The strategy of identifying which treatments are helpful for specific disorders has been formalized in several ways, including efforts to define empirically supported treatments (ESTs) (Chambless & Hollon, 1998). However, for most mental health disorders, multiple evidence-based treatments exist, and there are relatively few contexts in which a single specific treatment has been identified as superior to all others and other factors have been investigated.

Patient preference is one. This is appropriate, not only because it respects the patient's autonomy and dignity, but also due to the assumed relationship between a patient's preference and his or her willingness to initiate and engage with (or adhere to) a preferred treatment relative to a non-preferred treatment. To date, the relationship between patient preference and actual treatment outcomes is unclear, and it likely varies as a function of myriad contextual factors (e.g., patient's understanding of or exposure to the options; the necessity of the patient's active participation and commitment). In the clinical trials that have examined this association, researchers have reported results that are positive, negative, and equivocal (Cohen & DeRubeis, 2018). Regardless, practice guidelines are clear that respecting patient preference is an essential part of ethical clinical practice.

Clinician judgment also plays a significant role in treatment selection (Cohen & DeRubeis, 2018). Clinicians who attend to information about a specific patient's presentation can generate hypotheses about the patient's expected response to a given treatment (Lorenzo-Luaces, DeRubeis, & Bennett, 2015). For example, Raza and Holohan (2015) surveyed Veterans Affairs clinicians in the United States who had been trained in both CPT and prolonged exposure (PE) with regard to patient variables that they believed might inform the decision between CPT, PE, or alternative treatments. CPT was selected over PE for patients with strong guilt, strong shame, acts of perpetration, and dissociation history, whereas PE was preferred to CPT for patients with low literacy, low cognitive functioning, and moderate/severe traumatic brain injury. However, it should be noted that there is not an evidence base to support these selection criteria to date, and it is uncertain whether these are factors to which clinicians and patients should attend. Additionally, the complexity of the decision-making process in the context of numerous distinct factors suggests that there are opportunities for data-driven, multivariable prediction models to help inform the treatment selection process.

Individualized Metrics

Early research efforts to discover what works for whom largely revolved around subgroup analyses, in which differences between distinct subgroups (e.g., men vs. women, older vs. younger individuals, presence or absence of a history of childhood abuse) were examined. When these differences were detected and determined to be statistically significant, researchers would claim they had identified a potential moderator, meaning that a variable had been identified that was associated with differential response across different treatments. These factors have been labeled "prescriptive" variables. Statistically, this relationship was often detected[1] when predicting treatment response in the form of an interaction between a predictor variable and the treatment term (sometimes described as an "aptitude-by-treatment" interaction). These interactions could be "ordinal," which in subgroup analyses implies that the difference between expected treatment response exists in one subgroup but not the other (e.g., Treatment A is better than Treatment B for men, but no difference is expected between the two treatments for women). They could also be "disordinal," involving a full crossover effect (e.g., Treatment A is better than Treatment B for older individuals, and Treatment B is better than Treatment A for younger individuals). For example, Rizvi, Vogt, and Resick (2009) identified age as a disordinal prescriptive factor in an RCT comparing PE to CPT: older women had better outcomes in PE versus CPT and younger women had better outcomes in CPT relative to PE.

The more common and easily detected effects are prognostic. Prognostic variables are those for which associations with outcome exist either irrespective of treatment or for which the relationship is only known for a single treatment.[2] A prognostic relationship can be identified if a variable has been shown to predict treatment response in the same way across multiple treatments; for example, in an RCT comparing PE and CPT, Rizvi and colleagues (2009) found that, regardless of the treatment to which the women were randomized, those with higher pretreatment depression and guilt experienced larger improvements in PTSD symptoms than those with lower depression and guilt. Alternatively, when a predictive relationship is identified through the investigation of data from a sample of individuals in which everyone was provided with the same treatment, that relationship is also said to be prognostic. Importantly, prognostic relationships of this final type should not be *assumed* to provide information about what treatment an individual ought to

---

[1]It is important to note that prescriptive interaction effects can only be truly detected when data from two or more treatments are examined (Cohen & DeRubeis, 2018).

[2]It should be noted that although variables are often described as "being" prescriptive or prognostic, a given factor can have a prognostic relationship with outcome in one context and a prescriptive relationship in another. For example, if a study comparing Treatment A versus Treatment B found that individuals' levels on factor X had the same association with posttreatment outcome across both treatments, it would be accurate to describe factor X as prognostic in that study. However, an analysis of a separate study comparing Treatment A versus Treatment C might find that factor X predicted a differential response between those two treatments, and those authors would be justified in concluding that factor X was a prescriptive variable in their data. Both sets of authors would be correct.

receive. It is tempting to infer that a patient with a poor prognosis in a given treatment should be directed to seek an alternative. However, a patient who has a poor predicted outcome for a given treatment based on a prognostic model might be expected to have an equally poor or even worse response to an alternative treatment.

Despite the multitude of studies examining patient-specific characteristics of treatment outcomes in depression, anxiety, and to some extent PTSD, the uptake by clinicians has been minimal at best, due in part to the paucity of successful replications of the findings. For example, individual variables such as childhood abuse, depression, dissociation, and severity of symptoms that have been found to predict outcomes in some studies have been tested and not found predictive in others (see Cloitre, Petkova, Su, & Weiss, 2016, for a review). These conflicting results likely have many sources, including small sample sizes, inconsistent statistical methodology, treatment and sample heterogeniety, and weak effects of individual predictor variables (Cohen & DeRubeis, 2018).

Multivariable Prediction Models

Over the last decade, several different solutions for data-driven, evidence-based treatment selection have been described, including Kraemer's (2013) "M*" approach; Petkova, Tarpey, Su, and Ogden's (2016) composite moderator approach; and DeRubeis and colleagues' (2014) Personalized Advantage Index (PAI) approach. What these approaches have in common is their application of statistical modeling in longitudinal treatment datasets (that comprise pretreatment or baseline variables and posttreatment outcome data) to capture simultaneously the predictive signal from multiple prescriptive variables. By aggregating the effects of many small but reliable moderators, these approaches generate recommendations that could lead to clinically significant differences in patient outcomes.

The composite moderator approach has been used to assess treatment outcome in PTSD. Through this data-driven approach, Cloitre and colleagues (2016) identified patient characteristics that predicted differential outcome in three multimodular treatment conditions depending on the interventions included in the sequence. The three conditions included STAIR narrative therapy, a two-module treatment in which a skills module was followed by a trauma-focused module (the test condition) and two comparator treatments in which the content of each module was replaced by a nonspecific active comparator, present-centered therapy (PCT; called "supportive counseling" in the study). The two comparators resulted in a delivery of a predominantly trauma-focused therapy (PCT plus narrative therapy) and a predominantly skills-focused therapy (STAIR plus PCT). The moderator that most strongly differentiated outcomes was a ratio of patient burden (PTSD, depression, dissociation, interpersonal problems, and anger) relative to a patient strength (emotion regulation capacity). The participants in the STAIR narrative therapy condition showed the best outcomes regardless of ratio. However, participants with a low ratio of symptom severity relative to emotion regulation had better outcomes in the trauma-focused therapy than in the skills-focused treatment, whereas those with a high ratio of symptom severity relative to emotion regulation had better outcomes in the skills-focused treatment. If replicated, these results could be used to match patients with treatments whereby some patients would receive a trauma-focused treatment and others a skills-based or non-trauma-focused treatment based on a ratio identifying their symptom burden relative to strengths. This variable (a ratio of symptom burden to patient strengths) is an example of a prescriptive variable.

Another treatment selection approach that has been applied to PTSD is DeRubeis and colleagues' (2014) PAI approach. Using data from a study comparing CPT to PE in women with rape trauma PTSD, Keefe and colleagues (2018) identified four moderators that predicted differential risk of dropout between the two treatments: childhood physical abuse, current relationship conflict, anger, and race. All individuals in the study were randomized to either CPT or PE, which did not differ in their dropout rates. After creating a logistic regression model that tracked the interactions between all four variables and treatment, the risk of dropout for each individual in both conditions could be predicted, and the treatment associated with the highest likelihood of treatment completion identified. Patients who received their PAI-indicated treatment had a significantly lower dropout rate (19.7%) compared to those who received their nonindicated treatment (40.5%). If replicated, these findings combined with models designed to maximize symptom reduction could be used to minimize treatment dropout by helping match patients to the treatment most likely to result in treatment completion.

Prognostic models have also demonstrated potential utility for treatment selection when deciding between treatments that are not equivalent in their average treatment effect. Following the approach described by Lorenzo-Luaces, DeRubeis, van Straten, and Tiemens (2017), Wiltsey Stirman and colleagues (2020) constructed a single prognostic model for a combined sample of individuals with PTSD treated with either PE or PCT. They found that the patients with good prognoses who were randomized to receive PE experienced significantly more improvement than patients with good prognoses who received PCT, whereas patients with poor prognoses showed little to no advantage when receiving PE versus PCT. The patients predicted to have poor prognoses were those with higher symptom severity or case complexity, including worse mental and physical functioning, the presence of military sexual trauma, longer time since the trauma, and lower endorsement of treatment credibility. If replicated, these and other models could be used to inform the collaborative decision-making processing by which clinicians and patients determine the best path toward recovery from PTSD.

Nevertheless, one important criticism of these efforts is that the sample sizes available in the RCT datasets that have been used have been insufficient for the purpose of modeling interaction effects (Luedtke, Sadikova, & Kessler, 2019). This has led to recent proposals of alternative modeling approaches for informing treatment selection, including the use of prognostic models.

One solution proposed by Kessler, Bossarte, Luedtke, Zaslavsky, and Zubizarreta (2019) allows for researchers to move iteratively between more exploratory analyses using larger, inexpensive archival datasets and more controlled tests of precision medicine models in smaller clinical trial datasets that can accommodate more extensive measurement. A second solution (Kessler et al., 2017) is to construct independent prognostic models within each condition, and to then infer treatment recommendations by comparing the predictions for each treatment generated by the separate models. Deisenhofer and colleagues (2018) demonstrated this approach in a sample of individuals receiving TF-CBT or EMDR therapy for PTSD. Age, employment status, gender, and functional impairment were identified as predicting treatment response among the people receiving TF-CBT, and those four variables were used to construct a prognostic model for TF-CBT. A separate prognostic model that relied on only baseline depression and antidepressant prescription was constructed using data from the subset of the sample who received EMDR therapy. A new individual's values on the relevant factors would be fed into each prognostic model, thus generating separate predictions of treatment response from the two prognostic models (TF-CBT or EMDR therapy), and the recommended treatment would be identified by whichever treatment was predicted to lead to a better outcome.

Neurobiological Findings

Since the Institute of Medicine (2011) call for precision medicine specified for the development of personalized treatment strategies for mental disorders, research methodologies have been suggested to promote such development (Leon, 2011; Soliman, Aboharb, Zeltner, & Studer, 2017), with genetics (Smoller, 2014; Sullivan et al., 2018) and neuroimaging (Etkin, 2014) at the forefront. Genetic and epigenetic factors, and neuroimaging as well as neuroimmunological findings have made substantial contributions to the development of therapeutic algorithms that identify treatments likely to provide good outcome depending on patient characteristics. This approach has been applied successfully in various medical disciplines for a number of years, for example, in areas such as oncology (Bristow et al., 2018; Janiaud, Serghiou, & Ioannidis, 2019), guiding the therapeutic decision making of surgeons, medical oncologists, and radio-oncologists.

In mental health, personalized medicine appears to be in its infancy (Cohen & DeRubeis 2018; Ng & Weisz, 2016). The search for endophenotypes for major depression has long been suggested (Hasler, Drevets, Manji, & Charney, 2004). However, as Hellhammer, Meinlschmidt, and Pruessner (2018) pointed out in a recent review, "Psychobiological research has generated a tremendous amount of findings on the psychological, neuroen-docrine, molecular and environmental processes that are directly relevant for mental and physical health, but have overwhelmed our capacity to mean-ingfully absorb, integrate, and utilize this knowledge base" (p. 147).

In mood disorders, some progress has been made with regard to psy-chosocial risk factors as well as genetic and epigenetic factors, and neuroim-aging findings (Prendes-Alvarez & Nemeroff, 2018). For instance, increased gray matter density in the right inferior frontal gyrus (rIFG) was identified as a potential biomarker of bipolar disorder (Alda & Manchia, 2018). Further-more, greater pretreatment ventral and pregenual anterior cingulate cortex (ACC) activation may predict better antidepressant medication outcome but poorer psychotherapy outcome (Ball, Stein, & Paulus, 2014). In the field of anxiety disorders, only a few biological moderators of treatment outcome across disorders were identified (Schneider, Arch, & Wolitzky-Taylor, 2015). Again, genetics and neuroimaging seem to emerge as the most promising areas of research (Casey & Lee, 2015). As in depression, the ACC appears to play an important role (Ball et al., 2014).

In the area of trauma-related disorders, specifically PTSD, the literature to date on biological moderators of treatment outcome is even more scarce, and the majority of studies appear to suffer from methodological limita-tions (Schneider et al., 2015). Smoller (2016) emphasized the role of gene–environment interactions and the fact that stress-related disorders are poly-genic. Moreover, there appears to be genetic overlap among stress-related disorders including PTSD, major depressive disorder, and anxiety disorders.

Large-scale genome-wide association studies, epigenome-wide associa-tion studies, and other genomic analyses have demonstrated that the devel-opment of PTSD is strongly influenced by genetic and epigenetic factors. The Psychiatric Genomics Consortium PTSD Workgroup led by Karestan Koenen (Nievergelt et al., 2018) took a systematic approach to developing new knowledge about the genetic underpinnings of PTSD, using large datasets, up-to-date technologies, and novel analytic methodologies. For example, the consortium found that childhood trauma exposure and lifetime PTSD sever-ity are associated with accelerated DNA methylation age (Wolf et al., 2018). However, studies looking into genetic or epigenetic predictors of treatment outcome are still scarce. In a small pilot study of PE therapy with combat veterans suffering from PTSD, methylation of the GR gene (NR3C1) exon 1F promoter assessed at pretreatment predicted treatment outcome (Yehuda et al., 2013). More recently, Pape and colleagues (2018) identified pretreatment NR3C1 methylation levels as a potential marker to predict PTSD treatment outcome, independent of the type of therapy.

With regard to neuroimaging markers, the subgenual anterior cingulate cortex (sgACC), default mode network, and salience network seem to play an important role as outcome predictors of transcranial magnetic stimulation for PTSD (Philip et al., 2018).

Shvil, Rusch, Sullivan, and Neria (2013) reviewed neural, psychophysiological, and behavioral markers of fear processing in PTSD. It remains to be studied, however, to what degree markers of fear processing, such as hyperactivation of the amygdala, dorsal ACC, and insula, and hypoactivation in other brain areas, turn out to be sufficiently robust treatment outcome markers as well. The same applies to psychophysiological variables such as startle response, heart rate variability, or skin conductance response. In a recent small psychotherapy outcome study of a combination of CBT for substance use disorder with CPT for PTSD, Soder and colleagues (2019) identified baseline resting heart rate variability as a possible biomarker predicting PTSD treatment outcomes in adults with co-occurring substance use disorder and PTSD. The authors concluded that patients with poorer autonomic emotional regulation, as reflected by low heart rate variability, may not respond as well to psychotherapy in general.

Taken together, there is an emerging body of literature on putative biomarkers that might be used as predictors of PTSD treatment outcome. It can be expected that in the future, such biomarkers will be used to develop personalized treatment strategies for people with PTSD, and to inform collaborative processes of joint decision making among therapists and their patients. At this point in time, however, the development of therapeutic algorithms to optimize clinical outcomes of empirically supported therapies has a limited evidence base.

Conclusions

The goal of personalized therapy research is to generate a body of knowledge that will translate to clinical services such that therapists will be able to provide the most effective treatment in the most efficient manner to every patient based on their individual symptoms, characteristics, and preferences. This chapter has identified some of the conceptual and methodological building blocks that are contributing to the development of a science of personalized intervention. These include study designs that involve the systematic adaptation of treatments for specific populations, evaluation of flexible sequencing of modular interventions, and SMART designs that allow for the rapid testing and identification of adaptations likely to succeed. The building blocks also include statistical strategies and computer power that can analyze vast amounts of data to provide reliable information about which psychological, social, or genetic and other neurobiological characteristics are associated with what types of outcomes in which treatments, facilitating a match of patient to treatment to optimize outcome. Hopefully, these building blocks of treatment designs and statistical analyses can be productively stacked together to advance science and provide answers to the question that has long been asked: *What works for whom?* If successful, personalized intervention science will provide a research and treatment pathway that will markedly alter the nature of mental health care services.

REFERENCES

Alda, M., & Manchia, M. (2018). Personalized management of bipolar disorder. *Neuroscience Letters, 669*, 3–9.

Allon, M. (2015). EMDR group therapy with women who were sexually assaulted in the Congo. *Journal of EMDR Practice and Research, 9*, 28–34.

Ball, T. M., Stein, M. B., & Paulus, M. P. (2014). Toward the application of functional neuroimaging to individualized treatment for anxiety and depression. *Depression and Anxiety, 31*, 920–933.

Bass, J. K., Annan, J., McIvor Murray, S., Kaysen, D., Griffin, S., Cetinoglu, T., et al. (2013). Controlled trial of psychotherapy for Congolese survivors of sexual violence. *New England Journal of Medicine, 368*, 2182–2191.

Bernal, G., Jimenez-Chafey, M. I., & Domenech Rodríguez, M. M. (2009). Cultural adaptation of treatments: A resource for considering culture in evidence-based practice. *Professional Psychology: Research and Practice, 40*, 361–368.

Bolton, P., Bass, J. K., Zangana, G. A. S., Kamal, T., Murray, S. M., Kaysen, D., et al. (2014). A randomized controlled trial of mental health interventions for survivors of systematic violence in Kurdistan, Northern Iraq. *BMC Psychiatry, 14*, 360.

Borntrager, C. F., Chorpita, B. F., Higa-McMillan, C., & Weisz, J. R. (2009). Provider attitudes toward evidence-based practices: Are the concerns with the evidence or with the manuals? *Psychiatric Services, 60*, 677–681.

Bristow, R. G., Alexander, B., Baumann, M., Bratman, S. V., Brown, J. M., Camphausen, K., et al. (2018). Combining precision radiotherapy with molecular targeting and immunomodulatory agents: A guideline by the American Society for Radiation Oncology. *Lancet Oncology, 19*, e240–e251.

Casey, B. J., & Lee, F. S. (2015). Optimizing treatments for anxiety by age and genetics. *Annals of the New York Academy of Sciences, 1345*, 16–24.

Chambless, D. L., & Hollon, S. D. (1998). Defining empirically supported therapies. *Journal of Consulting and Clinical Psychology, 66*(1), 7.

Chorpita, B. F., Park, A., Tsai, K., Korathu-Larson, P., Higa-McMillan, C. K., Nakamura, B. J., et al. (2015). Balancing effectiveness with responsiveness: Therapist satisfaction across different treatment designs in the Child STEPs randomized effectiveness trial. *Journal of Consulting and Clinical Psychology, 83*, 709–718.

Chorpita, B. F., & Weisz, J. R. (2009). *MATCH-ADTC: Modular approach to therapy for children with anxiety, depression, trauma, or conduct problems*. Satellite Beach, FL: PracticeWise.

Cloitre, M., Petkova, E., Su, Z., & Weiss, B. (2016). Patient characteristics as a moderator of post-traumatic stress disorder treatment outcome: Combining symptom burden and strengths. *British Journal of Psychiatry Open, 2*, 101–106.

Cohen, Z. D., & DeRubeis, R. J. (2018). Treatment selection in depression. *Annual Review of Clinical Psychology, 14*, 15.1–15.28.

Collins, L. M., Murphy, S. A., & Strecher, V. (2007). The multiphase optimization strategy (MOST) and the sequential multiple assignment randomized trial

(SMART): New methods for more potent eHealth interventions. *American Journal of Preventive Medicine, 32*(5), S112–S118.

Daleiden, E. L., Chorpita, B. F., Donkervoet, C., Arensdorf, A. M., & Brogan, M. (2006). Getting better at getting them better: Health outcomes and evidence-based practice within a system of care. *Journal of the American Academy of Child and Adolescent Psychiatry, 45,* 749–756.

Deisenhofer, A. K., Delgadillo, J., Rubel, J. A., Böhnke, J. R., Zimmermann, D., Schwartz, B., et al. (2018). Individual treatment selection for patients with post-traumatic stress disorder. *Depression and Anxiety, 35,* 541–550.

DeRubeis, R. J., Cohen, Z. D., Forand, N. R., Fournier, J. C., Gelfand, L. A., & Lorenzo-Luaces, L. (2014). The Personalized Advantage Index: Translating research on prediction into individualized treatment recommendations. A demonstration. *PLOS ONE, 9*(1), e83875.

Dixon, L. E., Ahles, E., & Marques, L. (2016). Treating posttraumatic stress disorder in diverse settings: Recent advances and challenges for the future. *Current Psychiatry Reports, 18,* 108.

Etkin, A. (2014). Neuroimaging and the future of personalized treatment in psychiatry. *Depression and Anxiety, 31,* 899–901.

Hasler, G., Drevets, W. C., Manji, H., & Charney, D. S. (2004). Discovering endophenotypes for major depression. *Neuropsychopharmacology, 29,* 1765–1781.

Hellhammer, D., Meinlschmidt, G., & Pruessner, J. C. (2018). Conceptual endophenotypes: A strategy to advance the impact of psychoneuroendocrinology in precision medicine. *Psychoneuroendocrinology, 89,* 147–160.

Hijazi, A. M., Lumley, M. A., Ziadni, M. S., Haddad, L., Rapport, L. J., & Arnetz, B. B. (2014). Brief narrative exposure therapy for posttraumatic stress in Iraqi refugees: A preliminary randomized clinical trial. *Journal of Traumatic Stress, 27,* 314–322.

Hinton, D. E., Field, N. P., Nickerson, A., Bryant, R. A., & Simon, N. (2013). Dreams of the dead among Cambodian refugees: Frequency, phenomenology, and relationship to complicated grief and posttraumatic stress disorder. *Death Studies, 37,* 750–767.

Hinton, D. E., Rivera, E. I., Hofmann, S. G., Barlow, D. H., & Otto, M. W. (2012). Adapting CBT for traumatized refugees and ethnic minority patients: Examples from culturally adapted CBT (CA-CBT). *Transcultural Psychiatry, 49,* 340–365.

Institute of Medicine. (2011). *Toward precision medicine: Building a knowledge network for biomedical research and a new taxonomy of disease.* Washington, DC: National Academies Press.

Janiaud, P., Serghiou, S., & Ioannidis, J. P. A. (2019). New clinical trial designs in the era of precision medicine: An overview of definitions, strengths, weaknesses, and current use in oncology. *Cancer Treatment Review, 73,* 20–30.

Kaysen, D., Lindgren, K., Zangana, G. A. S., Murray, L., Bass, J., & Bolton, P. (2013). Adaptation of cognitive processing therapy for treatment of torture victims: Experience in Kurdistan, Iraq. *Psychological Trauma: Theory, Research, Practice, and Policy, 5,* 184.

Keefe, J. R., Wiltsey-Stirman, S., Cohen, Z. D., DeRubeis, R. J., Smith, B. N., & Resick, P. A. (2018). In rape trauma PTSD, patient characteristics indicate which trauma-focused treatment they are most likely to complete. *Depression and Anxiety, 35*(4), 330–338.

Kessler, R. C., Bossarte, R. M., Luedtke, A., Zaslavsky, A. M., & Zubizarreta, J. R. (2019). Machine learning methods for developing precision treatment rules with observational data. *Behaviour Research and Therapy, 120,* 103412.

Kessler, R. C., Van Loo, H. M., Wardenaar, K. J., Bossarte, R. M., Brenner, L. A., Ebert, D. D., et al. (2017). Using patient self-reports to study heterogeneity of treatment effects in major depressive disorder. *Epidemiology and Psychiatric Sciences, 26,* 22–36.

Kraemer, H. C. (2013). Discovering, comparing, and combining moderators of treatment on outcome after randomized clinical trials: A parametric approach. *Statistics in Medicine, 32,* 1964–1973.

Lei, H., Nahum-Shani, I., Lynch, K., Oslin, D., & Murphy, S. A. (2012). A "SMART" design for building individualized treatment sequences. *Association for Child and Adolescent Mental Health, 8,* 21–28.

Leon, A. C. (2011). Two clinical trial designs to examine personalized treatments for psychiatric disorders. *Journal of Clinical Psychiatry, 72,* 593–597.

Lorenzo-Luaces, L., DeRubeis, R. J., & Bennett, I. M. (2015). Primary care physician's selection of low intensity treatments for patients with depression. *Family Medicine, 47,* 511–516.

Lorenzo-Luaces, L., DeRubeis, R. J., van Straten, A., & Tiemens, B. (2017). A prognostic index (PI) as a moderator of outcomes in the treatment of depression: A proof of concept combining multiple variables to inform risk-stratified stepped care models. *Journal of Affective Disorders, 213,* 78–85.

Luborsky, L., Crits-Christoph, P., Mintz, J., & Auerbach, A. (1988). *Who will benefit from psychotherapy?: Predicting therapeutic outcomes.* New York: Basic Books.

Luedtke, A., Sadikova, E., & Kessler, R. C. (2019). Sample size requirements for multivariate models to predict between-patient differences in best treatments of major depressive disorder. *Clinical Psychological Science,* 2167702618815466.

Murphy, S. A. (2005). An experimental design for the development of adaptive treatment strategies. *Statistics in Medicine, 24,* 1455–1481.

Neuner, F., Onyut, P. L., Ertl, V., Odenwald, M., Schauer, E., & Elbert, T. (2008). Treatment of posttraumatic stress disorder by trained lay counselors in an African refugee settlement: A randomized controlled trial. *Journal of Clinical and Consulting Psychology, 76,* 686–694.

Neuner, F., Schauer, M., Klaschik, C., Karunakara, U., & Elbert, T. (2004). A comparison of narrative exposure therapy, supportive counseling, and psychoeducation for treating posttraumatic stress disorder in an African refugee settlement. *Journal of Consulting and Clinical Psychology, 72,* 579–587.

Ng, M. Y., & Weisz, J. R. (2016). Annual research review: Building a science of personalized intervention for youth mental health. *Journal of Child Psychology and Psychiatry, 57,* 216–236.

Nievergelt, C. M., Ashley-Koch, A. E., Dalvie, S., Hauser, M. A., Morey, R. A., Smith, A. K., et al. (2018). Genomic approaches to posttraumatic stress disorder: The psychiatric genomic consortium initiative. *Biological Psychiatry, 83,* 831–839.

O'Callaghan, P., McMullen, J., Shannon, C., Rafferty, H., & Black, A. (2013). A randomized controlled trial of trauma-focused cognitive behavioral therapy for sexually exploited, war-affected Congolese girls. *Journal of the American Academy of Child and Adolescent Psychiatry, 52,* 359–369.

Olthuis, J. V., Wozney, L., Asmundson, G. J., Cramm, H., Lingley-Pottie, P., &

McGrath, P. J. (2016). Distance-delivered interventions for PTSD: A systematic review and meta-analysis. *Journal of Anxiety Disorders, 44,* 9–26.

Pape, J. C., Carrillo-Roa, T., Rothbaum, B. O., Nemeroff, C. B., Czamara, D., Zannas, A. S., et al. (2018). DNA methylation levels are associated with CRF 1 receptor antagonist treatment outcome in women with post-traumatic stress disorder. *Clinical Epigenetics, 10,* 136.

Paul, G. L. (1967). Strategy of outcome research in psychotherapy. *Journal of Consulting Psychology, 31,* 109–118.

Petkova, E., Tarpey, T., Su, Z., & Ogden, R. T. (2016). Generated effect modifiers (GEM's) in randomized clinical trials. *Biostatistics, 18,* 105–118.

Philip, N. S., Barredo, J., van't Wout-Frank, M., Tyrka, A. R., Price, L. H., & Carpenter, L. L. (2018). Network mechanisms of clinical response to transcranial magnetic stimulation in posttraumatic stress disorder and major depressive disorder. *Biological Psychiatry, 83,* 263–272.

Prendes-Alvarez, S., & Nemeroff, C. B. (2018). Personalized medicine: Prediction of disease vulnerability in mood disorders. *Neuroscience Letters, 669,* 10–13.

Raza, G. T., & Holohan, D. R. (2015). Clinical treatment selection for posttraumatic stress disorder: Suggestions for researchers and clinical trainers. *Psychological Trauma: Theory, Research, Practice, and Policy, 7*(6), 547.

Rizvi, S. L., Vogt, D. S., & Resick, P. A. (2009). Cognitive and affective predictors of treatment outcome in cognitive processing therapy and prolonged exposure for posttraumatic stress disorder. *Behaviour Research and Therapy, 47,* 737–743.

Schneider, R. L., Arch, J. J., & Wolitzky-Taylor, K. B. (2015). The state of personalized treatment for anxiety disorders: A systematic review of treatment moderators. *Clinical Psychology Review, 38,* 39–54.

Schnyder, U., Ehlers, A., Elbert, T., Foa, E. B., Gersons, B. P., Resick, P. A., et al. (2015). Psychotherapies for PTSD: What do they have in common? *European Journal of Psychotraumatology, 6,* 28186.

Shvil, E., Rusch, H. L., Sullivan, G. M., & Neria, Y. (2013). Neural, psychophysiological, and behavioral markers of fear processing in PTSD: A review of the literature. *Current Psychiatry Reports, 15,* 358.

Smoller, J. W. (2014). Psychiatric genetics and the future of personalized treatment. *Depression and Anxiety, 3,* 893–898.

Smoller, J. W. (2016). The genetics of stress-related disorders: PTSD, depression, and anxiety disorders. *Neuropsychopharmacology, 41,* 297–319.

Soder, H. E., Wardle, M. C., Schmitz, J. M., Lane, S. D., Green, C., & Vujanovic, A. A. (2019). Baseline resting heart rate variability predicts post-traumatic stress disorder treatment outcomes in adults with co-occurring substance use disorders and post-traumatic stress. *Psychophysiology, 56,* e13377.

Soliman, M. A., Aboharb, F., Zeltner, N., & Studer, L. (2017). Pluripotent stem cells in neuropsychiatric disorders. *Molecular Psychiatry, 22,* 1241–1249.

Sullivan, P. F., Agrawal, A., Bulik, C. M., Andreassen, O. A., Børglum, A. D., Breen, G., et al. (2018). Psychiatric genomics: An update and an agenda. *American Journal of Psychiatry, 175,* 15–27.

Tay, A. K., & Silove, D. (2017). The ADAPT model: Bridging the gap between psychosocial and individual responses to mass violence and refugee trauma. *Epidemiology and Psychiatric Sciences, 26,* 142–145.

Valentine, S. E., Dixon, L., Borba, C. P., Shtasel, D. L., & Marques, L. (2016). Mental illness stigma and engagement in an implementation trial for cognitive processing therapy at a diverse community health center: A qualitative investigation. *International Journal of Culture and Mental Health, 9,* 139–150.

Weiss, W. M., Murray, L. K., Zangana, G. A. S., Mahmooth, Z., Kaysen, D., Dorsey, S., et al. (2015). Community-based mental health treatments for survivors of torture and militant attacks in Southern Iraq: A randomized control trial. *BMC Psychiatry, 15,* Article 249.

Weisz, J. R., Chorpita, B. F., Palinkas, L. A., Schoenwald, S. K., Miranda, J., Bearman, S. K., et al. (2012). Testing standard and modular designs for psychotherapy treating depression, anxiety, and conduct problems in youth: A randomized effectiveness trial. *Archives of General Psychiatry, 69,* 274–282.

Wiltsey Stirman, S., Cohen, Z., Lunney, C., DeRubeis, R., Wiley, J., & Schnurr, P. (2020). *A personalized index to inform selection of a trauma-focused or non-trauma-focused treatment for PTSD.* Manuscript submitted for publication.

Wolf, E. J., Maniates, H., Nugent, N., Maihofer, A. X., Armstrong, D., Ratanatharathorn, A., et al. (2018). Traumatic stress and accelerated DNA methylation age: A meta-analysis. *Psychoneuroendocrinology, 92,* 123–134.

Yehuda, R., Daskalakis, N. P., Desarnaud, F., Makotkine, I., Lehrner, A., Koch, E., et al. (2013). Epigenetic biomarkers as predictors and correlates of symptom improvement following psychotherapy in combat veterans with PTSD. *Frontiers in Psychiatry, 4,* 118.

CHAPTER 24

Training and Implementation of Evidence-Based Psychotherapies for PTSD

David S. Riggs, Maegan M. Paxton Willing, Sybil Mallonee, Craig Rosen, Shannon Wiltsey Stirman, and Shannon Dorsey

Despite strong empirical evidence for the effectiveness of evidence-based psychotherapies (EBPs) for posttraumatic stress disorder (PTSD; American Psychological Association, 2017; International Society for Traumatic Stress Studies [ISTSS], 2018), they are not commonly available in clinical care settings (e.g., Chorpita et al., 2015; Weisz, Doss, & Hawley, 2005). To better understand the low rates of EBP utilization, it is important to examine current training and implementation efforts. A number of training programs have been developed to instruct clinicians, often across widely dispersed health care systems, in the use of these treatments with the goal of increasing their utilization (Chorpita et al., 2015; Karlin et al., 2010; McHugh & Barlow, 2010). In high-income countries, large-scale efforts have been made to implement EBPs, including the large-scale implementation efforts by the U.S. Department of Veterans Affairs (VA) (Eftekhari et al., 2013; Karlin et al., 2010), Department of Defense (DoD) (Borah et al., 2013; Wilk et al., 2013), and international efforts such as the Improving Access to Psychological Therapies (IAPT) Program in England (Clark, 2018). In addition, mandates, incentives, and promotional efforts have been put in place to facilitate implementation of EBPs (McHugh & Barlow, 2010). Although several programs have proven successful at training large numbers of clinicians, even when providers are adequately trained to use a treatment, successful implementation of EBPs in client-serving settings has been much slower than expected (e.g., Chorpita et al., 2015; Weisz et al., 2005). A growing body of research from the field of implementation science demonstrates that dissemination and training alone do not ensure that EBPs will be adopted and effectively delivered. In this chapter, we review efforts and challenges in the implementation of EBPs for PTSD and provide some suggestions for overcoming the apparent barriers to their use.

Teaching Providers Treatments That Work

Training is a necessary but not sufficient strategy for EBP implementation. Historically, EBP training focused on training clinicians with advanced degrees (i.e., doctoral or master's level) and occurred within extended training programs (i.e., graduate training, postdoctoral fellowships). Initially, efforts to disseminate EBPs to practicing clinicians largely relied on providers' self-study of published treatment manuals to learn protocols and techniques (Mallonee, Phillips, Holloway, & Riggs, 2018). However, with growing research and experience, it became clear that this method of dissemination was not effective (e.g., Fixsen, Naoom, Blase, Friedman, & Wallace, 2005). In response, dissemination efforts that combine treatment manuals with in-person training by experts have become the most widely used method of dissemination (Dimeff et al., 2009).

A recent review by RAND (Hepner, Holliday, Sousa, & Tanielian, 2018) of 57 studies on training identified the key components of effective EBP training programs associated with greater treatment fidelity. In conjunction with its report, RAND developed a Training in Psychotherapy (TIP) tool (Hepner et al., 2018) that may be useful in evaluating various training programs. According to the RAND report, effective training typically includes a didactic element to teach and demonstrate the skills as well as a consultation or supervision period. Certification is available for some EBP training programs; however, there is a dearth of evidence regarding its role in strengthening fidelity (Hepner et al., 2018). Currently, no broadly accepted certification guidelines or requirements exist, and certification is commonly left to the determination of the trainer or treatment developer. Certification may be a useful tool to encourage trainees to reach utilization benchmarks outlined in the certification requirements, but that has not been established empirically.

Didactic Training Components

In-person workshops are generally effective at increasing trainee knowledge about and attitudes toward an EBP, but do not always result in trainee behavioral change (Beidas & Kendall, 2010; Herschell, Kolko, Baumann, & Davis, 2010). However, didactic trainings vary widely in format (e.g., workshop training or manual-based learning) and time (e.g., self-paced, massed over a multiday period, or spaced out over time). The training associated with increased EBP fidelity typically consisted of workshops lasting at least

2 days and integrated written materials (e.g., training manuals, handouts) with didactic presentations (Hepner et al., 2018). Training that included skills demonstration and/or interactive components like role plays or behavioral rehearsal (see Beidas, Cross, & Dorsey, 2014, for guidance on use) were associated with greater adherence to, and competence in, the EBP. However, the specific methods of demonstrating skills or promoting learner interaction varied widely (Hepner et al., 2018). Feedback offered to learners (comments on role plays or responses to homework assignments) during training appears useful to clarify and correct trainee perceptions while increasing their skills and understanding. Because feedback commonly occurs in conjunction with interactive trainings, it is unclear which contributes more to fidelity (Hepner et al., 2018). In terms of content, training programs typically present information on the theory underlying the EBP, empirical support for its use, key components of the treatment, and clinical decision making in applying the EBP (Hepner et al., 2018). The depth and modality with which each of these elements is covered vary widely across programs. To date, there are no studies that explore the relative value of these elements or various teaching methods in the dissemination of EBPs.

Remote Delivery of Didactic Training

In-person workshops represent the most common form of EBP training for professionals, but they are not without challenges. Providers may be unable to travel to workshops due to financial or logistical restrictions (see Mallonee et al., 2018). In addition, the limited availability of qualified trainers combined with a limited capacity in the workshop constrains the ability to widely disseminate EBPs.

To address some of these barriers, online training has become an alternative method of disseminating EBPs for PTSD. There are multiple online platforms and approaches differing with regard to factors such as learner control and involvement that may impact training effectiveness (Dalgarno & Lee, 2010; Harned, Korslund, & Linehan, 2014; Weingardt, 2004). Asynchronous online training (e.g., CPTweb, PEWeb, TF-CBTweb) is self-paced and designed to be completed at a time convenient for the learner. Studies have found asynchronous training produces knowledge gains equivalent to in-person training, although often gains in knowledge, EBP adherence, and EBP skill for any training conditions are modest (Beidas, Edmunds, Marcus, & Kendall, 2012). Dimeff and colleagues (2015) determined that online training produced greater knowledge gains than an in-person workshop, but the workshop produced greater increases in self-efficacy and motivation than did online training. Although asynchronous training is available at clinicians' convenience, the lack of a defined schedule may make it more difficult for some clinicians to dedicate time for training.

Alternatively, synchronous online platforms offer the opportunity for instructor-led, live workshops (Mallonee et al., 2018). We are aware of two such platforms that have been used in disseminating PTSD treatments to date: (1) video conferencing (Rakovshik, McManus, Vazquez-Montes, Muse, & Ougrin, 2016) and (2) SecondLife, a three-dimensional avatar-based e-learning platform (Mallonee et al., 2018; Paxton Willing et al., 2018; Ruzek et al., 2014). The existing research of online training, though limited, suggests that it is at least equally as effective as in-person training (Dimeff et al., 2015; German et al., 2017; Mallonee et al., 2018; Stein et al., 2015), is less expensive, and can reach multiple providers at a distance (Harned et al., 2014; Weingardt, 2004). One recent study focused on teaching prolonged exposure (PE) and cognitive processing therapy (CPT) found that Second-Life learners had similar gains in knowledge and a similar or greater sense of readiness than did learners attending in-person workshops; indeed, the SecondLife CPT learners reported larger increases in readiness than did the in-person CPT learners (Paxton et al., 2018). However, learners were significantly more satisfied with the teaching methods used in the in-person workshop than those used in SecondLife, perhaps due to their greater familiarity (Paxton Willing et al., 2018). Notably, positive outcomes like knowledge, attitudes, or readiness do not ensure provider behavioral change (e.g., EBP adoption, EBP delivery with fidelity).

Consultation

Although in-person workshops or virtual training appear effective at imparting knowledge, it has been demonstrated that some form of applied learning in which the provider is evaluated and given advice from a qualified clinician while using the EBP is an essential aspect of developing skills and competence (Hepner et al., 2018; Herschell et al., 2010; Nadeem, Gleacher, & Beidas, 2013). Such training, typically considered clinical supervision, is an integral part of professional training programs (Nadeem et al., 2013). When disseminating EBPs through workforce education, the applied portion of the training is commonly referred to as consultation. Consultation provided following initial workshop training has been shown to improve provider attitudes toward the EBP (Barnett et al., 2017; Ruzek et al., 2016), to strengthen adherence and competence (Hepner et al., 2018; Rakovshik et al., 2016), to improve patient outcomes (Monson et al., 2018), and to increase learners' subsequent use of the EBP in practice (Charney et al., 2019). Nonetheless, there may be significant challenges in getting providers to dedicate the necessary time for posttraining consultation (Smith, 2017). For reviews of consultation and its relationship to implementation, see Edmunds, Beidas, and Kendall (2013) and McLeod and colleagues (2018).

   Although it is generally agreed that some form of consultation following workshop training is valuable, there is a scarcity of empirical data on the optimal format or amount of consultation (Hepner et al., 2018). Feedback may be offered in person, via telephone, or via video-teleconference. Consultation is sometimes offered one-to-one but more often provided in a group with one expert and several learners. In one nonrandomized study, Stirman and colleagues (2017) found that providers who received group consultation with audio review showed increased competence with the EBP, whereas those receiving individual supervision and audio review decreased in competence 2 years after consultation ended. Some EBPs for PTSD (e.g., trauma-focused cognitive-behavioral therapy [TF-CBT]; Cohen, Mannarino, & Deblinger, 2006) require a period of consultation following the initial training as part of the certification. One study examining implementation of multiple EBPs, some of which required consultation following training and some of which did not, found that clinicians appreciated the posttraining consultation (Barnett et al., 2017).

Consultation typically, but not always, incorporates material from learners' own cases (Hepner et al., 2018). At the most resource-intensive level, this involves having the consultant listen to audio or view video recordings of EBP sessions to provide feedback to the learner on the content and quality of the EBP delivery (e.g., Eftekhari et al., 2013; Stirman et al., 2017). Recognizing the cost of this approach, other consultation programs review case materials (Chard, Ricksecker, Healy, Karlin, & Resick, 2012), discuss case conceptualization (Waltman, Hall, McFarr, & Creed, 2018), or review a limited number of recorded sessions (Charney et al., 2019) or segments of recorded sessions (Monson et al., 2018; Stirman et al., 2017). There are few data that address questions of whether and how much material needs to be reviewed for consultation to be effective. In a randomized trial, Monson and colleagues (2018) found that CPT workshop training plus standard consultation (without audio review) produced better patient outcomes than workshop training only. Yet contrary to predictions, CPT consultation with audio review of session content produced poorer patient outcomes than did standard CPT consultation.

In our experience, the provision of consultation is one of the primary rate-limiting factors for efforts to disseminate and promote the implementation of EBPs for PTSD. The expenses associated with providing consultation are high in terms of expert and learner time as well as the logistical requirements. Broad, effective implementation of EBPs will likely require new, less resource-intensive models for providing consultation that still promote competency and confidence in the delivery of the protocols (e.g., German et al., 2017). Developing more efficient training models is especially important because frequent staff turnover (Mor Barak, Nissley, & Levin, 2001) and role changes often necessitate repeated training events to maintain a trained staff (Beidas, Marcus, et al., 2016; German et al., 2017).

Training Staff in Low-Resource Countries

Most programs aimed at training individuals to deliver EBPs for PTSD have focused on training mental health professionals. However, in low-resource countries with few mental health professionals, it is possible to train lay counselors or paraprofessionals to deliver EBPs. Studies in low-resource countries have shown that lay personnel can be trained to effectively deliver narrative exposure therapy (Neuner et al., 2008), CPT (Bass et al., 2013; Bolton, Bass, et al., 2014), trauma-focused CBT (Murray et al., 2015), and the Common Elements Treatment Approach (CETA; Bolton, Lee, et al., 2014; Weiss et al., 2015). Such efforts require adapting treatments for local culture and literacy levels, more extended training, building a local cadre of supervisors for the EBP, and connections to mental health professionals for addressing safety concerns and other mental health issues (e.g., psychosis; Murray et al., 2011; Patel, Chowdhary, Rahman, & Verdeli, 2011). Low-resource countries often face additional implementation challenges that we cannot fully address here. These may include limited funding for social services, lack of mental health infrastructure, and sociopolitical instability (Chen, Olin, Stirman, & Kaysen, 2017).

Examples of Large-Scale Training Efforts

In high-income countries, large-scale efforts to implement EBPs for PTSD have been under way over the last decade. In the United States, the VA's dissemination efforts began in 2006 by conducting regular national in-person workshops and weekly phone call consultation posttraining (Karlin et al., 2010). These efforts continue, although they now have transitioned to a decentralized model, with workshops and consultations conducted at regional levels. The Department of Defense (DoD) also began training efforts in 2006 using somewhat different processes than the VA. The most notable difference is that DoD did not mandate consultation following workshop training, choosing instead to offer voluntary telephonic consultation. These efforts resulted in a large number of providers trained in PE and/or CPT, but barriers to delivering these treatments remain (Borah et al., 2013; Finley et al., 2015; Wilk et al., 2013), despite additional policy activities to support implementation (Karlin & Cross, 2014).

Efforts within civilian communities to increase implementation have typically been slower and more heterogeneous in nature. Often these efforts are driven by treatment developers or groups of early adopters who conduct workshops and provide consultation as an extension of the development of the treatment. Over time, networks of trainers and communities of trained providers may emerge. Examples of this can be seen in the dissemination of eye movement desensitization and reprocessing (EMDR) therapy and CPT (with its foundation in the VA implementation effort). Other efforts to disseminate evidence-based treatments among civilian providers reflect the work of government agencies. For example, although focused on the treatment of serious mental illness rather than PTSD specifically, individual states have implemented policies to increase the delivery of EBPs. Many of these include the development of state training programs in various EBPs (Bruns et al., 2016).

Over 17 states have developed TF-CBT training initiatives to better equip child- and adolescent-serving providers to address trauma-exposure sequelae (Sigel, Benton, Lynch, & Kramer, 2013). These initiatives have received widely varying financial support by states or grants, and all have included posttraining consultation or clinician coaching. They also have included a range of implementation supports to supplement in-person training, including assessment of organizational readiness to adopt and use quality assurance procedures to address implementation barriers, engagement of important stakeholders (e.g., child welfare, court representatives), and supervisor-specific trainings and supports (Sigel et al., 2013). The Washington State Initiative builds on work by Weisz and colleagues (2012) and extends beyond TF-CBT (Dorsey, Berliner, Lyon, Pullmann, & Murray, 2016) to include CBT for the other most commonly presenting child mental health problems. With supervisors and organizational leaders in community mental health, this group has developed three practical guides that organizations can access on their website, to provide guidance on implementing EBPs (*http://depts.washington.edu/hcsats/PDF/TF-%20CBT/pages/therapist_resources.html#*; Berliner, Dorsey, Merchant, Jungbluth, & Sedlar, 2013; Berliner, Dorsey, Sedlar, Jungbluth, & Merchant, 2013).

In addition, the National Child Traumatic Stress Network (NCTSN) supported the development of an asynchronous online training program, developed by the Medical University of South Carolina, that has been successful at increasing the spread of TF-CBT (Amaya-Jackson, Ebert, Forrester, & Deblinger, 2008). It aimed to create assessments and EBPs that were both developmentally and culturally appropriate that would be disseminated across diverse clinical settings. The NCTSN works to develop "state-of-the-art training platforms and to disseminate, implement, and adapt evidence-based treatments into community practices across the network" (Amaya-Jackson et al., 2008, p. 393). By utilizing a collaborative learning model, the NCTSN has been able to disseminate and implement EBPs within a number of diverse sites.

The United States is not the only country with large-scale efforts for EBP dissemination. For example, England has developed the IAPT Program whose mission is to minimize the gap between research and practice. This program was initiated by a coalition of clinical researchers and economists who emphasized to the public and to policymakers both the economic and social benefits of such a program (Gyani, Shafran, Layard, & Clark, 2013). The program includes the recommendation of CBT in the National Institute for Health and Care Excellence (NICE) treatment guidelines, of transparency in publishing outcome data on a quarterly basis, and also has included cost analyses to demonstrate the return on investment in training and dissemination. Upon approval, the program established a goal to train over 10,500 new therapists in the use of EBPs for a variety of disorders, including PTSD, by 2021. Although the program had a slow start when it began in 2008, it has gradually increased and is on target to meet its 2021 goal (Clark, 2018).

Within the IATP, training of providers in EBPs is conducted over the course of a year, during which they attend lectures on the EBPs at local universities, workshops, and case supervision 2 days a week. During the rest of the week, they see patients at local IAPT agencies, while receiving additional regular supervision and the opportunity to observe more experienced staff (Clark, 2011). The transparency of this program has allowed detailed research to be conducted on clinical outcomes both to monitor the effectiveness of the program as a whole and also to gain additional information to maximize clinical outcomes. For example, in one study early in the development of this program, researchers determined recovery rates of around 40%, improvement rates of approximately 64%, and deterioration rates of 6.6% (Gyani et al., 2013). Of note, despite the fact that the 40% recovery rate is about 10% less than IATP's recovery rate goal, the program exceeded its goal of moving people off of sick pay and/or state benefits due to their mental illness by more than 2,000 individuals (Clark, 2011). However, it was also found that these rates were impacted by the efficacy of practitioners to the NICE guidelines, with those following the guidelines more closely having better outcomes (Gyani et al., 2013).

In addition, the evidence-based practice task force of the Canadian Psychological Association (CPA; 2012) recommended a tridirectorate approach to dissemination to include the Education, Practice, and Science directorates. It advised these committees to use annual conventions, symposia, seminars, and continuing education opportunities to disseminate EBPs to providers. Together for Mental Health details an approach to improving the psychological health of the people of Wales as well as encouraging the use of EBPs (Welsh Government, 2012). In this endeavor, a number of initiatives to improve mental health have been established along with efforts by organizations within Wales to offer training for protocols such as Mental Health First Aid. For example, the All Wales Mental Health Promotion Network works to assemble and disseminate evidence in support of mental health improvement. The network recommends that providers continually monitor their practice, including patient outcomes and quality of care.

Contextual Factors in Implementation

As noted in earlier sections, dissemination and training are necessary but insufficient for ensuring that EBPs are actually delivered to individuals with PTSD (e.g., Herschell et al., 2010; Hershcell, Reed, Person Mecca, & Kolko, 2014; Monson et al., 2018). For example, despite training and policy directives, within the VA, it is estimated that 80% of patients with PTSD do not receive an EBP (Maguen et al., 2018). Recent research has shown that even behavioral health providers trained in the use of EBPs for PTSD are choosing not to use them (Borah et al., 2013), use them for only a small proportion of their patients (Finley et al., 2015; Rosen et al., 2017), or use them with low fidelity to the EBP protocol (Thompson, Simiola, Schnurr, Stirman, & Cook, 2018; Wilk et al., 2013).

A number of studies have begun to explore factors that limit the implementation of EBPs for PTSD within health care systems. In the United States, much of this work has been focused on the VA and DoD health care systems for adults and in community mental health settings for children and adolescents. Rosen and colleagues (2016) reviewed 32 papers that examined aspects of the dissemination and implementation of PE and CPT within the VA and identified three important determinants of EBP use: clinician confidence in the effectiveness of the treatment, facility/organizational support for the delivery of the EBP, and overcoming challenges in patient engagement with the treatment (Rosen et al., 2016). Similarly, Borah, Holder, Chen, and Gray (2017) identified clinician and organizational factors that limit the use of EBPs among DoD clinicians. Researchers at the Center for Deployment Psychology (CDP; 2015) have worked to identify barriers to EBP implementation based on their work to increase EBP use in the DoD health care system. The result of this effort is a list of more than 35 potential barriers that includes clinician factors (e.g., confidence in their ability to deliver EBP, belief in the efficacy of the treatment), patient characteristics (e.g., knowledge about EBP), and clinic factors (e.g., resource requirements) similar to those found in other studies (Borah et al., 2017; Rosen et al., 2016). However, a number of the barriers to EBP implementation were broader and more far-reaching (e.g., inability to schedule appointments around duty requirements). These were termed systemic barriers and are similar to contextual factors that have been found to impact the delivery of EBPs (Beidas & Kendall, 2010; Glisson & Williams, 2015). Yet, existing dissemination/implementation programs have largely focused on training providers and thus not adequately addressed other barriers to implementation.

Strategies to Address Barriers to Dissemination and Implementation

As discussed previously, multiple factors function to limit the implementation of EBPs for PTSD. These include provider knowledge and beliefs, patient beliefs about EBPs, and clinic climate, resources, and policies. The implementation literature has identified a number of strategies to overcoming barriers. It is beyond the scope of this chapter to identify specific approaches to overcoming the myriad of organizational barriers to EBP implementation. However, we will offer several broad approaches that may prove helpful in promoting EBP use. First, comprehensive approaches to preparing and supporting organizations and clinicians to implement EBPs are needed. Although the best approaches are still being identified, multifaceted approaches such as learning collaboratives (LoSavio et al., 2019) and tailored combinations of implementation strategies show promise.

Waltz and colleagues (2015) detail a six-point approach that includes planning, education, financing, restructuring, managing quality, and attending to policy context. In conjunction with a needs assessment that involves multiple stakeholder perspectives and, if possible, evaluation data, appropriate strategies can be mapped onto identified barriers and facilitators at the individual (provider, patient), organizational, system/outer context, and intervention levels (Lewis et al., 2018; Powell et al., 2017). The recommendations below leverage these categories to provide a framework for a multifaceted, flexible approach to overcoming implementation barriers.

System- and Policy-Level Approaches

Efforts to promote implementation are often impacted by large-scale changes in policy or process (Stirman, Gutner, Langdon, & Graham, 2016). For example, the VA's EBP for PTSD implementation efforts involved the expansion of their mental health care workforce as well as mandates stating that CPT or PE must be a treatment option at all facilities (Karlin et al., 2010; Karlin & Cross, 2014). Significant efforts to encourage the use of EBPs, including changes in policies and fiscal incentives, have been made by individual U.S. states (Bruns et al., 2016). The treatments studied by Bruns and colleagues were geared toward care for serious mental illness rather than PTSD specifically. However, their research raises an important concern in that their analyses suggest the trend of increased EBP implementation observed in the early 2000s has flattened or even begun to decline (Bruns et al., 2016), pointing to challenges in the sustainability of implementation efforts that have not yet garnered much attention in the literature.

There have been large-scale pushes for implementation EBPs in general (Bond & Drake, 2019). For instance, policy changes and mandates have occurred in many countries, as illustrated by the Mental Health Policy in England briefing paper that emphasized the need for the utilization of EBPs (Parkin, 2018). Additionally, the National Health and Medical Research Council of Australia has stated that treatment guidelines should utilize evidence to form their recommendations (Silagy, Rubin, Henderson-Smart, & Gross, 1998). Several psychological societies, such as the Canadian Psychological Association (2012) and Australian Psychological Society (2018), have provided treatment guidelines that focus on the need for EBPs. Even grander efforts are being undertaken to promote the use of EBPs. For example, the Programme for Improving Mental Health Care (PRIME) was designed to increase the implementation of EBPs in primary care and maternal health care centers in countries like India, Nepal, Ethiopia, Uganda, and South Africa (Lund et al., 2012).

Treatment guidelines and policy statements supporting the application of EBPs are positive developments, but they merely encourage their use; they do not mandate, reward, or resource use of these treatments. More powerful policy changes to support the spread of EBPs would require more serious social commitments. In low-resource countries, this would require advocacy to increase funding for mental health services (Chen et al., 2017) or a redesign of EBPs to be more inherently sustainable. In high-resource countries, shifts to incentivize the use of EBPs could include professional accreditation bodies requiring that clinicians have EBP trainings, health care organization or funders requiring that providers have the capacity to deliver EBPs, making the provision of EBPs part of health care quality or performance measures, billing and reimbursement policies that incentivize the provision of EBPs, routine measurement and reporting of patient outcomes, and/or payment policies based in part on patient improvement. To date, there has been limited research on how such economic incentives impact EBP use and patient outcomes in mental health (Stewart, Lareef, Hadley, & Mandell, 2017; Yuan, He, Meng, & Jia, 2017).

Local Organizational Context

In addition to being influenced by forces at the societal and policy levels, the implementation of EBPs is also strongly impacted by factors at the clinic or practice levels (inner context). EBP clinic-level organizational factors are often critical to the successful implementation of EBP protocols (Aarons, Hurlburt, & Horwitz, 2011; Damschroder et al., 2009; Sayer et al., 2017). In our experience, if clinic policies focus on efficiency (throughput) rather than effectiveness (outcomes), provide no ability to compare clinic outcomes, and do not offer opportunities/support for posttraining consultation, then the culture of the clinic is not encouraging the use of EBPs (Glisson et al., 2008), and research further supports this experience (Glisson & Williams, 2015; Sayer et al., 2017).

Factors at the organizational level also impact clinician attitudes and willingness to deliver EBPs. A positive organizational climate has been associated with more positive attitudes toward EBPs (Aarons & Sawitsky, 2006). Other studies have indicated that leadership support and characteristics are also associated with more positive attitudes (Aarons, 2004; Aarons, Ehrhart, Farahnak, & Hurlburt, 2015; Aarons & Sommerfeld, 2012). Clinic managers and/or clinical supervisors can promote EBP use by offering incentives or rewards for indications of EBP adoption, such as meeting implementation goals, offering peer education or supervision, conducting chart reviews to assess and support EBP use, or highlighting improvement in patient outcomes (Aarons, Ehrhart, Farahnak, & Sklar, 2014). In a study examining workplace-based supervision of TF-CBT (i.e., supervision delivered by supervisors already employed in the clinic), supervisors in clinics that had a more positive implementation climate were more likely to spend a higher percentage of their supervision time on EBP-relevant clinical content (i.e., case conceptualization, interventions; Dorsey et al., 2018). A more positive implementation climate was also associated with supervisors' greater coverage of TF-CBT elements (Lucid et al., 2018; Pullmann et al., 2018).

Thus, facilitating a supportive implementation climate and preparing clinic leaders to facilitate and reinforce EBP use may be at least as important as directly addressing clinician attitudes through training or motivational interventions. Clinics can also support EBP implementation by prioritizing the hiring of applicants with EBP interest and experience, and by providing support for training inexperienced clinicians. One of the Washington State organizational practical guides focuses specifically on orienting new providers to EBP given the ongoing challenge of workforce turnover (Berliner, Dorsey, Merchant, et al., 2013).

Another important organizational factor is alignment of resources to support EBP delivery. Studies comparing VA clinics and residential programs that were more and less successful in implementing EBPs suggest prioritization is key. Successful programs not only created a culture that values EBPs, they also aligned staff time and adjusted the workflow to support their implementation (Cook et al., 2015; Sayer et al., 2017). Clinics may explore the possibility of restructuring or simplifying administrative tasks to improve provider productivity or aligning documentation requirements with EBP reporting standards. Transferring some tasks to administrative staff or behavioral technicians (Matsuzaka et al., 2017) and reducing or eliminating ineffective interventions (e.g., open-ended support groups) can increase providers' time to learn and deliver EBPs. EBP implementation may benefit from more substantial changes to policy and processes, such as procedures for scheduling appointments, patient referral processes, case management procedures, or other clinic operations (Sayer et al., 2017).

Fidelity Support

Within the dissemination and implementation literature for PTSD treatments, the question of how well providers maintain treatment fidelity and competence over time has received relatively little attention. Data that suggest providers fail to deliver the treatment with fidelity (e.g., Wilk et al., 2013) are often interpreted to mean the initial training was inadequate. However, it is also possible that providers did learn to deliver the EBP in line with the protocol but subsequently drifted away from the manual (Center for Deployment Psychology, 2015). It may be necessary to incorporate strategies to assess provider fidelity/competence over time and provide additional guidance (e.g., refresher training, additional consultation) if drift is detected. There is a need for both effective (e.g., accurate assessment) and efficient (low-cost, low-burden) strategies to assess fidelity so that organizations can better assess when drift is occurring (Beidas, Maclean, et al., 2016; Schoenwald et al., 2010).

Ensuring that providers have ongoing access to expert consultation (at least on an ad hoc basis), peer consultation, or workplace-based supervision that focuses specifically on the EBP may be particularly useful when they are faced with complicated cases (Edmunds et al., 2013). Despite evidence that EBPs for PTSD often produce improvements for comorbid problems as well (see Riggs, Tate, Chrestman, & Foa, Chapter 12, this volume), clinicians may assume that the treatment will be ineffective, or even harmful for clients who have complex needs (Center for Deployment Psychology, 2015). Clinic case conferences or provider testimonials that share successes and lessons learned in implementing EBPs with complex cases can help colleagues adapt rather than abandon EBPs with such patients (Center for Deployment Psychology, 2015). To better tailor the techniques used to address concerns and skepticism, it is also important to understand clinicians' worldviews and approach toward practice, to determine whether their concerns about EBPs are more deeply rooted or motivated (Hornsey & Fielding, 2017).

A potentially important tool for addressing clinicians' concerns about the impact of EBP implementation on their clients is the adoption of measurement-based care practices (Fortney et al., 2016). Acknowledging that this often kicks off an entirely new implementation exercise, the integration and use of outcome measures (e.g., PTSD Checklist [PCL-5]; Blevins, Weathers, Davis, Witte, & Domino, 2015) in treatment planning and evaluation can help address many provider concerns. For example, it will allow the evaluation of (1) comparative outcome of clients treated with the EBP and those receiving other treatment, (2) treatment safety, and (3) the impact of modifying the EBP protocol (Center for Deployment Psychology, 2015). The clinicwide use of measurement-based care can also contribute to improved treatment response (Fortney et al., 2016).

Patient Engagement

Some providers may be hesitant to utilize EBTs due to beliefs that patients will not be receptive to the protocol (Center for Deployment Psychology, 2015; Rosen et al., 2017). However, patient receptivity is often a function of how they are educated about treatments. Providers should be trained on best practices in describing EBPs and provided with tools to increase patient buy-in while targeting their safety concerns and misconceptions. Tools for joint decision making around the treatment of PTSD have been shown to improve patient engagement and retention in EBPs (Mott, Stanley, Street, Grady, & Teng, 2014; Watts et al., 2015). Online resources for comparing treatment approaches (*www.ptsd.va.gov/apps/decisionaid*) can be used to support a collaborative approach to deciding which treatment approach to pursue with a particular client. Evidence-based engagement strategies can also be paired with EBPs, such as those developed by Mary McKay and colleagues, that help providers address both perception issues (e.g., stigma, negative past experiences with mental health care) and barriers to engagement (Dorsey et al., 2014; McKay & Bannon, 2004). In a small randomized controlled trial focused on engaging youth and foster parents, TF-CBT supplemented with McKay's evidence-based engagement strategies outperformed standard TF-CBT in preventing early treatment dropout (Dorsey et al., 2014).

Conclusions

For implementation efforts to be effective, one must allow sufficient time, leadership and policy support, and allotment of resources. Given the large number of factors that can inhibit EBP implementation efforts (Center for Deployment Psychology, 2015), no single approach is likely to resolve all the dissemination and implementation problems. Any successful approach likely needs to be flexible and multifaceted to address the unique and diverse challenges each clinic faces when endeavoring to integrate EBPs for the treatment of PTSD (Stirman et al., 2016). To improve efficiency, interventions designed to increase implementation should address multiple barriers rather than only one.

A participatory approach can be effective: working closely with clinic leadership and providers to identify their specific barriers and goals. Additionally, setting goals and monitoring progress are important throughout implementation efforts (e.g., Kirchner et al., 2014). In larger networks, such as the VA or military treatment facilities (MTFs), efforts would probably benefit from beginning small rather than making large, far-reaching changes. These focused efforts can be used to show that implementation efforts are feasible and effective. Clinics and providers should work to create an implementation plan that will be effective in their setting, building on their strengths and addressing their most significant barriers. Finally, it is imperative that as programs work to disseminate and implement EBPs for PTSD, they share their successes and lessons learned with other clinics and programs to expand and improve access to EBPs more generally.

As mentioned, follow-up studies of providers trained to use EBPs for PTSD suggest that they do not implement them universally (Borah et al., 2013; Finley et al., 2015; Rosen et al., 2017) or with complete fidelity (Thompson et al., 2018; Wilk et al., 2013). Furthermore, the study of Bruns and colleagues (2016) raises the broader challenge of sustaining implementation gains. As discussed, a number of efforts face many barriers that must be overcome to successfully implement EBPs. However, relatively little work has addressed the factors that interfere with sustainment of implementation gains once they have been made. It is highly likely that the reasons a clinic or provider fails to maintain the use of EBPs overlap with the barriers to initial implementation. That is, if a clinic needed to make organizational changes to implement treatments, then it is likely that the use of EBPs will be reduced as a result, should the organizational changes reverse due to a change in leadership or higher-level policy. However, it is also possible that factors not yet identified as barriers to initial implementation can contribute to failures to sustain the use of EBPS once they have been implemented. Research to identify these factors and understand how they might function to reduce the use of EBPs is needed.

Within the PTSD field, the challenges involved in the implementation and sustainment of EBP use raise additional questions about the nature of the treatments that are identified as first-line therapies for PTSD. On the whole, these therapies tend to be technique-driven (e.g., PE, CPT, EMDR therapy), with delivery following a relatively structured format over a number of in-person sessions. None of the individual techniques is particularly complicated, and the recommended number of sessions is typically limited. However, the existing treatments that work do require therapists to learn a new set of skills, patients to commit substantial time and resources to therapy, and both therapists and patients to approach the emotionally stressful aftereffects of trauma. In short, the nature of the psychotherapeutic approaches to treating PTSD may make them difficult to sustain. This raises a challenge as the field of PTSD treatment development progresses. Perhaps it is important to consider alternative treatment approaches and delivery strategies (e.g., online therapy) that are designed with questions of implementation and sustainment in mind as well as their efficacy in treating PTSD.

REFERENCES

Aarons, G. A. (2004). Mental health provider attitudes toward adoption of evidence-based practice: The Evidence-Based Practice Attitude Scale (EBPAS). *Mental Health Services Research, 6,* 61–74.

Aarons, G. A., Ehrhart, M. G., Farahnak, L. R., & Hurlburt, M. S. (2015). Leadership and organizational change for implementation (LOCI): A randomized mixed method pilot study of a leadership and organization development intervention for evidence-based practice implementation. *Implementation Science, 10*(11), 45.

Aarons, G. A., Ehrhart, M. G., Farahnak, L. R., & Sklar, M. (2014). Aligning leadership across systems and organizations to develop a strategic climate for evidence-based practice implementation. *Annual Review of Public Health, 35,* 255–274.

Aarons, G. A., Hurlburt, M., & Horwitz, S. M. (2011). Advancing a conceptual model of evidence-based practice implementation in public service sectors. *Administration and Policy in Mental Health and Health Services Research, 38,* 4–23.

Aarons, G. A., & Sawitzky, A. C. (2006). Organizational culture and climate and mental health provider attitudes toward evidence-based practice. *Psychological Services, 3,* 61–72.

Aarons, G. A., & Sommerfeld, D. H. (2012). Leadership, innovation climate, and attitudes toward evidence-based practice during a statewide implementation. *Journal of the American Academy of Child and Adolscent Psychiatry, 51,* 423–431.

Amaya-Jackson, L., Ebert, L., Forrester, A., & Deblinger, E. (2008). *Fidelity to the learning collaborative model: Essential elements of a methodology for the adoption and implementation of evidence-based practices.* Paper presented at annual meeting of the National Child Traumatic Stress Network, Anaheim, CA.

American Psychological Association. (2017). *Clinical practice guideline for the treatment of posttraumatic stress disorder (PTSD) in adults.* Washington, DC: Author. Retrieved from *www.apa.org/ptsd-guideline/ptsd.pdf.*

Australian Psychological Society. (2018). Evidence-based psychological interventions in the treatment of mental disorders: A review of the literature. Retrieved from *www.psychology.org.au/getmedia/23c6a11b-2600-4e19-9a1d-6ff9c2f26fae/Evidence-based-psych-interventions.pdf.*

Barnett, M., Brookman-Frazee, L., Regan, J., Saifan, D., Stadnick, N., & Lau, A. (2017). How intervention and implementation characteristics relate to community therapists' attitudes toward evidence-based practices: A mixed methods study. *Administration and Policy in Mental Health and Mental Health Services Research, 44*(6), 824–837.

Bass, J. K., Annan, J., McIvor Murray, S., Kaysen, D., Griffiths, S., Cetinoglu, T., et al. (2013). Controlled trial of psychotherapy for Congolese survivors of sexual violence. *New England Journal of Medicine, 368*(23), 2182–2191.

Beidas, R. S., Cross, W. F., & Dorsey, S. (2014). Show me don't tell me: Behavioral rehearsal as a training and fidelity tool. *Cognitive and Behavioral Practice, 21*(1), 1–11.

Beidas, R. S., Edmunds, J. M., Marcus, S. C., & Kendall, P. C. (2012). Training and consultation to promote implementation of an empirically supported treatment: A randomized trial. *Psychiatric Services, 63*(7), 660–665.

Beidas, R. S., & Kendall, P. C. (2010). Training therapists in evidence-based practice: A critical review of studies from a systems-contextual perspective. *Clinical Psychology: Science and Practice, 17*(1), 1–30.

Beidas, R. S., Maclean, J. C., Fishman, J., Dorsey, S., Schoenwald, S. K., Mandell, D. S., et al. (2016). A randomized trial to identify accurate and cost-effective fidelity measurement methods for cognitive-behavioral therapy: Project FACTS study protocol. *BMC Psychiatry, 16*(1), 323.

Beidas, R. S., Marcus, S., Wolk, C. B., Powell, B., Aarons, G. A., Evans, A. C., et al. (2016). A prospective examination of clinician and supervisor turnover within the context of implementation of evidence-based practices in a publicly-funded mental health system. *Administration and Policy in Mental Health and Mental Health Services Research, 43*(5), 640–649.

Berliner, L., Dorsey, S., Merchant, L., Jungbluth, N., & Sedlar, G. (2013). Practical guide for EBP implementation in public health. Retrieved from *http://depts.washington.edu/hcsats/PDF/TF-%20CBT/pages/Theoretical%20Perspective/EBP%20Organization%20Practical%20Guide%202013%20Version.pdf.*

Berliner, L., Dorsey, S., Sedlar, G., Jungbluth, N., & Merchant, L. (2013). Everyday competence and fidelity for EBP organizations: Practical guide. Retrieved from *http://depts.washington.edu/hcsats/PDF/TF-%20CBT/pages/Theoretical%20Perspective/Everyday%20Competence%20and%20Fidelity%20Guide-2013.pdf.*

Blevins, C. A., Weathers, F. W., Davis, M. T., Witte, T. K., & Domino, J. L. (2015). The posttraumatic stress disorder checklist for DSM-5 (PCL-5): Development and initial psychometric evaluation. *Journal of Traumatic Stress, 28*(6), 489–498.

Bolton, P., Bass, J. K., Zangana, G. A. S., Kamal, T., Murray, S. M., Kaysen, D., et al. (2014). A randomized controlled trial of mental health interventions for survivors of systematic violence in Kurdistan, Northern Iraq. *BMC Psychiatry, 14*(1), 360.

Bolton, P., Lee, C., Haroz, E. E., Murray, L. K., Dorsey, S., Robinson, C., et al. (2014). A transdiagnostic community-based mental health treatment for comorbid disorders: Development and outcomes of a randomized controlled trial among Burmese refugees in Thailand. *PLOS Medicine, 11*(11), e1001757.

Bond, G. R., & Drake, R. E. (2019). Assessing the fidelity of evidence-based practices:

History and current status of a standardized measurement methodology. *Administration and Policy in Mental Health and Mental Health Services Research.* [Epub ahead of print]

Borah, E. V., Holder, N., Chen, K., & Gray, S. (2017). Military behavioral health providers' attitudes, training and organizational barriers related to their use of evidence-based treatments for PTSD. *Best Practices in Mental Health, 13*(1), 34–46.

Borah, E. V., Wright, E. C., Donahue, D. A., Cedillos, E. M., Riggs, D. S., Isler, W. C., et al. (2013). Implementation outcomes of military provider training in cognitive processing therapy and prolonged exposure therapy for post-traumatic stress disorder. *Military Medicine, 178*(9), 939–944.

Bruns, E. J., Kerns, S. E., Pullmann, M. D., Hensley, S. W., Lutterman, T., & Hoagwood, K. E. (2016). Research, data, and evidence-based treatment use in state behavioral health systems, 2001–2012. *Psychiatric Services, 67*(5), 496–503.

Canadian Psychological Association. (2012). *Evidence-based practice of psychological treatments: A Canadian perspective.* Quebec City, Canada: CPA Task Force on Evidence-Based Practice of Psychological Treatments. Retrieved from *www.cpa.ca/docs/File/Practice/Report_of_the_EBP_Task_Force_FINAL_Board_ Approved_2012.pdf.*

Center for Deployment Psychology. (2015). Lessons learned manual: A framework for addressing barriers to evidence-based psychotherapy utilization in the Defense Department. Retrieved from *https://deploymentpsych.org/system/files/ member_resource/Lessons_Learned_Manual_0.pdf.*

Chard, K. M., Ricksecker, E. G., Healy, E. T., Karlin, B. E., & Resick, P. A. (2012). Dissemination and experience with cognitive processing therapy. *Journal of Rehabilitation Research and Development, 49*(5), 667–678.

Charney, M. E., Chow, L., Jakubovic, R. J., Federico, L. E., Goetter, E. M., Baier, A. L., et al. (2019). Training community providers in evidence-based treatment for PTSD: Outcomes of a novel consultation program. *Psychological Trauma: Theory, Research, Practice, and Policy, 11*(7), 793–801.

Chen, J. A., Olin, C. C., Stirman, S. W., & Kaysen, D. (2017). The role of context in the implementation of trauma-focused treatments: Effectiveness research and implementation in higher and lower income settings. *Current Opinion in Psychology, 14,* 61–66.

Chorpita, B. F., Park, A., Tsai, K., Korathu-Larson, P., Higa-McMillan, C. K., Nakamura, B. J., et al. (2015). Balancing effectiveness with responsiveness: Therapist satisfaction across different treatment designs in the Child STEPs randomized effectiveness trial. *Journal of Consulting and Clinical Psychology, 83*(4), 709–718.

Clark, D. M. (2011). Implementing NICE guidelines for psychological treatment of depression and anxiety disorders: The IAPT experience. *International Review of Psychiatry, 23*(4), 318–327.

Clark, D. M. (2018). Realizing the mass public benefit of evidence-based psychological therapies: The IAPT program. *Annual Review of Clinical Psychology, 14,* 159–183.

Cohen, J. A., Mannarino, A. P., & Deblinger, E. (2006). *Treating trauma and traumatic grief in children and adolescents.* New York: Guilford Press.

Cook, J. M., Dinnen, S., Thompson, R., Ruzek, J., Coyne, J. C., & Schnurr, P. P. (2015). A quantitative test of an implementation framework in 38 VA residential PTSD programs. *Administration and Policy in Mental Health and Mental Health Services Research, 42*(4), 462–473.

Dalgarno, B., & Lee, M. J. (2010). What are the learning affordances of 3-D virtual environments? *British Journal of Educational Technology, 41*(1), 10–32.

Damschroder, L. J., Aron, D. C., Keith, R. E., Kirsh, S. R., Alexander, J. A., & Lowery, J. C. (2009). Fostering implementation of health services research findings into practice: A consolidated framework for advancing implementation science. *Implementation Science, 4*(1), 50.

Dimeff, L. A., Harned, M. S., Woodcock, E. A., Skutch, J. M., Koerner, K., & Linehan, M. M. (2015). Investigating bang for your training buck: A randomized controlled trial comparing three methods of training clinicians in two core strategies of dialectical behavior therapy. *Behavior Therapy, 46*(3), 283–295.

Dimeff, L. A., Koerner, K., Woodcock, E. A., Beadnell, B., Brown, M. Z., Skutch, J. M., et al. (2009). Which training method works best?: A randomized controlled trial comparing three methods of training clinicians in dialectical behavior therapy skills. *Behaviour Research and Therapy, 47*(11), 921–930.

Dorsey, S., Berliner, L., Lyon, A. R., Pullmann, M. D., & Murray, L. K. (2016). A statewide common elements initiative for children's mental health. *Journal of Behavioral Health Services and Research, 43*(2), 246–261.

Dorsey, S., Kerns, S. E. U., Lucid, L., Pullmann, M. D., Harrison, J. P., Berliner, L., et al. (2018). Objective coding of content and techniques in workplace-based supervision of an EBT in public mental health. *Implementation Science, 13*(19).

Dorsey, S., Pullmann, M., Berliner, L., Koschmann, E. F., McKay, M., & Deblinger, E. (2014). Engaging foster parents in treatment: A randomized trial of supplementing trauma-focused cognitive behavioral therapy with evidence-based engagement strategies. *Child Abuse and Neglect, 38*(9), 1508–1520.

Edmunds, J. M., Beidas, R. S., & Kendall, P. C. (2013). Dissemination and implementation of evidence-based practices: Training and consultation as implementation strategies. *Clinical Psychology: Science and Practice, 20*(2), 152–165.

Eftekhari, A., Ruzek, J. I., Crowley, J. J., Rosen, C. S., Greenbaum, M. A., & Karlin, B. E. (2013). Effectiveness of national implementation of prolonged exposure therapy in Veterans Affairs care. *JAMA Psychiatry, 70*(9), 949–955.

Finley, E. P., Garcia, H. A., Ketchum, N. S., McGeary, D. D., McGeary, C. A., Stirman, S. W., et al. (2015). Utilization of evidence-based psychotherapies in Veterans Affairs posttraumatic stress disorder outpatient clinics. *Psychological Services, 12*(1), 73–82.

Fixsen, D. L., Naoom, S. F., Blase, K. A., Friedman, R. M., & Wallace, F. (2005). *Implementation research: A synthesis of the literature* (Publication No. 231). Tampa: University of South Florida, Louis de la Parte Florida Mental Health Institute, National Implementation Research Network.

Fortney, J. C., Unützer, J., Wrenn, G., Pyne, J. M., Smith, G. R., Schoenbaum, M., et al. (2016). A tipping point for measurement-based care. *Psychiatric Services, 68*(2), 179–188.

German, R. E., Adler, A., Frankel, S. A., Stirman, S. W., Pinedo, P., Evans, A. C., et al. (2017). Testing a web-based, trained-peer model to build capacity for evidence-based practices in community mental health systems. *Psychiatric Services, 69*(3), 286–292.

Glisson, C., Schoenwald, S. K., Kelleher, K., Landsverk, J., Hoagwood, K. E.,

Mayberg, S., et al. (2008). Therapist turnover and new program sustainability in mental health clinics as a function of organizational culture, climate, and service structure. *Administration and Policy in Mental Health and Mental Health Services Research, 35*(1-2), 124–133.

Glisson, C., & Williams, N. J. (2015). Assessing and changing organizational social contexts for effective mental health services. *Annual Review of Public Health, 36,* 507–523.

Gyani, A., Shafran, R., Layard, R., & Clark, D. M. (2013). Enhancing recovery rates: Lessons from year one of IAPT. *Behaviour Research and Therapy, 51*(9), 597–606.

Harned, M. S., Korslund, K. E., & Linehan, M. M. (2014). A pilot randomized controlled trial of dialectical behavior therapy with and without the dialectical behavior therapy prolonged exposure protocol for suicidal and self-injuring women with borderline personality disorder and PTSD. *Behaviour Research and Therapy, 55,* 7–17.

Hepner, K. A., Holliday, S. B., Sousa, J., & Tanielian, T. (2018). Training clinicians to deliver evidence-based psychotherapy. Retrieved from *www.rand.org/content/dam/rand/pubs/tools/TL300/TL306/RAND_TL306.pdf.*

Herschell, A. D., Kolko, D. J., Baumann, B. L., & Davis, A. C. (2010). The role of therapist training in the implementation of psychosocial treatments: A review and critique with recommendations. *Clinical Psychology Review, 30*(4), 448–466.

Herschell, A. D., Reed, A. J., Person Mecca, L., & Kolko, D. J. (2014). Community-based clinicians' preferences for training in evidence-based practices: A mixed-method study. *Professional Psychology: Research and Practice, 45,* 188–199.

Hornsey, M. J., & Fielding, K. S. (2017). Attitude roots and Jiu Jitsu persuasion: Understanding and overcoming the motivated rejection of science. *American Psychologist, 72*(5), 459.

International Society for Traumatic Stress Studies. (2018). New ISTSS prevention and treatment guidelines. Retrieved from *www.istss.org/treating-trauma/new-istss-prevention-and-treatment-guidelines.aspx.*

Karlin, B. E., & Cross, G., (2014). From the laboratory to the therapy room: National dissemination and implementation of evidence-based psychotherapies in the U.S. Department of Veterans Affairs Health Care System. *American Psychologist, 69*(1), 19–33.

Karlin, B. E., Ruzek, J. I., Chard, K. M., Eftekhari, A., Monson, C. M., Hembree, E. A., et al. (2010). Dissemination of evidence-based psychological treatments for posttraumatic stress disorder in the Veterans Health Administration. *Journal of Traumatic Stress, 23*(6), 663–673.

Kirchner, J. E., Ritchie, M. J., Pitcock, J. A., Parker, L. E., Curran, G. M., & Fortney, J. C. (2014). Outcomes of a partnered facilitation strategy to implement primary care–mental health. *Journal of General Internal Medicine, 29*(4), 904–912.

Lewis, C. C., Puspitasari, A., Boyd, M. R., Scott, K., Marriott, B. R., Hoffman, M., et al. (2018). Implementing measurement based care in community mental health: A description of tailored and standardized methods. *BMC Research Notes, 11*(1), 76.

LoSavio, S. T., Dillon, K. H., Murphy, R. A., Goetz, K., Houston, F., & Resick, P. A. (2019). Using a Learning Collaborative Model to Disseminate Cognitive Processing Therapy to Community-Based Agencies. *Behavior Therapy, 50*(1), 36–49.

Lucid, L., Meza, R. D., Pullmann, M. D., Jungbluth, N., Deblinger, E., & Dorsey, S.

(2018). Supervision in community mental health: Understanding intensity of EBT focus. *Behavior Therapy, 49,* 481–493.

Lund, C., Tomlinson, M., De Silva, M., Fekadu, A., Shidhaye, R., Jordans, M., et al. (2012). PRIME: A programme to reduce the treatment gap for mental disorders in five low- and middle-income countries. *PLOS Medicine, 9*(12), e1001359.

Maguen, S., Madden, E., Patterson, O. V., DuVall, S. L., Goldstein, L. A., Burkman, K., et al. (2018). Measuring use of evidence based psychotherapy for posttraumatic stress disorder in a large national healthcare system. *Administration and Policy in Mental Health and Mental Health Services Research, 45*(4), 519–529.

Mallonee, S., Phillips, J., Holloway, K., & Riggs, D. (2018). Training providers in the use of evidence-based treatments: A comparison of in-person and online delivery modes. *Psychology Learning and Teaching, 17*(1), 61–72.

Matsuzaka, C. T., Wainberg, M., Pala, A. N., Hoffmann, E. V., Coimbra, B. M., Braga, R. F., et al. (2017). Task shifting interpersonal counseling for depression: A pragmatic randomized controlled trial in primary care. *BMC Psychiatry, 17*(1), 225.

McHugh, R. K., & Barlow, D. H. (2010). The dissemination and implementation of evidence-based psychological treatments: A review of current efforts. *American Psychologist, 65*(2), 73–84.

McKay, M. M., & Bannon, W. M. (2004). Engaging families in child mental health services. *Child and Adolescent Psychiatry Clinics of North America, 13,* 905–921.

McLeod, B. D., Cox, J. R., Jensen-Doss, A., Herschell, A., Ehrenreich-May, J., & Wood, J. J. (2018). Proposing a mechanistic model of clinician training and consultation. *Clinical Psychology: Science and Practice, 25*(3), e12260.

Monson, C. M., Shields, N., Suvak, M. K., Lane, J. E., Shnaider, P., Landy, M. S., et al. (2018). A randomized controlled effectiveness trial of training strategies in cognitive processing therapy for posttraumatic stress disorder: Impact on patient outcomes. *Behaviour Research and Therapy, 110,* 31–40.

Mor Barak, M. E., Nissley, J. A., & Levin, A. (2001). Antecedents to retention and turnover among child welfare, social work, and other human service employees: What can we learn from past research?: A review and meta-analysis. *Administration and Policy in Mental Health and Mental Health Services Research, 39*(5), 341–352.

Mott, J. M., Stanley, M. A., Street, R. L., Jr., Grady, R. H., & Teng, E. J. (2014). Increasing engagement in evidence-based PTSD treatment through shared decision-making: A pilot study. *Military Medicine, 179*(2), 143–149.

Murray, L. K., Dorsey, S., Bolton, P., Jordans, M. J. D., Rahman, A., Bass, J., et al. (2011). Building capacity in mental health interventions in low resource countries: An apprenticeship model for training local providers. *Journal of Mental Health Systems, 5*(30).

Murray, L. K., Skavenski, S., Kane, J. C., Mayeya, J., Dorsey, S., Cohen, J. A., et al. (2015). Effectiveness of trauma-focused cognitive behavioral therapy among trauma-affected children in Lusaka, Zambia: A randomized clinical trial. *JAMA Pediatrics, 169*(8), 761–769.

Nadeem, E., Gleacher, A., & Beidas, R. S. (2013). Consultation as an implementation strategy for evidence-based practices across multiple contexts: Unpacking the black box. *Administration and Policy in Mental Health and Mental Health Services Research, 40*(6), 439–450.

Neuner, F., Onyut, P. L., Ertl, V., Odenwald, M., Schauer, E., & Elbert, T. (2008).

Treatment of posttraumatic stress disorder by trained lay counselors in an African refugee settlement: A randomized controlled trial. *Journal of Consulting and Clinical Psychology, 76*(4), 686.

Parkin, E. (2018). Mental health policy in England (Briefing paper no. CBP 07547). Retrieved from *http://researchbriefings.files.parliament.uk/documents/CBP-7547/ CBP-7547.pdf.*

Patel, V., Chowdhary, N., Rahman, A., & Verdeli, H. (2011). Improving access to psychological treatments: Lessons from developing countries. *Behavioral Research and Therapy, 49*(9), 523–528.

Paxton, M. M., Mallonee, S., Reo, G., Phillips, J., Martin, R., & Riggs, D. S. (2018, November). *Using online technology to disseminate evidence-based treatments for PTSD.* Poster presented at the annual meeting of the International Society for Traumatic Stress Studies, Washington, DC.

Paxton Willing, M. M., Mallonee, S., Reo, G., Phillips, J., Carrier, D. L., & Riggs, D. S. (2018). *Training providers in the use of evidenced-based practices.* Manuscript submitted for publication.

Powell, B. J., Beidas, R. S., Lewis, C. C., Aarons, G. A., McMillen, J. C., Proctor, E. K., et al. (2017). Methods to improve the selection and tailoring of implementation strategies. *Journal of Behavioral Health Services and Research, 44*(2), 177–194.

Pullmann, M. D., Lucid, L., Harrison, J., Martin, P., Deblinger, E., Benjamin, K. S., et al. (2018). Implementation climate and time predict intensity of supervision content related to evidence based treatment. *Frontiers in Public Health: Public Health Education and Promotion, 6*(280).

Rakovshik, S. G., McManus, F., Vazquez-Montes, M., Muse, K., & Ougrin, D. (2016). Is supervision necessary?: Examining the effects of Internet-based CBT training with and without supervision. *Journal of Consulting and Clinical Psychology, 84*(3), 191.

Rosen, C. S., Eftekhari, A., Crowley, J. J., Smith, B. N., Kuhn, E., Trent, L., et al. (2017). Maintenance and reach of exposure psychotherapy for posttraumatic stress disorder 18 months after training. *Journal of Traumatic Stress, 30*(1), 63–70.

Rosen, C. S., Matthieu, M. M., Cook, J. M., Stirman, S. W., Landes, S. J., Bernardy, N. C., et al. (2016). A review of studies on the system-wide implementation of evidence-based psychotherapies for posttraumatic stress disorder in the Veterans Health Administration. *Administration and Policy in Mental Health and Mental Health Services Research, 43*(6), 957–977.

Ruzek, J. I., Eftekhari, A., Rosen, C. S., Crowley, J. J., Kuhn, E., Foa, E. B., et al. (2016). Effects of a comprehensive training program on clinician beliefs about and intention to use prolonged exposure therapy for PTSD. *Psychological Trauma: Theory, Research, Practice, and Policy, 8*(3), 348.

Ruzek, J. I., Rosen, R. C., Garvert, D. W., Smith, L. D., Sears, K. C., Marceau, L., et al. (2014). Online self-administered training of PTSD treatment providers in cognitive–behavioral intervention skills: Results of a randomized controlled trial. *Journal of Traumatic Stress, 27*(6), 703–711.

Sayer, N. A., Rosen, C. S., Bernardy, N. C., Cook, J. M., Orazem, R. J., Chard, K. M., et al. (2017). Context matters: Team and organizational factors associated with reach of evidence-based psychotherapies for PTSD in the Veterans Health Administration. *Administration and Policy in Mental Health and Mental Health Services Research, 44*(6), 904–918.

Schoenwald, S. K., Garland, A. F., Chapman, J. E., Frazier, S. L., Sheidow, A. J., &

Southam-Gerow, M. A. (2010). Toward the effective and efficient measurement of implementation fidelity. *Administration and Policy in Mental Health and Mental Health Services Research, 38*(1), 32–43.

Sigel, B. A., Benton, A. H., Lynch, C. E., & Kramer, T. L. (2013). Characteristics of 17 statewides initiatives to disseminate trauma-focused cognitive-behavioral therapy (TF-CBT). *Psychological Trauma: Theory, Research, Practice, and Policy, 5*(4), 323–333.

Silagy, C., Rubin, G., Henderson-Smart, D., & Gross, P. (1998). *A guide to the development, implementation and evaluation of clinical practice guidelines.* Canberra: National Health and Medical Research Council, Commonwealth of Australia.

Smith, A. M. (2017). *An examination of the content of and engagement in ongoing consultation following training in trauma focused cognitive-behavioral therapy.* Unpublished doctoral dissertation, University of Miami.

Stein, B. D., Celedonia, K. L., Swartz, H. A., DeRosier, M. E., Sorbero, M. J., Brindley, R. A., et al. (2015). Implementing a web-based intervention to train community clinicians in an evidence-based psychotherapy: A pilot study. *Psychiatric Services, 66*(9), 988–991.

Stewart, R. E., Lareef, I., Hadley, T. R., & Mandell, D. S. (2017). Can we pay for performance in behavioral health care? *Psychiatric Services, 68*(2), 109–111.

Stirman, S. W., Gutner, C. A., Langdon, K., & Graham, J. R. (2016). Bridging the gap between research and practice in mental health service settings: An overview of developments in implementation theory and research. *Behavior Therapy, 47*(6), 920–936.

Stirman, S. W., Pontoski, K., Creed, T., Xhezo, R., Evans, A. C., Beck, A. T., et al. (2017). A non-randomized comparison of strategies for consultation in a community-academic training program to implement an evidence-based psychotherapy. *Administration and Policy in Mental Health and Mental Health Services Research, 44*(1), 55–66.

Thompson, R., Simiola, V., Schnurr, P. P., Stirman, S. W., & Cook, J. M. (2018). VA residential treatment providers' use of two evidence-based psychotherapies for PTSD: Global endorsement versus specific components. *Psychological Trauma: Theory, Research, Practice, and Policy, 10*(2), 131–139.

Waltman, S. H., Hall, B. C., McFarr, L. M., & Creed, T. A. (2018). Clinical case consultation and experiential learning in cognitive behavioral therapy implementation: Brief qualitative investigation. *Journal of Cognitive Psychotherapy, 32*(2), 112–126.

Waltz, T. J., Powell, B. J., Matthieu, M. M., Damschroder, L. J., Chinman, M. J., Smith, J. L., et al. (2015). Use of concept mapping to characterize relationships among implementation strategies and assess their feasibility and importance: Results from the Expert Recommendations for Implementing Change (ERIC) study. *Implementation Science, 10*(1), 1.

Watts, B. V., Schnurr, P. P., Zayed, M., Yinong, Y., Stender, P., & Llewellyn-Thomas, H. (2015). A randomized controlled clinical trial of a patient decision aid for posttraumatic stress disorder. *Psychiatric Services, 66*(2), 149–154.

Weingardt, K. R. (2004). The role of instructional design and technology in the dissemination of empirically supported, manual-based therapies. *Clinical Psychology: Science and Practice, 11*(3), 313–331.

Weisz, J. R., Chorpita, B. F., Palinkas, L. A., Schoenwald, S. K., Miranda, J., Bearman, S. K., et al. (2012). Testing standard and modular designs for psychotherapy treating depression, anxiety, and conduct problems in youth: A randomized effectiveness trial. *Archives of General Psychiatry, 69,* 274–282.

Weisz, J. R., Doss, A. J., & Hawley, K. M. (2005). Youth psychotherapy outcome research: A review and critique of the evidence base. *Annual Review of Psychology, 56,* 337–363.

Weiss, W. M., Murray, L. K., Zangana, G. A. S., Mahmooth, Z., Kaysen, D., Dorsey, S., et al. (2015). Community-based mental health treatments for survivors of torture and militant attacks in Southern Iraq: A randomized control trial. *BMC Psychiatry, 15*(1), 249.

Welsh Government. (2012). Together for Mental Health: A strategy for mental health and wellbeing in Wales. Retrieved from *https://gov.wales/sites/default/files/publications/2019-04/together-for-mental-health-summary.pdf.*

Wilk, J. E., West, J. C., Duffy, F. F., Herrell, R. K., Rae, D. S., & Hoge, C. W. (2013). Use of evidence-based treatment for posttraumatic stress disorder in Army behavioral healthcare. *Psychiatry: Interpersonal and Biological Processes, 76*(4), 336–348.

Yuan, B., He, L., Meng, Q., & Jia, L. (2017). Payment methods for outpatient care facilities. *Cochrane Database of Systematic Reviews,* Issue 3, Article No. CD011153.

CHAPTER 25

A Health Economics View

Ifigeneia Mavranezouli and Cathrine Mihalopoulos

According to the World Health Organization (WHO) World Mental Health Surveys, posttraumatic stress disorder (PTSD) has a lifetime prevalence of 3.9% in the general population, and 5.6% among those exposed to trauma (Koenen et al., 2017). The mean duration of PTSD symptoms is approximately 6 years, ranging from about 1 year for symptoms developed following exposure to a natural disaster to over 13 years following traumas involving combat experience (Kessler et al., 2017). These data suggest a mean number of 12.9 PTSD episodes per 100 people in the general population, which translate into a burden of 77.7 years lived with PTSD per 100 people (Kessler et al., 2017).

PTSD is associated with substantial levels of disability, loss of quality of life, and reduced productivity (Alonso et al., 2004). It is often comorbid with other mental disorders such as depression, substance abuse, other anxiety disorders (Kessler, Sonnega, Bromet, Hughes, & Nelson, 1995), and has been associated with cardiovascular and metabolic disease (Ahmadi et al., 2011; Dedert, Calhoun, Watkins, Sherwood, & Beckham, 2010). Despite the burden associated with PTSD, only a small proportion of people with PTSD seek treatment for their symptoms, ranging from 23% in low-/lower-middle-income countries to 54% in high-income countries (Koenen et al., 2017). Nevertheless, wide literature suggests that people with PTSD consume a considerable amount of health care resources.

People with posttraumatic stress symptoms incur significantly higher health care costs compared with people without such symptoms, including costs associated with outpatient visits, emergency department visits, mental health inpatient stays, physician contacts, and medication (Chan, Medicine, Air, & McFarlane, 2003; Lamoureux-Lamarche, Vasiliadis, Preville, & Berbiche, 2016; Walker et al., 2003). A U.S. study on Department of Veterans

Affairs patients with depression showed that those with comorbid PTSD symptoms had more frequent mental health specialty and other outpatient visits compared with patients with depression without PTSD (Chan, Cheadle, Reiber, Unutzer, & Chaney, 2009). In another U.S. study, patients with PTSD were found to incur significantly higher mental health and total health care costs than those incurred by patients with depression, after adjusting for baseline characteristics (Ivanova et al., 2011). Using data from the Nationwide Inpatient Sample (NIS), the largest all-payer inpatient care database in the United States, Haviland, Banta, Sonne, and Przekop (2016) estimated that between 2002 and 2011 there were 1,477,944 hospitalizations with either a primary or secondary PTSD diagnosis in the United States, costing $34.9 billion (2011 U.S. dollars). In Europe, in 2010 there were an estimated 7.7 million patients with PTSD, incurring health care costs of €8.24 million (2010 euros) (Gustavsson et al., 2011).

In addition to health care resources, people with PTSD may use social services and incur costs associated with social worker contacts, rehabilitation, housing, and social benefits. They are also likely to have PTSD-related out-of-pocket expenses and bear costs relating to absenteeism and unemployment. A study conducted in Northern Ireland estimated that in 2008 there were 74,935 individuals with PTSD in Northern Ireland, who incurred approximately £27.3 million in service costs (including hospitalizations and visits to health care professionals), £5.7 million in medication costs, and £139.8 million in reduced productivity (associated with either days of incapacity or reduced productivity while at work) (Ferry et al., 2015). These findings suggest that PTSD imposes a considerable burden on individuals, their carers and family, health and social care services, and the broader society.

Basic Concepts in Economic Evaluation of Health Care Interventions

The principle underpinning the development of health economics is the scarcity of health care resources and the choices that need to be made on how to best use these limited resources. When resources are used in one way to provide some form of health benefit, other benefits are forgone by not using resources in an alternative way (opportunity cost). Economic evaluation compares both costs and consequences of alternative courses of action to identify cost-effective strategies to inform decision making. The aim of economic evaluation is to achieve optimal allocation of resources in order to maximize the benefits for the population (Drummnod, Schulpher, Claxton, Stoddart, & Torrance, 2015). A number of regulatory and advisory bodies worldwide, such as the National Institute for Health and Care Excellence (NICE) in England (*www.nice.org.uk*), the Dutch National Health Care Institute (*https://english.zorginstituutnederland.nl*), the Norwegian Medicine Agency (*https://legemiddelverket.no/English*), the Canadian Agency for

Drugs and Technologies in Health (CADTH; *www.cadth.ca*), and the Pharmaceutical Benefits Advisory Committee (PBAC) in Australia (*https://pbac. pbs.gov.au*), incorporate cost-effectiveness considerations in their appraisals of health technologies and programs.

Depending on the measure of health outcome used, four broad types of economic evaluation can be identified: cost-effectiveness analysis, cost–consequence analysis, cost–benefit analysis, and cost–utility analysis (Drummnod et al., 2015). In cost-effectiveness analysis, a single outcome measure is used that is expressed in physical, clinically meaningful units (e.g., number of lives saved, mean change score on a PTSD symptom scale). In cost–consequence analysis, there is no summary measure of health outcome. Instead, various outcomes associated with the health care strategies assessed, such as clinical symptoms, acceptability, functioning, and quality of life, are considered alongside costs. In cost–benefit analysis, health outcomes are given a monetary value; this can be determined, for example, by asking individuals to state the maximum amount of money they are willing to pay to gain the health benefits accrued by the assessed strategy. Finally, in cost–utility analysis, a single summary measure of health outcome is used, capturing both mortality and morbidity aspects of health. Common examples of such outcome measures include the quality-adjusted life year (QALY), the disability-adjusted life year (DALY), and the health-adjusted life expectancy (HALE). The most commonly used metric is the QALY (Weinstein, Torrance, & McGuire, 2009).

QALYs express the amount of time spent by an individual in a health state, weighted by a utility value representing the "value" of the health-related quality of life (HRQoL) relating to this state. Utility values reflect people's preferences for health; they measure HRQoL on a scale from 0 (death) to 1 (perfect health). For example, 2 years of life with a HRQoL valued at 0.8 provide $2 \times 0.8 = 1.6$ QALYs. By incorporating quantity and quality of life in a single summary measure, QALYs allow broad cost-effectiveness comparisons across strategies aimed at different disease areas and patient populations (Brazier, Ratcliffe, Salomon, & Tsuchiya, 2017). For this reason, the QALY is the preferred summary outcome measure for economic evaluation by many regulatory bodies worldwide that have incorporated cost-effectiveness considerations in their decision-making processes (Sassi, 2006). Several studies, using a variety of validated methods, have translated the HRQoL of people with PTSD into "preference-based" utility values that can be used for the estimation of QALYs (Doctor, Zoellner, & Feeny, 2011; Freed et al., 2009; Gospodarevskaya, 2013; Haagsma et al., 2012; Mancino et al., 2006).

An alternative measure to the QALY is the DALY, a measure that has been widely used by the WHO and Institute of Health Metrics in their evaluation of the global burden of disease (Murray et al., 2012). DALYs express the number of years lost due to premature mortality or due to disability (World Health Organization, 2018). The use of DALYs in economic evaluation of health care interventions is less common than the use of QALYs; nevertheless, DALYs are being used in WHO Generalized Cost-Effectiveness Analysis studies (Murray, Evans, Acharya, & Baltussen, 2000) and studies aiming at priority setting in the Australian health care system (Carter et al., 2008).

The first step in estimating the total costs (that may be incurred or saved) associated with a health care strategy, service, or intervention is to determine the perspective of the economic evaluation (Byford & Raftery, 1998). Quite commonly, the adopted perspective is that of the providers (health service) or payers (e.g., health insurance) of health care; these perspectives take into account costs such as medication, health care staff time, hospitalization, laboratory testing, and the like. Depending on the stakeholders' interests and the bodies and individuals affected by the evaluated strategies, broader perspectives can be used that may include social care costs, costs falling onto other public bodies (e.g., the criminal justice system), out-of-pocket expenses for patients and families/carers, as well as indirect costs relating to productivity losses, for example, due to disability, unemployment, or time off from work (Drummnod et al., 2015). The broadest perspective is the societal one; this perspective measures the impact of an intervention or program on the welfare of the whole society, including both direct (health care and non-health care) costs and productivity losses (Byford & Raftery, 1998). Although adoption of a societal perspective is broadly advocated (Jonsson, 2009), it has been argued that incorporation of productivity losses may have equity implications (as it disfavors older adults, children, and people with disabilities); furthermore, it raises methodological issues in terms of quantifying and valuing productivity effects (Knies, Severens, Ament, & Evers, 2010; Schulper, 2001).

To determine the cost-effectiveness of a strategy, it is necessary to compare both costs and health outcomes between the strategy and its comparator. When a strategy has lower total costs and higher total benefits than its comparator, then it is clearly more cost-effective and is called "dominant." In contrast, when a strategy has higher total costs and lower total benefits than its comparator, it is less cost-effective and "dominated." When total costs and benefits are both higher or both lower than the comparator's, then they can be combined in an Incremental Cost-Effectiveness Ratio (ICER), which is the difference in costs (ΔC) divided by the difference in benefits (ΔB) between the two strategies, so that

$$ICER = \Delta C / \Delta B$$

The decision maker then needs to judge whether the additional (incremental) benefits are worth the incremental costs to determine whether the evaluated strategy is cost-effective. For example, NICE in England generally considers strategies as being cost-effective when they have an ICER of up to £20,000–£30,000/QALY (National Institute for Health and Care Excellence, 2013). In Canada, CADTH has not determined an explicit cost-effectiveness threshold (Canadian Agency for Drugs and Technologies in Health, 2017). In Australia, PBAC has also not set an explicit threshold; however, an implicit threshold of Aus$45,000–$50,000/QALY (or DALY) is effectively being used (Carter et al., 2008; Edney, Haji Ali, Cheng, & Karnon, 2018), whereas in the United States, the American College of Cardiology and American Heart Association consider interventions with an ICER below US$50,000/QALY as highly cost-effective (Dubois, 2016).

An economic analysis should include all options relevant to a decision problem, including standard care, and adopt an incremental approach of analysis, where each option is compared to the next most effective nondominated option. The option with the highest ICER below the cost-effectiveness threshold is the most cost-effective option.

Economic evaluations can be conducted alongside clinical trials or observational clinical studies, where the health outcomes and resources consumed by the study samples are measured in parallel, or by undertaking decision-analytic economic modeling. Decision-analytic models are simulations of alternative care pathways onto hypothetical cohorts of people (ranging from a single "average" person to an entire population) that allow the estimation of the relative cost-effectiveness of different programs over long time horizons by synthesizing clinical and cost data derived from various sources, such as clinical trials, observational studies, patient notes, and expert opinion (Petrou & Gray, 2011). The robustness of the results of economic modeling should be tested in sensitivity analysis, which explores the impact of different assumptions and of the uncertainty in the model input parameters on the results and conclusions of the economic analysis (Briggs, Sculpher, & Buxton, 1994). Probabilistic analysis enables concurrent consideration of uncertainty across all input parameters (Briggs, 1999) and allows estimation of the probability that an intervention is cost-effective at different cost-effectiveness thresholds (Fenwick, Claxton, & Sculpher, 2001).

Cost-Effectiveness of Interventions for PTSD

Several studies have assessed the cost-effectiveness of interventions for people with PTSD. The majority of economic evaluations have assessed treatments for adults, but more recently there has been emerging literature on the cost-effectiveness of treatments for children and adolescents with PTSD. The economic studies of treatments for PTSD described in this chapter were identified by a systematic literature search in the MEDLINE, Embase, and HTA databases for the period between January 2000 and November 2018, using combined terms to capture the target condition (PTSD) and terms relating to economic evaluation. The search did not attempt to identify gray literature. In addition, we have included a description of the primary economic analyses undertaken to inform the NICE 2018 PTSD guideline update (National Institute for Health and Care Excellence, 2018a). These analyses were based on clinical data gathered by NICE and therefore may have taken into account different clinical data from those considered for the International Society for Traumatic Stress Studies (ISTSS) guidelines update, due to differences in inclusion criteria and the overall methodology adopted between the two guidelines. It is thus important to recognize that this has led to some subtle differences between the NICE recommendations and those of ISTSS.

An overview of the methods and results of economic studies assessing treatments for PTSD in adults and children/adolescents is provided in Tables 25.1 and 25.2, respectively.

Interpretation of Economic Evidence: Implications for Policy and Practice

Summary of Cost-Effectiveness Findings

Treatments for Adults with PTSD

Limited evidence suggests that a stepped-care case-finding intervention may be cost-effective for adults after large-scale trauma. Cognitive-behavioral therapy with a trauma focus (CBT-T), prolonged exposure (PE), cognitive processing therapy (CPT), virtual reality exposure (VRE), and selective serotonin reuptake inhibitors (SSRIs) appear to be cost-effective relative to no treatment or treatment as usual (TAU) for adults with PTSD. On the other hand, collaborative care, group self-management therapy that includes a direct behavioral component, and CBT tailored for adults with PTSD and co-occurring severe mental illness have been shown to be no more cost-effective than either TAU or psychoeducation. PE appears to be more cost-effective than sertraline.

According to the only study that explored the relative cost-effectiveness across multiple treatment options, brief individual CBT-T (<8 sessions), psychoeducation, eye motion desensitization and reprocessing (EMDR) therapy, combined somatic and cognitive therapies, and self-help with support appear to be among the most cost-effective treatment options for adults with PTSD. In contrast, individual CBT-T >12 sessions, counseling, combined individual CBT-T and SSRIs, group CBT-T, and present-centered therapy appear to be the least cost-effective options relative to other active treatments. Counseling and individual CBT-T >12 sessions may be less cost-effective than no treatment. In between, there are other, "moderately" cost-effective options such as SSRIs, individual CBT-T 8–12 sessions, self-help without support, CBT without a trauma focus, and interpersonal psychotherapy (IPT).

TABLE 25.1. Overview of the Methods and Results of Economic Evaluations of Interventions for Adults with PTSD

Study Country	Type of economic evaluation Measure of outcome Study design and source of efficacy data Time horizon	Study population	Interventions compared	Perspective Cost elements Currency and cost year	Cost-effectiveness results Uncertainty
Cohen et al. (2017) U.S.	Cost-effectiveness and cost-utility analysis Number of PTSD-free days and DALY Decision-analytic modeling; diagnostic characteristics: assumption; efficacy: published studies 10 yr	Hypothetical cohort of individuals living in hurricane-affected areas of New York City	• Stepped-care case-finding intervention and early treatment: cases were referred to CBT; noncases were referred to SPR, an evidence-informed therapy that aims to reduce distress and improve coping and functioning • TAU; all patients were referred to SPR	Health care sector Therapists' time U.S. dollars, likely 2012	*Stepped care vs. TAU:* $0.80–1.61/PTSD-free day $3,429–6,858/DALY averted (Ranges derived from different assumptions regarding costs of CBT and SPR.) Results robust to use of a range of values for sensitivity and specificity (0.80–1).
Dunn et al. (2007) U.S.	Cost-consequence analysis PTSD symptoms measured by CAPS and DTSS; depressive symptoms measured by the 18-item HAMD and BDI-II, treatment compliance, satisfaction with treatment, treatment-targeted constructs, functioning measured by the BSI and ASI RCT (N = 101) 12 mon	Male veterans with chronic combat-related PTSD and depressive disorder	• Group self-management therapy that included a direct behavioral component • Group psychoeducation	Health service Psychiatric, medical, and surgical care; medication U.S. dollars, 1999	Self-management therapy resulted in similar costs and outcomes with psychoeducation.

Le, Doctor, Zoellner, & Feeny (2014) U.S.	Cost-utility analysis; QALY; RCT (N = 103) and preference trial (N = 97); 12 mon	Adults with PTSD	• Prolonged exposure • Sertraline	Societal; Therapists' time, medication, outpatient care and inpatient care, emergency department, pharmacy and other supportive services, productivity losses due to time spent in treatment and travel time to/from clinic; U.S. dollars, 2012	Prolonged exposure was dominant over sertraline in both RCT and preference trial (better outcomes, lower costs). Probability of prolonged exposure being cost-effective at a cost-effectiveness threshold of $100,000/QALY: 0.93 (range 0.91–0.95, for use of highest and lowest estimates of unit costs, respectively); at zero WTP, 0.60.
Meyers et al. (2013) U.S.	Cost-effectiveness analysis; PCL–military version score and BDI-II; Before–after study (N = 70); 12 mon	Veterans with combat-related PTSD or symptoms of PTSD	• Prolonged exposure or CPT • No treatment	Health service; Mental health care, primary care, emergency department; U.S. dollars, cost year not reported	Prolonged exposure or CPT was dominant over no treatment (better outcomes, lower costs). Difference in costs and outcomes was statistically significant.
Mihalopoulos et al. (2015) Australia	Cost-utility analysis; QALY and DALY; Decision-analytic economic modeling; systematic review and meta-analysis of RCTs; 5 yr	Prevalent cases of adults with PTSD in Australia in 2012, in receipt of non-evidence-based care	*1st comparison:* • CBT-T replacing or added on TAU • TAU (non-evidence-based care comprising consultation with health care professionals)	Health sector (government and patients' out-of-pocket expenses); Psychologists' and GPs' time; medication; Australian dollars, 2012	*1st comparison:* CBT-T vs. TAU: $19,000/QALY; $16,000/DALY averted. Probability of CBT-T being cost-effective: 1.00 at a cost-effectiveness threshold of $50,000/QALY

(continued)

TABLE 25.1. *(continued)*

Study / Country	Type of economic evaluation / Measure of outcome / Study design and source of efficacy data / Time horizon	Study population	Interventions compared	Perspective / Cost elements / Currency and cost year	Cost-effectiveness results / Uncertainty
Mihalopoulos et al. (2015) *(continued)*			*2nd comparison:* • SSRIs replacing or added on TAU • TAU (non-evidence-based medication)		Results most sensitive to changes in utility scores, participation rates, adherence to treatment, likelihood of being offered CBT and effectiveness *2nd comparison:* SSRIs vs. TAU: $230/QALY; ICER for DALYs averted not reported Probability of SSRIs being dominant: 0.27 Results most sensitive to changes in utility scores and participation rates
National Institute for Health and Care Excellence (2018c) UK	Cost-utility analysis QALY Decision-analytic economic modeling; systematic review and NMA of RCTs 3 yr	Adults with PTSD or clinically important symptoms of PTSD	• Combined somatic and cognitive therapies • Counseling • EMDR therapy • CBT without a trauma focus • IPT • Present-centered therapy	NHS and PSS Psychologists' time, inpatient and outpatient care, primary and community care, social services, medication GBP, 2017	All interventions except CBT-T individual <8 sessions and psychoeducation were dominated by one or more interventions. CBT-T individual <8 sessions vs. psychoeducation £9,208/QALY

* Psychoeducation
* Self-help with support
* Self-help without support
* SSRI
* CBT-T individual <8 sessions
* CBT-T individual 8–12 sessions
* CBT-T individual >12 sessions
* CBT-T group 8–12 sessions
* CBT-T individual 8–12 sessions + SSRI
* No treatment

CBT-T class included a range of interventions, such as cognitive processing therapy, CBT-T, cognitive therapy for PTSD, cognitive restructuring and imagery modification, narrative exposure, and prolonged exposure

Ranking of interventions by cost effectiveness (at a cost-effectiveness threshold of £20,000/QALY):
* CBT-T individual <8 sessions
* Psychoeducation
* EMDR therapy
* Combined somatic and cognitive therapies
* Self-help with support
* SSRI
* SH without support
* CBT-T individual 8–12 sessions
* IPT
* CBT without a trauma focus
* Present-centered therapy
* CBT-T group 8–12 sessions
* CBT-T individual 8–12 sessions + SSRI
* No treatment
* CBT-T individual >12 sessions
* Counseling
* Probability of CBT-T individual <8 sessions being the most cost-effective option: 0.28

Results robust to changes in the risk of relapse, changes in PTSD costs, use of alternative utility values, and different assumptions on the effect beyond 3 mon posttreatment

(continued)

TABLE 25.1. (*continued*)

Study / Country	Type of economic evaluation / Measure of outcome / Study design and source of efficacy data / Time horizon	Study population	Interventions compared	Perspective / Cost elements / Currency and cost year	Cost-effectiveness results / Uncertainty
Schmurr et al. (2013) U.S.	Cost-consequence analysis Primary: PTSD symptom severity, measured using the PDS Secondary: depression measured using the HSCL-20; functioning using the SF-12; perceived quality of PTSD care and overall care RCT (N = 195) 6 mon	Veterans with PTSD	• Collaborative care • TAU	Health service Outpatient visits including intervention, outpatient pharmacy, inpatient care (including pharmacy), and fee-for-service care U.S. dollars, 2010	Collaborative care was dominated by standard care (higher costs and similar or worse outcomes). No significant differences in outcomes, except in perceived quality of PTSD care, where collaborative care had a worse rating than TAU.
Slade et al. (2017) U.S.	Cost-effectiveness analysis Rate of PTSD remission (loss of clinical criteria for PTSD based on CAPS) RCT (N = 201) 12 mon	Adults with severe PTSD and co-occurring severe mental illness (major mood disorder, schizophrenia, or schizoaffective disorder)	• CBT tailored for adults with PTSD and co-occurring severe mental illness • Breathing retraining and psychoeducation	Public mental health system Therapists' time, mental health inpatient, outpatient, and emergency department care, psychotropic medication U.S. dollars, 2010	CBT vs. breathing retraining and psychoeducation: $36,893/PTSD remission Probability of CBT being cost-effective at a cost-effectiveness threshold of $50,000/PTSD remission: approx. 0.52

Study/Country	Analysis/Outcome measures	Population	Interventions	Perspective/Costs	Results
Tuerk et al. (2013) U.S.	Cost-effectiveness analysis PCL–military version score Before–after study (*N* = 60) 12 mon	Veterans with combat-related PTSD	• Prolonged exposure • No treatment	Mental health service Mental health care including intervention, medicine management, psychotherapy, supportive counseling, motivational interviewing, case management, and other relevant resource use; primary care costs were excluded U.S. dollars, 2009	Prolonged exposure was dominant over no treatment (better outcomes, lower costs). Difference in outcomes was statistically significant; level of significance of difference in costs not reported.
Wood et al. (2009) U.S.	Cost-consequence analysis PCL–military version score; PHQ-9; BAI Synthesis of data from multiple sources; noncomparative study (*N* = 12) for intervention effects; no modeling conducted 2 yr	Military staff with combat-related PTSD	• Virtual reality exposure therapy • TAU	Military system Therapists' time (assessment and intervention), military staff training (required to replace staff who would be medically discharged from duty due to the severity of their PTSD, if nonrecovered)	Virtual reality exposure therapy was dominant over TAU (better outcomes, lower costs).

Note: ASI, Addiction Severity Index; BAI, Beck Anxiety Inventory; BDI, Beck Depression Inventory; BSI, Brief Symptom Inventory; CAPS, clinician-administered PTSD Scale; CBT, cognitive-behavioral therapy; CBT-T, cognitive-behavioral therapy with a trauma focus; CPT, cognitive processing therapy; DALY, disability-adjusted life year; DTSS, Davidson Traumatic Stress Scale; EMDR, eye movement desensitization and reprocessing therapy; HAMD, Hamilton Depression Rating Scale; HSCL, Hopkins Symptom Checklist; ICER, incremental cost-effectiveness ratio; NHS, National Health Service; NMA, network meta-analysis; PCL, PTSD Check List; PDS, Posttraumatic Diagnostic Scale; PHQ, Patient Health Questionnaire; PSS, personal social services; QALY, quality-adjusted life year; RCT, randomized clinical trial; SF, short form; SPR, Skills for Psychological Recovery; SSRI, selective serotonin reuptake inhibitor; TAU, treatment as usual.

TABLE 25.2. Overview of the Methods and Results of Economic Evaluations of Interventions for Children and Adolescents with PTSD

Study Country	Type of economic evaluation Measure of outcome Study design and source of efficacy data Time horizon	Interventions compared	Study population	Perspective Cost elements Currency and cost year	Cost-effectiveness results Uncertainty
Aas, Iversen, Holt, Ormhaug, & Jensen (2018) Norway	Cost-utility analysis QALY RCT (N = 156) 2 yr	• CBT-T • TAU	Young people (10–18 years of age) presenting with symptoms of PTS	Health service Therapists' time Norwegian krone, 2018	CBT-T was dominant over TAU (more effective and less costly). Probability of CBT-T being cost-effective at a zero cost-effectiveness threshold: 0.96
Gospodarevskaya & Segal (2012) Australia	Cost-utility analysis QALY Decision-analytic economic modeling; meta-analysis of RCTs and indirect comparisons 31 yr	• CBT-T • CBT-T + SSRI • Nondirective supportive counseling • No treatment	Children who met all or most of the DSM-IV PTSD diagnostic criteria including at least one symptom of avoidance or reexperiencing; some had comorbid depression	Mental health service Therapists' time (psychologist, psychiatrist, GP, social worker), medication, parental group, or psychoeducational sessions Australian dollars, 2011	Counseling was dominated by CBT-T (less effective and more costly). CBT-T + SSRI vs. CBT-T $2,901/QALY CBT-T vs. no treatment $1,650/QALY Results sensitive to variation in clinical effectiveness

Study	Methods	Population	Interventions	Perspective / Costs	Results
McCrone et al. (2005) UK	Cost-consequence analysis Symptoms of PTSD using Orvaschel's PTSD scale; global impairment of functioning using the K-SADs and K-GAS RCT (N = 75) 2 yr	Sexually abused girls (6–14 years old) with symptoms of emotional or behavioral disturbance, 73% of whom had PTSD	• Individual psychoanalytical psychotherapy + support to parents • Group psychotherapy (with psychotherapeutic and psychoeducational components) + support to parents	Mental health services Therapists' time GBP, 1999	Individual therapy was significantly more costly than group therapy. No statistically significant difference in PTSD symptomatology or in global impairment of functioning between interventions; individual therapy showed significantly greater improvements in manifestations of PTSD compared with group therapy.
Mihalopoulos et al. (2015) Australia	Cost-utility analysis QALY and DALY Decision-analytic economic modeling; systematic review and meta-analysis of RCTs 5 yr	Prevalent cases of children and adolescents with PTSD in Australia in 2012, in receipt of non-evidence-based care	• CBT-T replacing or added on TAU • TAU (non-evidence-based care comprising consultation with health care professionals)	Health sector (government and patients' out-of-pocket expenses) Psychologists' and GPs' time Australian dollars, 2012	CBT-T vs. TAU: $8,900/QALY; $8,000/DALY averted Probability of CBT-T being cost-effective at a cost-effectiveness threshold of $50,000/QALY: 0.99 Results most sensitive to PTSD prevalence, effectiveness, adherence, and the likelihood of being considered eligible for CBT-T

(continued)

TABLE 25.2. (continued)

	National Institute for Health and Care Excellence (2018b)
Study	
Country	UK
Type of economic evaluation	Cost-utility analysis
Measure of outcome	QALY
Study design and source of efficacy data	Decision-analytic economic modeling; systematic review and NMA of RCTs
Time horizon	3 yr
Study population	Children and adolescents with PTSD or clinically important symptoms of PTSD
Interventions compared	• Cohen CBT-T/CPT (CBT-T) • CT-PTSD (CBT-T) • EMDR therapy • Family therapy • Group CBT-T (CBT-T) • Narrative exposure (CBT-T) • Parent training • Play therapy • Prolonged exposure (CBT-T) • Supportive counseling • No treatment
Perspective	
Cost elements	NHS and PSS Psychologists' time, inpatient and outpatient care, ambulance, emergency department, community staff, advice service, social services, medication
Currency and cost year	GBP, 2017
Cost-effectiveness results	
Uncertainty	CT-PTSD was dominant over all other interventions (less costly and more effective). Ranking of interventions by cost effectiveness (at a cost-effectiveness threshold of £20,000/QALY): • CT-PTSD • Narrative exposure • Play therapy • Prolonged exposure • Cohen CBT-T/CPT • EMDR therapy • Parent training • Group CBT • Family therapy • Support counseling • No treatment Probability of CT-PTSD being the most cost-effective option: 0.78 Results robust to changes in the risk of relapse and use of alternative utility data

Study	Analysis / outcomes / design / time horizon	Population	Interventions	Perspective / cost components / currency	Results / conclusions
Salloum et al. (2016) U.S.	Cost-consequence analysis Primary: trauma symptoms measured using the TSCYC, PTS subscale Secondary: CGI-S; CGI-I; CBCL; DIPA; treatment credibility and satisfaction; parents' assessment of PTSD diagnosis RCT ($N = 53$) 3 mon	Young children (aged 3–7 years) experiencing PTS symptoms	• Stepped-care CBT-T • Standard CBT-T	Societal (health care system and parents' productivity losses) Therapists' time, parents' productivity losses U.S. dollars, likely 2011	Stepped-care CBT-T similar to standard CBT-T regarding outcomes (less effective in CBCL externalizing T-scores) and less costly
Shearer et al. (2018) UK	Cost-utility analysis QALY RCT ($N = 29$) and extrapolation using decision-analytic economic modeling 3 yr	Children and adolescents aged 8–17 years, who had experienced a single traumatic event in the previous 2–6 mon and met age-appropriate diagnosis of PTSD	• CT-PTSD • Wait list	NHS and PSS Psychologists' time, inpatient and outpatient care, ambulance, emergency department, community staff, advice service, social services, medication GBP, 2014	CT-PTSD vs. wait list: £2,205/QALY Probability of CT-PTSD being cost-effective at a cost-effectiveness threshold of £20,000–30,000/QALY, respectively: 0.60–0.69 Conclusions on cost-effectiveness robust to completer case analysis and to inclusion of psychologist training costs

Note: CBCL, Child Behavior Checklist; CBT-T, cognitive-behavioral therapy with a trauma focus; CGI-I, Clinical Global Impression—Improvement; CGI-S, Clinical Global Impression—Severity; CPT, cognitive processing therapy; CT-PTSD, cognitive therapy for PTSD; DALY, disability-adjusted life year; DIPA, Diagnostic Infant and Preschool Assessment; EMDR, eye movement desensitization and reprocessing therapy; K-GAS, Kiddie Global Assessment Scale; K-SADs, Kiddie Schedule for Affective Disorders and Schizophrenia scale; NHS, National Health Service; NMA, network meta-analysis; PTS, posttraumatic stress; PSS, personal social services; QALY, quality-adjusted life year; RCT, randomized clinical trial; SSRI, selective serotonin reuptake inhibitor; TAU, treatment as usual; TSCYC, Trauma Symptom Checklist for Young Children.

Treatments for Children and Adolescents with PTSD

For children and adolescents with PTSD, evidence indicates that CBT-T, stepped-care CBT-T, and cognitive therapy for PTSD (CT-PTSD) are likely to be cost-effective compared with no treatment or TAU. Group psychotherapy may be more cost-effective than individual psychotherapy. Combination therapy consisting of CBT-T and SSRIs appears to be more cost-effective than CBT-T alone in children with PTSD and possible comorbid depression.

Regarding the relative cost-effectiveness across multiple treatment options, individual forms of CBT-T and, to a lesser degree, play therapy appear to be most cost-effective in the treatment of children and adolescents with PTSD, followed by EMDR therapy, parent training, and group CBT-T, with family therapy and supportive counseling being the least cost-effective treatments. Nevertheless, all these treatments are likely to be more cost-effective than no treatment for children and adolescents with PTSD.

Limitations of the Existing Evidence Base

Current economic evidence covers primarily the cost-effectiveness of treatments for adults, children, and young people with PTSD. There is very limited or nonexistent economic evidence for prevention and early intervention. Moreover, the evidence comes from a small number of developed countries (primarily the United States, but also the United Kingdom, Norway, and Australia); no evidence is available on the cost-effectiveness of treatments for people with PTSD in developing countries.

The majority of reviewed economic evaluations have included a limited number of treatment options, with a focus on CBT-T and its various forms, with other evidence-based treatments having been largely ignored in this literature. For example, the cost-effectiveness of EMDR therapy in adults and children/adolescents with PTSD has been assessed only in two analyses that informed national guidance in England (National Institute for Health and Care Excellence, 2018b, 2018c), despite the relatively wide evidence base on its clinical effectiveness, in particular among adults. Moreover, the vast majority of economic studies made comparisons of one active intervention with no treatment or TAU, or they made comparisons among a very limited number of active treatments. Although this may be reasonable in a single-intervention decision context (particularly when the comparator is TAU, which should theoretically include the mix of options currently being used), it can lead to a suboptimal allocation of resources if the new intervention is likely to displace another intervention that has not been formally considered in the evaluation.

To ensure efficient use of available resources, economic evaluations should assess the relative cost-effectiveness of the interventions or care likely to be displaced by adoption of the new intervention. The most appropriate comparator is likely to change in different decision contexts, and one of the hallmarks of good economic evaluations is ensuring that the appropriate comparators are used for each decision problem. If no interventions or care is likely to be displaced, then an appropriate comparator may be "no treatment." Unfortunately, many studies do not explicitly address whether the comparator is the mix of services likely to be displaced. Ideally, the assessment of the cost-effectiveness of a new intervention should also take into account any other new interventions that could, in principle, replace the mix of options currently forming TAU, by being implemented in addition to, or instead of, the new intervention of interest.

As can be seen from Tables 25.1 and 25.2, a large number of economic studies were conducted alongside randomized clinical trials (RCTs; 4/10 in adults and 4/7 in children/adolescents). Although these studies were of reasonable quality as suggested by their study design, most of them included a small number of participants and had relatively short time horizons that did not allow long-term outcomes and costs further down the care pathway to be considered and incorporated into the cost-effectiveness estimates. Therefore, their results should be replicated before robust conclusions can be drawn. However, one trial-based analysis extrapolated results beyond the trial endpoint, using decision-analytic modeling, and considered costs and benefits over a period of 3 years (Shearer et al., 2018). More important limitations characterize three economic studies in adults that used a before–after or noncomparative study design, as these designs are subject to bias.

Regarding model-based studies (3/10 in adults and 3/7 in children/adolescents), their quality depends on the assumptions used to structure and populate the models, sources of data, and methods of evidence synthesis, as well as the time horizon and ability to incorporate longer-term costs and outcomes. All model-based economic studies that assessed treatments for people with PTSD derived efficacy data from a review and meta-analysis of RCTs and had long time horizons, ranging from 3 to 31 years. The economic analyses that were conducted to inform national guidelines in England (National Institute for Health and Care Excellence, 2018b, 2018c) employed network meta-analytic (NMA) techniques for synthesis of the efficacy data. This approach considers information from both direct and indirect comparisons between interventions and allows simultaneous inference on multiple treatment options examined in RCTs while preserving randomization (Caldwell, Ades, & Higgins, 2005; Mavridis, Giannatsi, Cipriani, & Salanti, 2015). The simulation study on the stepped-care early intervention (Cohen et al., 2017) derived clinical data from a mixture of published studies and assumptions, and therefore results should be interpreted with greater caution, although sensitivity analysis examined the impact of different assumptions on the results.

Most of the studies utilized a health care perspective, often focusing on mental health care costs. The studies conducted in the United Kingdom included personal social service costs in their assessment and another two studies reported adopting a societal perspective, which, in addition to health care costs, included productivity losses. A number of studies considered only intervention costs as part of the health care perspective; however, people with PTSD may consume additional health care resources, such as emergency department, outpatient, and day care, which may be reduced following provision of effective interventions. Moreover, none of the studies included wider public-sector costs, such as those relating to rehabilitation, housing, and social benefits. However, it is likely that more effective interventions for PTSD improve social functioning and generate broader benefits for people with PTSD that are likely to create cost savings in other sectors beyond health care. Therefore, it is possible that the cost-effectiveness of effective treatments for PTSD has been underestimated in the current literature. Future research should address limitations and gaps in existing economic evidence.

Cost-Effectiveness of Providing Evidence-Based Treatments

One of the economic studies considered the cost-effectiveness of the implementation of Australian guidelines on the treatment of PTSD relative to TAU, which consisted of non-evidence-based care (Mihalopoulos et al., 2015). People receiving evidence-based interventions (who made up only a small part of the population receiving care for PTSD) were not considered in this analysis, as the decision context was to evaluate the costs and benefits of moving from non-evidence-based to evidence-based treatment at a population level. The study concluded that all evidence-based interventions that had been recommended in the Australian guidelines and were assessed in the analysis, that is, CBT-T and SSRIs for the treatment of PTSD in adults and CBT-T for the treatment of PTSD in children, were cost-effective compared to non-evidence-based TAU in Australia. This finding is in line with the findings of similar modeling studies concluding that the optimal, evidence-based treatment of anxiety disorders, including PTSD, would be cost-effective compared with TAU in Australia (Issakidis, Sanderson, Corry, Andrews, & Lapsley, 2004) and that universal access to evidence-based treatment for veterans with PTSD or depression would lead to substantial benefits and associated cost savings (Kilmer, Eibner, Ringel, & Pacula, 2011).

The Role of Economic Evidence in the Context of Guideline Development

Two of the analyses that evaluated the relative cost-effectiveness of treatments for PTSD in adults, as well as in children and adolescents (National Institute for Health and Care Excellence, 2018b, 2018c), informed the development of national clinical guidelines in England (National Institute for Health and Care Excellence, 2018a). NICE guidelines consider explicitly cost-effectiveness as one of the criteria for making practice recommendations. Economic analyses conducted within the NICE decision-making context should include, when possible, comparisons of all relevant alternatives and employ an incremental approach (National Institute for Health and Care Excellence, 2014). Therefore, the economic analyses undertaken to support the development of NICE PTSD guidelines included the entire spectrum of interventions available for PTSD, for which adequate evidence was available to inform economic modeling. The committee that developed the NICE PTSD practice recommendations considered the cost-effectiveness results and additional factors when formulating those recommendations, such as the quality and breadth of the evidence base across a variety of clinical outcomes for each intervention; the uncertainty characterizing some of the findings; the range of the severity of PTSD and the type of trauma in participants in the RCTs that informed the economic analysis; any populations for which interventions were ineffective or unsuitable; and patient preferences. Subsequently, the committee made strong ("offer") recommendations for the most cost-effective treatments that had a robust clinical evidence base (CBT-T for adults and children; EMDR therapy for adults); weaker ("consider") recommendations (supported computerized CBT-T, CBT without a trauma focus, and SSRIs for adults; EMDR therapy for children) or a research recommendation (emotional freedom technique for adults) for treatments that were relatively less cost-effective and/or had a more limited clinical evidence base; and no recommendations for treatments that were shown to be the least cost-effective in the guidelines' economic analysis and/or had a very limited clinical evidence base. Some of the treatments were recommended for specific subgroups, following interpretation of available clinical and economic evidence and the committee's considerations on the suitability of interventions:

- EMDR therapy was recommended for adults with non-combat-related trauma only.
- "Consider" recommendations were made for:
  - EMDR therapy in children and adolescents ages 7–17 years who do not respond to or engage with CBT-T.
  - Supported computerized CBT-T in adults who prefer it to face-to-face CBT-T or EMDR therapy as long as they do not have severe PTSD symptoms, in particular dissociative symptoms, and are not at risk of harm to themselves or others.
  - CBT without a trauma focus targeted at specific symptoms such as sleep disturbance or anger in adults who are unable or unwilling to engage in a trauma-focused intervention or have residual symptoms after a trauma-focused intervention (National Institute for Health and Care Excellence, 2018a).

In conclusion, economic evidence played an important role in supporting the development of NICE guideline recommendations but was considered alongside the quality and limitations of the clinical evidence base as well as patient-related issues. More generally, a wider range of issues underpin NICE guideline recommendations, such as ethical issues, equity considerations, policy imperatives, and equality legislation (National Institute for Health and Care Excellence, 2014).

Cost-Effectiveness Considerations in the Context of the ISTSS Guidelines: Generalizability and Transferability of Existing Cost-Effectiveness Findings to Other Settings

Cost-effectiveness was not explicitly considered in the development of ISTSS guidelines. Nevertheless, existing economic evidence supports all ISTSS strong recommendations on treatments for adults (CPT, CT, EMDR therapy, CBT-T, PE), children and adolescents (CBT-T and EMDR therapy), and most ISTSS standard recommendations on treatments for adults (CBT without a trauma focus, guided Internet-based CBT-T, narrative exposure therapy), with the exception of group CBT-T and present-centered therapy, which are recommended as options in the ISTSS guidelines but have been found to be less cost-effective than other active interventions (but nevertheless have been shown to be more cost-effective than no treatment). Current cost-effectiveness findings also support the ISTSS low effect recommendation for SSRIs in adults. Interestingly, but perhaps not unexpectedly, interventions with emerging or insufficient evidence are generally not cost-effective according to existing evidence. Overall, the implementation of ISTSS guidelines appears to ensure efficient use of resources and thus can be expected to be cost-effective, although determining an intervention's cost-effectiveness depends on the setting in which the intervention is provided and the adopted perspective (e.g., that of the provider, payer, government, or society).

Available studies indicate the cost-effectiveness of interventions in the specific settings within which the studies were conducted. To judge whether results are transferable to different countries and settings, one needs to consider the similarities and differences across settings regarding the study population characteristics, the funding arrangements and structure of the services for people with PTSD including access to treatment and designated care pathways, the intensity of resource use and unit prices, and wider implementation issues. Another issue to consider is the range of treatment options available in different settings, as the availability of different options may alter the relative cost-effectiveness of interventions, and also the similarities and differences of TAU, which was the comparator in many of the studies. An evidence-based intervention may be cost-effective relative to TAU that comprises basic, non-evidence-based care, but may not be so in a setting where TAU consists of alternative effective interventions. Moreover, assessing the cost-effectiveness of an intervention depends on the perspective adopted: for example, a health care intervention with benefits beyond health (e.g., a rehabilitation program that improves social functioning and reduces the need for costly social care interventions) may not be cost-effective from a pure health care perspective, but may be cost-effective from a wider health and social services perspective. Finally, conclusions on cost-effectiveness rely on the cost-effectiveness threshold adopted by policymakers, and this depends on the policymakers' willingness to pay for treatment benefits, which may vary across countries and health systems.

Conclusions

PTSD is associated with significant psychological and financial burdens for the patients, their family and carers, and wider society. Assessment of cost-effectiveness contributes to optimal allocation of health care resources and maximization of the benefits for the population. Available evidence suggests that a range of interventions are cost-effective in the treatment of people with PTSD. However, existing evidence is characterized by limitations and gaps that should be addressed in future research. In addition to clinical and cost-effectiveness considerations, other factors such as ethical issues, equity, legislation, policy, and implementation aspects should be considered when making decisions on the allocation of health care resources.

REFERENCES

Aas, E., Iversen, T., Holt, T., Ormhaug, S. M., & Jensen, T. K. (2018). Cost-effectiveness analysis of trauma-focused cognitive behavioral therapy: A randomized control trial among Norwegian youth. *Journal of Clinical Child and Adolescent Psychology, 48*(Suppl. 1), 1–14.

Ahmadi, N., Hajsadeghi, F., Mirshkarlo, H. B., Budoff, M., Yehuda, R., & Ebrahimi, R. (2011). Post-traumatic stress disorder, coronary atherosclerosis, and mortality. *American Journal of Cardiology, 108,* 29–33.

Alonso, J., Angermeyer, M. C., Bernert, S., Bruffaerts, R., Brugha, T. S., Bryson, H., et al. (2004). Disability and quality of life impact of mental disorders in Europe: Results from the European Study of the Epidemiology of Mental Disorders (ESEMeD) project. *Acta Psychiatrica Scandinavica Supplement, 420,* 38–46.

Brazier, J., Ratcliffe, J., Salomon, J. A., & Tsuchiya, A. (2017). *Measuring and valuing health benefits for economic evaluation* (2nd ed.). Oxford, UK: Oxford University Press.

Briggs, A. (1999). Economics notes: Handling uncertainty in economic evaluation. *British Medical Journal, 319,* 120.

Briggs, A., Sculpher, M., & Buxton, M. (1994). Uncertainty in the economic evaluation of health care technologies: The role of sensitivity analysis. *Health Economics, 3,* 95–104.

Byford, S., & Raftery, J. (1998). Perspectives in economic evaluation. *British Medical Journal, 316,* 1529–1530.

Caldwell, D. M., Ades, A. E., & Higgins, J. P. (2005). Simultaneous comparison of multiple treatments: Combining direct and indirect evidence. *British Medical Journal, 331,* 897–900.

Canadian Agency for Drugs and Technologies in Health. (2017). *Guidelines for the economic evaluation of health technologies: Canada* (4th ed.). Ottawa, ON, Canada: Author.

Carter, R., Vos, T., Moodie, M., Haby, M., Magnus, A., & Mihalopoulos, C. (2008). Priority setting in health: Origins, description and application of the Australian Assessing Cost-Effectiveness initiative. *Expert Review of Pharmacoeconomics and Outcomes Research, 8,* 593–617.

Chan, A. O., Medicine, M., Air, T. M., & McFarlane, A. C. (2003). Posttraumatic stress disorder and its impact on the economic and health costs of motor vehicle accidents in South Australia. *Journal of Clinical Psychiatry, 64,* 175–181.

Chan, D., Cheadle, A. D., Reiber, G., Unutzer, J., & Chaney, E. F. (2009). Health care utilization and its costs for depressed veterans with and without comorbid PTSD symptoms. *Psychiatric Services, 60,* 1612–1617.

Cohen, G. H., Tamrakar, S., Lowe, S., Sampson, L., Ettman, C., Linas, B., et al. (2017). Comparison of simulated treatment and cost-effectiveness of a stepped care case-finding intervention vs usual care for posttraumatic stress disorder after a natural disaster. *JAMA Psychiatry, 74,* 1251–1258.

Dedert, E. A., Calhoun, P. S., Watkins, L. L., Sherwood, A., & Beckham, J. C. (2010). Posttraumatic stress disorder, cardiovascular, and metabolic disease: A review of the evidence. *Annals of Behavioral Medicine, 39,* 61–78.

Doctor, J. N., Zoellner, L. A., & Feeny, N. C. (2011). Predictors of health-related quality-of-life utilities among persons with posttraumatic stress disorder. *Psychiatric Services, 62,* 272–277.

Drummnod, M. F., Schulpher, M. J., Claxton, K., Stoddart, G. L., & Torrance, G. W. (2015). *Methods for the economic evaluation of health care programmes* (4th ed.). Oxford, UK: Oxford University Press.

Dubois, R. W. (2016). Cost-effectiveness thresholds in the USA: Are they coming? Are they already here? *Journal of Comparative Effectiveness Research, 5,* 9–11.

Dunn, N. J., Rehm, L. P., Schillaci, J., Souchek, J., Mehta, P., Ashton, C. M., et al. (2007). A randomized trial of self-management and psychoeducational group therapies for comorbid chronic posttraumatic stress disorder and depressive disorder. *Journal of Traumatic Stress, 20,* 221–237.

Edney, L. C., Haji Ali, A. H., Cheng, T. C., & Karnon, J. (2018). Estimating the reference Incremental Cost-Effectiveness Ratio for the Australian health system. *Pharmacoeconomics, 36,* 239–252.

Fenwick, E., Claxton, K., & Sculpher, M. (2001). Representing uncertainty: The role of cost-effectiveness acceptability curves. *Health Economics, 10,* 779–787.

Ferry, F. R., Brady, S. E., Bunting, B. P., Murphy, S. D., Bolton, D., & O'Neill, S. M. (2015). The economic burden of PTSD in Northern Ireland. *Journal of Traumatic Stress, 28,* 191–197.

Freed, M. C., Yeager, D. E., Liu, X., Gore, K. L., Engel, C. C., & Magruder, K. M. (2009). Preference-weighted health status of PTSD among veterans: An outcome for cost-effectiveness analysis using clinical data. *Psychiatric Services, 60,* 1230–1238.

Gospodarevskaya, E. (2013). Post-traumatic stress disorder and quality of life in sexually abused Australian children. *Journal of Child Sexual Abuse, 22,* 277–296.

Gospodarevskaya, E., & Segal, L. (2012). Cost-utility analysis of different treatments for post-traumatic stress disorder in sexually abused children. *Child and Adolescent Psychiatry and Mental Health, 6*(15).

Gustavsson, A., Svensson, M., Jacobi, F., Allgulander, C., Alonso, J., Beghi, E., et al. (2011). Cost of disorders of the brain in Europe 2010. *European Neuropsychopharmacology, 21,* 718–779.

Haagsma, J. A., Polinder, S., Olff, M., Toet, H., Bonsel, G. J., & van Beeck, E. F. (2012). Posttraumatic stress symptoms and health-related quality of life: A two year follow up study of injury treated at the emergency department. *BMC Psychiatry, 12*(1).

Haviland, M. G., Banta, J. E., Sonne, J. L., & Przekop, P. (2016). Posttraumatic stress disorder-related hospitalizations in the United States (2002–2011): Rates, co-occurring illnesses, suicidal ideation/self-harm, and hospital charges. *Journal of Nervous and Mental Disease, 204,* 78–86.

Issakidis, C., Sanderson, K., Corry, J., Andrews, G., & Lapsley, H. (2004). Modelling the population cost-effectiveness of current and evidence-based optimal treatment for anxiety disorders. *Psychological Medicine, 34,* 19–35.

Ivanova, J. I., Birnbaum, H. G., Chen, L., Duhig, A. M., Dayoub, E. J., Kantor, E. S., et al. (2011). Cost of post-traumatic stress disorder vs major depressive disorder among patients covered by medicaid or private insurance. *American Journal of Managed Care, 17,* e314–e323.

Jonsson, B. (2009). Ten arguments for a societal perspective in the economic evaluation of medical innovations. *European Journal of Health Economics, 10,* 357–359.

Kessler, R. C., Aguilar-Gaxiola, S., Alonso, J., Benjet, C., Bromet, E. J., Cardoso, G., et al. (2017). Trauma and PTSD in the WHO World Mental Health Surveys. *European Journal of Psychotraumatology, 8,* 1353383.

Kessler, R. C., Sonnega, A., Bromet, E., Hughes, M., & Nelson, C. B. (1995). Posttraumatic stress disorder in the National Comorbidity Survey. *Archives of General Psychiatry, 52,* 1048–1060.

Kilmer, B., Eibner, C., Ringel, J. S., & Pacula, R. L. (2011). Invisible wounds, visible savings?: Using microsimulation to estimate the costs and savings associated with providing evidence-based treatment for PTSD and depression to veterans of Operation Enduring Freedom and Operation Iraqi Freedom. *Psychological Trauma: Theory, Research, Practice, and Policy, 3,* 201–211.

Knies, S., Severens, J. L., Ament, A. J., & Evers, S. M. (2010). The transferability of valuing lost productivity across jurisdictions: Differences between national pharmacoeconomic guidelines. *Value in Health, 13,* 519–527.

Koenen, K. C., Ratanatharathorn, A., Ng, L., McLaughlin, K. A., Bromet, E. J., Stein, D. J., et al. (2017). Posttraumatic stress disorder in the World Mental Health Surveys. *Psychological Medicine, 47,* 2260–2274.

Lamoureux-Lamarche, C., Vasiliadis, H. M., Preville, M., & Berbiche, D. (2016). Healthcare use and costs associated with post-traumatic stress syndrome in a community sample of older adults: Results from the ESA-Services study. *International Psychogeriatrics, 28,* 903–911.

Le, Q. A., Doctor, J. N., Zoellner, L. A., & Feeny, N. C. (2014). Cost-effectiveness of prolonged exposure therapy versus pharmacotherapy and treatment choice in posttraumatic stress disorder (the optimizing PTSD treatment trial): A doubly randomized preference trial. *Journal of Clinical Psychiatry, 75,* 222–230.

Mancino, M. J., Pyne, J. M., Tripathi, S., Constans, J., Roca, V., & Freeman, T. (2006). Quality-adjusted health status in veterans with posttraumatic stress disorder. *Journal of Nervous and Mental Disease, 194,* 877–879.

Mavridis, D., Giannatsi, M., Cipriani, A., & Salanti, G. (2015). A primer on network meta-analysis with emphasis on mental health. *Evidence-Based Mental Health, 18*, 40–46.

McCrone, P., Weeramanthri, T., Knapp, M., Rushton, A., Trowell, J., Miles, G., et al. (2005). Cost-effectiveness of individual versus group psychotherapy for sexually abused girls. *Child and Adolescent Mental Health, 10*, 26–31.

Meyers, L. L., Strom, T. Q., Leskela, J., Thuras, P., Kehle-Forbes, S. M., & Curry, K. T. (2013). Service utilization following participation in cognitive processing therapy or prolonged exposure therapy for post-traumatic stress disorder. *Military Medicine, 178*, 95–99.

Mihalopoulos, C., Magnus, A., Lal, A., Dell, L., Forbes, D., & Phelps, A. (2015). Is implementation of the 2013 Australian treatment guidelines for posttraumatic stress disorder cost-effective compared to current practice?: A cost-utility analysis using QALYs and DALYs. *Australian and New Zealand Journal of Psychiatry, 49*, 360–376.

Murray, C. J., Evans, D. B., Acharya, A., & Baltussen, R. M. (2000). Development of WHO guidelines on generalized cost-effectiveness analysis. *Health Economics, 9*, 235–251.

Murray, C. J., Vos, T., Lozano, R., Naghavi, M., Flaxman, A. D., Michaud, C., et al. (2012). Disability-adjusted life years (DALYs) for 291 diseases and injuries in 21 regions, 1990–2010: A systematic analysis for the Global Burden of Disease Study 2010. *Lancet, 380*, 2197–2223.

National Institute for Health and Care Excellence. (2013). *Guide to the methods of technology appraisal 2013*. London: Author.

National Institute for Health and Care Excellence. (2014). Developing NICE guidelines: The manual. Last updated October 2018. Retrieved from *www.nice.org.uk/process/pmg20*.

National Institute for Health and Care Excellence. (2018a). Post-traumatic stress disorder: Management. Retrieved from *www.nice.org.uk/guidance/ng116*.

National Institute for Health and Care Excellence. (2018b). Post-traumatic stress disorder: Management (update). Evidence report B: Evidence reviews for psychological, psychosocial and other non-pharmacological interventions for the treatment of PTSD in children. Retrieved from *www.nice.org.uk/guidance/ng116/evidence*.

National Institute for Health and Care Excellence. (2018c). Post-traumatic stress disorder: Management (update). Evidence report D: Evidence reviews for psychological, psychosocial and other non-pharmacological interventions for the treatment of PTSD in adults. Retrieved from *www.nice.org.uk/guidance/ng116/evidence*.

Petrou, S., & Gray, A. (2011). Economic evaluation using decision analytical modelling: Design, conduct, analysis, and reporting. *British Medical Journal, 342*, d1766.

Salloum, A., Wang, W., Robst, J., Murphy, T. K., Scheeringa, M. S., Cohen, J. A., et al. (2016). Stepped care versus standard trauma-focused cognitive behavioral therapy for young children. *Journal of Child Psychology and Psychiatry, 57*, 614–622.

Sassi, F. (2006). Calculating QALYs, comparing QALY and DALY calculations. *Health Policy and Planning, 21*, 402–408.

Schnurr, P. P., Friedman, M. J., Oxman, T. E., Dietrich, A. J., Smith, M. W., Shiner, B., et al. (2013). RESPECT-PTSD: Re-engineering systems for the primary care treatment of PTSD, a randomized controlled trial. *Journal of General Internal Medicine, 28,* 32–40.

Schulper, M. (2001). The role and estimation of productivity costs in economic evaluation. In F. Drummond & A. McGuire (Eds.), *Economic evaluation in health care: Merging theory with practice* (pp. 94–112). New York: Oxford University Press.

Shearer, J., Papanikolaou, N., Meiser-Stedman, R., McKinnon, A., Dalgleish, T., Smith, P., et al. (2018). Cost-effectiveness of cognitive therapy as an early intervention for post-traumatic stress disorder in children and adolescents: A trial based evaluation and model. *Journal of Child Psychology and Psychiatry, 59,* 773–780.

Slade, E. P., Gottlieb, J. D., Lu, W., Yanos, P. T., Rosenberg, S., Silverstein, S. M., et al. (2017). Cost-effectiveness of a PTSD intervention tailored for individuals with severe mental illness. *Psychiatric Services, 68,* 1225–1231.

Tuerk, P. W., Wangelin, B., Rauch, S. A. M., Dismuke, C. E., Yoder, M., Myrick, H., et al. (2013). Health service utilization before and after evidence-based treatment for PTSD. *Psychological Services, 10,* 401–409.

Walker, E. A., Katon, W., Russo, J., Ciechanowski, P., Newman, E., & Wagner, A. W. (2003). Health care costs associated with posttraumatic stress disorder symptoms in women. *Archives of General Psychiatry, 60,* 369–374.

Weinstein, M. C., Torrance, G., & McGuire, A. (2009). QALYs: The basics. *Value in Health, 12*(Suppl. 1), S5–S9.

Wood, D. P., Murphy, J., McLay, R., Koffman, R., Spira, J., Obrecht, R. E., et al. (2009). Cost effectiveness of virtual reality graded exposure therapy with physiological monitoring for the treatment of combat related post traumatic stress disorder. *Studies in Health Technology and Informatics, 144,* 223–229.

World Health Organization. (2018). Metrics: Disability-adjusted life year (DALY). Retrieved January 11, 2018, from *www.who.int/healthinfo/global_burden_disease/metrics_daly/en.*

CHAPTER 26

The Future of Traumatic Stress Treatments
Time to Grasp the Opportunity

David Forbes, Jonathan I. Bisson, Candice M. Monson, and Lucy Berliner

The *Posttraumatic Stress Disorder Prevention and Treatment Guidelines* advanced by the International Society for Traumatic Stress Studies (ISTSS) in 2018 represent a substantial step forward in our understanding of the most effective strategies to assist people whose lives have been affected by the experience of trauma and disaster. The chapters in this book have taken those guidelines to the next level, focusing on what they mean for mental health providers in clinical practice, how to implement the recommendations, what to do when treatment does not go as planned, and what the future may hold in each area. Although the research data provide much cause for optimism, it is also clear that substantial gaps in our knowledge still exist. Building on the platform of our solid knowledge base, it is now time for the field to grasp this opportunity and to confront the challenges raised in the preceding chapters in this volume. While retaining a solid commitment to evidence-based practice, we need to take the field beyond studies of a small number of specific interventions with defined populations to explore the broad critical underlying issues. A better understanding of these underpinnings will drive future developments in an integrated and coherent manner, increasing our chances of further enhancing improvements in the prevention and management of posttraumatic stress disorder (PTSD) and related conditions.

This chapter explores some of the themes raised in the preceding chapters, attempting to elucidate what they mean for our understanding of the field and the key research, clinical, and systemic implications for the coming years. The themes include the need for more sophisticated approaches to understanding the nature and course of human response to trauma, the mechanisms underlying those different trajectories, how best to improve our treatments, and challenges for implementing best-practice interventions. Running across all those themes is the crucial question of how to better match specific interventions to the unique needs of each individual.

The Nature and Course of Traumatic Stress Reactions

Several of the preceding chapters highlight the need for a better understanding of the many ways in which human beings respond to the experience of a potentially traumatic event, both within and beyond the construct of PTSD. Increased computing power through machine learning and artificial intelligence (AI) provides the opportunity to explore different trajectories in large populations exposed to the same or similar traumatic events. It is clear that some people show little or no adverse reaction, whereas others appear to develop problems immediately following the experience that, if left untreated, remain over the long term. Although those two groups are relatively easily identified, alternative trajectories present a greater challenge. Some people exposed to potentially traumatic events, for example, develop clinically significant acute reactions but appear to recover over the coming months, apparently with little or no external assistance. Others may report low levels of symptomatology, but steadily recruit symptoms over time to end up crossing the diagnostic threshold; for others, the course fluctuates and some experience symptoms with a delayed onset. It is reasonable to assume that each trajectory would benefit from a different approach to intervention in terms of, for example, timing, dose, type, and mode of delivery, but we can only tailor that assistance to individual need if we can predict the likely course and maintain active surveillance.

The initial chapters of this volume discuss the challenges ahead for epidemiology in developing tools to improve our ability to identify persons at risk of PTSD and related conditions, not only in the acute phases but also over the longer term. At present, we know that early PTSD symptom severity is a strong predictor of later PTSD, but we still cannot confidently predict which trajectory a trauma survivor will take. Our current screening instruments struggle at identifying those on other trajectories, including those who may remain "subsyndromal" but nevertheless experience substantial distress and functional impairment. If we can reliably determine the predictors of different trajectories—the risk factors, risk indicators, and protective factors—we will have the capacity to develop more effective screening and assessment strategies to ensure that adults, youth, and children are identified appropriately and offered the level and type of intervention they require at the appropriate juncture.

Not only are there substantial differences across individuals in the course of response and recovery following trauma, but also in the nature of the clinical presentation. As discussed in Chapter 22, mental health problems following trauma exposure are by no means limited to PTSD, with a range of comorbid conditions and personality factors commonly present. Indeed, many of these conditions, such as depression, anxiety, and substance use disorders, may develop in the aftermath of trauma independently of, and in the absence of, PTSD. Although much research has explored the impact of those comorbidities on PTSD treatment response following specific evidence-based interventions, the field has room to grow in addressing the question of how to adapt treatment when other conditions, or symptoms, are present. This may not simply be a question of adding or integrating another treatment (e.g., in substance use disorder) alongside the standard PTSD intervention. Rather, it may be about developing a more personalized and integrated approach to treatment designed to treat the specific constellations of symptoms (possibly networks of symptoms) with which the individual presents across a series of co-occurring conditions and associated features.

Recent developments in the diagnostic classification systems offer a specific example of this dilemma. The DSM-5 diagnosis takes a broad approach to describing the clinical picture of PTSD, with a wide variety of presentations all potentially coming under the same rubric. While the diagnosis provides a comprehensive clinical description, it is reasonable to assume that different variations of the disorder subsumed within this single diagnosis may respond differently to a specific treatment. ICD-11 has taken an alternative approach, adopting a very narrow definition of PTSD and introducing the new diagnosis of complex PTSD (CPTSD). This divergence in the diagnostic criteria for PTSD is discussed in Chapter 4, which highlights the fact that the two classification systems are no longer interchangeable and discusses the implications. Certainly, it provides an intriguing basis for future research. There are now therefore effectively three PTSD diagnoses across ICD and DSM, albeit one CPTSD. Do the DSM-5 and ICD-11 PTSD diagnoses represent different constructs, or is one subsumed within the other? Do they show different trajectories? How do each of these two PTSD diagnoses differentially interdigitate with the CPTSD diagnosis? Do they respond differently to our existing treatments and do they require different approaches?

Putting all this together, it is clear that, to more accurately tailor interventions to the specific needs of the individual, we need a more sophisticated understanding of the range of responses to trauma, both in terms of clinical presentation and recovery trajectories. As discussed further, we need to ascertain who is likely to respond to which kind of treatment and why. In practical terms, we need a better knowledge base of the relevant risk and protective factors for the development of disorder, the course of disorder, and response to treatment to improve our predictive capacity and tailor our interventions accordingly. These predictors will, of course, need to take into account pretrauma, peritrauma, and posttrauma variables in biological, psychological, and social domains.

Underlying Mechanisms

Great progress has been made in developing, and improving on, evidence-based treatments for PTSD and related conditions. This has resulted in four core treatments for adults and three core treatments for children being given the highest recommendation, and several others slightly lower recommendations, in the ISTSS guidelines. Each of these has, or has the potential for, variations in components and how it is delivered. For example, Chapters 11–15 discuss variations to standard versions of the treatments in terms of lengths of session, with and without writing components, massed versus spaced versions, adaptations to service delivery context, and so on. Although it is tempting to go down each of these pathways, conducting randomized controlled trials (RCTs) to determine whether this or that particular nuance results in a better outcome, this approach alone, even if more adaptive study designs are adopted, will result in slow progress. It also risks the potential to fail to identify more fundamental principles that should be driving our understanding of the field. To use an old quote, we risk "missing the wood for the trees." While not suggesting that the field should abandon that approach—it will always remain the core of good science and core to expanding our evidence base—the time has also come to increase our focus on the underlying mechanisms. This focus on underlying mechanisms needs to consider both the processes underlying disorder development in addition to the mechanisms of treatment effectiveness. Hence, this requires attention to the interactions between biological, psychological, and social factors that explain the development of, and recovery from, traumatic stress reactions.

One starting point in this search for core mechanisms involves identifying common elements of successful treatments. Are our successful treatments all doing the same thing, targeting the same underlying mechanisms? Chapter 11 has attempted to extract the core components that are shared by the treatments with the highest recommendations for adults: prolonged exposure (PE), cognitive processing therapy (CPT), cognitive therapy for PTSD (CT-PTSD), eye movement desensitization and reprocessing (EMDR) therapy, and undifferentiated trauma-focused cognitive-behavioral therapy (CBT). Three common elements are identified: addressing trauma-related cognitions, engaging with the traumatic memory, and addressing experiential avoidance. Similarly, these same three common elements appear in the child treatments with the highest recommendations (CBT-based trauma-focused therapy approaches targeting mainly the child, CBT-based trauma-focused therapy that is both child- and caregiver-focused, and EMDR therapy).

The authors in Chapter 11 speculated that information-processing paradigms (along with changing the personal meaning of the trauma) may go some way in explaining the mechanisms underlying those elements. We will use the information-processing paradigm to illustrate this discussion about mechanisms of treatment action and their corresponding treatment interventions designed to directly or indirectly intervene on those mechanisms. Those models broadly assume that the traumatic memory drives the cognitive, physiological, behavioral, and affective symptoms associated with PTSD and related conditions. For recovery to occur, that memory must be modified. That is, the person first needs to activate and engage with the traumatic memory to make it accessible for modification. Then the person needs to engage with, process, and incorporate information that is inconsistent with that contained in the memory. By doing so, links between trauma-related memories and responses in physiological, behavioral, and affective domains are weakened. In addition, advances in theory and neuroscience research suggest that original maladaptive trauma appraisals associated with the memory are weakened by competing alternative cognitions (vs. restructuring of them). It is assumed that, while PE, CPT, CT-PTSD, EMDR therapy, and undifferentiated trauma-focused CBT may use different treatment means to manipulate these mechanisms, they are all achieving the same ends by operating through these same underlying mechanisms.

Are there additional core elements of intervention that are shared by most, if not all, successful treatments? Many approaches include, formally or informally, at least some kind of attention to arousal reduction, anxiety management, and broader emotion regulation. The research suggests these approaches in isolation are not as efficacious in the treatment of PTSD—they help the person to manage the symptoms but do not address the underlying drivers. Nevertheless, as the authors of Chapter 19 note, a person's ability to reduce and control his or her reactivity to internal experience, to moderate arousal, and to control attentional focus may be important agents of change. If so, what is the mechanism? Perhaps they operate purely to facilitate the underlying mechanism of change—activation and modification of the traumatic memory or alternatively to make the underlying mechanisms highlighted more amenable to change by the common core elements previously cited. Relatedly, it is also important to acknowledge the role, across all of these treatments, of the nonspecific therapeutic alliance factors (therapeutic relationship, empathy, support, shared goals) that have demonstrated efficacy in their own right. Nevertheless, it is important to remain open to the potential benefit of basic lifestyle interventions (e.g., aerobic exercise, diet, sleep, hygiene, social engagement, enjoyable activities). There is a risk that, in our desire to maximize our clinical and/or theoretical sophistication, we may neglect these basic issues that have the potential to substantially improve the person's quality of life. Some clinicians may believe that addressing those issues might be interpreted as minimizing or avoiding addressing the traumatic experience. It is important to remember, however, that although they may not directly address the underlying traumatic stress mechanisms, the resulting improved mental state will make that work much easier.

The discussion thus far has focused on psychological treatments because they are supported by the strongest body of evidence. As noted in Chapter 16, however, pharmacological interventions also have an important role to play in the treatment of PTSD and related conditions. To the extent that they are successful, do they operate through the same mechanisms? Is their role primarily one of symptom management, reducing arousal and affective distress to the point that the person is able to engage—with or without a therapist—in the process of modifying traumatic memories? If so, perhaps the reason for the slightly disappointing rate of success of pharmacotherapy in PTSD is that these drugs are not directly targeting the core mechanisms that underpin the disorder. The future, however, may be different. While pharmacotherapy for PTSD to date has relied on drugs developed for other reasons—notably, antidepressants—there is increasing interest in drugs that may selectively target the traumatic memory directly, as well as drugs that may facilitate modification of the memories when administered during a trauma-focused therapy approach. Either way, the important message is to improve our understanding of the mechanisms by which successful treatments work so that they can be targeted directly.

A second potential body of evidence in the search for underlying mechanisms, beyond the commonalities of successful treatments, may lie in closer examination of the natural course of traumatic stress reactions. We need a better understanding of the mechanisms involved in long-term adverse outcomes: Why do some people have problems, whereas others do not? Why do some people show good recovery (without the need for professional assistance), while others do not? The field has made good progress in discovering risk indicators (i.e., characteristics of those subgroups in which PTSD is more common, such as gender) and risk factors (i.e., for which there is clear evidence of causal effect, such as exposure to further trauma). Some progress has been made in identifying potential protective factors, for example, cognitive flexibility and social support (although negative support is a stronger risk predictor). What the field has done less well to date is to use this information about risk to generate hypotheses about the underlying mechanisms that explain variations in human response to trauma. It is reasonable to assume that these risk variables operate through similar mechanisms to those discussed. That is, that there will be strong similarities between the mechanisms that underpin healthy recovery in the absence of treatment and those that underpin therapist-assisted recovery. To use the information processing paradigm discussed previously as an example, it may be that those people who recover without treatment are able to access the traumatic memory often enough and for long enough to allow it to be modified. This mechanism of change is facilitated by a therapist in the case of treatment. In those who do not receive treatment, it may be that risk and protective factors operate by facilitating or mitigating against activation and modification of the trauma memory. A strong social support network, for example, may make it easier to talk about what happened, whereas subsequent life stressors may reduce the person's capacity to address the original trauma.

In summary, while we continue RCT investigations of promising treatments, we are likely to accelerate progress if we are able to identify more accurately the specific mechanisms that explain the development of, and recovery from, disorder and target our treatments accordingly. In line with the discussions in the previous section, this will require recognition of different trauma responses—trajectories and clinical presentations—to determine which mechanisms best explain each response type. Only by understanding these different mechanisms can we effectively design treatment tailored to the many different ways in which humans respond to trauma.

Improving Treatment Effectiveness

Moving on from mechanisms, the preceding chapters highlight the substantial opportunities that exist to build on and improve existing treatments. As discussed in Chapter 16, there is great potential to develop novel pharmacotherapies that target the specific neurobiological characteristics of PTSD, thereby addressing the physiological and biological mechanisms that help to explain the clinical picture. Beyond traditional pharmacotherapy, the ISTSS guidelines for PTSD for the first time provide preliminary support for herbal remedies based on traditional medicines. Other biological treatments such as neurofeedback and transcranial magnetic stimulation also show promise for further development. Chapter 18 discusses the considerable potential that now exists and will continue to develop with advances in computing and artificial intelligence for online and other technologically based treatment approaches. Given the complex clinical picture of many PTSD presentations, particularly in the context of the broad approach taken by DSM-5, further research is required on the potential benefits of combining two or more existing treatments. This may, for example, include acute-acting pharmacological and other augmentation agents to enhance specific components of psychotherapy, such as 3,4-methylenedioxy-methamphetamine (MDMA) and similar trials discussed in Chapter 17. There has also been important progress in research focused on bolstering effectiveness through active engagement of supportive and significant others in treatment such as couples- or family-focused PTSD treatments. Chapter 19 also points the way to emerging interventions in the alternative and complementary approaches including meditation, yoga, and mindfulness-based interventions, which, although not designed for the treatment of PTSD specifically, are starting to demonstrate impact on PTSD symptomatology. The inclusion of complex PTSD as a recognized diagnostic category in ICD-11 will drive the exploration of treatments that target the specific profile of that disorder. In light of the high level of comorbidity highlighted in Chapter 22, transdiagnostic approaches may be beneficial in addressing underlying shared core vulnerabilities in PTSD and the common conditions.

While new and improved treatments for PTSD and related conditions must be developed through a rigorous empirical approach, the field needs to pay greater attention to their applicability in practical real-world applications. That is, can they be delivered effectively by clinicians across the community in their mental health clinics and consulting rooms? Furthermore, can these treatments be delivered beyond these mental health settings to include, for example, primary care settings and, for children and adolescents, potentially in school settings? We need to consider who will be engaged in the treatment process and how. With young children, for example, to what extent should we just work with parents rather than also actively involving the child in treatment? With adults, what difference does partner involvement make, and how and when should a partner be involved? We need to continue to expand our treatment trials with different populations in different settings, outside of specialized university clinics with first-class training and supervision. To enhance this broader applicability, researchers should aim to include end-user input and validation throughout the development process. We need to further promote clinical evaluation as part of routine care, with better collection of these data to inform development of future interventions applicable to real-world settings beyond traditional RCT designs. In this context, research also needs to explore how much a given treatment can be simplified or "degraded" and still maintain its efficacy. With which populations and clinical presentations will the "degraded" versions of treatment be sufficient, and who will continue to require the full protocol to achieve the desired results?

Beyond simply developing new or improved treatments, a major challenge for the field is developing our capacity to match the timing, type, and intensity of treatment to specific risk profiles and clinical presentations. This work will need to build on both a better understanding of the range of trajectories and symptom profiles following trauma exposure, and a greater focus on the mechanisms. Although the concept of personalized medicine is not new, it has yet to be systematically adopted in our approach to trauma treatment. Any suggestion that "one size fits all" when it comes to PTSD and related conditions is not borne out by the relatively modest treatment outcomes for some people with PTSD. The transdiagnostic approaches to treatment that focus more on dimensions or themes, rather than specific diagnoses, make it easier to design individual treatments to match specific clinical profiles. This concept of designing treatment to the specific needs of the patient applies not only to psychological constructs but also to pharmacological and other biological factors. A more sophisticated knowledge of genetic influences on trauma recovery, for example, may help guide decision making about which drugs (or psychological therapies) might have the best chance of success with different patients. In short, we need to do better at matching specific treatments (alone or in combination), as well as their dose, timing, and mode of delivery, to different subgroups of the affected population and different subtypes of clinical presentation.

Improving treatment may also involve paying greater attention to the desired outcomes. RCTs traditionally, and with good reason, focus primarily on symptom reduction with the main focus on PTSD. In real-world settings, however, the person's needs and goals are often much broader and, indeed, PTSD symptoms may not be the dominant concern. Being cognizant of that, it is important that the field stay open to a wide range of potential outcomes and that we strive to measure recovery in a more holistic way. This should, of course, critically include symptom reduction across PTSD and any comorbid conditions, but ought to also include attention to social relationships, occupational functioning (in the broadest sense), and quality of life. Symptom reduction without improvements in those other areas is likely to be of limited benefit to our patients. Equally, improvements in those other areas may go some way in reducing the severity of core symptoms or, at least, make treatment or self-management of those symptoms easier.

In this context, it is important to differentiate between those interventions that are designed primarily to reduce core symptoms, hopefully by addressing the underlying mechanisms, and those that are designed to improve quality of life and assist the client to manage his or her condition. Recent years have seen a substantial growth in interest around broader activities, approaches, and interventions such as a range of pet therapies (particularly stratifications in the sophistication of canine therapies) and outdoor physical challenges. These interventions clearly have the potential to be beneficial for some people with the disorder, enhancing broader quality of life and well-being in different ways. Rather than ruling them out on the grounds of lack of data in reliably reducing PTSD symptoms, the field needs to engage with these approaches by rigorously defining what they are designed to achieve. There is scope for some of them to become useful adjuncts to mainstream PTSD treatments in the search for more holistic outcomes. It also may be that over time these approaches and interventions demonstrate direct impact on PTSD symptoms. On a related theme, there is scope to improve our differentiation between active treatment and "maintenance." Although it is often suggested that the latter is superfluous and does not require a mental health professional, many clinicians would argue that a small proportion of their people with PTSD do require regular, albeit infrequent, contact to minimize the chance of relapse. This is a legitimate area for study: Who needs it and what should it comprise?

A final consideration in striving to improve our treatments is a better analysis of who does not respond to treatment and why. Several of the preceding chapters attempt to address this issue, with Chapter 13 suggesting that, at least for CPT, two common themes that emerge are lack of therapist fidelity to the protocol and problems with homework compliance. The first is potentially addressed through better training and more consistent supervision—not always easy for practitioners to arrange in routine clinical practice. The second, difficulties with compliance, is by no means unique to trauma treatments and has been the focus of considerable interest in the behavioral field. Here, we also need to consider the role of measurement-based care, where results and outcomes are actually used collaboratively and clinically with the patient. It may not only be helpful in guiding personalized approaches to treatment but also a very compelling process to aid practitioners in remaining "on course." It is a complex issue, and we need to understand the multiple potential contributing factors if we are to address it effectively. Although it may be tempting at times for some clinicians, it is not sufficient to "blame" the client for not working hard enough or not being committed to treatment. Rather, the subtle contingencies that are operating need to be examined. We need to acknowledge that even if delivered with perfect fidelity and full patient compliance to protocol and homework, it remains unlikely that everyone with PTSD would be "cured" with the current treatments. More broadly, the field needs to gain a better understanding of treatment moderators—those factors that facilitate or mitigate against a good treatment outcome. One simple example provided in Chapter 13 is patient preference: clients who are actively engaged in treatment planning and who have a say in which treatment they undergo are likely to respond better. This highlights the importance of taking a collaborative approach in the early stages of treatment planning. Ultimately, we seek to progress to a future where we are able to offer people with PTSD the choice of equally effective treatments that involve different techniques/paradigms that sit within a personalized medicine framework.

Challenges in Implementing Best Practice

Following from the discussion above regarding the importance of ensuring that our recommended treatments are applicable in real-world settings, continued efforts need to be devoted to implementation issues. These challenges are discussed in detail in Chapter 24: How best can we disseminate those treatments that have demonstrable effectiveness? How do we train and support clinicians as they work to implement those treatments? It is clear that our approach to this complex challenge needs to be flexible and multifaceted to address the unique and diverse challenges that each treatment setting faces when endeavoring to deliver evidence-based treatments to survivors of trauma. Several barriers to care have been identified including patient-based (e.g., stigma, personal beliefs about mental health treatment, readiness to change), clinician-based (e.g., poor training, low confidence, lack of understanding about effective treatments, lack of commitment to evidence-based care), and structural/organizational barriers (e.g., accessibility, complex service systems to negotiate, service gaps). Effective implementation of best-practice treatments needs to take into account, and address, these multiple barriers in a coherent and systematic way rather than focusing on only one or two.

Resource allocation is often a challenge for mental health providers. Although it is important to advocate for greater resources in responding to the mental health effects of trauma, the reality is that many clinicians will be working in underresourced areas. It is incumbent on the field to explore delivery options that make optimal use of limited resources while not compromising treatment efficacy. Considerations may include, for example, ensuring that interventions following trauma are delivered at the optimum time, neither too early nor too late to achieve the best outcomes in the most efficient manner. Indeed, determining this represents a research question in its own right. Dosing is important: How much treatment is required and at what frequency? Are "therapy breaks" useful? Similarly, with the ISTSS guidelines reporting increasing evidence from several recommended interventions suggesting that massed treatment (e.g., several hours daily over 2 weeks) may be as effective as more traditional therapy models, it is worth considering which might be the most efficient in any given setting. For clients in rural and remote areas, as well as those who find it hard to get to a clinic for other reasons, delivery via video technology holds considerable promise and may be a cheaper but equally effective alternative in some cases. The model proposed for CPT in Chapter 13 that uses a combination of self-study modules with therapist sessions appears to reduce the practitioner resources required without loss of treatment efficacy. All of these efficiency measures, however, must be supported with appropriate research evidence. Although many are, some of the suggestions still require empirical support. This discussion has been oriented primarily toward mental health services in high-income countries. While increasing attention has been devoted to the delivery of evidence-based treatments for trauma survivors in low- and middle-income countries, the challenges in those settings are, of course, substantially greater.

It is clear from Chapter 25 that providing evidence-based treatments for PTSD and related conditions is cost-effective. This is vital evidence to bring to the attention of governments and other purchasers of services (such as third-party insurers) as well as to senior management in service delivery organizations. Although it may require greater commitment from consumers, clinicians, health agencies, and purchasers, the long-term benefits in terms of both cost savings and quality of life are now clearly demonstrable. In implementing evidence-based treatments for PTSD in health care settings across the community, however, other factors in addition to clinical and cost-effectiveness require consideration. Ethical issues, equity, and legislative aspects should be also considered when making decisions on the allocation of health care resources.

Conclusions: Future Research Directions

The previous sections have proposed many areas for future research. In short, we need to better understand the nature and course of traumatic stress reactions—the different trajectories and clinical presentations—as well as improving our identification and prediction of these various responses to traumatic experiences. We need to increase our research focus on the mechanisms that underlie recovery from trauma exposure, both within and beyond the therapeutic context. We need to continue our efforts to develop new treatments and improve our existing interventions, while also ensuring that they are applicable to real-world settings and that they pay attention to a broad range of therapeutic outcomes. Finally, we need to place a greater emphasis on empirically supported strategies for dissemination and implementation, while recognizing the constraints inherent in many mental health service settings.

Many of these research questions can only be addressed in a limited fashion with modest, single-site studies. While there will always be a place for that research, the time has come to take traumatic stress research to the next level. We now have the computing capacity to deal with extremely large bodies of data. By combining multiple data sets from different sites and using newly developed sophisticated data analytic techniques, we have the potential to answer many of the complex questions raised in this discussion. The challenge now is to find ways to engage the international research community in collaborative efforts to solve these issues confronting the field. This will require not only commitment and funding, but also the development of appropriate structures within which these research collaborations can flourish.

The future for the field of traumatic stress has never looked more promising. Although there is much work still to do, the 2018 ISTSS guidelines and the preceding chapters attest to the enormous gains that have been made over the last 20 years. We now have a range of effective treatments for PTSD and related conditions that are constantly evolving to improve outcomes and meet the various challenges. A host of opportunities now present themselves to clinicians, researchers, and policymakers, all of whom share the same goal of improving outcomes for people affected by trauma.

Author Index

Subject Index

Note. Page numbers followed by an *f* or a *t* indicate a figure or a table.